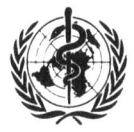

WORLD HEALTH ORGANIZATION

INTERNATIONAL AGENCY FOR RESEARCH ON CANCER

IARC MONOGRAPHS
ON THE
EVALUATION OF CARCINOGENIC RISKS TO HUMANS

Beryllium, Cadmium, Mercury, and Exposures in the Glass Manufacturing Industry

VOLUME 58

This publication represents the views and expert opinions
of an IARC Working Group on the
Evaluation of Carcinogenic Risks to Humans,
which met in Lyon,

9–16 February 1993

1993

IARC MONOGRAPHS

In 1969, the International Agency for Research on Cancer (IARC) initiated a programme on the evaluation of the carcinogenic risk of chemicals to humans involving the production of critically evaluated monographs on individual chemicals. In 1980 and 1986, the programme was expanded to include evaluations of carcinogenic risks associated with exposures to complex mixtures and other agents.

The objective of the programme is to elaborate and publish in the form of monographs critical reviews of data on carcinogenicity for agents to which humans are known to be exposed, and on specific exposure situations; to evaluate these data in terms of human risk with the help of international working groups of experts in chemical carcinogenesis and related fields; and to indicate where additional research efforts are needed.

This project is supported by PHS Grant No. 5-UO1 CA33193-11 awarded by the US National Cancer Institute, Department of Health and Human Services. Additional support has been provided since 1986 by the Commission of the European Communities.

©International Agency for Research on Cancer 1993

ISBN 92 832 1258 4

ISSN 0250-9555

Publications of the World Health Organization enjoy copyright protection in accordance with the provisions of Protocol 2 of the Universal Copyright Convention.

All rights reserved. Application for rights of reproduction or translation, in part or *in toto*, should be made to the International Agency for Research on Cancer.

Distributed for the International Agency for Research on Cancer
by the Secretariat of the World Health Organization, Geneva

PRINTED IN THE UNITED KINGDOM

CONTENTS

NOTE TO THE READER 5

LIST OF PARTICIPANTS 7

PREAMBLE 13
    Background 13
    Objective and Scope 13
    Selection of Topics for Monographs 14
    Data for Monographs 15
    The Working Group 15
    Working Procedures 15
    Exposure Data 16
    Studies of Cancer in Humans 17
    Studies of Cancer in Experimental Animals 21
    Other Relevant Data 23
    Summary of Data Reported 24
    Evaluation 26
    References 30

GENERAL REMARKS ON THE AGENTS CONSIDERED 35

THE MONOGRAPHS
    Beryllium 41
    Cadmium 119
    Mercury 239
    Exposures in the Glass Manufacturing Industry 347

SUMMARY OF FINAL EVALUATIONS 377

APPENDIX 1. SUMMARY TABLES OF GENETIC AND RELATED EFFECTS . 381

APPENDIX 2. ACTIVITY PROFILES FOR GENETIC AND RELATED
    EFFECTS 389

CUMULATIVE INDEX TO THE *MONOGRAPHS* SERIES 417

NOTE TO THE READER

The term 'carcinogenic risk' in the *IARC Monographs* series is taken to mean the probability that exposure to an agent will lead to cancer in humans.

Inclusion of an agent in the *Monographs* does not imply that it is a carcinogen, only that the published data have been examined. Equally, the fact that an agent has not yet been evaluated in a monograph does not mean that it is not carcinogenic.

The evaluations of carcinogenic risk are made by international working groups of independent scientists and are qualitative in nature. No recommendation is given for regulation or legislation.

Anyone who is aware of published data that may alter the evaluation of the carcinogenic risk of an agent to humans is encouraged to make this information available to the Unit of Carcinogen Identification and Evaluation, International Agency for Research on Cancer, 150 cours Albert Thomas, 69372 Lyon Cedex 08, France, in order that the agent may be considered for re-evaluation by a future Working Group.

Although every effort is made to prepare the monographs as accurately as possible, mistakes may occur. Readers are requested to communicate any errors to the Unit of Carcinogen Identification and Evaluation, so that corrections can be reported in future volumes.

IARC WORKING GROUP ON THE EVALUATION OF CARCINOGENIC RISKS TO HUMANS: BERYLLIUM, CADMIUM, MERCURY, AND EXPOSURES IN THE GLASS MANUFACTURING INDUSTRY

Lyon, 9–16 February 1993

LIST OF PARTICIPANTS

Members[1]

A. Aitio, Biomonitoring Laboratory, Institute of Occupational Health, Arinatie 3, 00370 Helsinki, Finland

L. Alessio, Institute of Occupational Medicine, Piazzale Spedali Civili 1, 25123 Brescia, Italy

O. Axelson, Department of Occupational Medicine, University Hospital, 581 85, Linköping, Sweden (*Vice-Chairman*)

J. Coenen, Institute for Environmental Hygiene, Heinrich Heine University of Düsseldorf, Postfach 103751, 4000 Düsseldorf, Germany

S. De Flora, Institute of Hygiene and Preventive Medicine, University of Genoa, via Pastore 1, 16132 Genoa, Italy

P. Grandjean, Department of Environmental Medicine, Institute of Community Health, Odense University, Winsløwparken 17, 5000 Odense C, Denmark (*Chairman*)

U. Heinrich, Department of Experimental and Environmental Hygiene, Fraunhofer Institute of Toxicology and Aerosol Research, Nikolai-Fuchs-Strasse 1, 3000 Hanover 61, Germany

J.E. Huff, Environmental Carcinogenesis Program, National Institute of Environmental Health Sciences, PO Box 12233, Research Triangle Park, NC 27709, USA

M. Ikeda, Department of Public Health, Kyoto University Faculty of Medicine, Kyoto 606, Japan

R. Kavlock, Developmental Toxicology Division, Health Effects Research Laboratory, US Environmental Protection Agency (MD-71), Research Triangle Park, NC 27711, USA

---

[1]Unable to attend: F. Pott, Institute for Environmental Hygiene, Heinrich Heine University of Düsseldorf, Postfach 103751, 4000 Düsseldorf, Germany

G. Kazantzis, Environmental Geochemistry Research, Royal School of Mines, Imperial College of Science, Technology and Medicine, Prince Consort Road, London W7 2BP, United Kingdom

S. Langård, Telemark Central Hospital, Department of Occupational Medicine, Olavsgt 26, 39000 Postgrunn, Norway

L.S. Levy, Institute of Occupational Health, University of Birmingham, Edgbaston, Birmingham B15 2TT, United Kingdom

G. Oberdörster, Department of Environmental Medicine, School of Medicine and Dentistry, 575 Elmwood Avenue, Box EHSC, Rochester, NY 14642, USA

S. Olin, ILSI Risk Science Institute, 1126 Sixteenth Street NW, Washington DC 20036, USA

N.E. Pearce, Department of Medicine, Wellington School of Medicine, University of Otago, PO Box 7343, Wellington South, New Zealand

T.G. Rossman, Institute of Environmental Medicine, New York University Medical Center, Long Meadow, Tuxedo, NY 10987, USA

K.H. Schaller, Institute of Labour and Social Medicine and Polyclinic of Occupational Diseases, University of Erlangen-Nürnberg, Schillerstrasse 25/29, 8520 Erlangen, Germany

C. Shy, Department of Epidemiology, School of Public Health, University of North Carolina, CB 7400, Chapel Hill, NC 27599, USA

S. Skerfving, Department of Occupational and Environmental Medicine, University Hospital, 22185 Lund, Sweden

S. Swierenga, Drugs Directorate, Health and Welfare Canada, Tunney's Pasture, Ottawa, Ontario, Canada K1A 012

M.J. Thun, American Cancer Society, 1599 Clifton Road NE, Atlanta, GA 30329, USA

M.P. Waalkes, Laboratory of Comparative Carcinogenesis, National Cancer Institute, Frederick Cancer Research Development Center, Building 538, Room 205E, Frederick, MD 21702, USA

Representatives/observers

Commission of the European Communities

G. Aresini, Health and Safety Directorate, Industrial Medicine and Hygiene Unit, Commission of the European Communities, Bâtiment Jean Monnet, 2920 Luxembourg, Grand Duchy of Luxembourg

Eurométaux (Association européenne des Métaux)

P. Kotin, University of Colorado Medical School, Department of Microbiology, Colorado State University, 4505 South Yosemite, 330, Denver, CO 80237, USA

International Council on Metals and the Environment

T. Sorahan, Department of Public Health and Epidemiology, University of Birmingham, PO Box 363, Edgbaston, Birmingham B15 2TT, United Kingdom

National Center for Toxicological Research

W. Allaben, National Center for Toxicological Research, Jefferson, AR 72079-9502, USA

Occupational Safety and Health Administration

P.F. Infante, Occupational Safety and Health Administration, US Department of Labor, Room N-3718, 200 Constitution Avenue NW, Washington DC 20210, USA

Primary Glass Manufacturers' Confederation

J. Blackburn, 40 Carlton Avenue, Upholland, Skelmersdale, Lancashire WN8 0AE, United Kingdom

Secretariat

International Programme on Chemical Safety

E. Smith, International Programme on Chemical Safety, World Health Organization, 1211 Geneva 27, Switzerland

IARC

P. Boffetta, Unit of Analytical Epidemiology
S. Cordier, Unit of Analytical Epidemiology
P. Demers, Unit of Analytical Epidemiology
M. Friesen, Unit of Environmental Carcinogenesis and Host Factors
M.-J. Ghess, Unit of Carcinogen Identification and Evaluation
E. Heseltine, 24290 St Léon-sur-Vézère, France
C. Malaveille, Unit of Environmental Carcinogenesis and Host Factors
D. McGregor, Unit of Carcinogen Identification and Evaluation
D. Mietton, Unit of Carcinogen Identification and Evaluation
H. Møller, Unit of Carcinogen Identification and Evaluation
C. Partensky, Unit of Carcinogen Identification and Evaluation
I. Peterschmitt, Unit of Carcinogen Identification and Evaluation, Geneva, Switzerland
L. Tomatis, Director
H. Vainio, Unit of Carcinogen Identification and Evaluation
J. Wilbourn, Unit of Carcinogen Identification and Evaluation

Secretarial assistance

M. Lézère
J. Mitchell
S. Reynaud

PREAMBLE

IARC MONOGRAPHS PROGRAMME ON THE EVALUATION OF CARCINOGENIC RISKS TO HUMANS[1]

PREAMBLE

1. BACKGROUND

In 1969, the International Agency for Research on Cancer (IARC) initiated a programme to evaluate the carcinogenic risk of chemicals to humans and to produce monographs on individual chemicals. The *Monographs* programme has since been expanded to include consideration of exposures to complex mixtures of chemicals (which occur, for example, in some occupations and as a result of human habits) and of exposures to other agents, such as radiation and viruses. With Supplement 6 (IARC, 1987a), the title of the series was modified from *IARC Monographs on the Evaluation of the Carcinogenic Risk of Chemicals to Humans* to *IARC Monographs on the Evaluation of Carcinogenic Risks to Humans*, in order to reflect the widened scope of the programme.

The criteria established in 1971 to evaluate carcinogenic risk to humans were adopted by the working groups whose deliberations resulted in the first 16 volumes of the *IARC Monographs* series. Those criteria were subsequently updated by further ad-hoc working groups (IARC, 1977, 1978, 1979, 1982, 1983, 1987b, 1988, 1991a; Vainio *et al.*, 1992).

2. OBJECTIVE AND SCOPE

The objective of the programme is to prepare, with the help of international working groups of experts, and to publish in the form of monographs, critical reviews and evaluations of evidence on the carcinogenicity of a wide range of human exposures. The *Monographs* may also indicate where additional research efforts are needed.

The *Monographs* represent the first step in carcinogenic risk assessment, which involves examination of all relevant information in order to assess the strength of the available evidence that certain exposures could alter the incidence of cancer in humans. The second step is quantitative risk estimation. Detailed, quantitative evaluations of epidemiological data may be made in the *Monographs*, but without extrapolation beyond the range of the data

---

[1]This project is supported by PHS Grant No. 5-UO1 CA33193-11 awarded by the US National Cancer Institute, Department of Health and Human Services. Since 1986, the programme has also been supported by the Commission of the European Communities.

available. Quantitative extrapolation from experimental data to the human situation is not undertaken.

The term 'carcinogen' is used in these monographs to denote an exposure that is capable of increasing the incidence of malignant neoplasms; the induction of benign neoplasms may in some circumstances (see p. 22) contribute to the judgement that the exposure is carcinogenic. The terms 'neoplasm' and 'tumour' are used interchangeably.

Some epidemiological and experimental studies indicate that different agents may act at different stages in the carcinogenic process, and several different mechanisms may be involved. The aim of the *Monographs* has been, from their inception, to evaluate evidence of carcinogenicity at any stage in the carcinogenesis process, independently of the underlying mechanisms. Information on mechanisms may, however, be used in making the overall evaluation (IARC, 1991a; Vainio *et al*., 1992; see also pp. 28-30).

The *Monographs* may assist national and international authorities in making risk assessments and in formulating decisions concerning any necessary preventive measures. The evaluations of IARC working groups are scientific, qualitative judgements about the evidence for or against carcinogenicity provided by the available data. These evaluations represent only one part of the body of information on which regulatory measures may be based. Other components of regulatory decisions may vary from one situation to another and from country to country, responding to different socioeconomic and national priorities. **Therefore, no recommendation is given with regard to regulation or legislation, which are the responsibility of individual governments and/or other international organizations.**

The *IARC Monographs* are recognized as an authoritative source of information on the carcinogenicity of a wide range of human exposures. A users' survey, made in 1988, indicated that the *Monographs* are consulted by various agencies in 57 countries. Each volume is generally printed in 4000 copies for distribution to governments, regulatory bodies and interested scientists. The *Monographs* are also available *via* the Distribution and Sales Service of the World Health Organization.

3. SELECTION OF TOPICS FOR MONOGRAPHS

Topics are selected on the basis of two main criteria: (a) there is evidence of human exposure, and (b) there is some evidence or suspicion of carcinogenicity. The term 'agent' is used to include individual chemical compounds, groups of related chemical compounds, physical agents (such as radiation) and biological factors (such as viruses). Exposures to mixtures of agents may occur in occupational exposures and as a result of personal and cultural habits (like smoking and dietary practices). Chemical analogues and compounds with biological or physical characteristics similar to those of suspected carcinogens may also be considered, even in the absence of data on a possible carcinogenic effect in humans or experimental animals.

The scientific literature is surveyed for published data relevant to an assessment of carcinogenicity. The IARC surveys of chemicals being tested for carcinogenicity (IARC, 1973-1992) and directories of on-going research in cancer epidemiology (IARC, 1976-1992) often indicate those exposures that may be scheduled for future meetings. Ad-hoc working groups convened by IARC in 1984, 1989 and 1991 gave recommendations as to which agents should be evaluated in the *IARC Monographs* series (IARC, 1984, 1989, 1991b).

As significant new data on subjects on which monographs have already been prepared become available, re-evaluations are made at subsequent meetings, and revised monographs are published.

4. DATA FOR MONOGRAPHS

The *Monographs* do not necessarily cite all the literature concerning the subject of an evaluation. Only those data considered by the Working Group to be relevant to making the evaluation are included.

With regard to biological and epidemiological data, only reports that have been published or accepted for publication in the openly available scientific literature are reviewed by the working groups. In certain instances, government agency reports that have undergone peer review and are widely available are considered. Exceptions may be made on an ad-hoc basis to include unpublished reports that are in their final form and publicly available, if their inclusion is considered pertinent to making a final evaluation (see pp. 26 *et seq.*). In the sections on chemical and physical properties, on analysis, on production and use and on occurrence, unpublished sources of information may be used.

5. THE WORKING GROUP

Reviews and evaluations are formulated by a working group of experts. The tasks of the group are: (i) to ascertain that all appropriate data have been collected; (ii) to select the data relevant for the evaluation on the basis of scientific merit; (iii) to prepare accurate summaries of the data to enable the reader to follow the reasoning of the Working Group; (iv) to evaluate the results of epidemiological and experimental studies on cancer; (v) to evaluate data relevant to the understanding of mechanism of action; and (vi) to make an overall evaluation of the carcinogenicity of the exposure to humans.

Working Group participants who contributed to the considerations and evaluations within a particular volume are listed, with their addresses, at the beginning of each publication. Each participant who is a member of a working group serves as an individual scientist and not as a representative of any organization, government or industry. In addition, nominees of national and international agencies and industrial associations may be invited as observers.

6. WORKING PROCEDURES

Approximately one year in advance of a meeting of a working group, the topics of the monographs are announced and participants are selected by IARC staff in consultation with other experts. Subsequently, relevant biological and epidemiological data are collected by IARC from recognized sources of information on carcinogenesis, including data storage and retrieval systems such as BIOSIS, Chemical Abstracts, CANCERLIT, MEDLINE and TOXLINE—including EMIC and ETIC for data on genetic and related effects and reproductive and developmental effects, respectively.

For chemicals and some complex mixtures, the major collection of data and the preparation of first drafts of the sections on chemical and physical properties, on analysis, on production and use and on occurrence are carried out under a separate contract funded by the US National Cancer Institute. Representatives from industrial associations may assist in the preparation of sections on production and use. Information on production and trade is obtained from governmental and trade publications and, in some cases, by direct contact with industries. Separate production data on some agents may not be available because their publication could disclose confidential information. Information on uses may be obtained from published sources but is often complemented by direct contact with manufacturers. Efforts are made to supplement this information with data from other national and international sources.

Six months before the meeting, the material obtained is sent to meeting participants, or is used by IARC staff, to prepare sections for the first drafts of monographs. The first drafts are compiled by IARC staff and sent, prior to the meeting, to all participants of the Working Group for review.

The Working Group meets in Lyon for seven to eight days to discuss and finalize the texts of the monographs and to formulate the evaluations. After the meeting, the master copy of each monograph is verified by consulting the original literature, edited and prepared for publication. The aim is to publish monographs within nine months of the Working Group meeting.

The available studies are summarized by the Working Group, with particular regard to the qualitative aspects discussed below. In general, numerical findings are indicated as they appear in the original report; units are converted when necessary for easier comparison. The Working Group may conduct additional analyses of the published data and use them in their assessment of the evidence; the results of such supplementary analyses are given in square brackets. When an important aspect of a study, directly impinging on its interpretation, should be brought to the attention of the reader, a comment is given in square brackets.

7. EXPOSURE DATA

Sections that indicate the extent of past and present human exposure, the sources of exposure, the people most likely to be exposed and the factors that contribute to the exposure are included at the beginning of each monograph.

Most monographs on individual chemicals, groups of chemicals or complex mixtures include sections on chemical and physical data, on analysis, on production and use and on occurrence. In monographs on, for example, physical agents, biological factors, occupational exposures and cultural habits, other sections may be included, such as: historical perspectives, description of an industry or habit, chemistry of the complex mixture or taxonomy.

For chemical exposures, the Chemical Abstracts Services Registry Number, the latest Chemical Abstracts Primary Name and the IUPAC Systematic Name are recorded; other synonyms are given, but the list is not necessarily comprehensive. For biological agents, taxonomy and structure are described, and the degree of variability is given, when applicable.

Information on chemical and physical properties and, in particular, data relevant to identification, occurrence and biological activity are included. For biological agents, mode of replication, life cycle, target cells, persistence and latency, host response and description of nonmalignant disease caused by them are given. A description of technical products of chemicals includes trades names, relevant specifications and available information on composition and impurities. Some of the trade names given may be those of mixtures in which the agent being evaluated is only one of the ingredients.

The purpose of the section on analysis is to give the reader an overview of current methods, with emphasis on those widely used for regulatory purposes. Methods for monitoring human exposure are also given, when available. No critical evaluation or recommendation of any of the methods is meant or implied. The IARC publishes a series of volumes, *Environmental Carcinogens: Methods of Analysis and Exposure Measurement* (IARC, 1978–92), that describe validated methods for analysing a wide variety of chemicals and mixtures. For biological agents, methods of detection and exposure assessment are described, including their sensitivity, specificity and reproducibility.

The dates of first synthesis and of first commercial production of a chemical or mixture are provided; for agents which do not occur naturally, this information may allow a reasonable estimate to be made of the date before which no human exposure to the agent could have occurred. The dates of first reported occurrence of an exposure are also provided. In addition, methods of synthesis used in past and present commercial production and different methods of production which may give rise to different impurities are described.

Data on production, international trade and uses are obtained for representative regions, which usually include Europe, Japan and the USA. It should not, however, be inferred that those areas or nations are necessarily the sole or major sources or users of the agent. Some identified uses may not be current or major applications, and the coverage is not necessarily comprehensive. In the case of drugs, mention of their therapeutic uses does not necessarily represent current practice nor does it imply judgement as to their therapeutic efficacy.

Information on the occurrence of an agent or mixture in the environment is obtained from data derived from the monitoring and surveillance of levels in occupational environments, air, water, soil, foods and animal and human tissues. When available, data on the generation, persistence and bioaccumulation of the agent are also included. In the case of mixtures, industries, occupations or processes, information is given about all agents present. For processes, industries and occupations, a historical description is also given, noting variations in chemical composition, physical properties and levels of occupational exposure with time and place. For biological agents, the epidemiology of infection is described.

Statements concerning regulations and guidelines (e.g., pesticide registrations, maximal levels permitted in foods, occupational exposure limits) are included for some countries as indications of potential exposures, but they may not reflect the most recent situation, since such limits are continuously reviewed and modified. The absence of information on regulatory status for a country should not be taken to imply that that country does not have regulations with regard to the exposure. For biological agents, legislation and control, including vaccines and therapy, are described.

8. STUDIES OF CANCER IN HUMANS

(a) *Types of studies considered*

Three types of epidemiological studies of cancer contribute to the assessment of carcinogenicity in humans—cohort studies, case–control studies and correlation (or ecological) studies. Rarely, results from randomized trials may be available. Case reports of cancer in humans may also be reviewed.

Cohort and case–control studies relate individual exposures under study to the occurrence of cancer in individuals and provide an estimate of relative risk (ratio of incidence in those exposed to incidence in those not exposed) as the main measure of association.

In correlation studies, the units of investigation are usually whole populations (e.g., in particular geographical areas or at particular times), and cancer frequency is related to a summary measure of the exposure of the population to the agent, mixture or exposure circumstance under study. Because individual exposure is not documented, however, a causal relationship is less easy to infer from correlation studies than from cohort and case–control studies. Case reports generally arise from a suspicion, based on clinical experience, that the concurrence of two events—that is, a particular exposure and occurrence of a cancer—has happened rather more frequently than would be expected by chance. Case reports usually lack complete ascertainment of cases in any population, definition or enumeration of the population at risk and estimation of the expected number of cases in the absence of exposure. The uncertainties surrounding interpretation of case reports and correlation studies make them inadequate, except in rare instances, to form the sole basis for inferring a causal relationship. When taken together with case–control and cohort studies, however, relevant case reports or correlation studies may add materially to the judgement that a causal relationship is present.

Epidemiological studies of benign neoplasms, presumed preneoplastic lesions and other end-points thought to be relevant to cancer are also reviewed by working groups. They may, in some instances, strengthen inferences drawn from studies of cancer itself.

(b) Quality of studies considered

The *Monographs* are not intended to summarize all published studies. Those that are judged to be inadequate or irrelevant to the evaluation are generally omitted. They may be mentioned briefly, particularly when the information is considered to be a useful supplement to that in other reports or when they provide the only data available. Their inclusion does not imply acceptance of the adequacy of the study design or of the analysis and interpretation of the results, and limitations are clearly outlined in square brackets at the end of the study description.

It is necessary to take into account the possible roles of bias, confounding and chance in the interpretation of epidemiological studies. By 'bias' is meant the operation of factors in study design or execution that lead erroneously to a stronger or weaker association than in fact exists between disease and an agent, mixture or exposure circumstance. By 'confounding' is meant a situation in which the relationship with disease is made to appear stronger or to appear weaker than it truly is as a result of an association between the apparent causal factor and another factor that is associated with either an increase or decrease in the incidence of the disease. In evaluating the extent to which these factors have been minimized in an individual study, working groups consider a number of aspects of design and analysis as described in the report of the study. Most of these considerations apply equally to case–control, cohort and correlation studies. Lack of clarity of any of these aspects in the reporting of a study can decrease its credibility and the weight given to it in the final evaluation of the exposure.

Firstly, the study population, disease (or diseases) and exposure should have been well defined by the authors. Cases of disease in the study population should have been identified in a way that was independent of the exposure of interest, and exposure should have been assessed in a way that was not related to disease status.

Secondly, the authors should have taken account in the study design and analysis of other variables that can influence the risk of disease and may have been related to the exposure of interest. Potential confounding by such variables should have been dealt with either in the design of the study, such as by matching, or in the analysis, by statistical adjustment. In cohort studies, comparisons with local rates of disease may be more appropriate than those with national rates. Internal comparisons of disease frequency among individuals at different levels of exposure should also have been made in the study.

Thirdly, the authors should have reported the basic data on which the conclusions are founded, even if sophisticated statistical analyses were employed. At the very least, they should have given the numbers of exposed and unexposed cases and controls in a case–control study and the numbers of cases observed and expected in a cohort study. Further tabulations by time since exposure began and other temporal factors are also important. In a cohort study, data on all cancer sites and all causes of death should have been given, to reveal the possibility of reporting bias. In a case–control study, the effects of investigated factors other than the exposure of interest should have been reported.

Finally, the statistical methods used to obtain estimates of relative risk, absolute rates of cancer, confidence intervals and significance tests, and to adjust for confounding should have been clearly stated by the authors. The methods used should preferably have been the generally accepted techniques that have been refined since the mid-1970s. These methods have been reviewed for case–control studies (Breslow & Day, 1980) and for cohort studies (Breslow & Day, 1987).

(c) *Inferences about mechanism of action*

Detailed analyses of both relative and absolute risks in relation to temporal variables, such as age at first exposure, time since first exposure, duration of exposure, cumulative exposure and time since exposure ceased, are reviewed and summarized when available. The analysis of temporal relationships can be useful in formulating models of carcinogenesis. In particular, such analyses may suggest whether a carcinogen acts early or late in the process of carcinogenesis, although at best they allow only indirect inferences about the mechanism of action. Special attention is given to measurements of biological markers of carcinogen exposure or action, such as DNA or protein adducts, as well as markers of early steps in the carcinogenic process, such as proto-oncogene mutation, when these are incorporated into epidemiological studies focused on cancer incidence or mortality. Such measurements may allow inferences to be made about putative mechanisms of action (IARC, 1991a; Vainio *et al.*, 1992).

(d) *Criteria for causality*

After the quality of individual epidemiological studies of cancer has been summarized and assessed, a judgement is made concerning the strength of evidence that the agent, mixture or exposure circumstance in question is carcinogenic for humans. In making their judgement, the Working Group considers several criteria for causality. A strong association (i.e., a large relative risk) is more likely to indicate causality than a weak association, although it is recognized that relative risks of small magnitude do not imply lack of causality and may be important if the disease is common. Associations that are replicated in several studies of the same design or using different epidemiological approaches or under different circumstances of exposure are more likely to represent a causal relationship than isolated observations from single studies. If there are inconsistent results among investigations, possible reasons are sought (such as differences in amount of exposure), and results of studies judged to be of high quality are given more weight than those from studies judged to be methodologically less sound. When suspicion of carcinogenicity arises largely from a single study, these data are not combined with those from later studies in any subsequent reassessment of the strength of the evidence.

If the risk of the disease in question increases with the amount of exposure, this is considered to be a strong indication of causality, although absence of a graded response is not necessarily evidence against a causal relationship. Demonstration of a decline in risk after cessation of or reduction in exposure in individuals or in whole populations also supports a causal interpretation of the findings.

Although a carcinogen may act upon more than one target, the specificity of an association (i.e., an increased occurrence of cancer at one anatomical site or of one morphological type) adds plausibility to a causal relationship, particularly when excess cancer occurrence is limited to one morphological type within the same organ.

Although rarely available, results from randomized trials showing different rates among exposed and unexposed individuals provide particularly strong evidence for causality.

When several epidemiological studies show little or no indication of an association between an exposure and cancer, the judgement may be made that, in the aggregate, they show evidence of lack of carcinogenicity. Such a judgement requires first of all that the studies giving rise to it meet, to a sufficient degree, the standards of design and analysis described above. Specifically, the possibility that bias, confounding or misclassification of exposure or outcome could explain the observed results should be considered and excluded with reasonable certainty. In addition, all studies that are judged to be methodologically sound should be consistent with a relative risk of unity for any observed level of exposure and, when considered together, should provide a pooled estimate of relative risk which is at or near unity and has a narrow confidence interval, due to sufficient population size. Moreover, no individual study nor the pooled results of all the studies should show any consistent tendency for relative risk of cancer to increase with increasing level of exposure. It is important to note that evidence of lack of carcinogenicity obtained in this way from several epidemiological studies can apply only to the type(s) of cancer studied and to dose levels and intervals between first exposure and observation of disease that are the same as or less than those observed in all the studies. Experience with human cancer indicates that, in some cases, the period from first exposure to the development of clinical cancer is seldom less than 20 years; latent periods substantially shorter than 30 years cannot provide evidence for lack of carcinogenicity.

9. STUDIES OF CANCER IN EXPERIMENTAL ANIMALS

All known human carcinogens that have been studied adequately in experimental animals have produced positive results in one or more animal species (Wilbourn *et al.*, 1986; Tomatis *et al.*, 1989). For several agents (aflatoxins, 4-aminobiphenyl, azathioprine, betel quid with tobacco, BCME and CMME (technical grade), chlorambucil, chlornaphazine, ciclosporin, coal-tar pitches, coal-tars, combined oral contraceptives, cyclophosphamide, diethylstilboestrol, melphalan, 8-methoxypsoralen plus UVA, mustard gas, myleran, 2-naphthylamine, nonsteroidal oestrogens, oestrogen replacement therapy/steroidal oestrogens, solar radiation, thiotepa and vinyl chloride), carcinogenicity in experimental animals was established or highly suspected before epidemiological studies confirmed the carcinogenicity in humans (Vainio *et al.*, 1993). Although this association cannot establish that all agents and mixtures that cause cancer in experimental animals also cause cancer in humans, nevertheless, **in the absence of adequate data on humans, it is biologically plausible and prudent to regard agents and mixtures for which there is sufficient evidence (see p. 27) of carcinogenicity in experimental animals as if they presented a carcinogenic risk to humans.** The possibility that a given agent may cause cancer through a species-specific mechanism which does not operate in humans, see p. 28, should also be taken into consideration.

The nature and extent of impurities or contaminants present in the chemical or mixture being evaluated are given when available. Animal strain, sex, numbers per group, age at start of treatment and survival are reported.

Other types of studies summarized include: experiments in which the agent or mixture was administered in conjunction with known carcinogens or factors that modify carcinogenic effects; studies in which the end-point was not cancer but a defined precancerous lesion; and experiments on the carcinogenicity of known metabolites and derivatives.

For experimental studies of mixtures, consideration is given to the possibility of changes in the physicochemical properties of the test substance during collection, storage, extraction, concentration and delivery. Chemical and toxicological interactions of the components of mixtures may result in nonlinear dose–response relationships.

An assessment is made as to the relevance to human exposure of samples tested in experimental animals, which may involve consideration of: (i) physical and chemical characteristics, (ii) constituent substances that indicate the presence of a class of substances, (iii) the results of tests for genetic and related effects, including genetic activity profiles, DNA adduct profiles, proto-oncogene mutation and expression and suppressor gene inactivation. The relevance of results obtained with viral strains analogous to that being evaluated in the monograph must also be considered.

(a) Qualitative aspects

An assessment of carcinogenicity involves several considerations of qualitative importance, including (i) the experimental conditions under which the test was performed, including route and schedule of exposure, species, strain, sex, age, duration of follow-up; (ii) the consistency of the results, for example, across species and target organ(s); (iii) the spectrum of neoplastic response, from preneoplastic lesions and benign tumours to malignant neoplasms; and (iv) the possible role of modifying factors.

As mentioned earlier (p. 15), the *Monographs* are not intended to summarize all published studies. Those studies in experimental animals that are inadequate (e.g., too short a duration, too few animals, poor survival; see below) or are judged irrelevant to the evaluation are generally omitted. Guidelines for conducting adequate long-term carcinogenicity experiments have been outlined (e.g., Montesano *et al.*, 1986).

Considerations of importance to the Working Group in the interpretation and evaluation of a particular study include: (i) how clearly the agent was defined and, in the case of mixtures, how adequately the sample characterization was reported; (ii) whether the dose was adequately monitored, particularly in inhalation experiments; (iii) whether the doses and duration of treatment were appropriate and whether the survival of treated animals was similar to that of controls; (iv) whether there were adequate numbers of animals per group; (v) whether animals of both sexes were used; (vi) whether animals were allocated randomly to groups; (vii) whether the duration of observation was adequate; and (viii) whether the data were adequately reported. If available, recent data on the incidence of specific tumours in historical controls, as well as in concurrent controls, should be taken into account in the evaluation of tumour response.

When benign tumours occur together with and originate from the same cell type in an organ or tissue as malignant tumours in a particular study and appear to represent a stage in the progression to malignancy, it may be valid to combine them in assessing tumour incidence (Huff *et al.*, 1989). The occurrence of lesions presumed to be preneoplastic may in certain instances aid in assessing the biological plausibility of any neoplastic response observed. If an agent or mixture induces only benign neoplasms that appear to be end-points that do not readily undergo transition to malignancy, it should nevertheless be suspected of being a carcinogen and it requires further investigation.

(b) Quantitative aspects

The probability that tumours will occur may depend on the species, sex, strain and age of the animal, the dose of the carcinogen and the route and length of exposure. Evidence of an increased incidence of neoplasms with increased level of exposure strengthens the inference of a causal association between the exposure and the development of neoplasms.

The form of the dose–response relationship can vary widely, depending on the particular agent under study and the target organ. Both DNA damage and increased cell division are important aspects of carcinogenesis, and cell proliferation is a strong determinant of dose–response relationships for some carcinogens (Cohen & Ellwein, 1990). Since many chemicals require metabolic activation before being converted into their reactive intermediates, both metabolic and pharmacokinetic aspects are important in determining the dose–response pattern. Saturation of steps such as absorption, activation, inactivation and elimination may produce nonlinearity in the dose–response relationship, as could saturation of processes such as DNA repair (Hoel *et al.*, 1983; Gart *et al.*, 1986).

(c) Statistical analysis of long-term experiments in animals

Factors considered by the Working Group include the adequacy of the information given for each treatment group: (i) the number of animals studied and the number examined histologically, (ii) the number of animals with a given tumour type and (iii) length of survival. The statistical methods used should be clearly stated and should be the generally accepted techniques refined for this purpose (Peto et al., 1980; Gart et al., 1986). When there is no difference in survival between control and treatment groups, the Working Group usually compares the proportions of animals developing each tumour type in each of the groups. Otherwise, consideration is given as to whether or not appropriate adjustments have been made for differences in survival. These adjustments can include: comparisons of the proportions of tumour-bearing animals among the effective number of animals (alive at the time the first tumour is discovered), in the case where most differences in survival occur before tumours appear; life-table methods, when tumours are visible or when they may be considered 'fatal' because mortality rapidly follows tumour development; and the Mantel-Haenszel test or logistic regression, when occult tumours do not affect the animals' risk of dying but are 'incidental' findings at autopsy.

In practice, classifying tumours as fatal or incidental may be difficult. Several survival-adjusted methods have been developed that do not require this distinction (Gart et al., 1986), although they have not been fully evaluated.

10. OTHER RELEVANT DATA

(a) Absorption, distribution, metabolism and excretion

Concise information is given on absorption, distribution (including placental transfer) and excretion in both humans and experimental animals. Kinetic factors that may affect the dose–response relationship, such as saturation of uptake, protein binding, metabolic activation, detoxification and DNA repair processes, are mentioned. Studies that indicate the metabolic fate of the agent in humans and in experimental animals are summarized briefly, and comparisons of data from humans and animals are made when possible. Comparative information on the relationship between exposure and the dose that reaches the target site may be of particular importance for extrapolation between species.

(b) Toxic effects

Data are given on acute and chronic toxic effects (other than cancer), such as organ toxicity, increased cell proliferation, immunotoxicity and endocrine effects. The presence and toxicological significance of cellular receptors is described.

(c) Reproductive and developmental effects

Effects on reproduction, teratogenicity, fetotoxicity and embryotoxicity are also summarized briefly.

(d) Genetic and related effects

Tests of genetic and related effects are described in view of the relevance of gene mutation and chromosomal damage to carcinogenesis (Vainio et al., 1992).

The adequacy of the reporting of sample characterization is considered and, where necessary, commented upon; with regard to complex mixtures, such comments are similar to those described for animal carcinogenicity tests on p. 21. The available data are interpreted critically by phylogenetic group according to the end-points detected, which may include DNA damage, gene mutation, sister chromatid exchange, micronucleus formation, chromosomal aberrations, aneuploidy and cell transformation. The concentrations employed are given, and mention is made of whether use of an exogenous metabolic system *in vitro* affected the test result. These data are given as listings of test systems, data and references; bar graphs (activity profiles) and corresponding summary tables with detailed information on the preparation of the profiles (Waters *et al.*, 1987) are given in appendices.

Positive results in tests using prokaryotes, lower eukaryotes, plants, insects and cultured mammalian cells suggest that genetic and related effects could occur in mammals. Results from such tests may also give information about the types of genetic effect produced and about the involvement of metabolic activation. Some end-points described are clearly genetic in nature (e.g., gene mutations and chromosomal aberrations), while others are to a greater or lesser degree associated with genetic effects (e.g., unscheduled DNA synthesis). In-vitro tests for tumour-promoting activity and for cell transformation may be sensitive to changes that are not necessarily the result of genetic alterations but that may have specific relevance to the process of carcinogenesis. A critical appraisal of these tests has been published (Montesano *et al.*, 1986).

Genetic or other activity manifest in experimental mammals and humans is regarded as being of greater relevance than that in other organisms. The demonstration that an agent or mixture can induce gene and chromosomal mutations in whole mammals indicates that it may have carcinogenic activity, although this activity may not be detectably expressed in any or all species. Relative potency in tests for mutagenicity and related effects is not a reliable indicator of carcinogenic potency. Negative results in tests for mutagenicity in selected tissues from animals treated *in vivo* provide less weight, partly because they do not exclude the possibility of an effect in tissues other than those examined. Moreover, negative results in short-term tests with genetic end-points cannot be considered to provide evidence to rule out carcinogenicity of agents or mixtures that act through other mechanisms (e.g., receptor-mediated effects, cellular toxicity with regenerative proliferation, peroxisome proliferation) (Vainio *et al.*, 1992). Factors that may lead to misleading results in short-term tests have been discussed in detail elsewhere (Montesano *et al.*, 1986).

When available, data relevant to mechanisms of carcinogenesis that do not involve structural changes at the level of the gene are also described.

The adequacy of epidemiological studies of reproductive outcome and genetic and related effects in humans is evaluated by the same criteria as are applied to epidemiological studies of cancer.

(*e*) *Structure–activity considerations*

This section describes structure–activity relationships that may be relevant to an evaluation of the carcinogenicity of an agent.

11. SUMMARY OF DATA REPORTED

In this section, the relevant epidemiological and experimental data are summarized. Only reports, other than in abstract form, that meet the criteria outlined on p. 15 are considered for evaluating carcinogenicity. Inadequate studies are generally not summarized: such studies are usually identified by a square-bracketed comment in the preceding text.

(a) *Exposures*

Human exposure is summarized on the basis of elements such as production, use, occurrence in the environment and determinations in human tissues and body fluids. Quantitative data are given when available.

(b) *Carcinogenicity in humans*

Results of epidemiological studies that are considered to be pertinent to an assessment of human carcinogenicity are summarized. When relevant, case reports and correlation studies are also summarized.

(c) *Carcinogenicity in experimental animals*

Data relevant to an evaluation of carcinogenicity in animals are summarized. For each animal species and route of administration, it is stated whether an increased incidence of neoplasms or preneoplastic lesions was observed, and the tumour sites are indicated. If the agent or mixture produced tumours after prenatal exposure or in single-dose experiments, this is also indicated. Negative findings are also summarized. Dose–response and other quantitative data may be given when available.

(d) *Other data relevant to an evaluation of carcinogenicity and its mechanisms*

Data on biological effects in humans that are of particular relevance are summarized. These may include toxicological, kinetic and metabolic considerations and evidence of DNA binding, persistence of DNA lesions or genetic damage in exposed humans. Toxicological information, such as that on cytotoxicity and regeneration, receptor binding and hormonal and immunological effects, and data on kinetics and metabolism in experimental animals are given when considered relevant to the possible mechanism of the carcinogenic action of the agent. The results of tests for genetic and related effects are summarized for whole mammals, cultured mammalian cells and nonmammalian systems.

When available, comparisons of such data for humans and for animals, and particularly animals that have developed cancer, are described.

Structure–activity relationships are mentioned when relevant.

For the agent, mixture or exposure circumstance being evaluated, the available data on end-points or other phenomena relevant to mechanisms of carcinogenesis from studies in humans, experimental animals and tissue and cell test systems are summarized within one or more of the following descriptive dimensions:

(i) Evidence of genotoxicity (i.e., structural changes at the level of the gene): for example, structure–activity considerations, adduct formation, mutagenicity (effect on specific genes), chromosomal mutation/aneuploidy

(ii) Evidence of effects on the expression of relevant genes (i.e., functional changes at the intracellular level): for example, alterations to the structure or quantity of the product of a proto-oncogene or tumour suppressor gene, alterations to metabolic activation/-inactivation/DNA repair

(iii) Evidence of relevant effects on cell behaviour (i.e., morphological or behavioural changes at the cellular or tissue level): for example, induction of mitogenesis, compensatory cell proliferation, preneoplasia and hyperplasia, survival of premalignant or malignant cells (immortalization, immunosuppression), effects on metastatic potential

(iv) Evidence from dose and time relationships of carcinogenic effects and interactions between agents: for example, early/late stage, as inferred from epidemiological studies; initiation/promotion/progression/malignant conversion, as defined in animal carcinogenicity experiments; toxicokinetics

These dimensions are not mutually exclusive, and an agent may fall within more than one of them. Thus, for example, the action of an agent on the expression of relevant genes could be summarized under both the first and second dimension, even if it were known with reasonable certainty that those effects resulted from genotoxicity.

12. EVALUATION

Evaluations of the strength of the evidence for carcinogenicity arising from human and experimental animal data are made, using standard terms.

It is recognized that the criteria for these evaluations, described below, cannot encompass all of the factors that may be relevant to an evaluation of carcinogenicity. In considering all of the relevant data, the Working Group may assign the agent, mixture or exposure circumstance to a higher or lower category than a strict interpretation of these criteria would indicate.

(a) Degrees of evidence for carcinogenicity in humans and in experimental animals and supporting evidence

These categories refer only to the strength of the evidence that an exposure is carcinogenic and not to the extent of its carcinogenic activity (potency) nor to the mechanisms involved. A classification may change as new information becomes available.

An evaluation of degree of evidence, whether for a single agent or a mixture, is limited to the materials tested, as defined physically, chemically or biologically. When the agents evaluated are considered by the Working Group to be sufficiently closely related, they may be grouped together for the purpose of a single evaluation of degree of evidence.

(i) *Carcinogenicity in humans*

The applicability of an evaluation of the carcinogenicity of a mixture, process, occupation or industry on the basis of evidence from epidemiological studies depends on the variability over time and place of the mixtures, processes, occupations and industries. The Working Group seeks to identify the specific exposure, process or activity which is considered most likely to be responsible for any excess risk. The evaluation is focused as narrowly as the available data on exposure and other aspects permit.

The evidence relevant to carcinogenicity from studies in humans is classified into one of the following categories:

Sufficient evidence of carcinogenicity: The Working Group considers that a causal relationship has been established between exposure to the agent, mixture or exposure circumstance and human cancer. That is, a positive relationship has been observed between the exposure and cancer in studies in which chance, bias and confounding could be ruled out with reasonable confidence.

Limited evidence of carcinogenicity: A positive association has been observed between exposure to the agent, mixture or exposure circumstance and cancer for which a causal interpretation is considered by the Working Group to be credible, but chance, bias or confounding could not be ruled out with reasonable confidence.

Inadequate evidence of carcinogenicity: The available studies are of insufficient quality, consistency or statistical power to permit a conclusion regarding the presence or absence of a causal association, or no data on cancer in humans are available.

Evidence suggesting lack of carcinogenicity: There are several adequate studies covering the full range of levels of exposure that human beings are known to encounter, which are mutually consistent in not showing a positive association between exposure to the agent, mixture or exposure circumstance and any studied cancer at any observed level of exposure. A conclusion of 'evidence suggesting lack of carcinogenicity' is inevitably limited to the cancer sites, conditions and levels of exposure and length of observation covered by the available studies. In addition, the possibility of a very small risk at the levels of exposure studied can never be excluded.

In some instances, the above categories may be used to classify the degree of evidence related to carcinogenicity in specific organs or tissues.

(ii) *Carcinogenicity in experimental animals*

The evidence relevant to carcinogenicity in experimental animals is classified into one of the following categories:

Sufficient evidence of carcinogenicity: The Working Group considers that a causal relationship has been established between the agent or mixture and an increased incidence of malignant neoplasms or of an appropriate combination of benign and malignant neoplasms in (a) two or more species of animals or (b) in two or more independent studies in one species carried out at different times or in different laboratories or under different protocols.

Exceptionally, a single study in one species might be considered to provide sufficient evidence of carcinogenicity when malignant neoplasms occur to an unusual degree with regard to incidence, site, type of tumour or age at onset.

Limited evidence of carcinogenicity: The data suggest a carcinogenic effect but are limited for making a definitive evaluation because, e.g., (a) the evidence of carcinogenicity is restricted to a single experiment; or (b) there are unresolved questions regarding the adequacy of the design, conduct or interpretation of the study; or (c) the agent or mixture increases the incidence only of benign neoplasms or lesions of uncertain neoplastic potential, or of certain neoplasms which may occur spontaneously in high incidences in certain strains.

Inadequate evidence of carcinogenicity: The studies cannot be interpreted as showing either the presence or absence of a carcinogenic effect because of major qualitative or quantitative limitations, or no data on cancer in experimental animals are available.

Evidence suggesting lack of carcinogenicity: Adequate studies involving at least two species are available which show that, within the limits of the tests used, the agent or mixture is not carcinogenic. A conclusion of evidence suggesting lack of carcinogenicity is inevitably limited to the species, tumour sites and levels of exposure studied.

(b) *Other data relevant to the evaluation of carcinogenicity*

Other evidence judged to be relevant to an evaluation of carcinogenicity and of sufficient importance to affect the overall evaluation is then described. This may include data on preneoplastic lesions, tumour pathology, genetic and related effects, structure–activity relationships, metabolism and pharmacokinetics, and physicochemical parameters.

Data relevant to mechanisms of the carcinogenic action are also evaluated. The strength of the evidence that any carcinogenic effect observed is due to a particular mechanism is assessed, using terms such as weak, moderate or strong. Then, the Working Group assesses if that particular mechanism is likely to be operative in humans. The strongest indications that a particular mechanism operates in humans come from data on humans or biological specimens obtained from exposed humans. The data may be considered to be especially relevant if they show that the agent in question has caused changes in exposed humans that are on the causal pathway to carcinogenesis. Such data may, however, never become available, because it is at least conceivable that certain compounds may be kept from human use solely on the basis of evidence of their toxicity and/or carcinogenicity in experimental systems.

For complex exposures, including occupational and industrial exposures, chemical composition and the potential contribution of carcinogens known to be present are considered by the Working Group in its overall evaluation of human carcinogenicity. The Working Group also determines the extent to which the materials tested in experimental systems are related to those to which humans are exposed.

(c) Overall evaluation

Finally, the body of evidence is considered as a whole, in order to reach an overall evaluation of the carcinogenicity to humans of an agent, mixture or circumstance of exposure.

An evaluation may be made for a group of chemical compounds that have been evaluated by the Working Group. In addition, when supporting data indicate that other, related compounds for which there is no direct evidence of capacity to induce cancer in humans or in animals may also be carcinogenic, a statement describing the rationale for this conclusion is added to the evaluation narrative; an additional evaluation may be made for this broader group of compounds if the strength of the evidence warrants it.

The agent, mixture or exposure circumstance is described according to the wording of one of the following categories, and the designated group is given. The categorization of an agent, mixture or exposure circumstance is a matter of scientific judgement, reflecting the strength of the evidence derived from studies in humans and in experimental animals and from other relevant data.

Group 1—The agent (mixture) is carcinogenic to humans.
The exposure circumstance entails exposures that are carcinogenic to hur:. ns.

This category is used when there is *sufficient evidence* of carcinogenicity in humans. Exceptionally, an agent (mixture) may be placed in this category when evidence in humans is less than sufficient but there is *sufficient evidence* of carcinogenicity in experimental animals and strong evidence in exposed humans that the agent (mixture) acts through a relevant mechanism of carcinogenicity.

Group 2

This category includes agents, mixtures and exposure circumstances for which, at one extreme, the degree of evidence of carcinogenicity in humans is almost sufficient, as well as those for which, at the other extreme, there are no human data but for which there is evidence of carcinogenicity in experimental animals. Agents, mixtures and exposure circumstances are assigned to either group 2A (probably carcinogenic to humans) or group 2B (possibly carcinogenic to humans) on the basis of epidemiological and experimental evidence of carcinogenicity and other relevant data.

Group 2A — The agent (mixture) is probably carcinogenic to humans.
The exposure circumstance entails exposures that are probably carcinogenic to humans.

This category is used when there is *limited evidence* of carcinogenicity in humans and *sufficient evidence* of carcinogenicity in experimental animals. In some cases, an agent (mixture) may be classified in this category when there is *inadequate evidence* of carcinogenicity in humans and *sufficient evidence* of carcinogenicity in experimental animals and strong evidence that the carcinogenesis is mediated by a mechanism that also operates in humans. Exceptionally, an agent, mixture or exposure circumstance may be classified in this category solely on the basis of *limited evidence* of carcinogenicity in humans.

Group 2B — The agent (mixture) is possibly carcinogenic to humans.
The exposure circumstance entails exposures that are possibly carcinogenic to humans.

This category is used for agents, mixtures and exposure circumstances for which there is *limited evidence* of carcinogenicity in humans and less than *sufficient evidence* of carcinogenicity in experimental animals. It may also be used when there is *inadequate evidence* of carcinogenicity in humans but there is *sufficient evidence* of carcinogenicity in experimental animals. In some instances, an agent, mixture or exposure circumstance for which there is *inadequate evidence* of carcinogenicity in humans but *limited evidence* of carcinogenicity in experimental animals together with supporting evidence from other relevant data may be placed in this group.

Group 3 — The agent (mixture or exposure circumstance) is not classifiable as to its carcinogenicity to humans.

This category is used most commonly for agents, mixtures and exposure circumstances for which the evidence of carcinogenicity is inadequate in humans and inadequate or limited in experimental animals.

Exceptionally, agents (mixtures) for which the evidence of carcinogenicity is inadequate in humans but sufficient in experimental animals may be placed in this category when there is strong evidence that the mechanism of carcinogenicity in experimental animals does not operate in humans.

Agents, mixtures and exposure circumstances that do not fall into any other group are also placed in this category.

Group 4 — The agent (mixture) is probably not carcinogenic to humans.

This category is used for agents or mixtures for which there is *evidence suggesting lack of carcinogenicity* in humans and in experimental animals. In some instances, agents or mixtures for which there is *inadequate evidence* of carcinogenicity in humans but *evidence suggesting lack of carcinogenicity* in experimental animals, consistently and strongly supported by a broad range of other relevant data, may be classified in this group.

References

Breslow, N.E. & Day, N.E. (1980) *Statistical Methods in Cancer Research*, Vol. 1, *The Analysis of Case-control Studies* (IARC Scientific Publications No. 32), Lyon, IARC

Breslow, N.E. & Day, N.E. (1987) *Statistical Methods in Cancer Research*, Vol. 2, *The Design and Analysis of Cohort Studies* (IARC Scientific Publications No. 82), Lyon, IARC

Cohen, S.M. & Ellwein, L.B. (1990) Cell proliferation in carcinogenesis. *Science*, 249, 1007–1011

Gart, J.J., Krewski, D., Lee, P.N., Tarone, R.E. & Wahrendorf, J. (1986) *Statistical Methods in Cancer Research*, Vol. 3, *The Design and Analysis of Long-term Animal Experiments* (IARC Scientific Publications No. 79), Lyon, IARC

Hoel, D.G., Kaplan, N.L. & Anderson, M.W. (1983) Implication of nonlinear kinetics on risk estimation in carcinogenesis. *Science*, 219, 1032–1037

Huff, J.E., Eustis, S.L. & Haseman, J.K. (1989) Occurrence and relevance of chemically induced benign neoplasms in long-term carcinogenicity studies. *Cancer Metastasis Rev.*, 8, 1–21

IARC (1973–1992) *Information Bulletin on the Survey of Chemicals Being Tested for Carcinogenicity/Directory of Agents Being Tested for Carcinogenicity*, Numbers 1–15, Lyon

  Number 1 (1973)   52 pages
  Number 2 (1973)   77 pages
  Number 3 (1974)   67 pages
  Number 4 (1974)   97 pages
  Number 5 (1975)   88 pages
  Number 6 (1976)   360 pages
  Number 7 (1978)   460 pages
  Number 8 (1979)   604 pages
  Number 9 (1981)   294 pages
  Number 10 (1983) 326 pages
  Number 11 (1984) 370 pages
  Number 12 (1986) 385 pages
  Number 13 (1988) 404 pages
  Number 14 (1990) 369 pages
  Number 15 (1992) 317 pages

IARC (1976–1992)

  Directory of On-going Research in Cancer Epidemiology 1976. Edited by C.S. Muir & G. Wagner, Lyon

  Directory of On-going Research in Cancer Epidemiology 1977 (IARC Scientific Publications No. 17). Edited by C.S. Muir & G. Wagner, Lyon

  Directory of On-going Research in Cancer Epidemiology 1978 (IARC Scientific Publications No. 26). Edited by C.S. Muir & G. Wagner, Lyon

  Directory of On-going Research in Cancer Epidemiology 1979 (IARC Scientific Publications No. 28). Edited by C.S. Muir & G. Wagner, Lyon

  Directory of On-going Research in Cancer Epidemiology 1980 (IARC Scientific Publications No. 35). Edited by C.S. Muir & G. Wagner, Lyon

Directory of On-going Research in Cancer Epidemiology 1981 (IARC Scientific Publications No. 38). Edited by C.S. Muir & G. Wagner, Lyon

Directory of On-going Research in Cancer Epidemiology 1982 (IARC Scientific Publications No. 46). Edited by C.S. Muir & G. Wagner, Lyon

Directory of On-going Research in Cancer Epidemiology 1983 (IARC Scientific Publications No. 50). Edited by C.S. Muir & G. Wagner, Lyon

Directory of On-going Research in Cancer Epidemiology 1984 (IARC Scientific Publications No. 62). Edited by C.S. Muir & G. Wagner, Lyon

Directory of On-going Research in Cancer Epidemiology 1985 (IARC Scientific Publications No. 69). Edited by C.S. Muir & G. Wagner, Lyon

Directory of On-going Research in Cancer Epidemiology 1986 (IARC Scientific Publications No. 80). Edited by C.S. Muir & G. Wagner, Lyon

Directory of On-going Research in Cancer Epidemiology 1987 (IARC Scientific Publications No. 86). Edited by D.M. Parkin & J. Wahrendorf, Lyon

Directory of On-going Research in Cancer Epidemiology 1988 (IARC Scientific Publications No. 93). Edited by M. Coleman & J. Wahrendorf, Lyon

Directory of On-going Research in Cancer Epidemiology 1989/90 (IARC Scientific Publications No. 101). Edited by M. Coleman & J. Wahrendorf, Lyon

Directory of On-going Research in Cancer Epidemiology 1991 (IARC Scientific Publications No. 110). Edited by M. Coleman & J. Wahrendorf, Lyon

Directory of On-going Research in Cancer Epidemiology 1992 (IARC Scientific Publications No. 117). Edited by M. Coleman, J. Wahrendorf & E. Demaret, Lyon

IARC (1977) *IARC Monographs Programme on the Evaluation of the Carcinogenic Risk of Chemicals to Humans. Preamble* (IARC intern. tech. Rep. No. 77/002), Lyon

IARC (1978) *Chemicals with Sufficient Evidence of Carcinogenicity in Experimental Animals*—IARC Monographs *Volumes 1–17* (IARC intern. tech. Rep. No. 78/003), Lyon

IARC (1978–1993) *Environmental Carcinogens. Methods of Analysis and Exposure Measurement*:

   Vol. 1. *Analysis of Volatile Nitrosamines in Food* (IARC Scientific Publications No. 18). Edited by R. Preussmann, M. Castegnaro, E.A. Walker & A.E. Wasserman (1978)

   Vol. 2. *Methods for the Measurement of Vinyl Chloride in Poly(vinyl chloride), Air, Water and Foodstuffs* (IARC Scientific Publications No. 22). Edited by D.C.M. Squirrell & W. Thain (1978)

   Vol. 3. *Analysis of Polycyclic Aromatic Hydrocarbons in Environmental Samples* (IARC Scientific Publications No. 29). Edited by M. Castegnaro, P. Bogovski, H. Kunte & E.A. Walker (1979)

   Vol. 4. *Some Aromatic Amines and Azo Dyes in the General and Industrial Environment* (IARC Scientific Publications No. 40). Edited by L. Fishbein, M. Castegnaro, I.K. O'Neill & H. Bartsch (1981)

   Vol. 5. *Some Mycotoxins* (IARC Scientific Publications No. 44). Edited by L. Stoloff, M. Castegnaro, P. Scott, I.K. O'Neill & H. Bartsch (1983)

   Vol. 6. N-*Nitroso Compounds* (IARC Scientific Publications No. 45). Edited by R. Preussmann, I.K. O'Neill, G. Eisenbrand, B. Spiegelhalder & H. Bartsch (1983)

   Vol. 7. *Some Volatile Halogenated Hydrocarbons* (IARC Scientific Publications No. 68). Edited by L. Fishbein & I.K. O'Neill (1985)

   Vol. 8. *Some Metals: As, Be, Cd, Cr, Ni, Pb, Se, Zn* (IARC Scientific Publications No. 71). Edited by I.K. O'Neill, P. Schuller & L. Fishbein (1986)

Vol. 9. *Passive Smoking* (IARC Scientific Publications No. 81). Edited by I.K. O'Neill, K.D. Brunnemann, B. Dodet & D. Hoffmann (1987)

Vol. 10. *Benzene and Alkylated Benzenes* (IARC Scientific Publications No. 85). Edited by L. Fishbein & I.K. O'Neill (1988)

Vol. 11. *Polychlorinated Dioxins and Dibenzofurans* (IARC Scientific Publications No. 108). Edited by C. Rappe, H.R. Buser, B. Dodet & I.K. O'Neill (1991)

Vol. 12. *Indoor Air* (IARC Scientific Publications No. 109). Edited by B. Seifert, H. van de Wiel, B. Dodet & I.K. O'Neill (1993)

IARC (1979) *Criteria to Select Chemicals for* IARC Monographs (IARC intern. tech. Rep. No. 79/003), Lyon

IARC (1982) *IARC Monographs on the Evaluation of the Carcinogenic Risk of Chemicals to Humans, Supplement 4, Chemicals, Industrial Processes and Industries Associated with Cancer in Humans (IARC Monographs, Volumes 1 to 29)*, Lyon

IARC (1983) *Approaches to Classifying Chemical Carcinogens According to Mechanism of Action* (IARC intern. tech. Rep. No. 83/001), Lyon

IARC (1984) *Chemicals and Exposures to Complex Mixtures Recommended for Evaluation in* IARC Monographs *and Chemicals and Complex Mixtures Recommended for Long-term Carcinogenicity Testing* (IARC intern. tech. Rep. No. 84/002), Lyon

IARC (1987a) *IARC Monographs on the Evaluation of Carcinogenic Risks to Humans*, Supplement 6, *Genetic and Related Effects: An Updating of Selected* IARC Monographs *from Volumes 1 to 42*, Lyon

IARC (1987b) *IARC Monographs on the Evaluation of Carcinogenic Risks to Humans*, Supplement 7, *Overall Evaluations of Carcinogenicity: An Updating of* IARC Monographs *Volumes 1 to 42*, Lyon

IARC (1988) *Report of an IARC Working Group to Review the Approaches and Processes Used to Evaluate the Carcinogenicity of Mixtures and Groups of Chemicals* (IARC intern. tech. Rep. No. 88/002), Lyon

IARC (1989) *Chemicals, Groups of Chemicals, Mixtures and Exposure Circumstances to be Evaluated in Future IARC Monographs, Report of an ad hoc Working Group* (IARC intern. tech. Rep. No. 89/004), Lyon

IARC (1991a) *A Consensus Report of an* IARC Monographs *Working Group on the Use of Mechanims of Carcinogenesis in Risk Identification* (IARC intern. tech. Rep. No. 91/002), Lyon

IARC (1991b) *Report of an Ad-hoc* IARC Monographs *Advisory Group on Viruses and Other Biological Agents Such as Parasites* (IARC intern. tech. Rep. No. 91/001), Lyon

Montesano, R., Bartsch, H., Vainio, H., Wilbourn, J. & Yamasaki, H., eds (1986) *Long-term and Short-term Assays for Carcinogenesis—A Critical Appraisal* (IARC Scientific Publications No. 83), Lyon, IARC

Peto, R., Pike, M.C., Day, N.E., Gray, R.G., Lee, P.N., Parish, S., Peto, J., Richards, S. & Wahrendorf, J. (1980) Guidelines for simple, sensitive significance tests for carcinogenic effects in long-term animal experiments. In: *IARC Monographs on the Evaluation of the Carcinogenic Risk of Chemicals to Humans*, Supplement 2, *Long-term and Short-term Screening Assays for Carcinogens: A Critical Appraisal*, Lyon, pp. 311–426

Tomatis, L., Aitio, A., Wilbourn, J. & Shuker, L. (1989) Human carcinogens so far identified. *Jpn. J. Cancer Res.*, 80, 795–807

Vainio, H., Magee, P., McGregor, D. & McMichael, A., eds (1992) *Mechanisms of Carcinogenesis in Risk Identification* (IARC Scientific Publications No. 116), Lyon, IARC

Vainio, H., Wilbourn, J. & Tomatis, L. (1993) Identification of environmental carcinogens: the first step in risk assessment. In: Mehlman, M.A. & Upton, A., eds, *The Identification and Control of Environmental and Occupational Diseases*, Princeton, Princeton Scientific Publishing Company (in press)

Waters, M.D., Stack, H.F., Brady, A.L., Lohman, P.H.M., Haroun, L. & Vainio, H. (1987) Appendix 1. Activity profiles for genetic and related tests. In: *IARC Monographs on the Evaluation of Carcinogenic Risks to Humans*, Suppl. 6, *Genetic and Related Effects: An Updating of Selected IARC Monographs from Volumes 1 to 42*, Lyon, IARC, pp. 687–696

Wilbourn, J., Haroun, L., Heseltine, E., Kaldor, J., Partensky, C. & Vainio, H. (1986) Response of experimental animals to human carcinogens: an analysis based upon the IARC Monographs Programme. *Carcinogenesis*, 7, 1853–1863

GENERAL REMARKS ON THE AGENTS CONSIDERED

This fifty-eighth volume of *IARC Monographs* covers some metals and their compounds—beryllium and beryllium compounds, cadmium and cadmium compounds, mercury and inorganic and methylmercury compounds. Exposures in the glass manufacturing industry are also addressed, as several metallic salts and pigments may be used in manufacture and colouring of crystal and art glass and in the production of glass containers.

Beryllium compounds were used extensively in the past as phosphors in fluorescent lighting tubes; they are now widely used in solid-state computer and communication systems and in the aircraft and aerospace industries. Beryllium also occurs in coal, the burning of which results in some environmental exposure. Occupational exposure to beryllium and beryllium compounds has been reduced over the last 40 years, and low permissible exposure limits have been set in some countries. Beryllium and beryllium compounds were evaluated previously in the *Monographs* (IARC, 1972, 1980, 1987a). Extended analyses have been reported of mortality among cohorts of workers in beryllium plants and of those entered into the US Beryllium Case Registry, and it is mainly on the basis of those new studies that a re-evaluation was made.

Cadmium and cadmium compounds were also evaluated previously (IARC, 1973, 1976, 1987b). Occupational exposure to cadmium can occur in zinc smelting and cadmium refining, in cadmium alloy production, in nickel–cadmium battery manufacture and through the production and use of cadmium pigments. Environmental exposures to cadmium may occur owing to its presence as a pollutant in food and water. Exposure to cadmium can occur also through the smoking of tobacco. New analyses of epidemiological cohorts and the results of new studies of carcinogenicity in experimental animals were considered by the Working Group in making the re-evaluation reported here.

Mercury and mercury compounds are considered for the first time in the *IARC Monographs*. Metallic mercury and inorganic salts as well as some organomercury compounds are included. Organomercury salts and those used in organomercury fungicides and bactericides are mentioned, but commercial biocidal products are not included. Human exposure to mercury can occur *via* many sources, including mercury mining, chloralkali plants, manufacture of thermometers, maintenance of mercury-containing instruments and from dental amalgams. Exposure to methylmercury compounds has occurred from the consumption of mercury-contaminated fish, and mercury poisoning has resulted from eating bread accidentally made from seed treated with organomercury fungicides and intended for sowing.

The environmental occurrence of and exposures to cadmium and mercury compounds were reviewed within the International Programme on Chemical Safety (WHO, 1990, 1991, 1992a,b), and reference is made to those reviews throughout this volume. Cadmium and mercury were included by the International Register of Potentially Toxic Chemicals of the United Nations Environment Programme (UNEP, 1984, 1992) in its listing of dangerous chemical substances and processes of global significance.

A monograph on exposures in the glass manufacturing industry was prepared, as several epidemiological studies reported in the recent literature suggested an increased risk for cancer, mainly of the lung. Some of the studies were conducted in areas of northern Europe where crystal and art glass are made; in some studies, however, the type of glass industry involved is poorly defined. In particular, no epidemiological data were available that specifically addressed risks for workers employed in the automated manufacture of flat glass (Pilkington process), the most widely used process in the modern glass industry. A basic ingredient in the making of glass is silica, and exposures to lead, arsenic and several metallic pigments may occur, including cadmium and mercury salts. Cross-reference is made to relevant volumes of *IARC Monographs* in which evaluations of these components can be found. Occupational exposures in the production of glass fibres are not considered in this volume, because they have been evaluated previously (IARC, 1988)[1]: there is *sufficient evidence* for the carcinogenicity of glasswool in experimental animals; there is *inadequate evidence* for the carcinogenicity of glass filaments in experimental animals; there is *inadequate evidence* for the carcinogenicity of glasswool and of glass filaments in humans. **Overall evaluation:** glasswool is *possibly carcinogenic to humans (Group 2B)*; and glass filaments are *not classifiable as to their carcinogenicity to humans (Group 3)*.

Traditional analytical methods for determining exposure to metals, in particular to mercury and cadmium, provide only total concentrations of metal, and specific chemical compounds of the elements cannot be identified. Exposure limit values often refer to total concentrations of an element. Marked differences exist, however, in the deposition, absorption and distribution of the different compounds of each element, and particle size determines uptake through the lungs. Bioavailability and solubility in physiological fluids may also differ for different compounds.

Biological monitoring, by analysis of blood and urine, is often useful in determining exposure or body burden. The toxicological data available on cadmium and mercury are extensive; as the *Monographs* are not intended to provide a complete review of such information, unless it has a direct bearing on the evaluation of potential carcinogenicity, a selection of illustrative original references were summarized to provide an outline of the available evidence. Information on the toxicokinetics of beryllium in humans is very limited, and few data are available on concentrations of beryllium in biological fluids obtained from occupationally exposed and control populations. For agents that induce cancer at the site of entry, e.g., in the respiratory system, however, biological monitoring may not be predictive of individual risk in the absence of knowledge about toxicokinetic behaviour.

Although much research has been conducted on the metals covered in this volume, the molecular mechanisms of action that may lead to carcinogenic effects are still not completely understood. Involvement of the immune system in beryllium- and mercury-induced chronic diseases may complicate the dose-response patterns; it also raises the possibility of the

---

[1]For definition of the italicized terms, see Preamble, pp. 26–30.

existence of subpopulations who are susceptible to effects that may be related to carcinogenicity.

References

IARC (1972) *IARC Monographs on the Evaluation of Carcinogenic Risk of Chemicals to Man*, Vol. 1, *Some Inorganic Substances, Chlorinated Hydrocarbons, Aromatic Amines, N-Nitroso Compounds, and Natural Products*, Lyon, pp. 17–28

IARC (1973) *IARC Monographs on the Evaluation of Carcinogenic Risk of Chemicals to Man*, Vol. 2, *Some Inorganic and Organic Compounds*, Lyon, pp. 74–99

IARC (1976) *IARC Monographs on the Evaluation of Carcinogenic Risk of Chemicals to Man*, Vol. 11, *Cadmium, Nickel, Some Epoxides, Miscellaneous Industrial Chemicals and General Considerations on Volatile Anaesthetics*, Lyon, pp. 39–74

IARC (1980) IARC (1972) *IARC Monographs on the Evaluation of the Carcinogenic Risk of Chemicals to Humans*, Vol. 23, *Some Metals and Metallic Compounds*, Lyon, pp. 143–204

IARC (1987a) *IARC Monographs on the Evaluation of Carcinogenic Risks to Humans*, Suppl. 7, *Overall Evaluations of Carcinogenicity: An Updating of* IARC Monographs *Volumes 1 to 42*, Lyon, pp. 127–128

IARC (1987b) *IARC Monographs on the Evaluation of Carcinogenic Risks to Humans*, Suppl. 7, *Overall Evaluations of Carcinogenicity: An Updating of* IARC Monographs *Volumes 1 to 42*, Lyon, pp. 139–142

IARC (1988) *IARC Monographs on the Evaluation of Carcinogenic Risks to Humans*, Vol. 43, *Man-made Mineral Fibres and Radon*, Lyon, pp. 39–171

UNEP (1984) *List of Environmentally Dangerous Chemical Substances and Processes of Global Significance* (Report of the Executive Director of UNEP to the 12th Session of Its Governing Council), Geneva, International Register of Potentially Toxic Chemicals

UNEP (1992) *Chemical Pollution: A Global Overview*, Geneva

WHO (1990) *Methylmercury* (Environmental Health Criteria 101), Geneva

WHO (1991) *Inorganic Mercury* (Environmental Health Criteria 118), Geneva

WHO (1992a) *Cadmium* (Environmental Health Criteria 134), Geneva

WHO (1992b) *Cadmium—Environmental Aspects* (Environmental Health Criteria 135), Geneva

THE MONOGRAPHS

BERYLLIUM AND BERYLLIUM COMPOUNDS

Beryllium and beryllium compounds were considered by previous Working Groups, in 1971, 1979 and 1987 (IARC, 1972, 1980, 1987a). New data have since become available, and these are included in the present monograph and have been taken into consideration in the evaluation. The agents considered herein include (a) metallic beryllium, (b) beryllium–aluminium and –copper alloys and (c) some beryllium compounds.

1. Exposure Data

1.1 Chemical and physical data and analysis

1.1.1 *Synonyms, trade names and molecular formulae*

Synonyms, trade names and molecular formulae for beryllium, beryllium–aluminium and –copper alloys and certain beryllium compounds are presented in Table 1. The list is not exhaustive, nor does it comprise necessarily the most commercially important beryllium-containing substances; rather, it indicates the range of beryllium compounds available.

1.1.2 *Chemical and physical properties of the pure substances*

Selected chemical and physical properties of beryllium, beryllium–aluminium and –copper alloys and the beryllium compounds covered in this monograph are presented in Table 2.

The French chemist Vauquelin discovered beryllium in 1798 as the oxide, while analysing emerald to prove an analogous composition (Newland, 1984). The metallic element was first isolated in independent experiments by Wöhler (1828) and Bussy (1828), who called it 'glucinium' owing to the sweet taste of its salts; that name is still used in the French chemical literature. Wöhler's name 'beryllium' was officially recognized by IUPAC in 1957 (WHO, 1990). The atomic weight and common valence of beryllium were originally the subject of much controversy but were correctly predicted by Mendeleev to be 9 and +2, respectively (Everest, 1973).

Beryllium is the lightest of all solid, chemically stable substances and has an unusually high melting-point. It has a very low density and a very high strength-to-weight ratio. Beryllium is lighter than aluminium but is more than 40% more rigid than steel. It has excellent electrical and thermal conductivities. Its only markedly adverse feature is relatively pronounced brittleness, which has restricted the use of metallic beryllium to specialized applications (WHO, 1990).

Table 1. Synonyms (Chemical Abstracts Service (CAS) names are in italics), trade names and atomic or molecular formulae of beryllium and beryllium compounds

Chemical name	CAS Reg. No.[a]	Synonyms and trade names	Formula
Beryllium metal	7440-41-7	*Beryllium*; beryllium-9; beryllium element; beryllium metallic; glucinium; glucinum	Be
Beryllium–aluminium alloy[b]	12770-50-2	*Aluminium alloy, nonbase, Al,Be*; aluminium–beryllium alloy	Al.Be
Beryllium–copper alloy[c]	11133-98-5	*Copper alloy, base, Cu,Be*; copper–beryllium alloy	Be.Cu
Beryl	1302-52-9	Beryllium aluminosilicate; beryllium aluminium silicate	$Al_2Be_3(SiO_3)_6$
Beryllium chloride	7787-47-5	Beryllium dichloride	$BeCl_2$
Beryllium fluoride	7787-49-7 (12323-05-6)	Beryllium difluoride	BeF_2
Beryllium hydroxide	13327-32-7 (1304-49-0)	Beryllium dihydroxide	$Be(OH)_2$
Beryllium sulfate	13510-49-1	*Sulfuric acid, beryllium salt (1:1)*	$BeSO_4$
Beryllium sulfate tetrahydrate	7787-56-6	*Sulfuric acid, beryllium salt (1:1), tetrahydrate*	$BeSO_4.4H_2O$
Beryllium oxide	1304-56-9	Beryllia; beryllium monoxide Thermalox™	BeO
Beryllium carbonate basic[d]	1319-43-3	*Carbonic acid, beryllium salt, mixture with beryllium hydroxide (Be(OH)₂)*	$BeCO_3.Be(OH)_2$
Beryllium nitrate	13597-99-4	Beryllium dinitrate; *nitric acid, beryllium salt*	$Be(NO_3)_2$
Beryllium nitrate trihydrate	7787-55-5	*Nitric acid, beryllium salt, trihydrate*	$Be(NO_3)_2.3H_2O$
Beryllium nitrate tetrahydrate	13510-48-0	Beryllium dinitrate tetrahydrate; *nitric acid, beryllium salt, tetrahydrate*	$Be(NO_3)_2.4H_2O$
Beryllium phosphate	13598-15-7	*Phosphoric acid, beryllium salt (1:1)*	$BeHPO_4$
Beryllium silicate[e]	13598-00-0	Phenazite; *phenakite*	$Be_2(SiO_4)$
Zinc beryllium silicate	39413-47-3 (63089-82-7)	*Silicic acid, beryllium zinc salt*	Unspecified

[a]Replaced CAS Registry numbers are shown in parentheses.

[b]Related compound registered by CAS is beryllium alloy, base, Be,Al historically (Lockalloy), Al (24–44%).Be (56–76%) [12604-81-8; replaced Registry No., 12665-28-0]; 60 beryllium–aluminium alloys are registered with CAS numbers, with different percentages of the two elements.

[c]Related compound registered by CAS is beryllium alloy, base, Be,Cu [39348-30-6]; 111 beryllium–copper alloys are registered with CAS numbers, with different percentages of the two elements.

[d]CAS name and Registry number shown were selected as being closest to the formula given by Lide (1991). Related compounds registered by CAS are: bis[carbonato(2)]dihydroxytriberyllium, $(BeCO_3)_2.Be(OH)_2$ [66104-24-3]; carbonic acid, beryllium salt (1:1), tetra-hydrate, $BeCO_3.4H_2O$ [60883-64-9]; carbonic acid, beryllium salt (1:1), $BeCO_3$ [13106-47-3]; and bis[carbonato(2-)]oxodiberyllium, $(CO_3)_2Be_2O$ [66104-25-4].

[e]Related compounds registered by CAS are: bertrandite, $Be_4(OH)_2O(SiO_3)_2$ [12161-82-9]; beryllium silicate, formula unspecified [58500-38-2]; silicic acid (H_2SiO_3), beryllium salt (1:1), $Be(SiO_3)$ [14902-94-4]; silicic acid (H_4SiO_4), beryllium salt (1:2), $Be_2(SiO_4)$ [15191-85-2]

Table 2. Physical properties of pure beryllium and beryllium compounds

Chemical name	Relative atomic/molecular mass	Melting-point (°C)	Typical physical description	Density (g/cm^3)	Solubility
Beryllium metal	9.0122	1287	Grey, close-packed, hexagonal, brittle metal	1.85 (20 °C)	Soluble in most dilute acids and alkali; decomposes in hot water; insoluble in mercury and cold water
Beryllium chloride	79.92	399.2	Colourless to slightly yellow, orthorhombic, deliquescent crystal	1.899 (25 °C)	Soluble in water, ethanol, diethyl ether and pyridine; slightly soluble in benzene, carbon disulfide and chloroform; insoluble in acetone, ammonia and toluene
Beryllium fluoride	47.01	555	Colourless or white, amorphous, hygroscopic solid	1.986	Soluble in water, sulfuric acid, mixture of ethanol and diethyl ether; slightly soluble in ethanol; insoluble in hydrofluoric acid
Beryllium hydroxide	43.03	138 (dec.^{a})	White, amorphous, amphoteric powder	1.92	Soluble in hot concentrated acids and alkali; slightly soluble in dilute alkali; insoluble in water
Beryllium sulfate	105.07	550 (dec.)	Colourless crystal	2.443	Forms soluble tetrahydrate in hot water; insoluble in cold water
Beryllium sulfate tetrahydrate	177.14	NR	Colourless, tetragonal crystal	1.713	Soluble in water; slightly soluble in concentrated sulfuric acid; insoluble in ethanol
Beryllium oxide	25.01	2530	Colourless to white, hexagonal crystal or amorphous, amphoteric powder	3.01 (20 °C)	Soluble in concentrated acids and alkali; insoluble in water
Beryllium carbonate	69.02	NR	NR	NR	Soluble in acids and alkali; insoluble in cold water; decomposes in hot water
Beryllium carbonate, basic	112.05	NR	White powder		Soluble in acids and alkali; insoluble in cold water; decomposes in hot water
Beryllium nitrate, trihydrate	187.97	60	White to faintly yellowish, deliquescent mass	1.56	Very soluble in water and ethanol
Beryllium phosphate	104.99	NR	NR	NR	Slightly soluble in water

Table 2 (contd)

Chemical name	Relative atomic/molecular mass	Melting-point (°C)	Typical physical description	Density (g/cm³)	Solubility
Beryllium silicate	110.11	NR	Triclinic, colourless crystal	3.0	Insoluble in acids
Zinc beryllium silicate	Unspecified	NR	Crystalline solid	NR	NR

From Ballance et al. (1978); Walsh & Rees (1978); IARC (1980); Sax & Lewis (1987); Lewis (1988); Budavari (1989); Lide (1991); Aldrich Chemical Co. (1992). NR, not reported; dec., decomposes
^{a}Decomposes to beryllium oxide (Sax & Lewis, 1987).

Natural beryllium is 100% ^{9}Be isotope; four unstable isotopes with mass numbers of 6, 7, 8 and 10 have been made artificially. Because of its low atomic number, beryllium is very permeable to X-rays. Neutron emission after bombardment with α or γ rays is the most important of its nuclear physical properties, and beryllium can be used as a neutron source. Moreover, its low neutron absorptiveness and high-scattering cross-section make it a suitable moderator and reflector in structural materials in nuclear facilities; while most other metals absorb neutrons emitted during the fission of nuclear fuel, beryllium atoms only reduce the energy of such neutrons and reflect them back into the fission zone (Ballance *et al.*, 1978; Newland, 1984; WHO, 1990).

The chemical properties of beryllium differ considerably from those of the other alkaline earths, but it has a number of chemical properties in common with aluminium. Like aluminium, beryllium is amphoteric and shows very high affinity for oxygen; on exposure to air or water vapour, a thin film of beryllium oxide forms on the surface of the bare metal, rendering the metal highly resistant to corrosion, to hot and cold water and to oxidizing acids. Dichromate in water enhances this resistance by forming a protective film of chromate, similar to that formed on aluminium. In powder form, beryllium is readily oxidized in moist air and burns with a temperature of about 4500 °C when ignited in oxygen (Newland, 1984; Petzow *et al.*, 1985; WHO, 1990).

Cationic beryllium salts are hydrolysed in water; they form insoluble hydroxides or hydrated complexes at pH values between 5 and 8 and form beryllates above a pH of 8 (Reeves, 1986).

1.1.3 *Technical products and impurities*

Beryllium metal—purities: technical or nuclear grade, 98–> 99.5%; Grade A, 99.87%; Grade AA, 99.96%; distilled grade, > 99.99%; forms: single crystals, flakes, powders, plates, sheets, foils, wires, rods (Sax & Lewis, 1987; Alfa Products, 1990; CERAC, Inc., 1991; Aldrich Chemical Co., 1992; Atomergic Chemetals Corp., undated; D.F. Goldsmith Chemical & Metal Corp., undated); impurities vary with the production method (see section 1.2.1 and Tables 5 and 6).

Beryllium–aluminium alloy—composition limits for one alloy (%): Be, 4.5–6.0; Si, 0.2; Fe, 0.2; Mg, 0.5, Mn, 0.02; Cr, 0.02; Ni, 0.02; Ti, 0.02; Zn, 0.1; Cu, 0.05 (KBAlloys, 1985)

Beryllium–copper alloy—composition limits for one alloy (Alloy 20C or C82500) (%): Be, 2.0–2.25; Co, 0.35–0.65; total unnamed elements, 0.5 max; Cu, remainder (Stonehouse & Zenczak, 1991)

Beryllium chloride—purities: 97–99.5%; impurities (mg/kg): Al, 50; Fe, 100; Si, 30; Cd, 10; Ni, 120; Cu, 10; Co, 10; Zn, 10; Cr, 10; Mn, 10; Mg, 150 (Kawecki Berylco Industries, 1968; Alfa Products, 1990; CERAC, Inc., 1991; Strem Chemicals, 1992; Fluka Chemie AG, 1993)

Beryllium fluoride—purity: 99.5%; impurities (mg/kg): Al, 75; Fe, 75; Ni, 40; Cu, 10 (Kawecki Berylco Industries, 1968; CERAC, Inc., 1991; D.F. Goldsmith Chemical & Metal Corp., undated)

Beryllium hydroxide—contains different levels of several impurities depending on whether it is made from beryl ore or bertrandite ore (IARC, 1980)

Beryllium sulfate tetrahydrate—purities: 98.3–99.99%; impurities (%): chloride, Ca, Cd, Co, Cu, Fe, Ni, Pb and Zn, all < 0.005; K, Na, < 0.01 (Alfa Products, 1990; Aldrich Chemical Co., 1992; Fluka Chemie AG, 1993)

Beryllium oxide—purities: 99–99.99% (Alfa Products, 1990; CERAC, Inc., 1991; Aldrich Chemical Co., 1992; Strem Chemicals, 1992). The purity of beryllia is critical to its thermal conductivity: as the purity drops below 99.5%, thermal conductivity drops off rapidly. Impurities (mg/kg): Al, 46; Fe, 32; Cr, 8; Mn, < 2; Ni, 9; B, 2; Ca, 31; Co, < 1; Cu, 3; Si, 1861; Mg, 922; Li, 2; Zn, < 20; Ti, 5; Na, 173; Ag, < 1; Mo, < 3; Pb, 2. Silicon and magnesium silicates are added to beryllia powder as sintering aids (Brush Wellman, undated)

Beryllium carbonate—impurities (mg/kg): Al, 30; Fe, 100; Si, 150 (IARC, 1980)

Beryllium nitrate (trihydrate)—purity: 99.5% (D.F. Goldsmith Chemical & Metal Corp., undated); impurities (mg/kg): Al, 20; Fe, 30; Si, 50; Na, 20 (Kawecki Berylco Industries, 1968)

Impurities that occur in beryllium compounds that have been the subjects of previous monographs are: cadmium (IARC, 1987b), chromium (IARC, 1990a), cobalt (IARC, 1991), lead (IARC, 1987c), nickel (IARC, 1990b) and silica (IARC, 1987d).

1.1.4 Analysis

Beryllium metal

Selected methods for the determination of beryllium and beryllium compounds in various media are presented in Table 3. Other methods have been reviewed (IARC, 1980; Agency for Toxic Substances and Disease Registry, 1988; WHO, 1990).

Table 3. Methods for the analysis of beryllium and beryllium compounds (as Be)

Sample matrix	Sample preparation	Assay procedure	Limit of detection	Reference
Air[a]	Collect on membrane filter; dissolve in nitric acid	FLAA	0.08 µg/m^3; 0.002 µg/ml	Kleinman et al. (1989a)
	Collect sample on cellulose ester membrane filter; add nitric and sulfuric acids; heat; cool; evaporate to dryness; add sodium sulfate/sulfuric acid solution; heat	GFAA	0.005 µg/sample	Eller (1987) (Method 7102)
	Collect sample on cellulose ester membrane filter; ash with nitric:perchloric acid solution (4:1) v:v; heat; repeat; heat to dryness; dilute with nitric:perchloric acid solution (4:1)	ICP	1 µg/sample	Eller (1984) (Method 7300)
Water, ground- and surface	Acidify with nitric and hydrochloric acids (Method 3005)	FLAA ICP (313 nm)	0.005 mg/L 0.3 µg/L	US Environmental Protection Agency (1986a) (Method 6010)

Table 3 (contd)

Sample matrix	Sample preparation	Assay procedure	Limit of detection	Reference
Aqueous samples, extracts, wastes	Acidify with nitric acid; heat and evaporate to low volume; cool; add nitric acid; reheat and reflux with hydrochloric acid (Method 3010)	FLAA ICP (313 nm)	0.005 mg/L 0.3 µg/L	US Environmental Protection Agency (1986a,b) (Methods 6010 and 7090)
Oils, greases, waxes (organic extract)	Dissolve in xylene or methyl isobutyl ketone (Method 3040)	FLAA ICP (313 nm)	0.005 mg/L 0.3 µg/L	US Environmental Protection Agency (1986a) (Method 6010)
Sediments, sludges, soils	Digest with nitric acid and hydrogen peroxide; reflux with hydrochloric acid (Method 3050)	FLAA ICP (313 nm)	0.005 mg/L 0.3 µg/L	US Environmental Protection Agency (1986a) (Method 6010)
Aqueous samples, extracts, wastes	Acidify with nitric acid; evaporate to low volume; cool; add nitric acid; heat to complete digestion (Method 3020)	GFAA	0.2 µg/L	US Environmental Protection Agency (1986a,c) (Method 7091)
Sediments, sludges, soils	Digest with nitric acid and hydrogen peroxide; reflux with nitric acid (Method 3050)	GFAA	0.2 µg/L	US Environmental Protection Agency (1986a,c) (Method 7091)
Tissue samples	Ash in hot concentrated nitric acid	FLAA	2 µg/L	Kleinman et al. (1989b)
Urine	Inject untreated samples directly into a pretreated graphite tube; follow standard addition method	GFAA	0.5 µg/L	Angerer & Schaller (1985)
	Modify matrix with magnesium nitrate; follow platform technique	GFAA	0.05 µg/L	Paschal & Bailey (1986)

FLAA, flame atomic absorption spectrometry; GFAA, graphite furnace atomic absorption spectrometry; ICP, inductively coupled argon plasma emission spectrometry

^{a}[Digestion with a solution of nitric acid:perchloric acid:sulfuric acid and addition of several drops of hydrofluoric acid are currently recommended in sample preparation. Detection limits can be reduced to 0.001 µg/ml and sensitivity to 0.0001 µg/ml.]

Methods used up to the 1960s included spectroscopic, fluorometric, gamma activation, spectrophotometric and automatic titrimetric techniques (Ballance et al., 1978). The main deficiency of spectrophotometric methods lies in the nonspecificity of the complexing agents used to form coloured complexes with beryllium. The limit of detection of these methods was about 100 ng/sample. The fluorimetric method, which is based on fluorescent dyes (preferably morin), has a very low limit of detection, 0.02 ng/sample; its sensitivity is exceeded only by that of the gas chromatographic method. The fluorimetric method may, however, be subject to error unless several time-consuming, cumbersome processing steps are undertaken prior to analysis (WHO, 1990).

Atomic absorption spectrometry is a rapid, very convenient method for analysing biological and environmental samples. The limit of detection for the flame technique is 2–10 µg/L and lower when the sample is concentrated before analysis (WHO, 1990). The graphite furnace method is much more sensitive, with a detection limit of approximately 0.1 µg/L. Blood, urine and tissue samples can be analysed by this technique with or without digestion of the biological matrix (see Table 3).

Inductively coupled plasma atomic emission spectrometry has been introduced to determine beryllium directly in a variety of biological and environmental matrices, because of its high sensitivity and low level of interference. Owing to its high sensitivity and specificity, gas chromatography is also used for determining beryllium in environmental and biological media, particularly at ultratrace levels. Beryllium can be converted into a volatile form by chelation with trifluoroacetylacetone before injection into the chromatographic column (WHO, 1990).

1.2 Production and use

1.2.1 *Production*

More than 40 beryllium-bearing minerals are known, but only two are of economic significance. The first beryllium mineral to be exploited commercially was beryl ($3BeO.Al_2O_3.6SiO_2$), an aluminosilicate (WHO, 1990). The largest deposits of beryl are found in Brazil and the former USSR (Petkof, 1982; Stonehouse & Zenczak, 1991). Beryl ore contains about 11% beryllium oxide (up to 4% beryllium) and is often obtained as a by-product of feldspar quarrying (for typical ore composition, see Table 17). In addition to the other major components, aluminium oxide and silicon dioxide, the principal impurities in the ores include alkali metals, alkaline-earth metals, iron, manganese and phosphorus. In its purest gem quality, it occurs as emerald (chromium-containing beryl), aquamarine (iron-containing beryl) and some other semiprecious stones (Petzow *et al.*, 1985; WHO, 1990).

The other mineral of economic significance, bertrandite ($4BeO.2SiO_2.H_2O$), is a beryllium silicate hydrate. Although bertrandite ore contains less than 1% beryllium, it became economically important in the late 1960s because it can be processed to beryllium hydroxide highly efficiently. Bertrandite mined in the USA accounts for about 85% of US consumption of beryllium ore. The total world reserves of beryllium that can be recovered by mining bertrandite are estimated at 200 000 tonnes (Petzow *et al.*, 1985; WHO, 1990).

Known deposits of other beryllium-containing minerals are being studied for possible commercialization. Most notable among these are phenakite ($2BeO.SiO_2$) at Yellowknife, Northwest Territory, Canada, the chrysoberyl ($BeO.Al_2O_3$) deposits of the Seward Peninsula, Alaska, and the Sierra Blanca deposits near El Paso, Texas, USA (Stonehouse & Zenczak, 1991).

Beryllium production started in some industrialized countries around 1916. Beryllium gained commercial importance in the early 1930s, following the realization that beryllium–copper alloys are extraordinarily hard, resistant to corrosion, non-magnetic, do not spark and withstand high temperatures. In addition, the nuclear and thermal properties and high specific modulus of beryllium metal made it attractive for nuclear and aerospace applications, including weapons. The latter use is the main reason why reliable data on the production and consumption of beryllium have been scarce and incomplete. Considerable fluctuations in the supply and demand of beryllium result from variations in government programmes in armaments, nuclear energy and aerospace. For example, the demand for beryllium in the USA that was created by the programme for development of the atomic bomb was about equivalent to total world demand up to 1940 (WHO, 1990).

Production in the rest of the world paralleled those fluctuations in the beryllium market, with 222 tonnes produced in 1965, 320 tonnes in 1969 and 144 tonnes in 1974. Data on US production are now available, and world production of beryllium as beryl is shown in Table 4. If production from bertrandite is included, the USA appears to be the world's largest producer of beryllium raw materials (WHO, 1990).

(a) Processing of beryl and bertrandite

The first step in the processing of beryl ore is normally hand-sorting to select beryl crystals containing at least 10% beryllium oxide (Ballance *et al.*, 1978) on the basis of shape and colour (Powers, 1991).

Two commercial methods have been used to process beryl to beryllium hydroxide: the fluoride process and the sulfate process. In the *fluoride process*, which was discontinued in the 1970s, beryl was sintered together with sodium hexafluorosilicate, or the less expensive sodium fluoroferrate, at 700–800 °C to convert beryllium oxide to a water-soluble salt, sodium beryllium tetrafluoride (Na_2BeF_4). The reaction product was then leached with water at room temperature and precipitated from the purified solution with caustic soda as beryllium hydroxide (Petzow *et al.*, 1985; WHO, 1990).

The *sulfate process*, the only process currently used, involves either alkali or heat treatment of beryl. With alkali treatment, which was discontinued in the 1960s, finely ground beryl was heated until fusion or sintered below the melting-point with suitable alkalis, such as hydroxides and carbonates of sodium, potassium and calcium. With heat treatment, which has been used since the 1970s, beryl is melted without additives and quenched with water; the water insoluble portion, a solid solution with silicon dioxide, is reheated to 900 °C to render a total of 90–95% of the beryl soluble. Heat-treated or alkali-treated beryl is then extracted with sulfuric acid and carried through several additional purification steps to produce a fine-grained, readily filtered beryllium hydroxide (Petzow *et al.*, 1985; WHO, 1990).

The beryllium-poor bertrandite ores ($\leq$ 0.5–0.8% BeO) mined in the USA since 1960 cannot be smelted economically by conventional methods, and a less complicated procedure has been developed in which a very pure beryllium hydroxide is produced by liquid–liquid extraction. This so-called 'SX-carbonate process' involves direct leaching of bertrandite ore with sulfuric acid, extraction of the sulfuric acid leachate with di(2-ethylhexyl)phosphoric acid in kerosene, stripping of beryllium from the organic phase with aqueous ammonium carbonate, and, through a series of heat, hydrolysis and precipitation steps, production of beryllium hydroxide (Petzow *et al.*, 1985; WHO, 1990). Beryllium hydroxide is the starting material for the production of beryllium, beryllia and beryllium alloys. For further processing, it is ignited to form the oxide (BeO) or converted to the fluoride (BeF_2) (WHO, 1990).

Table 4. World production of beryl (tonnes)

Country	1980	1981	1982	1983	1984	1986	1987	1988	1989	1990	1991[a]
Argentina	31	7	6	24[b]	15[a]	50	46	39	89[c]	85[a]	80
Brazil[d]	550	854[c]	1062	1252[a,c]	1252	907[c]	1000	913	800	850[a]	850
Madagascar	10	10	10	10	10	50 kg	35 kg	3 kg	154 kg	150 kg[c]	3
Mozambique	20	18	15	15[a]	15	1	ND	ND	ND	ND	ND
Portugal	19	18	19	18	18	ND	4	4	4	4	4
Rwanda	108	59	69	33	36	ND	ND	ND	ND	ND	ND
Republic of South Africa	ND	122	58	22	ND	3	135 kg	72 kg	ND	1[c]	1
Russia[a]	1800	1800	1800	1900	1900	1900	2000	2000	2000	1600	1300
USA[e]	6756[c]	6653[c]	4945	6046	5470[c]	5927	5499	5313	4592	4548	4339[c]
Zimbabwe	9	42	52	50[a]	50	103	83	33	46	28[c]	30
World[f]	9319	9597	8051	9375	8772	8891	8632	8302	7532	7119	6607

From Kramer (1985a, 1991a, 1992a) [some figures are estimates]; beryl has also been produced in China, perhaps in Bolivia and Namibia and in small amounts in Nepal, but the available information is inadequate to formulate reliable estimates of production. ND, no data

[a]Estimated
[b]Preliminary
[c]Revised
[d]Export data for 1980–84
[e]Includes bertrandite ore calculated as equivalent to beryl containing 11% BeO
[f]Totals are not the sum of the columns, because world values are revised figures.

(b) Beryllium metal

The chief difficulties involved in the production of beryllium metal are the reactivity and high melting-point of the metal and the extreme stability of the oxide. Of the many possible methods of producing beryllium, two have been used in industry: fusion electrolysis and reduction of halides by metals. The only industrial process currently in use, developed in the 1930s, is reduction of beryllium fluoride with magnesium. The reaction is started by heating a mixture of relatively coarse-grained beryllium fluoride and magnesium in a graphite crucible. At a temperature of about 1300 °C, the reaction produces a mixture of beryllium pebbles and magnesium fluoride (Petzow *et al.*, 1985).

All practical electrolytic methods of production are based on decomposition of beryllium fluoride, beryllium oxide or beryllium chloride mixed with halides of the alkali metals or alkaline-earth metals. Several methods for the electrolysis of beryllium fluoride were developed in the 1920s. Electrolysis was carried out at above the melting-point of beryllium, at 1290–1400 °C; these methods are now obsolete. Electrolysis of beryllium chloride can be carried out at temperatures so low that the metal neither melts nor oxidizes. The beryllium is obtained as solid flakes, which are separated by washing out the electrolyte. This method was used in France, Japan, the United Kingdom and the former USSR (Petzow *et al.*, 1985).

Beryllium pebbles or flakes still contain many impurities and must be refined before they can be used to fabricate structural pieces. The main impurities in electrolytically produced beryllium are sodium and chloride; the main impurities in beryllium produced by the magnesium reduction process are magnesium and magnesium fluoride. Other impurities include beryllium oxide, carbon and metals, the most important being aluminium, iron and silicon (Petzow *et al.*, 1985). Beryllium is available mainly as block and rolled sheet and, to a lesser extent, as extruded bar, wire and near net shapes (Smugeresky, 1986).

Several commercial grades of beryllium are produced for specific uses: structural, nuclear, instrument, optical and electronic (Smugeresky, 1986). Commercial grades of beryllium are refined exclusively by vacuum melting in beryllium oxide or magnesium oxide crucibles and casting in graphite ingot moulds. The melting of magnesium-reduced beryllium in a high vacuum produces a metal of a purity comparable to that of electrolytic beryllium. Melting the electrolytic flakes in a vacuum further reduces the content of halides and low-boiling metals. A very pure grade of beryllium, particularly with respect to the content of oxide, aluminium, iron, silicon, carbon and halides, can be produced by electrolytic refining (SR flakes) (Ballance *et al.*, 1978; Petzow *et al.*, 1985).

(c) Beryllium–aluminium alloy

Beryllium–aluminium alloys (originally termed 'lockalloy' by the inventors, who were working for the Lockheed Co.) exhibit high bend ductility and high strength and are weldable and easy to machine. A major factor in their successful development was the preparation of a relatively fine, two-phase microstructure by a gas atomization process with quenching into water. The resultant powders are dried, then hot degassed, hot compacted and extruded to bars, from which thin sheet and thin-section extrusion are produced. Lockalloys were produced commercially from the late 1960s until 1975 (Lewis, 1988). The one remaining US manufacturer currently produces beryllium–aluminium alloys under the trade name AlBeMet™ (Brush Wellman, 1992).

(d) Beryllium–copper alloy

Alloys with copper are the most important beryllium alloys. Copper–beryllium master alloy is manufactured commercially by an arc-furnace method in which beryllium oxide is reduced by carbon in the presence of molten copper at 1800–2000 °C; the resulting alloy typically contains 4.0–4.25 wt % beryllium. The master alloy is then melted together with virgin copper or copper scrap to produce the desired alloy, which is usually cast into billets (Ballance *et al.*, 1978; Stonehouse & Zenczak, 1991).

(e) Beryllium chloride

Beryllium chloride can be prepared either directly from beryl by the chloride process or by chlorination of beryllium oxide under reducing conditions. Beryllium chloride is purified by distillation in a stream of hydrogen, followed by fractional condensation (Petzow *et al.*, 1985).

(f) Beryllium fluoride

In the production of beryllium fluoride, beryllium hydroxide is dissolved in an ammonium hydrogen fluoride solution to produce ammonium tetrafluoroberyllate. Impurities can be precipitated as hydroxides. Upon concentration, ammonium tetrafluoroberyllate crystallizes from solution and is separated; after heating, it dissociates into ammonium fluoride and beryllium fluoride (Petzow *et al.*, 1985).

(g) Beryllium hydroxide

Beryllium hydroxide exists in three forms. By adding alkali to a beryllium salt solution to make a slightly basic pH, a gelatinous beryllium hydroxide is produced. Aging of this amorphous product results in a metastable tetragonal crystalline form, which, after months of standing, is transformed into a stable, orthorhombic crystalline form. The orthorhombic modification is also precipitated by hydrolysis from a hot sodium beryllate solution containing more than 5 g/L beryllium. Granular beryllium hydroxide is the readily filtered product from sulfate extraction processing of beryl (Walsh & Rees, 1978).

(h) Beryllium sulfate

Beryllium sulfate can be obtained by heating beryllium sulfate dihydrate in air to 400 °C and from the reaction of beryl ore or beryllium oxide with sulfuric acid (Walsh & Rees, 1978; Petzow *et al.*, 1985).

(i) Beryllium sulfate tetrahydrate

Beryllium sulfate tetrahydrate is produced commercially in a highly purified state by fractional crystallization from a beryllium sulfate solution obtained by reacting beryllium hydroxide with sulfuric acid. The tetrahydrate crystallizes from the aqueous solution in well-developed crystals (Walsh & Rees, 1978; Petzow *et al.*, 1985).

(j) Beryllium oxide

Beryllium oxide is produced by the following processes: beryllium hydroxide is first converted to high-purity beryllium sulfate tetrahydrate, as described above. This salt is calcined at carefully controlled temperatures, between 1150 and 1450 °C, selected to give the properties of the beryllium oxide powders required by individual beryllia ceramic fabricators. Alternatively, beryllium hydroxide may be purified first and then calcined directly to beryllium oxide powder (Walsh & Rees, 1978). In another process, beryl ore is fused with sodium silicic fluoride at 700–800 °C, with conversion to sodium fluoroberyllate and precipitation by means of caustic soda from the purified leached solution as beryllium hydroxide, from which the anhydrous chloride can be obtained by reaction with carbon and chlorine at 800 °C (US National Library of Medicine, 1992).

Today, practically all of the beryllium oxide produced commercially is calcined at temperatures of 1000 °C or higher and is referred to as 'high-fired'. Beryllium oxide that is calcined at temperatures lower than 1000 °C is referred to as 'low-fired'; it consists of poorly crystallized, small particles which are more reactive and more soluble in dilute acid than those of high-fired beryllium oxide (Finch *et al.*, 1988).

(k) Beryllium carbonate

Basic beryllium carbonate is formed in the reaction of beryllium salt solutions with alkali metal or ammonium carbonate solutions. If excess ammonium carbonate is used, a readily filtered precipitate of variable composition is formed on boiling. This salt is a suitable starting material for the preparation of beryllium salts of all types. Gentle calcining causes ammonia to escape, leaving beryllium basic carbonate. Further heating drives off the carbon dioxide to produce beryllium hydroxide (Petzow *et al.*, 1985).

(l) Beryllium nitrate

Beryllium nitrate trihydrate is prepared by crystallizing a solution of beryllium hydroxide or carbonate that has been treated with a slight excess of concentrated nitric acid; the dihydrates and monohydrates are also formed, depending on the concentration of the acid used. The anhydrous form may be obtained by treating an ethyl acetate solution of beryllium chloride with dinitrogen tetroxide but not by dehydration of one of the hydrated species; the latter operation results in thermal decomposition of the nitrate, with evolution of nitrous fumes (Drury *et al.*, 1978).

(m) Beryllium phosphate

Beryllium phosphate can be produced by the reaction of disodium hydrophosphate with a beryllium salt solution or by reaction of beryllium hydroxide solution with phosphoric acid (Mellor, 1946).

(n) Beryllium silicate

No information was available to the Working Group.

(o) Zinc beryllium silicate

No information was available to the Working Group.

1.2.2 *Use*

Typical use patterns for beryllium, beryllium alloys and beryllium compounds in the USA are presented in Table 5.

Table 5. Use patterns for beryllium in the USA (%)

Use category	1985	1987	1990	1991	1992
Metal and alloy in nuclear reactors and in military and aerospace applications	40	40	23	29	29
Alloy and oxide in electrical equipment	36	35	17	19	20
Alloy and oxide in electronic components	17	17	35	47	45
Alloy, metal and oxide in other applications	7	8	25	5	6

From Kramer (1985b, 1987, 1990, 1991b, 1992b)

(a) Beryllium metal

Some of the typical uses of beryllium metal are: structural material in space technology; moderator and reflector of neutrons in nuclear reactors; source of neutrons when bombarded with α particles; special windows for X-ray tubes; in gyroscopes, computer parts, inertial guidance systems; additives in solid propellant rocket fuels; beryllium–copper alloys; heat-sink material in low-weight, high-performance aircraft brakes; scanning mirrors and large mirror components of satellite optical systems; hardening of copper; and in developmental brass alloys (Sax & Lewis, 1987; WHO, 1990).

(b) Beryllium–aluminium alloy

The use of beryllium in alloys is based on a combination of properties that beryllium confers on other metals. Low density combined with strength, high melting-point, resistance to oxidation and a high modulus of elasticity make beryllium alloys light-weight materials that can withstand high acceleration and centrifugal forces. Most metals, however, form very brittle compounds with beryllium, and this and the low solubility of most elements in solid beryllium are the reasons why beryllium-rich alloys have not found extensive use (WHO, 1990). Historically, the only alloy with a high beryllium content was lockalloy, which contained 62% beryllium and 38% aluminium (Petzow *et al.*, 1985). Recently, Brush Wellman (1992) introduced a family of beryllium–aluminium alloys containing 20–60% beryllium and sold as AlBeMet™.

Aluminium–beryllium alloys are used mainly to save weight, reduce life-cycle cost and increase reliability in aerospace structures of advanced design. Small additions of beryllium to aluminium impart high strength, thermal stability and unusual resistance to oxidation (Lewis, 1988; WHO, 1990). These alloys are also used in computer information storage devices.

(c) Beryllium–copper alloy

The principal uses of beryllium stem from the discovery in the 1920s that the addition of only 2% beryllium to copper results in an alloy six times stronger than copper. Beryllium–copper alloys withstand high temperatures, are extraordinarily hard, are resistant to corrosion, do not spark and are non-magnetic. These alloys are used in many critical moving parts of aircraft engines and in key components of precision instruments, electrical relays and switches. An alloy containing 25% beryllium has limited application in camera shutters. Beryllium–copper hammers, wrenches and other tools are used in petroleum refineries where sparks from steel against steel might cause explosions (Newland, 1984). A representative use for beryllium–copper alloys in the electronics industry is in integrated circuit sockets and electronic connectors (Stonehouse & Zenczak, 1991). These alloys are also used in sports equipment (e.g., golf clubs).

(d) Beryllium chloride

Beryllium chloride has been used as a raw material in the electrolytic production of beryllium and as the starting material for synthesis of organoberyllium compounds (Petzow et al., 1985).

(e) Beryllium fluoride

Beryllium floride is used as an intermediate in the preparation of beryllium and beryllium alloys. It was used as an additive to welding and soldering fluxes because it dissolves metal oxides readily; it was also used in nuclear reactors and glass manufacture (Petzow et al., 1985; Sax & Lewis, 1987). It is being investigated for use in fibre optic cables because of its low absorbance of ultraviolet radiation.

(f) Beryllium hydroxide

Beryllium hydroxide is used as an intermediate in the manufacture of beryllium and beryllium oxide (Budavari, 1989).

(g) Beryllium sulfate tetrahydrate

Beryllium sulfate tetrahydrate is used as an intermediate in the production of beryllium oxide powder for ceramics (Walsh & Rees, 1978).

(h) Beryllium oxide

Beryllium oxide has an extremely high melting-point, very high thermal conductivity, low thermal expansion and high electrical resistance. It can either be moulded or applied as a coating to a metal or other base; through the process of sintering (1480 °C), a hard, compact mass with a smooth glassy surface is formed. The ceramic properties of sintered beryllium oxide make it suitable for the production or protection of materials to be used at high temperatures in corrosive environments. Beryllium oxide ceramics have the highest thermal conductivity of the oxide ceramics (Newland, 1984; WHO, 1990). They are also used as dental materials (ceramic crowns).

Specific applications include: transistor mountings, semiconductor packages and microelectronic substrates. Transparency to microwaves has led to its use as windows, radomes and antennae in microwave devices; it is also used in high-power laser tubes. Its low density and other properties make it attractive for aerospace and military applications, such as gyroscopes and armour; general refractory uses include thermocouple sheaths and crucibles. It is also used as an additive to glass, ceramics and plastics; in the preparation of beryllium compounds; as a catalyst for organic reactions; and in nuclear reactor fuels and moderators (Livey, 1986; Sax & Lewis, 1987; US Environmental Protection Agency, 1987; Budavari, 1989).

(i) Beryllium nitrate

Beryllium nitrate was used until the late 1960s for stiffening incandescent gas mantles (Petzow *et al.*, 1985).

(j) Beryllium phosphate

Beryllium phosphate is not known to be produced commercially.

(k) Beryllium silicate

Beryllium silicate is not known to be produced commercially.

(l) Zinc beryllium silicate

Zinc beryllium silicate is not known to be produced or used commercially at present. It was used until about 1950 as a fluorescent lamp phosphor (WHO, 1990).

1.3 Occurrence

The environmental occurrence of beryllium has been reviewed extensively (Agency for Toxic Substances and Disease Registry, 1988; WHO, 1990).

1.3.1 *Natural occurrence*

Beryllium is the forty-fourth most abundant element in the Earth's crust (Drury *et al.*, 1978; Reeves, 1986), with an average content of about 6 mg/kg. It occurs in rocks and minerals (mica schist, granite, pegmatite and argillite) at concentrations of 0.038–11.4 mg/kg (Drury *et al.*, 1978). The most highly enriched beryllium deposits are found in granitic pegmatites, in which independent beryllium minerals crystallize (WHO, 1990).

Some 40 beryllium-containing minerals have been identified. Only ores containing beryl ($3BeO.Al_2O_3.6SiO_2$) and bertrandite ($4BeO.2SiO_2.H_2O$) have achieved commercial significance (Drury *et al.*, 1978). The most important environmental source of beryllium is the burning of coal. Coals contain 1.8–2.2 mg beryllium/kg dry weight (US Environmental Protection Agency, 1987), and beryllium occurs in the ash of many coals at concentrations of about 100 mg/kg (WHO, 1990). These waste products could represent an extensive beryllium reserve. The beryllium content of fuel oils has been estimated to be less than 0.1 ppm (Drury *et al.*, 1978).

1.3.2 *Occupational exposure*

The range of industrial processes in which occupational exposure to beryllium occurs has expanded over the past two decades: The number of uses has increased, and the occupational settings have diversified. It is used in many manufacturing industries (see above) and in a growing industry for recycling and processing. Nonsiliceous mineral slag used for sand blasting is also frequently contaminated with beryllium. Potential exposure settings are summarized in Table 6.

Table 6. Industries and trades in which there is potential exposure to beryllium

Ceramics
Electrical connectors
Nonferrous foundries
Nonferrous smelters
Sandblasting
Aerospace
Nuclear control equipment
Electronics
Refractories
Beryllium smelting or fabrication
Hazardous waste processing
Dental equipment and supplies
Engineering and scientific equipment
Mechanical measuring devices
Tool and die making
Soldering
Welding or flame cutting
Metal plating
Automotive parts
Telecommunication equipment
Golf club manufacture

From Cullen et al. (1986); WHO (1990)

The US Occupational Safety and Health Administration summarized data on occupational exposure to beryllium for the period 1 June 1979 to 31 January 1984 (Table 7), based on inspections of work places. Exposure levels in excess of the threshold limit value of 2 $\mu g/m^3$ were found mainly in the traditional beryllium industry but also in high technology industries.

(a) Processing and manufacturing

Substances to which potential exposure occurs during ore processing include ore dust, silicon dioxide fumes and acid mists and fumes of beryllium sulfate; those during beryllium oxide production include fumes of lead sulfide, copper sulfide and sulfur trioxide and dusts of beryllium oxide; those during production of beryllium metal include acid fluoride mists, fumes and dusts of beryllium ammonium fluoride, beryllium fluoride, hydrogen fluoride, ammonium fluoride, beryllium metal and beryllium oxide; and those during production of beryllium–copper alloy include beryllium oxide, copper and beryllium–copper alloy dusts and fumes. Machining potentially involves exposure to respirable particles of beryllium alloys in the absence of adequate controls (Laskin et al., 1950; Preuss, 1988). Exposure concentrations in various industries have been reviewed (WHO, 1990).

Table 7. Occupational exposure to beryllium compounds (1 June 1979 to 31 January 1984)

Type of industry	No. of samples in which beryllium is detected	No. of samples ≥ 0.5 µg/m³[a]	No. of samples ≥ 2 µg/m³[b]
Traditional[c]	25	16	9
High-technology[d]	3	3	2
Secondary process[e]	5	1	0
Dental laboratory	1	0	0
Total	34	20	11

From Cullen et al. (1986)
[a]Criterion of the US National Institute for Occupational Safety and Health
[b]Standard of the US Occupational Safety and Health Administration
[c]Including particulate blasting, shipbuilding and repair, nonferrous foundries, nonclay refractories, beryllium machining and fabrication and metalworking
[d]Including the semiconductor industry, precision electronics industry and spacecraft and missile manufacture
[e]Including secondary nonferrous smelters, nonferrous foundries and hazardous waste reclamation

Although there are few quantitative data on exposure to beryllium before 1947, there seems to be little doubt that extremely high concentrations were encountered in the work place (US National Institute for Occupational Safety and Health, 1972). In the USA, concentrations greater than 1000 µg/m³ were not uncommon in beryllium extraction facilities (Eisenbud & Lisson, 1983). Exposures measured in December 1946 (by the filter-paper dust sampler method) ranged from 110 to 4710 µg/m³ in the furnace area of a beryllium extraction plant (Laskin et al., 1950). Concentrations of 590–43 300 µg/m³ were found in a beryllium–copper alloy plant in Lorain, Ohio, USA, monitored by the Atomic Energy Commission in 1947 and 1948 (Zielinski, 1961). After institution of control measures in 1949 in a new beryllium-copper alloy production plant in Elmore, Ohio, the limit of 2 µg/m³ was considerably exceeded between 1953 and 1960, with time-weighted average values of 3.8–9.5 µg/m³ in 1953, 6.8–19.1 µg/m³ in 1956 and 23.1–54.6 µg/m³ in 1960 (Zielinski, 1961; US National Institute for Occupational Safety and Health, 1972). In the same beryllium–copper alloy plant, a new furnace was installed between 1960 and 1966. Concentrations ranged from < 0.1 µg/m³ in the mixing areas to 1050 µg/m³ in the oxide areas in 1960 and from 0.2 µg/m³ in the saw area to 249 µg/m³ in the arc furnace area in 1966. Five-day average beryllium concentrations in this plant were 60.3 µg/m³ in 1960 and 18.1 µg/m³ in 1966 (see Table 8) (Cholak et al., 1967).

In a summary of beryllium concentrations in 2627 air samples taken during 1950–57 in two US beryllium production plants, Breslin and Harris (1959) reported that 10–15% of workers were exposed to concentrations greater than 2 µg/m³ and that the average concentration in each plant in many operations was 10 µg/m³. Exposures may have been higher in plants that were not monitored by the Atomic Energy Commission (US National Institute for Occupational Safety and Health, 1972).

Table 8. Concentrations of beryllium in air at a number of locations in a beryllium–copper alloy plant in Ohio (USA) during two cycles of air monitoring six years apart

Location	Year	Beryllium concentration ($\mu g/m^3$) of air per 2-h period		
		Average	Median	Range
Oxide area	1960	149.4	72.5	0.4–1050.0
	1966	10.7	8.1	0.8–29.3
Arc furnace area	1960	87.6	50.0	22.1–502.0
	1966	25.9	36.9	7.7–249.0
Mixing area	1960	21.6	14.4	< 0.1–452.0
	1966	20.0	14.7	5.9–88.5
Casting area	1960	39.8	14.6	0.2–535.0
	1966	25.4	20.5	8.5–210.5
Fisher furnace area	1960	40.8	28.8	0.2–340.0
	1966	7.3	5.5	1.5–37.8
Saw area in rolling mill	1960	25.6	21.1	< 2.5–92.5
	1966	5.7	4.0	0.2–18.4
Cropping area	1960	52.8	33.6	14.0–399.0
Ajax furnace area[a]	1966	14.4	11.1	4.6–87.5
All areas	1960	60.3	28.4	< 0.1–1050.0
	1966	18.1	11.4	0.2–249.0

From Cholak et al. (1967)
[a]Approximately same area as cropping area in 1960

The US Atomic Energy Commission presented exposure data from five major beryllium-processing plants for various periods during 1950–61. Up to 40–75% of the daily weighted average exposures exceeded 2 $\mu g/m^3$ (US National Institute for Occupational Safety and Health, 1972).

[The Working Group noted the uncertainty of the representativeness for exposure of workers of air monitoring data obtained in the 1940s, 1950s and 1960s.]

In the early 1970s in a beryllium extraction and processing plant in northeastern USA, peak concentrations up to 1310 $\mu g/m^3$ were observed (Kanarek et al., 1973). Follow-up analyses in 1974 showed a significant decrease (Sprince et al., 1978).

The US National Institute for Occupational Safety and Health conducted several surveys of air in different beryllium plants in the USA. In a beryllium production plant, concentrations of 0.3–160 $\mu g/m^3$ were found in 1971, the high values occurring in powdering operations (H.M. Donaldson, 1971; cited in WHO, 1990). In another beryllium production plant, the concentrations of airborne beryllium in 1972 rarely exceeded the threshold limit value of 2 $\mu g/m^3$ (H.M. Donaldson & P.J. Shuler, 1972; cited in WHO, 1990). Beryllium concentrations in 50 personal samples collected at a secondary copper smelter in 1982–83 ranged between < 0.2 and 0.5 $\mu g/m^3$ (Cherniak & Kominsky, 1984). In 1983, the concentrations of beryllium in 121 personal air samples obtained in the refinery and manufacturing melt areas of a precious metals refinery ranged from 0.22 to 42 μg/m³ (mean, 1.4 μg/m³) (K.P. McManus *et al.*, 1986; cited in WHO, 1990). Concentrations in the beryllium shop of another plant in 1985 ranged from < 0.2 to 7.2 μg/m³ and exceeded 0.5 μg/m³ in 6/33 breathing-zone samples (Gunter & Thoburn, 1986).

Kriebel *et al.* (1988a) described the beryllium concentrations in a plant in which most of the beryllium refined in the USA since 1934 has been produced, the principal product always having been beryllium–copper alloys (containing ≤ 2–4% beryllium). Table 9 summarizes the daily weighted average concentrations in 16 departments in four periods. The concentrations were high for many years, with some estimated to have been in excess of 100 μg/m³; as late as 1975, average exposures to beryllium in some jobs were greater than 10 μg/m³. After about 1977, the levels were in compliance with the permissible exposure limit of 2 μg/m³. The median cumulative exposure of 297 white male workers surveyed in 1977 was 65 μg/m³-years; their median exposure was 0.4 μg/m³, and the mean number of years worked was 17. [The Working Group noted that there was some overlap in the plants surveyed.]

Table 9. Daily weighted average concentrations of beryllium (μg/m³) in 16 departments[a] in a US beryllium production plant in four periods

Department	Approximate no. of workers in 1943	No. of jobs in department	Period			
			1935–54	1955–64	1965–76	1977–83
Oxide	46	14	46	16	8.8	0.5
Arc furnace room	26	6	80	51	11	0.7
Detroit furnaces	24	4	51	51	33	NA
Foundry	27	5	19	19	13	NA
Melt and cast	105	6	18	18	7.6	1.1
Hot rolling	19	8	9.3	9.3	2.5	0.2
Cold rolling	29	8	9.2	5.7	2.5	0.2
Rod and wire	39	8	5.9	5.9	2.0	0.2
Annealing	10	5	13	13	5.7	0.1
Pickling	11	3	0.2	0.2	0.2	0.1
Machining, grinding	60	5	1.7	1.7	0.9	0.1
Maintenance	73	13	6.2	5.7	3.5	0.1
Inspection	12	7	1.6	1.6	0.9	0.1
Laundry	–	1	2.5	2.5	1.0	0.1
Laboratories, research and development	28	6	1.4	1.4	1.2	0.2
Stores, shipping	20	3	3.6	3.6	2.0	0.1
Total	529	102				

From Kriebel *et al.* (1988a); NA, not applicable; these departments were not operational during 1977–83.
[a]Smaller departments were grouped for presentation.

(b) Machining and use

Personal air samples taken at US factories in which machining of beryllium metal and alloys involved drilling, boring, cutting and sanding did not contain any detectable amount of beryllium (Gilles, 1976; Boiana, 1980; Lewis, 1980). In a US boat factory in which workers were engaged in grid blasting, beryllium concentrations of 6–134 µg/m^3 were measured (Love & Donohue, 1983). Breathing-zone air samples taken from workers during grinding, polishing, cutting and welding of beryllium-containing alloys in a German metal processing plant contained < 0.1–11.7 µg/m^3 beryllium in total dust; 0.1–10.0 µg/m^3 during hand cutting; 1.4–11.7 µg/m^3 during automatic cutting; 2.1–3.63 µg/m^3 during welding without exhaust extraction; and 1.12–1.34 µg/m^3 during welding with exhaust extraction (Minkwitz *et al.*, 1983; WHO, 1990).

Dental laboratory technicians were exposed to < 2 µg/m^3 beryllium in the breathing zone during the processing of beryllium-containing dental alloys in the USA when exhaust ventilation was used (Dvivedi & Shen, 1983). Air measurements in three dental laboratories in Italy where melting and finishing of dental prostheses were carried out revealed beryllium concentrations in the breathing area in the range of 0.04–1.7 µg/m^3. The mean concentration of beryllium in the urine of 46 dental technicians (0.34 µg/L; range, 0.05–1.7) was higher than that of non-occupationally exposed subjects (mean, 0.26 µg/L; range, < 0.03–0.8) (Apostoli *et al.*, 1989a). [The Working Group noted that the smoking habits of the technicians were not defined.]

1.3.3 *Air*

The major source of atmospheric beryllium is combustion of coal, and its most prevalent chemical form is probably beryllium oxide, mainly bound to particles smaller than 1 µm (WHO, 1990). In earlier reports, average atmospheric background concentrations of beryllium were reported to be less than 0.1 (Bowen, 1966) and 0.2 ng/m^3 (Sussmann *et al.*, 1959). The air of over 100 cities in the USA, sampled in 1964–65, did not contain detectable amounts of beryllium (detection limit, 0.1 ng/m^3) (Drury *et al.*, 1978). Annual average background concentrations during 1977–81 throughout the USA were around the detection limit of 0.03 ng/m^3. Annual averages at urban monitoring stations where concentrations exceeded 0.1 ng/m^3 ranged between 0.11 and 6.7 ng/m^3 during 1981–86 (US Environmental Protection Agency, 1987; WHO, 1990). These data are similar to those found in other countries: Ikebe *et al.* (1986) found an average of 0.042 ng/m^3 in 76 air samples collected in 17 Japanese cities between 1977 and 1980; the highest values were found in Tokyo (0.22 ng/m^3) and in an industrial area in Kitakyushu (0.21 ng/m^3). R. Freise and G.W. Israel (1987, cited in WHO, 1990) found annual mean values in Berlin (Germany) of 0.2–0.33 ng/m^3. A concentration of 0.06 ng/m^3 was measured in a residential area, an office area and the inner city area of Frankfurt, whereas 0.02 ng/m^3 was measured in a rural area near Frankfurt (Müller, 1979).

Atmospheric concentrations of beryllium in the vicinity of beryllium processing plants are often higher than those elsewhere. A mean concentration of 15.5 ng/m^3 and a maximum concentration of 82.7 ng/m^3 were reported near a Pennsylvania (USA) factory, whereas background levels in several locations in the area averaged only 0.2 ng/m^3 (Sussman *et al.*, 1959).

The average concentration of beryllium in air 400 m from a beryllium extracting and processing plant in the former USSR, which was not equipped with emission control devices, was 1 µg/m^3; at 1000 m, it was 10–100 ng/m^3. Between 500 and 1500 m from a mechanical beryllium-finishing plant with operational filter facilities, no beryllium was detected in air [detection limit not given] (Izmerov, 1985). Bencko et al. (1980) reported beryllium concentrations of 3.9–16.8 ng/m^3 (average, 8.4 ng/m^3) in the vicinity of a power (coal) plant in former Czechoslovakia.

1.3.4 Tobacco smoke

In a German study of three brands of cigarettes [origin of tobaccos and number of samples not given], 0.47–0.75 µg beryllium was found per cigarette. Less than 10% of the beryllium content (0.011–0.074 µg/cigarette) was released into mainstream smoke during smoking (Zorn & Diem, 1974).

1.3.5 Water

Beryllium concentrations in surface waters are usually in the range 0.01–0.1 µg/L (WHO, 1990). The concentrations in 15 major US river basins ranged from 0.01 to 1.22 µg/L, with a mean of 0.19 µg/L (Safe Drinking Water Committee, 1977). Water samples taken from various areas near the Seward Peninsula in Alaska contained beryllium concentrations of 0.034–2.4 µg/L (Gosink, 1976). Surface water in eastern USA and Siberia contained beryllium at concentrations ranging from 0.1 to 0.9 µg/L (Safe Drinking Water Committee, 1977). Groundwater samples from Germany contained < 5–9 ng/L, with a mean of 8 ng/L; beryllium concentrations in seawater were 10 times lower than those in surface water (Reichert, 1974). Concentrations of 0.2–0.9 ng/L (mean, 0.5) (Merrill et al., 1960) and 2 ng/L (Meehan & Smythe, 1967) were reported in the Pacific Ocean. Measures and Edmond (1982) found still lower concentrations, 0.04–0.06 ng/L, in the mixed layer—up to about 500 m.

In a survey of 380 US drinking-water sources in 1962–67, beryllium was found in only 1.1% of samples, at concentrations ranging from 20 to 170 ng/L (mean, 100) (Safe Drinking Water Committee, 1977). Sauer and Lieser (1986) found beryllium at 27 ± 8 ng/L in drinking-water samples from Germany.

1.3.6 Soils

Beryllium occurs in most soils. Drury et al. (1978) reported an average of 6 mg/kg (range, 0.1–4.0) worldwide and 0.04–1.45 mg/kg in Kenya. Of 847 samples of agricultural soils collected at a depth of 20 cm throughout the USA, 66% contained < 1 mg/kg, 22% between 1 and 2 mg/kg and 12% between 2 and 7 mg/kg (Shacklette et al., 1971). The mean beryllium concentration in 27 soil profiles (with 129 horizons) of uncontaminated soil from various locations in Japan was 1.31 mg/kg (Asami & Fukazawa, 1985).

In some small, unpolluted areas in which rocks contain large amounts of beryllium, the overlying soils show relatively high beryllium concentrations; e.g., soils in the Lost River Valley, Alaska, USA, contained up to 300 mg/kg, with an average of 60 mg/kg (WHO, 1990).

1.3.7 Food

Only limited, variable data are available on beryllium contents of food (WHO, 1990). The concentrations in various foods collected in New South Wales, Australia, ranged from 10 to 470 µg/kg ash weight (0.07–1175 µg/kg fresh weight); the highest concentrations were found in peanut shells (Meehan & Smythe, 1967).

Owing to the limited data, the daily human intake of beryllium from food has not been determined. In a study in the United Kingdom (Hamilton & Minsky, 1973), the average total dietary intake was estimated to be < 15 µg/day. The US Environmental Protection Agency (1987) estimated a total daily consumption of about 420 ng, most of which came from food (120 ng/day) and drinking-water (300 ng/day); air and dust reportedly contributed very little to the total intake of beryllium.

1.3.8 *Human tissues and secretions*

The measured concentrations of beryllium in body fluids and tissues have diminished substantially over the past 10 years, probably as a consequence of improved analytical techniques, including better procedures for minimizing beryllium contamination during collection and assay. The validity of the data reported in the older literature is therefore somewhat doubtful.

Sprince *et al.* (1976) analysed specimens taken at autopsy from patients without granulomatous disease and found less than 20 µg/kg dry weight of beryllium in lung tissue (mean, 5 µg/kg; range, 3–10; six cases) and mediastinal lymph nodes (mean, 11 µg/kg; range, 6–19; seven cases). These concentrations are within the range of 90% of the values of 2–30 µg/kg dry lung tissue found in 125 lung specimens obtained during thoracic surgery (Baumgardt *et al.*, 1986).

Caroli *et al.* (1988) analysed different parts of lung tissue from 12 subjects in an urban area of Rome (Italy), who were nonsmokers, 50 or more years old and had not been occupationally exposed to beryllium during their lifetime. The overall mean of 5 µg/kg fresh weight indicates a smaller concentration range than those above, which were expressed in dry weight.

In a survey of 66 patients with beryllium disease in the US Beryllium Case Registry, the concentrations of beryllium ranged from 4 to 45 700 µg/kg dried tissue; 82% of the patients had concentrations of more than 20 µg/kg dry weight. Peripheral lymph-node specimens from five patients contained 2–490 µg/kg beryllium and mediastinal specimens, 56–8500 µg/kg (Sprince *et al.*, 1976).

Beryllium concentrations in urine specimens from non-occupationally exposed subjects are summarized in Table 10. The mean beryllium concentration in blood from 20 non-occupationally exposed German subjects was 0.9 µg/L (SD, 0.5) (Stiefel *et al.*, 1980).

Smoking appears to influence the concentration beryllium in urine: the beryllium concentration in the urine of heavy smokers (0.31 ± 0.17 µg/L) was significantly greater than that of nonsmokers (0.20 ± 0.14 µg/L) (Apostoli *et al.*, 1989b).

An exposure concentration of 2 µg/m^3 beryllium in air was found to correspond to about 7 µg/L in urine and about 4 µg/L in blood (Zorn *et al.*, 1988).

Table 10. Urinary concentrations of beryllium, identified by graphite furnace atomic absorption, in specimens from non-occupationally exposed subjects

Country	No. of subjects	Concentration (µg/L; mean ± SD)	Reference
USA	120	0.9 ± 0.4	Grewal & Kearns (1977)
Italy	56	0.6 ± 0.2	C. Minoia et al. (1985; cited by Apostoli et al., 1989b)
USA	NR	0.13	Paschal & Bailey (1986)
Italy	163	0.24 ± 0.16 (range, < 0.03–0.8)	Apostoli et al. (1989b)
Italy	579	0.4 (range, < 0.02–0.82)	Minoia et al. (1990)

Modified from Apostoli et al. (1989b); NR, not reported

1.4 Regulatory status and guidelines

Occupational exposure limits and guidelines for beryllium and beryllium compounds established in different parts of the world are given in Table 11.

Table 11. Occupational exposure limits and guidelines for beryllium and beryllium compounds

Country or region	Year	Concentration (µg/m³)	Interpretation[a]
Argentina	1991	2	TWA, potential carcinogen
Australia	1990	2	TWA, probable human carcinogen
Belgium	1990	2	TWA, probable human carcinogen
Bulgaria	1984	1	TWA
China	1979	1	TWA
Denmark	1992	1	TWA[b]
Finland	1990	0	Suspected of having carcinogenic potential
France	1990	2	TWA, carcinogen
Germany	1992	0	A2[c]
Hungary	1990	1	STEL, probable human carcinogen, irritant, sensitizer
Indonesia	1978	2	TWA
Italy	1978	2	TWA
Japan	1991	2	TWA, probable human carcinogen
Korea, Republic of	1983	2	TWA
Mexico	1984	2	TWA
Netherlands	1986	2	TWA
Poland	1985	1	TWA

Table 11 (contd)

Country or region	Year	Concentration (μg/m³)	Interpretation[a]
Romania	1975	1	STEL
Sweden	1991	2	TWA, causes cancer, sensitizer
Switzerland	1990	2	TWA, inhalable dust, absorbed through skin
Taiwan	1981	2	TWA
United Kingdom	1994	2 (proposal)	STEL
USA[e]			
OSHA	1989	2	TWA (PEL)
		5	Ceiling
		25	Max
NIOSH	1990	0.5	TWA, carcinogen (REL)
ACGIH	1992	2	TWA, A2[d] (TLV)
Venezuela	1978	2	TWA
		25	Ceiling

From Arbeidsinspectie (1986); Cook (1987); US Occupational Safety and Health Administration (OSHA) (1989); Arbetarskyddsstyrelsens (1991); Institut National de Recherche et de Sécurité (1990); US National Institute for Occupational Safety and Health (1990); International Labour Office (1991); American Conference of Governmental Industrial Hygienists (ACGIH) (1992); Anon. (1992); Arbejdstilsynet (1992); Deutsche Forschungsgemeinschaft (1992); UNEP (1993).

[a]The concentrations given may or may not have regulatory or legal status in the various countries; for interpretation of the values, the original references or other authoritative sources should be consulted. TWA, time-weighted average; STEL, short-term exposure limit; Max, acceptable maximal peak (of 30-min maximal duration) above the acceptable ceiling concentration for an 8-h shift; PEL, proposed exposure limit; REL, recommended exposure limit; TLV, threshold limit value

[b]Beryllium and beryllium compounds are on a list of dangerous compounds but not classified for carcinogenic effect.

[c]Compounds which in the Commission's opinion have proven so far to be unmistakably carcinogenic in animal experimentation only; namely under conditions which are comparable to those for possible exposure of a human being at the workplace, or from which such comparability can be deduced

[d]Suspected human carcinogen; chemical substance, or substances associated with industrial processes, which are suspected of inducing cancer, on the basis of either limited epidemiological evidence or demonstration of carcinogenesis in one or more animal species by appropriate methods

Stationary sources (extraction plants, ceramic plants, foundries, incinerators and propellant plants for the processing of beryllium ore, beryllium, beryllium oxide, beryllium alloys and beryllium-containing waste; machine shops for the processing of beryllium, beryllium oxide and any alloy containing more than 5% beryllium by weight) are subject to the US national emission standard for beryllium, which is 0.01 μg/m³ (30-day average) in ambient air for those production facilities which qualify for regulation through ambient air monitoring. Other facilities must meet a total site emission limit of 10 g per 24 h (US Environmental Protection Agency, 1992).

In the European Economic Community, beryllium and beryllium compounds are not permitted in cosmetic products (Commission of the European Communities, 1991a, 1992). Waste (except domestic waste) containing or contaminated by beryllium and beryllium compounds is classified as hazardous waste (effective date, 12 December 1993) (Commission of the European Communities, 1991b). Member States must take the necessary steps to limit the introduction of beryllium and its compounds into groundwater (effective date, 26 January 1982) (Commission of the European Communities, 1980). Beryllium and beryllium compounds (except aluminium beryllium silicates) are classified as very toxic and irritant (effective date, 1 July 1992) (Commission of the European Communities, 1991c).

2. Studies of Cancer in Humans

Beryllium was considered previously by three working groups (IARC, 1972, 1980, 1987). The first group (IARC, 1972) found the four epidemiological studies available at that time (Hardy *et al.*, 1967; Stoeckle *et al.*, 1969; Mancuso & El-Attar, 1969; Mancuso, 1970) not to provide evidence of the existence of a possible relationship between exposure to beryllium compounds and the occurrence of cancer in man. The second working group (IARC, 1980) reviewed four subsequent cohort studies (Infante *et al.*, 1980; Mancuso, 1979, 1980; Wagoner *et al.*, 1980) and concluded that the evidence for an increased risk for lung cancer from occupational exposure to beryllium was limited. No new study was available at the time of the third review (IARC, 1987).

2.1 Cohort studies (see Table 12, p. 70)

Mancuso (1979) conducted a retrospective cohort mortality study of workers employed in two beryllium extraction, production and fabrication facilities in the USA: one in Lorain, Ohio, and the other in Reading, Pennsylvania (see Table 13, p. 71, for description). The cohort was limited to workers who had been employed for at least three months during 1942–48. Observed and expected numbers of deaths were compared using a modified life-table analysis. Expected deaths were calculated on the basis of five-year mortality rates for the general white male population of the USA, except that the author did not have access to the actual national mortality rates for 1968–75 and calculated expected deaths for that period by applying US mortality rates for 1965–67. As a consequence of this extrapolation, expected lung cancer death rates for the 1968–75 period were underestimated by a factor of 10% (Saracci, 1985). The standardized mortality ratio (SMR) for lung cancer among the 1222 workers in the Ohio plant was 2.00 (1.8 with Saracci's adjustment; 95% confidence interval [CI], 1.2–2.7); that among the 2044 workers at the Pennsylvania plant was 1.37 (1.25 with Saracci's adjustment; 95% CI, 0.9–1.7). The combined lung cancer SMR (with Saracci's adjustment) for the two plants was 1.42 (95% CI, 1.1–1.8). A consistently greater excess of lung cancer was seen in the two plants among workers who were followed for 15 or more years since first employment; the SMRs (with Saracci's adjustment) were 2.0 (95% CI, 1.3–3.1) for the Ohio plant and 1.5 (95% CI, 1.0–2.1) for the Pennsylvania plant. In the combined cohort, the excess of lung cancer was limited to workers who had been employed for less than five years and followed for 15 or more years since first employment. [The

Working Group noted that no analysis of risk by job title or exposure category was conducted. The period of initial employment of the study cohort preceded the imposition by the US Atomic Energy Commission in 1949 of a 2 μg/m³ 8-h time-weighted average limit for occupational exposure to beryllium and a ceiling limit of 25 μg/m³, applicable to all beryllium facilities under contract to the Commission (Preuss, 1988).] A study of the beryllium alloy plant in Lorain, Ohio, conducted in 1947–48 by the US Atomic Energy Commission (Zielinski, 1961), showed concentrations of beryllium ranging from 411 μg/m³ in the general air surrounding the mixing operation to 43 300 μg/m³ in the breathing zone of alloy operatives. Control measures were introduced throughout US plants after 1949, and exposure levels in beryllium facilities were reduced markedly. Extraction plants, for example, were able to maintain exposure levels of 2 μg/m³ or less, while certain foundry operations had air concentrations consistently in excess of 2 μg/m³, with maximal values greater than 1000 μg/m³ during the period 1968–72 in the Pennsylvania plant (Wagoner et al., 1980).

Mancuso (1980) re-analysed mortality in the same Ohio and Pennsylvania beryllium extraction and processing plants, but extended the period of employment of the study cohort to 1937–48 and used as a comparison group viscose rayon industry workers employed at one company during 1938–48. Mortality was followed up through 1976. Among the 3685 cohort members from the two beryllium plants, 80 lung cancer deaths were observed, whereas 57.1 were expected on the basis of the total mortality experience of the viscose rayon workers (SMR, 1.40; $p < 0.01$) and 50.6 deaths were expected on the basis of the mortality experience of viscose rayon workers employed in a single department of the industry (SMR, 1.58; $p < 0.01$). [The Working Group noted that use of the latter reference cohort may introduce a selection bias into the analysis, since the mortality experience of workers who never change departments while employed in the industry may differ from that of the total workforce of the industry, for non-occupational reasons.] Lung cancer SMRs were calculated by duration of employment in comparison with the entire group of viscose rayon employees; these values were 1.38 ($p < 0.05$; 52 observed deaths) for one year or less of employment, 1.06 (14 observed deaths) for more than one year to four years or less, and 2.22 ($p < 0.01$; 14 observed deaths) for more than four years' employment.

Wagoner et al. (1980) expanded the cohort mortality study of the same Pennsylvania plant analysed by Mancuso (1979, 1980) to include workers employed at some time during 1942–67 and followed them up to 1 January 1976. [This interval extends across the year 1949 when, as previously noted, the Atomic Energy Commission standard of 2 μg/m³ was introduced and a substantial reduction in exposure to beryllium subsequently occurred (US National Institute for Occupational Safety and Health, 1972).] They also used 1965–67 national lung cancer mortality rates to calculate expected lung cancer deaths for the period 1968–75. [The adjustment of Saracci (1985) is thus appropriate in considering these results.] Wagoner et al. (1980) observed 47 lung cancer deaths among the 3055 workers in the study cohort, whereas 37.7 were expected (with Saracci's adjustment) on the basis of national mortality experience, yielding an SMR of 1.25 (95% CI, 0.9–1.7). When lung cancer SMRs were calculated by latency, the SMRs were 0.88 (9 deaths) for < 15 years' latency, 1.16 (18 deaths) for 15–24 years' latency and 1.68 (20 deaths) for ≥ 25 years' latency, the 95% CI for latter SMR being 1.0–2.6. Within latency categories, there was no pattern of increasing (or decreasing) SMR by duration of employment, dichotomized into less than five and five years or more. Analysis by duration yields an unstable estimate for longer duration strata owing to small numbers: for ≥ 5 years, the SMR is 1.1 (seven deaths) and the 95% CI is 0.4–2.3 (Saracci, 1985). A decline in risk for death from chronic beryllium disease was seen in relation to the same categories of length of employment. The potential for confounding of the SMR by a different distribution of smoking habits in the US population and in the beryllium cohort was calculated on the basis of a 1968 medical survey, in which detailed smoking histories of workers at the Pennsylvania plant were obtained, and of the 1964–65 Health Interview Survey of a probability sample of the US population, in which current and past smoking habits were queried. The overall calculations suggest that reported differences in smoking habits were sufficient to increase the lung cancer risk among the beryllium workers by 14%, in the absence of beryllium exposure; however, as also discussed by Wagoner *et al*. (1980), the white male age-adjusted rate for lung cancer mortality in the county in which the Pennsylvania plant was located (31.8/100 000) was lower than the average annual white male age-adjusted mortality rate for the USA as a whole (38.0/100 000). Wagoner *et al*. (1980) calculated that the risk for mortality from lung cancer in the beryllium cohort, if adjusted for differences in mortality between the County and the USA and for residential stability of cohort members, was underestimated by a factor up to 19%. [The Working Group noted that these two factors—smoking distribution and lower regional lung cancer mortality—bias the SMR estimate in opposite directions.]

Infante *et al*. (1980) analysed the mortality experience of white males entered into the Beryllium Case Registry while alive, with a diagnosis of chronic beryllium disease or acute beryllium-related pneumonitis. The Beryllium Case Registry was established in 1952 to collect data on the epidemiology, diagnosis, clinical features, course and complications of beryllium-related diseases. Individuals who were entered into the Registry were categorized as having either acute beryllium-induced pneumonitis or chronic systemic beryllium diseases (Sprinze & Kazemi, 1980). Individuals who were referred to the Registry for evaluation of beryllium-related diseases were employed in a variety of occupations, but most worked in beryllium extraction and smelting, metal production and fluorescent tube production. A total of 421 white males who entered the Registry alive between July 1952 and December 1975 were followed through to 31 December 1975. Seven deaths from lung cancer were observed and 3.3 were expected, based on national mortality rates for the period 1952–67 (SMR, 2.12, not significant). Since published vital statistics were not available for the period 1968–75, national mortality rates for 1965–67 were applied to 1968–75. If the number of expected deaths is increased by 10%, the expected value becomes [3.63], and the adjusted SMR is [1.93; 95% CI, 0.8–4.0]. For men who were entered into the Registry with a diagnosis of beryllium-related acute pneumonitis, the SMR (with Saracci's adjustment) for lung cancer is 2.86 (95% CI, 1.0–6.2; six cases). For those who were entered with a diagnosis of chronic beryllium disease, one lung cancer death was observed, with 1.52 expected (SMR, 0.66; 95% CI, 0.1–3.7). [The Working Group noted the small expected number of lung cancer deaths, particularly among workers with chronic lung disease, and the relatively short follow-up time for those workers who were entered into the Registry after 1965 (≤ 10 years). Chronic beryllium disease results from hypersensitivity to beryllium and may occur at much lower exposures than acute beryllium pneumonitis. A small number of the cases occurred among people living near the plants but who were not occupationally exposed.]

An extended analysis of mortality among people entered into the Beryllium Case Registry was reported by Steenland and Ward (1991). The study cohort, which now included women (34% of the cohort) and men of all races, numbered 689 people who were alive at entry into the Registry between July 1952 and the end of 1980. Mortality follow-up was extended through 1988 [actual US death rates were available for comparison for all years, eliminating the need for Saracci's adjustment in this and the report of Ward et al. (1992)]. Excess mortality was found for all cancers (SMR, 1.51; 95% CI, 1.17–1.91; 70 observed deaths), due primarily to an excess of lung cancer (SMR, 2.00; 95% CI, 1.33–2.89; 28 observed deaths); there were also excess deaths from nonmalignant respiratory disease (SMR, 34.23; 95% CI, 29.1–40.0; 158 observed deaths) and all causes of deaths (SMR, 2.19; 95% CI, 1.17–1.91; 428 observed deaths). The SMR for lung cancer was greater among cohort members with acute beryllium pneumonitis (SMR, 2.32; 95% CI, 1.35–3.72; 17 cases) than among those with chronic beryllium disease (SMR, 1.57; 95% CI, 0.75–2.89; 10 cases) (one death was due to disease of unknown type). The SMRs for nonmalignant respiratory disease were 10 times higher in the chronic disease group (SMR, 68.6) than in the acute disease group (SMR, 6.6). The SMRs for lung cancer varied little by time since first exposure (SMR, 1.95; 95% CI, 0.94–3.59 for $\leq$ 20 years since first exposure; 2.03; 95% CI, 1.20–3.21 for > 20 years) or by duration of exposure. [The Working Group presumed that duration of exposure to beryllium was determined by duration of employment in a beryllium plant, although this is not specified in the published report.] Taking into account the distribution of smoking habits among 32% of the cohort members questioned in 1965 and from a national survey of the US population studied in 1965, Steenland and Ward (1991) concluded that the study cohort smoked less (current smokers, 26%) than the US referent population (39%) in 1965 and that, if the 32% sample were representative of the entire cohort, smoking was unlikely to be a confounder of the observed excess lung cancer. Selection bias was diminished in this study because: people who died before entry into the Registry were excluded; only five individuals who had cancer before entry into the Registry were found in a review of Registry records, and none of these had lung cancer; and if patients with lung cancer had entered the Registry preferentially, the follow-up interval on these subjects would have been short, whereas only three of the 28 observed lung cancer deaths occurred within five years of entry into the Registry. [The Working Group noted that the results of this Beryllium Case Registry cohort study yield a higher lung cancer SMR than was found in other studies of beryllium-exposed workers, particularly among those who were entered with acute beryllium pneumonitis and who could therefore be assumed to have had a higher intensity of exposure to beryllium. This finding is consistent with the assumption that the risk for lung cancer is proportional to the intensity of exposure to beryllium. Furthermore, it provides indirect evidence that beryllium, rather than smoking, explains the findings, as people with acute pneumonitis were unlikely to smoke more than workers with chronic beryllium disease.]

Ward et al. (1992) reported the results of a cohort mortality study of 9225 male workers (8905 white, 320 non-white) employed by two companies at seven beryllium plants in Ohio and Pennsylvania. The results are summarized in Tables 12–16 (pp. 70–73). [Two of these plants (in Lorain, OH, and Reading, PA) are the same as those studied by Mancuso (1979, 1980) and Wagoner et al. (1980) (see Table 13).] Workers had to have worked for at least two days between 1940 and 1969 to qualify for entry into the study cohort. Mortality follow-up

Table 12. Cohort studies of lung cancer in beryllium workers

Reference	Cohort or plant location	Period of employment	Termination of follow-up	Comparison population	SMR	95% CI	Lung cancers observed
Mancuso (1979)	Lorain, OH Reading, PA Combined	1942–48 1942–48	1974 1975	US white males	1.8[a] 1.25[a] 1.42[a]	1.2–2.7 0.9–1.7 1.1–1.8	25 40 65
Mancuso (1980)	Lorain, OH Reading, PA	1937–48	1976	Viscose rayon workers	1.40	[1.1–1.7]	80
Wagoner et al. (1980)	Reading, PA	1942–67	1975	US white males	1.25[a]	0.9–1.7	47
Infante et al. (1980)	Beryllium Case Registry	Entry into Registry 1952–75	1975	US white males Acute pneumonitis Chronic beryllium disease	[1.93] 2.86[a] 0.66[a]	[0.8–4.0] 1.0–6.2 0.1–3.7	7 6 1
Steenland & Ward (1991)	Beryllium Case Registry	Entry into Registry 1952–80	1988	US men and women (all races) Acute pneumonitis Chronic beryllium disease	2.00 2.32 1.57	1.33–2.89 1.35–3.72 0.75–2.89	28 17 10
Ward et al. (1992)	Seven beryllium processing plants	1940–69	1988	US males, all races	1.26	1.12–1.42	280

SMR, standardized mortality ratio; CI, confidence interval; [ ], calculated by the Working Group
[a]With Saracci's adjustment

was extended through to 1988 and was analysed using standard modified life-table methods. The influence of local differences in mortality was evaluated by comparing SMRs derived from national and from local county mortality rates. The effect of the dissimilar distribution of smoking habits between beryllium workers and the US population was also evaluated. In the total cohort of 9225 workers, there were 3240 deaths (35% of the total) and 269 235 person-years of follow-up, of which 52% were person-years at risk 15 years or more after first employment in the beryllium industry. The SMR for all causes was 1.05 (95% CI, 1.01–1.08), that for all cancers was 1.06 (95% CI, 0.99–1.44), and that for nonmalignant respiratory disease was 1.48 (95% CI, 1.21–1.80). With the exception of that for cancer of the respiratory system, none of the SMRs for cancers at specific sites was significantly different from 1.00. The overall SMR for lung cancer was 1.26 (95% CI, 1.12–1.42; 280 observed deaths, based on US rates). SMRs for cancers of the larynx and of the upper respiratory tract were below 1.00.

Table 13. Years during which major processes were used at the US beryllium plants in the study of Ward *et al.* (1992)

Plant location	Ore refining	Beryllium oxide production	Metal production	Beryllium–copper alloy production	Machining
Lorain, OH	1935–48	1935–48	1935–48	1935–47	–
Reading, PA	1935–66	1035–66	–	1935–present	1938–present
Lucky, OH	1950–58	1950–58	1950–58	–	–
Perkins (Cleveland), OH	1937–55	1937–62	1948–62	–	1941–63
St Clair (Cleveland), OH	–	–	–	–	1963–73
Elmore, OH	1958–77	1958–present	1958–present	1952–present	1958–present
Hazelton, PA	1958–78	1958–78	1958–78	1958–78	1958–78

The dates refer only to the processes and were not used to restrict the cohorts. For example, workers hired at the Lucky plant in 1949 were included in the study, as were a few individuals hired at the Lorain plant in 1949 and early 1950.

The SMRs for lung cancer at individual plants (Table 14) were greater than 1.00 at four of the six locations: two plants near Cleveland, OH—Perkins and St Clair—were combined into one cohort because records of the two plants could not be separately identified. The SMRs were significantly greater than 1.00 only at the Lorain, OH, and Reading, PA, plants [the same facilities studied by Mancuso (1979, 1980) and Wagoner *et al.* (1980)]. It is noteworthy that cohorts in which there was a high SMR for pneumoconiosis and other respiratory diseases, presumably indicating higher exposure to beryllium also consistently had elevated SMRs for lung cancer. When lung cancer SMRs were stratified by latency at each plant, three of the six locations showed higher SMRs for the 15–30-year and > 30-year latency categories compared with the < 15-year latency category (Table 15); however, for the total cohort, lung cancer SMRs increased stepwise with increasing latency (bottom row of Table 15). When SMRs were stratified by decade of hire (Table 16), values greater than 1.00 were seen for all three locations in which workers were hired before 1950 (the period when exposures to beryllium were also greater than subsequently), but SMRs were also greater than 1.00 in four of the five locations where workers were hired between 1950 and 1959.

Table 14. Mortality of workers employed in 1940–69 at the seven US beryllium processing plants in the study of Ward et al. (1992)

Plant location	Total no. of workers	Percentage of workers employed for		SMR			Pneumoconiosis and other respiratory disease (based on US rates)	No. of lung cancer deaths
		< 1 year	1–5 years	Lung cancer (based on US rates)	Lung cancer (based on county rates)			
Lorain, OH	1192	84.6	12.8	1.69**	1.60**		1.94**	57
Reading, PA	3569	53.8	22.3	1.24*	1.42**		1.34	120
Cleveland, OH (two plants)	1593	47.3	29.8	1.08	1.05		1.22	44
Lucky, OH	405	62.2	35.8	0.82	0.84		0.87	9
Elmore, OH	1323	29.0	24.9	0.99	1.06		0.69	15
Hazelton, PA	590	19.7	17.8	1.39	1.50		2.00	13
Multiple plants	257	0.8	12.1	1.67	–		2.60	13
Location unknown	296	49.3	41.6	1.33	–		3.47**	9
Total[a]	9225	49.7	23.4	1.26**	1.32*		1.48**	280

*$p < 0.05$; **$p < 0.01$
[a]See also Table 12

As seen in the bottom row of Table 16, decade of hire was one of the strongest correlates of lung cancer mortality risk in the total cohort. Poisson regression analysis, with control for age, race, calendar time and time since first employment, showed an independent effect of decade of hire on lung cancer SMRs in the total cohort. Duration of employment had no effect. [The Working Group noted that, given the much higher exposures to beryllium prior to 1950 and the fact that 73% of the total cohort worked for less than five years, duration of employment does not separate that segment of the cohort which received the highest exposures to beryllium.]

Table 15. Standardized mortality ratios (SMRs) for lung cancer by location of plants and latency since time of first employment in the US beryllium plants in the study of Ward *et al.* (1992)

Location	Latency < 15 years		Latency 15–30 years		Latency > 30 years	
	SMR	Observed deaths	SMR	Observed deaths	SMR	Observed deaths
Lorain, OH	0.38	1	2.09**	21	1.66*	35
Reading, PA	0.78	9	1.17	44	1.40*	67
Cleveland, OH	1.30	9	0.91	20	1.27	15
Lucky, OH	0.96	1	0.85	4	0.76	4
Elmore, OH	0.51	2	1.14	12	1.31	1
Hazelton, PA	1.91	4	1.26	9	–	0
Multiple plants	–	0	1.23	4	2.38*	9
Location unknown	0.64	1	1.28	5	2.30	3
Total	0.89	27	1.20	119	1.46**	134

*$p < 0.05$; **$p < 0.01$

Table 16. Standardized mortality ratios (SMRs) for lung cancer by location of plants and decade of hire in the US beryllium plants in the study of Ward *et al.* (1992)

Location	Hired before 1950		Hired 1950–59		Hired 1960–69	
	SMR	Observed deaths	SMR	Observed deaths	SMR	Observed deaths
Lorain, OH	1.69**	57	–	–	–	–
Reading, PA	1.26*	92	1.42	26	0.35	2
Cleveland, OH	1.06	12	1.32	26	0.63	6
Lucky, OH	–	–	0.82	9	–	–
Elmore, OH	–	–	1.42	12	0.45	3
Hazelton, PA	–	–	1.86	9	0.87	4
Multiple plants	2.53**	12	0.36	1	–	–
Location unknown	2.30	4	0.62	2	1.57	3
Total	1.42**	177	1.24	85	0.62	18

*$p < 0.05$; **$p < 0.01$

When lung cancer SMRs for each of the six locations were based on local county mortality rates (Ward *et al.*, 1992; see Table 14), the SMRs differed only slightly from those based on US rates. The largest difference occurred in the Reading, PA, cohort, in which the SMR based on US rates was 1.24 and that based on county rates was 1.42. For all six locations, the lung cancer SMR based on US rates was 1.26 (95%, 1.12-1.42), while that based on local county rates was 1.32 (95% CI, 1.19-1.46). When lung cancer SMRs were adjusted for the distribution of smoking habits at four of the plants in which a smoking survey was conducted in 1968 [covering 1466 (15.9%) of the 9225 members of the cohort], the SMR for the total cohort changed from 1.26 to 1.12, and the SMRs in two of the largest, oldest plants changed from 1.69 to 1.49 (Lorain, OH) and from 1.24 to 1.09 (Reading, PA). The authors noted that the major difficulty in interpreting the smoking-adjusted SMRs is that data on smoking were collected in the late 1960s, while most (94%) of the lung cancer cases occurred among workers hired in the 1940s and 1950s. Thus, the validity of the adjustment for smoking depends on the assumption that differences in smoking habits between the cohort and the US population were the same in the 1940s and 1950s as they were in the late 1960s and that smoking data obtained from 16% of the workers adequately represented the distribution of smoking in the entire cohort. The authors estimated the contribution of smoking to be 13%, i.e., smoking alone could account for a lung cancer SMR of 1.13 *versus* the 1.26 actually observed.

2.2 Case-control studies

Hinds *et al.* (1985) applied a computerized job-exposure matrix to data from a case-control study of lung cancer among males in Hawaii, USA. Between 1 September 1979 and 31 July 1982, 261 cases of newly diagnosed primary lung cancer among male residents of Oahu, Hawaii, were identified through a population-based tumour registry and a review of pathology records at all major hospitals and interviewed. Controls were identified by random-digit dialling and matched on sex and age. Information on occupation was obtained during the interview and applied to a job-exposure matrix to estimate exposure levels to various agents for each study subject. The job-exposure matrix was constructed from lists of occupational codes by Hoar *et al.* (1980), and these were used to code both the primary and secondary occupations of all subjects according to industry; each code was then linked to various levels of exposure to each agent. Each agent was grouped into three exposure levels (no exposure, low exposure, high exposure). The association of each agent with lung cancer risk was estimated by the odds ratio, which was determined by multiple logistic regression analysis and adjusted for age, ethnicity and smoking status. Excess risk for lung cancer was found to be associated with exposure to beryllium at both low (odds ratio, 1.62; 95% CI, 1.04-2.51) and high levels (1.57; 0.81-3.01). Other exposures considered in the analysis were coal-tar and pitch, petroleum, arsenic, chromium, asbestos and nickel. [The Working Group noted that it is not clear whether the odds ratio for beryllium was simultaneously controlled for the other exposures.]

Carpenter *et al.* (1988) conducted a nested case-control study of cancers of the central nervous system among workers employed at some time between 1973 and 1977 at two nuclear facilities in Oak Ridge, TN (USA); deaths of 72 white males and 17 white females from cancer of the central nervous system were identified from information on death certificates, and four controls were matched to each case for race, sex, facility at which initially employed, year of birth and year of hire. Each job title and department combination was subjectively evaluated for potential exposure to each of 26 chemicals, including beryllium. The evaluation took into account period of employment, literature on the processes used at each facility, quantities and toxicities of chemicals used in the processes, interviews with workers involved in processes at different time periods, and the results of urine analyses and air monitoring. Each job title/department combination was given a rank for potential exposure to each of the 26 chemicals; rank 0 had probably no exposure, rank 1 had low potential, rank 2 had moderate potential and rank 3 had high potential for exposure to the specified chemical. Matched conditional logistic regression analyses were conducted and included potential confounding factors such as socioeconomic status. On the basis of 26 cases ever exposed to beryllium, the odds ratio for cancers of the central nervous system was 1.5 (95% CI, 0.6–3.9). The matched analysis by highest rank ever held *versus* rank 0 yielded odds ratios of 1.26, 12.8 and 3.29 for ranks 1, 2 and 3, respectively (all odds ratios had a p value of 0.09 or greater). When risk estimates were calculated for a 10-year latency, the odds ratios were 1.13, 0.85 and 1.77 for ranks 1, 2 and 3, respectively. A further analysis based on time spent in ranks 2 and 3, assuming a 10-year latency, yielded odds ratios of 0.77, 0.90, 1.30 and 1.88 ($p > 0.5$) for workers with < 3 years, 3–10 years, 11–20 years and 21 years or more in ranks 2 and 3 compared with ranks 0 and 1. The authors concluded that their study does not support the hypothesis that occupational exposures to any of the 26 chemicals studied appreciably increase the risk for cancers of the central nervous system; they noted specifically that, although a weak association between exposure to beryllium and cancers of the central nervous system was observed, confidence intervals [not given for analyses by rank or latency] were wide and included the null value.

2.3 Childhood cancer

A case–control study on parental occupation and childhood cancer carried out in Denver, CO, USA (Feingold *et al.*, 1992), included 252 cases of childhood cancer diagnosed during 1976–83 and 222 population controls selected by random-digit dialling. A job-exposure matrix was used to assign parental exposures for six months or longer during the year prior to the child's birth on the basis of job titles. Odds ratios were estimated for all cancers, acute lymphocytic leukaemia and brain cancer, after adjusting for age at diagnosis, year of diagnosis, sex, mother's age at time of birth, maternal smoking during pregnancy, birth weight, birth order and indicators of social class. When all cancers were considered, no association was found between childhood cancer and exposure to beryllium or its compounds for either the mother or the father (odds ratio, 1.0; 95% CI, 0.1–7.1; based on two exposed cases; and 1.6; 0.6–4.4; based on 17 exposed cases, respectively). When the exposures of the fathers were analysed for specific types of cancer, an elevated odds ratio was found for brain cancer (2.1; 0.6–7.6; 5 cases) but not for acute lymphocytic leukaemia (1.3; 0.3–5.9; 5 cases). Most of the subjects considered to have been exposed to beryllium were electrical equipment assemblers and installers (67%), metal processes and welders (20%). [The Working Group noted that other occupational exposures were not considered in the analysis.]

3. Studies of Cancer in Experimental Animals

3.1 Beryllium ores

Inhalation exposure

(a) *Rat*

Groups of 60 and 33 male Charles River, caesarian-derived rats and 30 Greenacres Controlled Flora rats (more than four weeks old) were exposed by inhalation to **beryl ore** (geometric mean particle diameter, 0.64 μm) or **bertrandite ore** (geometric mean particle diameter, 0.27 μm) as 15 mg/m^3 dust (the threshold limit value for inert dust in 1968) for 6 h per day on five days a week for up to 17 months. A third group, serving as controls, was housed in an inhalation chamber without exposure. The bertrandite ore atmosphere in the inhalation chamber contained 210 μg/m^3 beryllium, and the beryl ore atmosphere contained 620 μg/m^3 beryllium (for chemical composition, see Table 17). The death rates of the animals exposed to the two ores exceeded that of controls by 13%. Of the animals killed after 12 months of exposure, 5/11 treated with beryl ore had foci of squamous metaplasia or small epidermoid tumours. Of those killed at 17 months, 18/19 had lung tumours (18 bronchiolar alveolar-cell tumours, 7 adenomas, 9 adenocarcinomas and 4 epidermoid tumours). No metastasis was observed. In the group treated with bertrandite ore, granulomatous lesions and some atypical proliferations in the lung were observed, but no bronchiolar alveolar-cell tumour or other lung tumour was found. Controls had no neoplastic or granulomatous pulmonary lesion (Wagner *et al.*, 1969). [The Working Group noted the high crystalline silica content of the bertrandite ore and the incomplete reporting of the study.]

(b) *Hamster*

Groups of 48 and 17 male Syrian golden hamsters (more than four weeks old) were exposed by inhalation to **beryl ore** (geometric mean particle diameter, 0.64 μm) or **bertrandite ore** (geometric mean particle diameter, 0.27 μm) as 15 mg/m^3 dust for 6 h per day, five days a week for up to 17 months. A third group, serving as controls, was housed in an inhalation chamber without exposure. The bertrandite ore atmosphere in the inhalation chamber contained 210 μg/m^3 beryllium, and the beryl ore atmosphere contained 620 μg/m^3 (for chemical composition, see Table 17). The mortality of the animals exposed to the two ores exceeded that of controls by 25%. Atypical proliferations, first seen at 12 months in both groups of exposed animals, and lesions considered by the authors to be bronchiolar alveolar-cell tumours, except for their size, occurred. The lesions in the beryl-exposed animals were reported to become larger and more adenomatous after 17 months. The control hamsters had no pulmonary lesion (Wagner *et al.*, 1969). [The Working Group noted the incomplete reporting of the study.]

(c) *Monkey*

Groups of 12 and 4 male squirrel monkeys (*Saimiri sciurea*) (more than four weeks old) were exposed by inhalation to **beryl ore** (geometric mean particle diameter, 0.64 μm) or **bertrandite ore** (geometric mean particle diameter, 0.27 μm) as 15 mg/m^3 dust for 6 h per day, five days a week for up to 23 months. A third group, serving as controls, was housed in an inhalation chamber without exposure. The bertrandite ore atmosphere in the inhalation chamber contained 210 μg/m^3 beryllium, and the beryl ore atmosphere contained 620 μg/m^3 (for chemical composition, see Table 17). The death rates of the animals exposed to the two ores exceeded that of controls by 11%. No tumour was found. Aggregates of dust-laden macrophages, lymphocytes and plasma cells were observed near respiratory bronchioles and small blood vessels in the lungs of exposed animals. Control monkeys had no similar change (Wagner et al., 1969). [The Working Group noted the incomplete reporting and the limited duration of the study.]

Table 17. Chemical composition (of constituents representing > 0.1%) of representative bertrandite and beryl ore samples

Chemical constituent	Analysis by weight (%)	
	Bertrandite	Beryl ore
Be[a]	1.4	4.14
Al_2O_3	9.8	18.1
SiO_2	63.9[b]	
SiO_2 (as silicates)		63.6
SiO_2 (as quartz)		1.9
Fe_2O_3	1.8	1.1
MnO_2	1.8	1.0
CaF_2	8.3	
CaO	0.2	
MgO	2.3	1.1
K_2O	1.2	
Na_2O	1.5	0.5
ZnO	0.7	
CO_2	0.2	
NiO		0.5

Modified from Wagner et al. (1969)
[a][Probably as the oxide]
[b]23.5% of the mineral constituents were crystalline quartz and 23.5%, cristobalite (crystalline silica); the remainder was other silicates.

3.2 Beryllium metal and alloys

3.2.1 Intratracheal instillation

Rat: Twelve groups of 35 female Wistar rats, three months old, were treated with a single intratracheal instillation of 0.5 or 2.5 mg **beryllium metal** (100% Be), **passivated beryllium metal** (99% Be, 0.26% Cr [as chromate]), **beryllium–aluminium alloy** (62% Be, 38% Al), **beryllium–copper alloy** (4% Be, 96% Cu), **beryllium–copper–cobalt alloy** (2.4% Be, 0.4%

Co, 96% Cu) or **beryllium–nickel alloy** (2.2% Be, 97.8% Ni), with geometric mean particle sizes of 1–2 μm, suspended in 0.4 ml isotonic saline, followed by 0.2 ml saline. Forty control animals were instilled with 0.6 ml saline. The rats were killed when moribund or 18 months after instillation. The first lung neoplasm appeared 8–10 months after instillation. Lung neoplasms, mostly adenocarcinomas and adenomas, were found in 2/21 rats treated with the low dose and in 9/16 rats given the high dose of beryllium metal, in 7/20 animals treated with the low dose and in 9/26 treated with the high dose of passivated beryllium metal, and in 1/21 treated with the low dose and in 4/24 given the high dose of beryllium–aluminium alloy. No lung tumour occurred in 39 controls or in the groups treated with other alloys. The incidence of lung neoplasms was significantly ($p < 0.008$) increased over that in controls (using Fisher's exact test, one-tailed) in the groups that received 2.5 mg beryllium metal or 0.5 mg and 2.5 mg passivated beryllium metal (Groth *et al.*, 1980). [The Working Group noted the low beryllium content of the beryllium–copper alloy, the beryllium–copper–cobalt alloy and the beryllium–nickel alloy.]

3.2.2 *Intravenous injection*

Rabbit: In a study reported as a letter to the Editor, 24 young rabbits [sex and strain unspecified] received a series of intravenous injections of a washed suspension of finely divided **beryllium metal** in water (total dose, 40 mg/animal). Nine animals had died with liver necrosis within seven days, and 10 more died with this condition during the next month. Two of the surviving five rabbits died from pulmonary infections, two developed characteristic bone sarcomata, and a single rabbit survived (Barnes, 1950).

3.3 Beryllium compounds

3.3.1 *Oral administration*

Rat: **Beryllium sulfate** was administered to 52 male and 52 female Long–Evans rats (BLU:LE) in the drinking-water at a concentration of 5 ppm [5 mg/L] from weaning until natural death. The water also contained 5 ppm chromium[III] acetate, 50 ppm zinc acetate and 5 ppm copper acetate; 10 ppm manganese chloride and 1 ppm cobalt chloride; and 1 ppm sodium molybdate. An equal number of animals treated with water served as controls. The life span of the treated rats did not differ significantly from that of controls, but 20–30% of rats in each group died from pneumonia. No significant difference in tumour incidence was observed between treated and control groups (Schroeder & Mitchener, 1975). [The Working Group noted that the dose was too low for an evaluation of carcinogenicity.]

3.3.2 *Inhalation*

(a) Rat

Twenty-seven male and female albino Wistar rats, weighing 140–210 g, and 109 male and female Sherman rats, weighing 80–110 g, were exposed by inhalation to **beryllium sulfate tetrahydrate** aerosol to give a concentration of 1 μg/ft^3 Be [35.8 μg/m^3], for 8 h per day on 5.5 days a week for 180 days. Control groups of 69 male and female Wistar and 70 male and female Sherman rats were maintained in normal air. In the 52 rats that survived the treatment, were transferred to 'normal air' and observed for periods of up to 18 months, 76 lung tumours were found, eight with metastases. The tumours included 18 adenomas, 5 squamous carcinomas, 24 acinous adenocarcinomas, 11 papillary adenocarcinomas and 7 alveolar-cell adenocarcinomas. None of the 139 control rats had lung tumours (Schepers *et al.*, 1957). [The Working Group noted the incomplete reporting of the study.]

A group of 75 male and 75 female Sprague–Dawley CD rats, six weeks of age, were exposed by inhalation to **beryllium sulfate tetrahydrate** aerosol for 7 h per day on five days a week for 72 weeks at a mean atmospheric concentration of 34.25 ± 23.66 $\mu g/m^3$ Be (average particle diameter, 0.118 μm). An equal number of control animals was exposed to an aerosol of distilled water. Subgroups of animals were killed each month up to the 56th week of exposure; 87% of all animals survived to their scheduled sacrifices. The first lung tumour was observed after nine months of exposure. All of the 43 rats that survived 13 months or more after the beginning of treatment had tumours, and all of the 56 tumours studied histologically were reported to be alveolar adenocarcinomas. No lung tumour was found in the control group (Reeves *et al.*, 1967). [The Working Group noted the incomplete reporting of the study.]

Groups of 30–50 female albino rats, weighing 155–160 g, received **beryllium oxide** or **beryllium chloride** by inhalation at concentrations of 0.8, 4, 30 or 400 $\mu g/m^3$ for 1 h per day on five days a week for four months. A group of 160 females served as controls. Only malignant epithelial lung tumours were considered: these occurred in 3/44, 4/39, 6/26 and 8/21 rats treated with beryllium oxide and in 1/44, 2/42, 8/24 and 11/19 treated with beryllium chloride, but in none of the controls (Litvinov *et al.* 1984) [The Working Group noted the incomplete reporting of the study.]

(b) Rabbit

Three groups of rabbits [sex, strain and age unspecified] were exposed by inhalation to aerosols of **beryllium oxide** (average particle diameter, 0.285 μm; range, 0.11–1.25) at doses of 1 (five rabbits), 6 (six rabbits) or 30 (eight rabbits) μg/L Be for 5 h per day on five days a week for 9–13 months. No control group was available. An osteogenic sarcoma in the left pubis with widespread visceral metastases was observed in one rabbit that had been exposed to 6 μg/L Be for 235 days over 11 months (Dutra *et al.*, 1951). [The Working Group noted the small number of animals and the short duration of exposure.]

(c) Monkey

In a study reported as an abstract, 16 rhesus monkeys (*Macaca mulatta*) were exposed daily by inhalation 'for a long period of time' to **beryllium sulfate** aerosol at a concentration of 35 $\mu g/m^3$ Be. Primary anaplastic pulmonary tumours with adenomatous and epidermoid patterns were observed in three monkeys between six months and eight years after the beginning of exposure (Vorwald, 1967).

3.3.3 *Intratracheal instillation*

(a) Rat

A group of 35 female Wistar-derived rats, three months old, received single intratracheal instillations of 50 μg Be as **beryllium hydroxide** suspended in distilled water, followed 10 months later by a second instillation of 25 μg. A group of 35 controls received a single intratracheal instillation of 2.5 mg chrysotile asbestos. Both materials were suspended in 0.4 ml distilled water, and the instillation was followed by 0.2 ml distilled water. Of the beryllium hydroxide-treated rats sacrificed at 19 months of age, 13/25 had pulmonary tumours (six adenomas and seven adenocarcinomas); one rat had both an epidermoid carcinoma and an adenocarcinoma. The lungs of all of the animals instilled with chrysotile had small and occasionally larger scars; adenomas occurred in two rats and an adenocarcinoma in a third. Metaplastic foci were found in the lungs of 5% of the chrysotile-treated group, whereas in 90% of the animals instilled with beryllium most of the normal lung tissue was replaced by metaplastic foci and tumours (Groth *et al.*, 1980). [The Working Group noted the lack of an appropriate control group.]

Two groups of 30 male Wistar rats, 10 weeks of age, were instilled intratracheally with **beryllium oxide** (low-temperature fired, 900 °C; 1 mg as Be) or arsenic trioxide (1 mg as As) once a week for 15 weeks. A group of 16 rats served as untreated controls. All rats in the beryllium-treated group, 19 in the arsenic-treated group and all of the controls survived the treatment period and were observed for life. Two malignant (one squamous-cell carcinoma and one adenocarcinoma) and four benign lung adenomas (three suspected of malignancy) were found in rats treated with beryllium, and one malignant lung tumour (a squamous-cell carcinoma) was found in those treated with arsenic; no lung tumour was observed in the control group (Ishinishi *et al.*, 1980).

Eight groups of inbred albino rats [initial number and sex unspecified], weighing 140–150 g, received single intratracheal instillations of **high-temperature fired beryllium oxide** (2000 °C) or **low-temperature fired beryllium oxide** (600 °C) at doses of 0.036, 0.36, 3.6 and 18 mg/kg bw. A group of 300 untreated rats served as controls. All animals were observed for life. Malignant epithelial lung tumours occurred in 0/76, 0/84, 2/77 and 2/103 rats treated with the high-temperature fired beryllium oxide and in 3/69, 7/81, 18/79 and 8/26 rats treated with the low-temperature fired compound. None were found in 104 controls (Litvinov *et al.*, 1983).

(*b*) *Monkey*

In a study reported as an abstract, a group of 20 rhesus monkeys (*Macaca mulatta*) received an intrabronchial intubation and/or a bronchomural injection [unspecified] of **beryllium oxide** particulates suspended in sterile physiological saline. The first bronchogenic tumour was detected about 4.5 years after first treatment. In the course of the following year, two additional monkeys developed tumours, which were highly anaplastic, with adenomatous and epidermoid patterns (Vorwald, 1967).

3.3.4 *Intravenous injection*

(*a*) *Mouse*

In a study reported as an abstract, three groups of mice received 20–22 intravenous injections (two/week) of either **zinc beryllium silicate** (8.36 mg Zn, 0.264 mg Be), zinc silicate (2.8 mg Zn) or **beryllium oxide** (1.54 mg Be). A fourth group was untreated. 'Some' mice given zinc beryllium silicate were reported to have developed malignant bone tumours (Cloudman *et al.*, 1949).

(b) *Rabbit*

In a study reported as an abstract, rabbits received synthetic **zinc beryllium silicate** and its ingredients, **beryllium oxide**, zinc oxide, silicic acid and zinc silicate, intravenously in 20 doses totalling 1 g of particles 3 μm or smaller, over a six-week period. All of the seven rabbits given zinc beryllium silicate which survived the injections for seven months or more developed malignant osteosarcomas, four with visceral metastases. One rabbit killed one year after injection of beryllium oxide had a malignant osteosarcoma. Such tumours were not induced by administration of 65 other minerals in the same way (Gardner & Heslington, 1946).

In a study reported as an abstract, three groups of rabbits received 20–22 intravenous injections (two/week) of either **zinc beryllium silicate** (550 mg Zn, 17 mg Be), zinc silicate (390 mg Zn) or **beryllium oxide** (390 mg Be). A fourth group was untreated. Four of five rabbits given zinc beryllium silicate which survived over one year from the start of injections had bone tumours, three with metastases (Cloudman *et al.*, 1949).

Six groups comprising 67 rabbits of different breeds and sexes were injected intravenously twice a week with various samples of **zinc beryllium silicate** (67% ZnO, 28% SiO_2, 2% BeO and 3% MnO; or 67% ZnO, 31% SiO_2 and 2% BeO), **beryllium silicate** or zinc silicate, with particle sizes of 5 μm or less as a 1 ml suspension in water at the dose schedule indicated in Table 18. Bone sarcomas developed in 7/21 rabbits injected with beryllium silicates that survived for 30 weeks or more. The earliest evidence of malignant change was observed at 32 weeks, and the latest tumour occurred 83 weeks after the last injection. No tumour was found in any of the animals injected with zinc silicate only (Barnes *et al.*, 1950). [The Working Group noted the poor survival.]

Table 18. Results of experiments in rabbits with beryllium silicates

Material injected	Conc. of suspension (%)	No. of injections	Total amount injected (g)	Initial no./group	No. of survivors	No. with osteosarcomas
Zinc beryllium silicate	10	10	1.0	10	3	0
Zinc beryllium silicate	30	6	2.1	12	3	2
Zinc beryllium silicate	10	10	1.0	12	11	4
Beryllium silicate	20	6	1.2	11	3	1
Beryllium silicate	10	10	1.0	12	8	0
Zinc silicate	20	6	1.2	10	8	0

From Barnes *et al.* (1950)

Young, adult, male and female white rabbits [number unspecified] were given intravenous injections of either a highly purified **beryllium oxide** or a **calcined phosphor** containing beryllium oxide, zinc oxide and silica mixed in a molar ratio of 1:1:1, as 1% suspensions in physiological saline. The particles of the powders were smaller than 1 μm. The beryllium oxide-treated group received a total of 360–700 mg Be/rabbit in 20–26 injections, and the phosphor group received 64–90 mg Be/rabbit in 17–25 injections. The compounds were given three times a week over approximately six to nine weeks. One year or more after the first injection, six animals given beryllium oxide and three given calcined phosphor were still alive. The first tumour was found 11.5 months after the start of the experiment. Osteosarcomas were found in all six beryllium oxide-treated rabbits (two were reported after the paper had been submitted for publication); some were metastases and some were multiple primary tumours. Osteosarcomas were found in 2/3 rabbits given the phosphor. About 50 untreated rabbits kept for similar or longer periods developed no malignant tumour (Dutra & Largent, 1950). [The Working Group noted the small group sizes, the limited reporting and the incomplete observations.]

A group of 13 female and 11 male rabbits of unselected strains, with an average initial body weight of 5.5 lbs [2.5 kg], received intravenous injections of insoluble beryllium compounds under sterile conditions at a dose of 5 ml at one-day or four-day intervals, in an attempt to administer a total of 1 g of the powder. Five animals received **beryllium phosphate**; six rabbits received a **zinc beryllium silicate** containing 60% ZnO, 30% SiO$_2$, 2% MnO and 2.3% BeO; four received another zinc beryllium silicate containing 14% **beryllium oxide** and 48% zinc oxide; and nine rabbits received **beryllium oxide** from different sources. Except for the beryllium phosphate, which was administered in a 0.1% suspension in saline, all substances were injected as 1% suspensions in saline. Eight animals died of various causes within three months of the start of treatment, and eight more rabbits died at 14–28 months from infectious diseases. Seven of the eight surviving rabbits developed osteogenic sarcomas: three in the group treated with zinc beryllium silicate containing 2.3% BeO, three in the group treated with zinc beryllium silicate containing 14% BeO and one treated with beryllium oxide. One animal that received 100 mg beryllium phosphate was still alive 2.5 years after injection (Hoagland et al., 1950). [The Working Group noted the small group size and the lack of appropriate controls.]

Osteosarcomas were found in 2/4 rabbits within 18 months after a single intravenous injection of 1 g **beryllium phosphate**; no tumour was found in three rabbits that received 1 g **beryllium oxide**. Of animals injected with beryllium oxide mixed with zinc oxide, manganese oxide and/or silicon oxide, 9/31 developed osteosarcomas (Araki et al., 1954). [The Working Group noted the small number of animals, the lack of an appropriate control group and the incomplete reporting.]

Ten adult, male rabbits received two intravenous injections per week for 10 weeks of 5 ml of a 1% suspension of **zinc beryllium silicate** containing 3.36% **beryllium oxide** (total dose, 1 g zinc beryllium silicate or 33.6 mg beryllium oxide). Five rabbits developed osteogenic sarcomas 9–11 months after the injection period (Janes et al., 1954). [The Working Group noted the lack of an appropriate control group and the small group size.]

Fourteen rabbits were injected intravenously with 5 ml of a 1% suspension of **zinc beryllium silicate** (size of particles, 1–3 µm) in physiological saline twice a week for 10 weeks (total dose, 1 g zinc beryllium silicate). The animals died or were killed 28–57 weeks after the last injection. Osteogenic sarcomas appeared in 10/14 rabbits 30–52 weeks after the last injection (Kelly et al., 1961). [The Working Group noted the lack of an appropriate control group and the small group size.]

Osteosarcomas were induced in 3/20 rabbits 15–18 months after single intravenous injections of **beryllium oxide** (total dose, 1 g/rabbit) as a 1% suspension in saline (Komitowski, 1968). [The Working Group noted the lack of an appropriate control group.]

Sixty rabbits, six months of age on average, were treated intravenously with a 1% **beryllium oxide** suspension in 5 ml physiological saline, once a week for 25 weeks. Of the 29 animals that survived until the end of the experiment, 21 developed sarcomas (Fodor, 1977). [The Working Group noted the lack of an appropriate control group and the incomplete reporting.]

3.3.5 Intraperitoneal injection

Mouse: In a screening assay based on the accelerated induction of lung adenomas in a strain highly susceptible to development of this neoplasm, three groups of 20 male A/J mice, five to six weeks old, were injected intraperitoneally three times a week for eight weeks with **beryllium sulfate tetrahydrate** (purity ≥ 99%) suspended in distilled water at doses of 0.02, 0.05 or 0.1 (maximum tolerated dose) mg/mouse per injection. An equal number of animals were treated with the vehicle only and served as controls. The authors stated that beryllium sulfate produced a significant (χ^2 analysis) increase in lung tumour incidence at total doses of 1.2 and 2.4 mg/mouse with no significant increase in lung tumour multiplicity (Ashby *et al.*, 1990). [The Working Group noted that the increases were not significant using Fisher's exact test.]

3.3.6 Implantation and/or injection into bone

Rabbit: Of 55 rabbits that received 1–43 injections of 10 mg **beryllium oxide** as a 1% suspension in isotonic saline into the marrow of the right femur twice weekly (20 mg/week), one developed a chondroma, three developed osteomas, 15 developed chondrosarcomas and seven developed osteochondrosarcomas. The average time between the last injection and the appearance of a tumour was 85 days. The period of observation was one to two years (Yamaguchi, 1963).

A group of 12 rabbits of mixed breeds and sexes, six weeks old, received 20 mg **zinc beryllium silicate powder** (particle diameter, ≤ 5 μm), suspended in 0.5 ml of water, as a single intramedullary injection into the upper end of the right tibia. A similar suspension of **zinc oxide** was injected into the left tibia as a control. All rabbits survived the injections for at least 12 months; four animals died of intercurrent infections. Osteogenic sarcomas were found in four rabbits at 12–15 months; three metastasized. The remaining four animals were killed at 15–20 months with no clinical or radiological evidence of tumours. No effect was seen with zinc oxide (Tapp, 1966).

Three groups of six rabbits of mixed breeds and sexes, six to eight weeks old, received implants of 10 mg **zinc beryllium silicate**, **beryllium oxide** or **beryllium silicate** under the periosteum of the upper end of the right tibia. Three animals from each group also received implants of zinc oxide or zinc silicate in a similar procedure into the left tibia and served as controls. Nine animals were killed between 2 and 18 months; the remaining animals lived for 25 months. Four of the animals developed central osteogenic sarcomas between 10 and 25 months after implantation; two occurred in animals treated with beryllium and metastasized, one occurred in an animal given zinc beryllium silicate and metastasized, and one occurred in an animal given beryllium silicate. No tumour occurred in the left tibia of the animals implanted with zinc oxide or zinc silicate (Tapp, 1969).

After intramedullary administration of **beryllium oxide** [purity, dose and dose schedule unspecified] (particle size, ~4 μm) in gelatin into the femur, 5/20 rabbits developed osteogenic sarcomas with lung metastases during an observation period of 24 months. The first tumour was observed 13 months after injection (Komitowski, 1974). [The Working Group noted the lack of an appropriate control group and the incomplete reporting.]

Rabbits were given intramedullary implantations of **beryllium carbonate** (173 rabbits), **beryllium acetate** (18 rabbits), **beryllium acetylacetonate** (10 rabbits), **beryllium laurate** (3 rabbits) or **beryllium stearate** (3 rabbits). Thirty animals given beryllium carbonate developed osteosarcomas 10–17 months after the first treatment; the tumours were detected radiologically between 10 and 21 months and confirmed histologically. One rabbit given beryllium acetylacetonate that survived 13 months developed an osteosarcoma (Matsuura, 1974). [The Working Group noted the incomplete reporting and the small numbers of animals in groups other than the group treated with beryllium carbonate.]

A group of 65 Fauve de Bourgogne rabbits [sex unspecified], 15–20 weeks old, received single intraosseous injections of 0.5 ml of a suspension prepared from 1 g **zinc beryllium silicate** in 15 ml distilled water and gelatin (33 mg Be) into the tibial or femoral metaphysis. Of the 65 rabbits that survived more than four months after the injection, 45 developed osteogenic sarcomas. Radiographic examination indicated that the first sarcomatous changes occurred after three months (Mazabraud, 1975). [The Working Group noted the lack of an appropriate control group.]

Three groups of 10 male rabbits [strain unspecified], six weeks of age, received implants of pellets of hydroxypropylcellulose mixed with **beryllium oxide** into the distal metaphysis of the right femur as follows: Group 1, into the internal callus one week after production of an artificial fracture at a dose of 300 mg; Group 2, into the bone-marrow cavity at a dose of 300 mg; and Group 3, into the bone-marrow cavity at a dose of 50 mg. A further group of 10 rabbits served as untreated controls. At 56 weeks, osteosarcomas had developed in 10/10 rabbits in Group 1, in 7/10 rabbits in Group 2 and in 1/10 rabbits in Group 3. Tumours appeared significantly earlier in Group 1 than in the other groups, and 80% of animals with osteosarcomas had lung metastases (Hiruma, 1991).

3.3.7 *Administration with known carcinogens*

Mouse: Five groups of 40 female and 40 male SENCAR mice, seven to nine weeks old, received a single intraperitoneal injection of 0, 0.01, 0.1, 1.0, 5.0 or 10.0 μg/mouse **beryllium sulfate** [purity unspecified]) in saline. One week after treatment, each animal received dermal applications of 2 μg 12-*O*-tetradecanoylphorbol 13-acetate (TPA) twice a week for 26 weeks. A positive control group received 50.5 μg/mouse benzo[*a*]pyrene followed by the TPA treatment. About 95% of the animals survived the treatment. Beryllium sulfate did not induce a significant number of mouse skin papillomas (Nesnow *et al.* 1985).

4. Other Relevant Data

4.1 Absorption, distribution, metabolism and excretion

The kinetics and effects of beryllium in humans and animals have been reviewed (Eisenbud, 1984; Skilleter, 1984; Cullen *et al.*, 1986; Reeves, 1986; Skilleter, 1986; Kriebel *et al.*, 1988b; Reeves, 1989; WHO, 1990; Deodhar & Barna, 1991; Haley, 1991).

4.1.1 *Humans*

After accidental exposure of 25 people to beryllium dust, the mean serum concentration of beryllium one day later was 3.5 ppb (μg/L); six days later, it had decreased to 2.4 ppb (Zorn *et al.*, 1986). In unexposed humans who had a mean blood beryllium concentration of 0.9 ng/g (ml), 33.2% of the beryllium in blood was associated with cellular constituents, 7.3% with low-molecular-weight compounds, 8.0% with prealbumin and 51.5% with γ-globulin (Stiefel *et al.*, 1980).

Subjects in the Beryllium Case Registry had elevated concentrations of beryllium in lung tissue (e.g. 0.32 μg/g in a metastinal node) more than 20 years after termination of short-term occupational exposure to beryllium (Sprince *et al.*, 1976).

4.1.2 *Experimental systems*

Retention of carrier-free ^{7}Be as chloride after oral dosage of RF mice, Sprague–Dawley rats, beagle dogs and *Macaca speciosa* monkeys was followed in urine excreted during the first two days. The authors estimated from counts in urine that the gastrointestinal absorption was about 0.6%; however, the urinary excretion of the three monkeys studied was reported to be 3.71% (Furchner *et al.*, 1973).

An early study on the kinetics of continuously inhaled beryllium sulfate in rats showed that the pulmonary burden of beryllium reached a plateau after about 36 weeks. After cessation of exposure, clearance was faster in males than in females. Beryllium was accumulated in tracheobronchial lymph nodes, where the concentration reached a peak at 52 weeks (Reeves & Vorwald, 1967). When rats were exposed to ^{7}Be as chloride and ^{4}Be as sulfate in aqueous aerosols by inhalation using nose-only exposure, 60% of the amount of beryllium deposited initially (the sum of the total body burden and the excreted amount) was found in the lungs and 13.5% in the skeleton (Zorn *et al.*, 1977).

When dogs inhaled aerosols of ^{7}Be as oxide calcined at 500 °C (low-fired) or 1000 °C (high-fired) through the nose, disappearance from the lungs followed first-order kinetics. The clearance half-time was 240 days for high-fired beryllium oxide and 64 days for the low-fired compound. Most of the beryllium in the body was located in the skeleton, tracheobronchial lymph nodes, liver and blood. During the first 32 days after exposure, 59% of the low-fired and 68% of the high-fired beryllium oxide was excreted through the gastrointestinal tract; by 180 days, 47% of the low-fired and 54% of the high-fired was excreted by that route and the balance *via* the kidneys (Finch *et al.*, 1990).

In rats, the clearance of inhaled beryllium oxide calcined at 1000 °C through the lungs showed two successive half-times: the first, comprising 30% of the initial lung burden, was

2.5 days, and the second (70%), 833 days. One to 63 days after exposure, a small fraction (0.58–1.73%) of the initial lung burden was observed in thoracic lymph nodes. About 15% was excreted in the faeces and 1.4% in the urine (Rhoads & Sanders, 1985). The clearance from the alveoli of inhaled beryllium oxide calcined at 1000 °C was faster in hamsters than in rats (Sanders et al., 1975).

The disappearance of beryllium from the lungs of rats 3–171 days after exposure to 800 mg/m^3 metallic beryllium aerosol (mass median aerodynamic diameter, 1.4 µm; geometric mean standard deviation, 1.9) by nose-only inhalation once for 50 min was reported to fit best a first-order kinetic model with a half-time of 240 days (Haley et al., 1990). In a carcinogenicity study (Wagner et al., 1969), described in detail in section 3.1, rats, hamsters and squirrel monkeys were exposed by inhalation to ore dusts containing beryllium, beryl (containing 4.14% beryllium) and bertrandite (containing 1.4% beryllium). Increased concentrations of beryllium were detected in the skeleton, liver and lung after 6–12 months of exposure to beryl or bertrandite; exposure to beryl led to higher tissue concentrations than did exposure to bertrandite.

The highest concentrations of beryllium after an intramuscular injection of carrier-free ^{7}Be as chloride to rats were observed initially in the skeleton, liver, kidney, lungs and spleen; 56.3% of the dose injected was still at the site of injection after one day. During a 64-day follow-up, the skeleton and, to a lesser degree, spleen showed a constant increase, while there was a gradual decrease in the other organs; 20.5% of the dose injected was still at the site of injection (Crowley et al., 1949). Accumulation in the liver, kidney, spleen and, especially, the skeleton was also observed seven days after an intravenous administration of ^{7}Be to rats and rabbits. In rats receiving ^{7}Be as sulfate, the liver and spleen contained appreciable amounts of beryllium; in animals receiving carrier-free ^{7}Be, a higher percentage was found in the skeleton. These differences were less marked in rabbits (Scott et al., 1950).

Accumulation of beryllium in compact bone, liver and kidney was observed in dairy cows given carrier-free ^{7}Be as chloride orally or intravenously (Mullen et al., 1972).

After intravenous injection of carrier-free ^{7}Be as chloride into rats in a solution at pH 2, 47% of the dose was excreted predominantly in the urine and 43% was detected in bone and bone marrow after 24 h; only 4% was detected in liver and 0.1% in spleen. When 1 µmol unlabelled beryllium chloride was added as carrier to the solution to be injected, the proportion found in the liver increased to 25% and that in spleen to 1%. At pH 6, 59% was found in the liver after administration of carrier-free ^{7}Be and 44% after addition of unlabelled beryllium chloride. Administration of labelled plus 0.15 µmol unlabelled beryllium chloride in citrate at pH 6 elicited similar responses to carrier-free ^{7}Be at pH 2, while labelled plus 0.3 µmol unlabelled beryllium hydroxide was accumulated strongly in the liver and spleen (Klemperer et al., 1952).

The uptake of intravenously administered (20–800 µg/kg bw) beryllium phosphate was much more extensive in the liver and spleen (approximately 55% of the dose) than that of beryllium sulfate or citrate in mouse; the same phenomenon was observed in rats given a single dose (200 µg/kg bw). The uptake of the two soluble compounds was practically nil at dose levels up to 50 µg/kg, while uptake of the phosphate was independent of dose (Vacher et al., 1974).

Beryllium phosphate and beryllium sulfate accumulated in both nonparenchymal and parenchymal cells of the liver after intravenous administration (Skilleter & Price, 1978). Beryllium oxide granules accumulated intracellularly in marrow throughout the skeletal system after intravenous administration to rabbits of beryllium oxide [method of preparation not given] (Fodor, 1977).

After an intraperitoneal or intravenous dose of carrier-free ^{7}Be as chloride, the disappearance of beryllium was best characterized by three consecutive half-times of 0.2–0.5, 6.3–21.7 and 50.9–52.4 days in mice, rats, dogs and *Macaca speciosa* monkeys (Furchner et al., 1973).

Transplacental transfer of beryllium was demonstrated in mice after intravenous injection of beryllium chloride (Bencko et al., 1979). Transport of ^{7}Be [chemical unspecified] across the rat placenta after intravenous injection was also reported (Schulert et al., 1969).

An estimated 1% of a single oral dose of carrier-free ^{7}Be as chloride to a dairy cow was excreted in the milk within 91 h (Mullen et al., 1972).

After an intravenous injection of beryllium sulfate to rats, most of the beryllium in plasma coeluted in Sephadex chromatography with phosphate and was attached to plasma globulins. A small part of the dose remained in a low-molecular-weight form (Vacher & Stoner, 1968). One-fourth to one-third of blood-borne beryllium in unexposed guinea-pigs and rats was bound to cellular constituents; this proportion was unchanged in animals exposed to beryllium by inhalation. In both exposed and unexposed guinea-pigs, the proportion bound to prealbumin was approximately 70%; in rats, it was 65% (Stiefel et al., 1980). When beryllium chloride (10^{-4} mol/L) was dissolved in different plasma constituents at their normal plasma concentrations, only a very small proportion (generally less than 2.5%) remained dialysable; only citrate (62%), maleate (30%) and bicarbonate (10%) were significantly dialysable. Phosphate decreased the dialysable part of beryllium to 0.2%, and 4% of the added beryllium remained dialysable. It was concluded that at beryllium concentrations in excess of about 10^{-7} mol/L, most of the beryllium in plasma is nondialysable phosphate, and the small dialysable part is mainly citrate (Feldman et al., 1953). In line with this finding, only 3% of beryllium sulfate added to serum *in vitro* traversed a dialysis membrane within 24 h (Reeves & Vorwald, 1961). A low-affinity binding site for beryllium was observed on the outer cell surface of human and guinea-pig lymphocytes; a binding site with a higher affinity was detected in the cell nucleus (Skilleter & Price, 1984).

After repeated intraperitoneal administrations to rats of beryllum sulfate, beryllium was concentrated in nuclei in the cells of the proximal convoluted tubuli (Berry et al., 1987, 1989). In hepatocytes, beryllium was accumulated in lysosomes and nuclei (Levi-Setti et al., 1988). After intravenous administration, the highest concentrations were observed in lysosomes; only at doses approaching the LD_{50} (corresponding to 2–83 μmol/kg bw beryllium sulfate) was there also accumulation in the nuclei in the liver (Witschi & Aldridge, 1968).

Beryllium showed affinity to nuclei isolated from rat liver *in vitro* (Witschi & Aldridge, 1968); it was not bound to DNA or histones (Witschi & Aldridge, 1968; Parker & Stevens, 1979) but to a highly phosphorylated non-histone protein fraction (Parker & Stevens, 1979).

4.2. Toxic effects

4.2.1 *Humans*

Exposure to beryllium compounds may cause an acute chemical pneumonitis, tracheobronchitis, conjunctivitis, dermatitis and chronic granulomatous pulmonary disease with systemic manifestations (Hardy & Tepper, 1959; Freiman & Hardy, 1970). The acute pulmonary disease was first described in Germany in 1933 (Weber & Engelhardt, 1933) and the chronic form in the USA in 1946 (Hardy & Tabershaw, 1946).

Acute beryllium disease, most frequently related to intense but brief exposure, consists of respiratory tract irritation and dermatitis, sometimes with conjunctivitis. The respiratory tract symptoms range from mild nasopharyngitis to a severe chemical pulmonitis, which may be fatal (Hardy & Tepper, 1959; Kriebel *et al.*, 1988b). In fatal cases, histopathological findings in the lungs have included interstitial oedema, cellular infiltration, elevated numbers of plasma cells, alveolar cell proliferation or desquamation and, sometimes, interalveolar oedema, hyaline membranes and organizing pneumonia (Freiman & Hardy, 1970).

Chronic beryllium disease is a systemic disorder with primary manifestations in the lung, characterized by a decrease in transfer factor with restrictive and obstructive ventilatory function. Histopathologically, the disease is characterized by non-caseating granuloma formation with giant cells, as in sarcoidosis, primarily seen in the lungs but also in other tissues. Chest radiography usually shows diffuse infiltrates and hilar adenopathy (Hardy & Tepper, 1959; Freiman & Hardy, 1970; Jones Williams, 1977; Kriebel *et al.*, 1988b). An improvement in lung function and even in lung radiographic findings was reported after a significant decrease in the air concentration of beryllium due to improved engineering and ventilation in plants (Sprince *et al.*, 1978).

Beryllium compounds known to cause beryllium-induced diseases include metallic beryllium (Jones Williams, 1977), beryllium alloys (Lieben *et al.*, 1964) and beryllium oxide fumes (Cullen *et al.*, 1987). The first cases of beryllium disease were identified in the fluorescent light-bulb industry (Hardy & Tabershaw, 1946), in which beryllium-containing phosphors (zinc beryllium manganese silicate), prepared by firing the individual oxides with silica, were used (Eisenbud & Lisson, 1983).

Although chronic beryllium disease has become rare since the adoption of stringent industrial hygiene measures, sporadic cases are still reported (Karkinen-Jääskeläinen *et al.*, 1982; Cullen *et al.*, 1987; Rossman *et al.*, 1988; Kreiss *et al.*, 1989; Newman *et al.*, 1989), e.g., among workers in a precious metal refinery, where exposure to beryllium did not exceed 2 $\mu g/m^3$ (Cullen *et al.*, 1987). A conspicuous feature of chronic beryllium disease is its occasional occurrence outside facilities in which beryllium compounds are used: Sterner and Eisenbud (1951) reported 10 cases among people who had never worked in a beryllium plant but who lived within 1 km of one; the best estimate of beryllium concentrations in the air in the area was 0.01–0.1 $\mu g/m^3$. In 1983, when the US registry for beryllium diseases contained 622 cases of chronic beryllium disease, 65 had had no occupational exposure to beryllium, 42 could be attributed to air pollution (41 occurred in the vicinity of two large production plants and one in a woman living near a fluorescent-lamp plant) and 23 to household exposure to dust brought home on work clothes (Eisenbud & Lisson, 1983).

In the cohort study based on the Beryllium Case Registry, reported in detail in section 2 (p. 68), the SMR for non-neoplastic respiratory diseases was 16.4 ($p < 0.001$) and that for non-neoplastic respiratory diseases (other than influenza and pneumonia), 32.1 ($p < 0.001$) (Infante et al., 1980). In an updating of the cohort (Steenland & Ward, 1991), described in detail in section 2, the SMR for nonmalignant lung disease was 26.3 (95% CI, 20.6–33.1) for workers with less than four years of exposure and 45.8 (95% CI, 36.6–56.5) for workers with longer exposure.

In a cohort study of 9225 male workers employed in seven beryllium processing facilities in the USA (Ward et al., 1992; described in section 2, p. 69), the SMR for pneumoconiosis and other respiratory diseases was 1.48 (95% CI, 1.21–1.80), that for diseases of the heart was 1.06 (1.00–1.12) and that for chronic and unspecified nephritis, renal failure and other renal sclerosis, 1.49 (1.00–2.12).

A nonsymptomatic form of chronic beryllium disease—typical granulomatous changes in transbronchial biopsy specimens with positive lymphocyte transformation tests—has been reported (Newman et al., 1989).

Beryllium dermatitis may be a typical contact dermatitis, localized dermal ulceration or a subcutaneous granuloma. Ulceration of granulomas develops after a particle of a beryllium-containing substance is introduced into an abrasion, laceration or cut (Hardy & Tepper, 1959). People with beryllium-induced contact dermatitis react to patch testing (Curtis, 1951; DeNardi et al., 1952). Patch testing may cause a flare of the dermatitis in sensitized people; it may also induce beryllium sensitivity (Curtis, 1951)

A role of immunological mechanisms in beryllium-induced chronic disease was originally proposed by Sterner and Eisenbud (1951). The condition has the features of a type IV cell-mediated hypersensitivity disorder, the beryllium acting as a hapten (Dayan et al., 1990). Cell-free extracts of blood lymphocytes from people with experimentally induced, localized, dermal granulomatous beryllium lesions cultured in the presence of beryllium oxide contained migration inhibition factor, which inhibits the migration of guinea-pig peritoneal exudate cells (Henderson et al., 1972). The factor was also produced by cell cultures originating from the blood of patients with chronic beryllium disease (Jones Williams et al., 1972; Marx & Burrell, 1973). Lymphocytes from such patients responded to a beryllium oxide or beryllium sulfate challenge by blast transformation and increased thymidine incorporation (Hanifin et al., 1970; Deodhar et al., 1973). Proliferation of lymphocytes from patients with chronic beryllium disease in response to a challenge with beryllium sulfate or fluoride was more marked in lymphocytes obtained by bronchoalveolar lavage than in those harvested from circulating blood (Epstein et al., 1982; Cullen et al., 1987; Saltini et al., 1989). The only lymphocytes obtained from bronchoalveolar lavage which proliferated were CD4+ (helper/inducer) T cells (Saltini et al., 1989).

4.2.2 Experimental systems

When beryllium (as lactate or sulfate) was given intravenously to rats or rabbits at a dose of 0.5 or 0.75 mg/kg Be, death invariably followed within four days; the primary cause of death was liver damage and ensuing hypoglycaemia. In rabbits, but not in rats, convulsions were observed before death (Aldridge et al., 1950).

A granulomatous lung disease, morphologically and immunologically similar to chronic beryllium disease in humans, was induced in beagle dogs by inhalation of beryllium oxide calcined at 500 °C, but not with beryllium oxide calcined at 1000 °C (Haley et al., 1989).

Intratracheal instillation of 10 mg beryllium oxide (calcined at 560 °C) into male Hartley guinea-pigs of an inbred strain caused focal interstitial lymphomononuclear infiltrates in the lungs, which progressed to granulomatous lung lesions with fibrosis. Lymphocytes from the blood of these animals responded to beryllium sulfate *in vitro* by increased incorporation of tritiated thymidine (lymphocyte transformation test). The animals exhibited a positive reaction to intradermal beryllium sulfate. Intravenous or oral administration of beryllium sulfate before intratracheal instillation of beryllium oxide decreased the intensity of the pulmonary reaction; a similar effect was observed when the animals were treated with prednisone, L-asparaginase or cyclophosphamide. Splenic cells from animals with beryllium-induced lung disease given intraperitoneally to another group of animals of the same strain caused a similar disease and skin reactivity to beryllium sulfate. No lung disease, skin reactivity or reaction in the lymphocyte transformation test was induced by similar treatment of another inbred strain of guinea-pigs (Barna et al., 1981).

In another study using the same responsive guinea-pig strain, lymphokine production by isolated lymph node cells from animals treated with beryllium oxide endotracheally and challenged with beryllium sulfate was demonstrated *in vitro*. The cells also secreted a factor that inhibited the migration of macrophages (Barna et al., 1984).

Strain A (H-2^a haplotype) mice given an intratracheal instillation challenge of beryllium sulfate or beryllium oxide (calcined at 550 and 1100 °C) after immunization with beryllium sulfate had increased numbers of lymphocytes in bronchoalveolar lavage fluids two, four and eight weeks (months for the oxide) after the challenge. The cells were mainly CD4+ T lymphocytes. By four weeks, microgranulomas were observed in the lungs, which had developed into granulomatous lesions by eight weeks in the case of the sulfate. Such changes were not observed in mice not immunized with beryllium sulfate or in pretreated mice that were not challenged, nor in two strains of mice with different H-2 haplotypes [C57Bl/6(H-2^b) and BALB/c(H-2^d)] (Huang et al., 1992).

In a descriptive toxicity study (see p. 86), male Fischer 344/N rats were exposed by nose only to 800 mg/m^3 metallic beryllium dust (mass median aerodynamic diameter, 1.4 µm) for 50 min, to give an initial lung burden of 625 µg. The animals were then followed for 171 days with timed terminations at 3, 7, 10, 14, 31, 59 and 115 days. Necrotizing, haemorrhagic pulmonitis and intra-alveolar fibrosis, followed by chronic inflammatory changes, were observed. The prevailing cell type obtained by bronchoalveolar lavage was neutrophils; few lymphocytes and no granulomas were observed (Haley et al., 1990). Similarly, after a 1-h exposure of rats to 4.05 mg/m^3 Be as beryllium sulfate (mass median aerodynamic diameter, 1.9 µm), progressive focal interstitial pneumonitis, but no granulomatous disease, was observed; the gross histological picture was similar three weeks and 3, 6 and 12 months after the exposure (Sendelbach et al., 1989).

Intratracheal instillation of beryllium sulfate after immunization with a subcutaneous injection of beryllium sulfate fortified with ovalbumin and Freund's adjuvant resulted in granulomatous pulmonary disease in Fischer 344 rats within six weeks, accompanied by accumulation of both T and B lymphocytes in the lung tissue (Votto et al., 1987).

In a carcinogenicity study (Wagner et al., 1969; see section 3.1, p. 76), granulomatous lung lesions were observed in hamsters and rats exposed to bertrandite but not in those exposed to beryl ore. [It is not clear if the granulomas were morphologically similar to those observed in humans with chronic beryllium disease or to those in dogs and guinea-pigs after short-term exposure to beryllium oxide.]

The effect of beryllium sulfate (1-h exposure by inhalation; 13 mg/m^3 Be; particle mass median aerodynamic diameter, 1.9 μm) on cell kinetics was studied in rats and mice by autoradiographic determination of the proportion of tritium-labelled cells 90 min after intraperitoneal administration of tritiated thymidine (Sendelbach et al., 1986). In rats, a strong proliferative response was seen, involving type II alveolar epithelial cells and interstitial and capillary endothelial cells. In mice, the proliferative response was weaker and was limited to alveolar macrophages and interstitial and endothelial cells.

Dietary administration of beryllium carbonate at 0.125-1% caused changes typical of rachitis in the skeleton of rats (Guyatt et al., 1933).

Exposure of female rats by nose-only inhalation to beryllium oxide aerosol (mass median aerodynamic diameter, 1.10 μm; calcined at approximately 1000 °C [dust concentration and length of exposure not given]), to give an initial alveolar deposition of 30 μg beryllium, decreased alveolar clearance of subsequently administered plutonium oxide by up to 40% (Sanders et al., 1975).

The concentration of beryllium sulfate required to decrease the viability of canine pulmonary alveolar macrophages in vitro by 50% was 0.11 mmol/L; the corresponding concentration for beryllium oxide calcined at 500 °C was 1.4 mmol/L, and that for beryllium oxide calcined at 1000 °C was 3.3 mmol/L. [Because of the limited solubility of beryllium sulfate in tissue culture media, it is not clear what proportion was truly in solution.] The solubility of the high-fired beryllium oxide in 100 ml 0.1 N hydrochloric acid was considerably lower than that of the low-fired compound. There was a similar tendency for differential solubility in simulated serum ultrafiltrate, which was not, however, significant (Finch et al., 1988). Similar results were obtained in a study of cultured rat tracheal epithelial cells (Steele et al., 1989).

Intravenous administration of beryllium sulfate at 30 μmol/kg bw to rats decreased the stimulation of thymidine incorporation into liver DNA after partial hepatectomy (Witschi, 1968); the decrease was accompanied by decreased activities of thymidine kinase, thymidylate kinase, thymidylate synthetase, deoxycytidylate deaminase and DNA polymerase (Witschi, 1970). No effect was observed on the incorporation of ^{14}C-orotic acid into RNA, the activity of RNA polymerase, incorporation of ^{14}C-leucine into histones or acetylation of histones (Marcotte & Witschi, 1972).

Addition of beryllium sulfate at 1-5 μmol/L increased ^{3}H-thymidine incorporation into splenic lymphocyte DNA by two to three fold (Price & Skilleter, 1985). This weak mitogenic effect was limited to B lymphocytes (Newman & Campbell, 1987). Beryllium sulfate, brought into solution as a sulfosalicylic acid complex, inhibited the growth of mouse fibroblasts in culture at concentrations higher than 10^{-5} mol/L (Rössner & Bencko, 1980).

Be^{2+} at a concentration of 0.1 mmol/L inhibited the proliferation of rat hepatocytes in culture induced by epidermal growth factor by 72%, but it did not affect the binding of growth factor to its receptors on the hepatocytes (Skilleter & Legg, 1989).

Beryllium fluoride complexes were bound to microtubules polymerized in the presence of glycerol from tubulin isolated from pig brain and stabilized the polymer formed (Carlier *et al.*, 1988, 1989). Divalent beryllium ($BeSO_4$), but not beryllium fluoride, stimulated microtubule-associated protein-dependent polymerization of tubulin purified from bovine brain and stabilized the polymer formed (Hamel *et al.*, 1991, 1992).

4.3 Reproductive and developmental effects

4.3.1 *Humans*

Kline *et al.* (1951) described the pregnancy of a 25-year-old woman who worked in a fluorescent-tube factory in 1942–44. She displayed signs of radiographic changes in lungs, cyanosis and dyspnoea in the seventh month of her second pregnancy in 1950. No beryllium was detected in a lung biopsy. The woman was treated with adrenocorticotrophic hormone and steroids and delivered a 2.75-kg child seven weeks later. Twenty-four-hour specimens of the urine of the infant collected on the second and third day after birth contained 0.4 and 0.015 µg Be. The child became severely hypoglycaemic after 48 h but was subsequently released from hospital.

Savitz *et al.* (1989) examined a subset of people covered by the 1980 US National Natality and Fetal Mortality Surveys for indications of adverse effects related to maternal or paternal occupational exposures to beryllium, as assessed from a job–exposure matrix. Paternal occupational exposure was associated with 3170 stillbirths, 552 preterm deliveries and 371 babies small for gestational age; the corresponding odds ratios (with 95% CI) were: 1.0 (0.7–1.3), 1.0 (0.5–2.0) and 0.9 (0.5–1.7), respectively. Maternal exposure to beryllium was not associated with these end-points.

4.3.2 *Experimental systems*

The effects of beryllium compounds on reproduction and prenatal development have been reviewed (Barlow & Sullivan, 1982). After oral exposure of male and female rats to a single intratracheal dose of 0.2 mg beryllium oxide (fired at 960 °C in one study and 500 °C in a second), no effect was noted in repeated breeding trials on fertility, postnatal viability or growth over 15 months. In fact, beryllium-treated rats tended to produce more litters over time than did controls (Clary *et al.*, 1975).

All offspring of Sprague–Dawley rats exposed intravenously to 0.316 mg/kg bw beryllium nitrate (one-tenth of the reported LD_{50}) on gestation day 1 died within two to three days after birth. Exposure to beryllium on day 11, but not on day 12, 13, 15 or 17 of gestation, resulted in death *in utero*; all pups in the other groups died within two to three days of delivery (Mathur *et al.*, 1987). [The Working Group noted the potential confounding effect of anaesthesia and surgery in the experimental design.]

4.4 Genetic and related effects

4.4.1 *Humans*

No data were available to the Working Group.

4.4.2 *Experimental systems* (see also Table 19 and Appendices 1 and 2)

(a) *Beryllium salts*

Beryllium sulfate was mutagenic to *Bacillus subtilis* in the *rec* assay, but no effect was seen using a higher dose of beryllium chloride. [The latter was actually a null effect, as no zone of inhibition was seen.] Both beryllium chloride and beryllium nitrate were mutagenic in a *rec* assay using spores of *B. subtilis*.

A null effect was also seen with beryllium sulfate in *Escherichia coli* in the pol^+/pol^- assay for DNA modifying effects. In a spot test using four strains of *E. coli* with different repair capacities, beryllium sulfate caused zones of inhibition of growth only in repair-deficient strains. The inhibition decreased with increasing pH, with little effect above pH 5–6. The authors suggested that beryllium interferes with use of exogenous orthophosphate rather than with DNA repair.

Beryllium chloride did not induce SOS repair, measured as λ prophage induction; no inhibition of growth was seen with continuous exposure to up to 5 mM, however, suggesting lack of uptake.

Beryllium sulfate was inactive in most bacterial mutagenesis assays. It did not induce point mutations in *Salmonella typhimurium* in the absence of metabolic activation in four laboratories. Negative results were found in the presence of various metabolizing systems, except in strain TA1535, in which equivocal results were obtained in the presence of some Aroclor-induced liver enzymes; however, no toxicity was seen, even at doses up to 5 mg/plate. Beryllium chloride and beryllium nitrate at similarly high doses were not mutagenic to *S. typhimurium*. Beryllium sulfate was not mutagenic to *S. typhimurium* in a plate incorporation assay, but it gave positive results in single fluctuation tests with *E. coli* and with one strain of *S. typhimurium*. Beryllium chloride induced a modest increase in the number of mutations in the *lac*I gene when grown with *E. coli*, but no clear dose–response relationship. It did not enhance the mutagenicity of ultraviolet radiation to *E. coli*, but it enhanced the mutagenicity of 9-aminoacridine to *S. typhimurium*.

Beryllium sulfate was not mutagenic when injected intraperitoneally to adult male Swiss–Webster mice in a host-mediated assay using *S. typhimurium* strains. It did not induce mitotic recombination in *Saccharomyces cerevisiae* D3 in the presence or absence of metabolic activation, and did not induce mutation in a host-mediated assay using the same strain.

Beryllium sulfate tetrahydrate did not induce unscheduled DNA synthesis in primary hepatocytes, as measured by autoradiographic light nuclear labelling; however, a dose of 10 mg/ml was reported to be toxic.

In the only study available, beryllium chloride was reported to increase the frequency of 8-azaguanine-resistant mutants in Chinese hamster V79 cells by a factor of about 6.

Beryllium chloride and beryllium nitrate induced sister chromatid exchange in the same cells. Beryllium sulfate also increased the frequency of sister chromatid exchange in cultured human lymphocytes and in Syrian hamster embryo cells. Studies on the ability of beryllium salts to induce chromosomal aberrations *in vitro* have had mixed results. Beryllium sulfate increased the frequency of chromatid aberrations in human lymphocytes in one of two studies, and a 21-fold increase was seen in the same study with Syrian hamster embryo cells. Higher doses of beryllium sulfate were nonclastogenic to Chinese hamster lung cells; however, toxicity was seen only at 2.5 mg/ml. It had little effect on chromosomes in Chinese hamster ovary cells, but fairly high concentrations enhanced the frequency of X-ray-induced chromatid-type exchanges. Extremely high concentrations of beryllium chloride caused chromosomal 'stickiness' in cultured peripheral lymphocytes of domestic pigs; chromosomal breakage was rare, whereas chromatid breaks were frequent.

Beryllium sulfate induced morphological transformation of Syrian hamster embryo cells and enhanced the transformation of the cells by simian adenovirus SA7 [no dose–response given]. In a comparative evaluation of in-vitro transformation systems, beryllium sulfate induced morphological transformation in BALB/3T3 cells, in Syrian hamster embryo cells and in Rauscher murine leukaemia virus-infected Fischer 344 rat embryo cells. [In none of the studies were transformed cells injected into suitable hosts to verify the occurrence of malignant transformation.]

In the only report of exposure *in vivo*, beryllium sulfate given by gavage at 50 and 80% of the four-day maximal tolerated dose did not induce micronuclei in the bone marrow of mice. A marked depression of bone-marrow erythropoiesis was observed, suggesting a toxic effect to the marrow.

(b) *Beryllium oxide*

This sparingly soluble compound did not induce differential toxicity in *B. subtilis*, mutation in two strains of *S. typhimurium* or sister chromatid exchange in Chinese hamster V79 cells.

Both single-strand breaks and morphological cell transformation were reported to be induced by low-fired beryllium oxide, but conflicting results were obtained for both end-points with high-fired beryllium oxide. [The data were not particularly convincing.]

Considerations with regard to genotoxic mechanisms

As pointed out in a review, beryllium is uniquely amphoteric among the alkaline earth elements. It can form positive and negative ions in acidic and basic media but not at neutrality, at which it forms poorly soluble particulates. Beryllium salts are readily precipitated in the tissues and are transported in blood predominantly as colloidal phosphate–hydroxide complexes weakly associated with plasma globulins; these may be taken up by macrophages. Cultured cells essentially accumulate only colloidal or particulate beryllium, by a temperature-dependent process deduced to be endocytosis. Macrophages, the cells most active in the endocytosis of particulate materials, appear to be those most sensitive to the cytotoxicity of beryllium (reviewed by Skilleter, 1984). Beryllium was toxic to mammalian cells only at concentrations at which a precipitate was seen in the culture

Table 19. Genetic and related effects of beryllium compounds

Test system	Result		Dose[a] (LED/HID)	Reference
	Without exogenous metabolic system	With exogenous metabolic system		
Beryllium chloride				
PRB, λ Prophage induction, *Escherichia coli*	–[b]	0	45	Rossman *et al.* (1984)
BSD, *Bacillus subtilis* rec assay, differential toxicity	–	0	22.5	Nishioka (1975)
BSD, *Bacillus subtilis* (spores) rec assay, differential toxicity	+	0	84	Kuroda *et al.* (1991)
SA0, *Salmonella typhimurium* TA100, reverse mutation	–	0	NR	Ogawa *et al.* (1987)
SA0, *Salmonella typhimurium* TA100, reverse mutation	–	–	280	Kuroda *et al.* (1991)
SA2, *Salmonella typhimurium* TA102, reverse mutation	–	0	NR	Ogawa *et al.* (1987)
SA7, *Salmonella typhimurium* TA1537, reverse mutation	–	0	NR	Ogawa *et al.* (1987)
SA7, *Salmonella typhimurium* TA1537, reverse mutation	+[c]	0	450	Ogawa *et al.* (1987)
SA9, *Salmonella typhimurium* TA98, reverse mutation	–	0	NR	Kuroda *et al.* (1991)
SA9, *Salmonella typhimurium* TA98, reverse mutation	–	–	280	Ogawa *et al.* (1987)
SAS, *Salmonella typhimurium* TA2637, reverse mutation	–	0	NR	Ogawa *et al.* (1987)
SAS, *Salmonella typhimurium* TA2637, reverse mutation	+[c]	0	450	Ogawa *et al.* (1987)
ECK, *Escherichia coli* KMBL 3835 (*lacI* gene), forward mutation	+	0	0.09	Zakour & Glickman (1984)
EC2, *Escherichia coli* WP2, reverse mutation	–[d]	0	18	Rossman & Molina (1986)
G9H, Gene mutation, Chinese hamster lung V79 cells, *hprt* locus, *in vitro*	+	0	18	Miyaki *et al.* (1979)
SIC, Sister chromatid exchange, Chinese hamster lung V79 cells, *in vitro*	+	0	3.5	Kuroda *et al.* (1991)
CIA, Chromosomal aberrations, swine lymphocytes, *in vitro*	+	0	1.8	Vegni Talluri & Guiggiani (1967)
Beryllium nitrate				
BSD, *Bacillus subtilis* (spores) rec assay, differential toxicity	+	0	51	Kuroda *et al.* (1991)
SA0, *Salmonella typhimurium* TA100, reverse mutation (spot test)	–	0	900	Tso & Fung (1981)
SA0, *Salmonella typhimurium* TA100, reverse mutation	–	–	170	Kuroda *et al.* (1991)

Table 19 (contd)

Test system	Result Without exogenous metabolic system	Result With exogenous metabolic system	Dose[a] (LED/HID)	Reference
Beryllium nitrate (contd)				
SA9, *Salmonella typhimurium* TA98, reverse mutation	?	0	NR	Arlauskas *et al.* (1985)
SA9, *Salmonella typhimurium* TA98, reverse mutation	–	–	170	Kuroda *et al.* (1991)
SIC, Sister chromatid exchange, Chinese hamster lung V79 cells, *in vitro*	+	0	2.0	Kuroda *et al.* (1991)
Beryllium sulfate				
ECD, *Escherichia coli pol* A, differential toxicity (spot test)	–	0	28	Rosenkranz & Poirier (1979)
BSD, *Bacillus subtilis rec* assay, differential toxicity	+	0	90	Kada *et al.* (1980); Kanematsu *et al.* (1980)
ERD, *Escherichia coli rec* strains, differential toxicity	+	0	2.25	Dylevoi (1990)
SA0, *Salmonella typhimurium* TA100, reverse mutation	–	–	6	Simmon (1979a)
SA0, *Salmonella typhimurium* TA100, reverse mutation	–	–	14	Dunkel *et al.* (1984)[e]
SA0, *Salmonella typhimurium* TA100, reverse mutation	–	0	NR	Arlauskas *et al.* (1985)
***Salmonella typhimurium* TA100, reverse mutation (fluctuation)	+	0	4.5	Arlauskas *et al.* (1985)
SA0, *Salmonella typhimurium* TA100, reverse mutation	–	–	127	Ashby *et al.* (1990)
SA5, *Salmonella typhimurium* TA1535, reverse mutation	–	–	10	Rosenkranz & Poirier (1979)
SA5, *Salmonella typhimurium* TA1535, reverse mutation	–	–	6	Simmon (1979a)
SA5, *Salmonella typhimurium* TA1535, reverse mutation	–	?[f]	0.9	Dunkel *et al.* (1984)[e]
SA5, *Salmonella typhimurium* TA1535, reverse mutation	–	0	NR	Arlauskas *et al.* (1985)
SA5, *Salmonella typhimurium* TA1535, reverse mutation	–	–	127	Ashby *et al.* (1990)
SA7, *Salmonella typhimurium* TA1537, reverse mutation	–	–	6	Simmon (1979a)
SA7, *Salmonella typhimurium* TA1537, reverse mutation	–	–	14	Dunkel *et al.* (1984)[e]
SA7, *Salmonella typhimurium* TA1537, reverse mutation	–	0	NR	Arlauskas *et al.* (1985)
SA7, *Salmonella typhimurium* TA1537, reverse mutation	–	–	127	Ashby *et al.* (1990)
SA8, *Salmonella typhimurium* TA1538, reverse mutation	–	–	10	Rosenkranz & Poirier (1979)
SA8, *Salmonella typhimurium* TA1538, reverse mutation	–	–	6	Simmon (1979a)

Table 19 (contd)

Test system	Result		Dose[a] (LED/HID)	Reference
	Without exogenous metabolic system	With exogenous metabolic system		
Beryllium sulfate (contd)				
SA8, *Salmonella typhimurium* TA1538, reverse mutation	–		14	Dunkel *et al.* (1984)[c]
SA8, *Salmonella typhimurium* TA1538, reverse mutation	–	0	NR	Arlauskas *et al.* (1985)
SA8, *Salmonella typhimurium* TA1538, reverse mutation	–	–	127	Ashby *et al.* (1990)
SA8, *Salmonella typhimurium* TA1538, reverse mutation	–		6	Simmon (1979a)
SA9, *Salmonella typhimurium* TA98, reverse mutation	–		14	Dunkel *et al.* (1984)[c]
SA9, *Salmonella typhimurium* TA98, reverse mutation	–	0	NR	Arlauskas *et al.* (1985)
SA9, *Salmonella typhimurium* TA98, reverse mutation	–	–	127	Ashby *et al.* (1990)
SA9, *Salmonella typhimurium* TA98, reverse mutation	–		6	Simmon (1979a)
SAS, *Salmonella typhimurium* TA1536, reverse mutation	–		14	Dunkel *et al.* (1984)[c]
ECW, *Escherichia coli* WP2 *uvr*A, reverse mutation	?	0	NR	Arlauskas *et al.* (1985)
***, *Escherichia coli* WP2 *uvr*A, reverse mutation (fluctuation test)				
SCH, *Saccharomyces cerevisiae* D3, mitotic recombination	–		430	Simmon (1979b)
URP, Unscheduled DNA synthesis, primary rat hepatocytes		0	86	Williams *et al.* (1982)
SIS, Sister chromatid exchange, Syrian hamster embryo cells *in vitro*	+	0	0.05	Larramendy *et al.* (1981)
CIC, Chromosomal aberrations, Chinese golden hamster ovary cells *in vitro*	–	0	9	Brooks *et al.* (1989)
CIC, Chromosomal aberrations, Chinese hamster ovary cells *in vitro*	+[g]	0	9	Brooks *et al.* (1989)
CIC, Chromosomal aberrations, Chinese hamster lung cells *in vitro*	–		64	Ashby *et al.* (1990)
CIS, Chromosomal aberrations, Syrian hamster embryo cells *in vitro*	+	0	0.25	Larramendy *et al.* (1981)
TBM, Cell transformation, BALB/c 3T3 mouse cells *in vitro*	+	0	0.05	Dunkel *et al.* (1981)
TCS, Cell transformation, Syrian golden hamster embryo cells *in vitro*	+	0	0.016	Pienta *et al.* (1977)
TCS, Cell transformation, Syrian hamster embryo cells *in vitro*	+	0	0.13	DiPaolo & Casto (1979)

Table 19 (contd)

Test system	Result		Dose[a] (LED/HID)	Reference
	Without exogenous metabolic system	With exogenous metabolic system		
Beryllium sulfate (contd)				
TRR, Cell transformation, RLV/Fischer rat embryo cells in vitro	+	0	0.005	Dunkel et al. (1981)
T7S, Cell transformation SA7/Syrian hamster embryo cells in vitro	+	0	5	Casto et al. (1979)
SHL, Sister chromatid exchange, human lymphocytes in vitro	+	0	0.05	Larramendy et al. (1981)
CHF, Chromosomal aberrations, human MRC5 fibroblasts in vitro	–	0	0.005	Paton & Allison (1972)
CHL, Chromosomal aberrations, human lymphocytes in vitro	+	0	0.25	Larramendy et al. (1981)
CHL, Chromosomal aberrations, human WI38 lymphocytes in vitro	–	0	0.009	Paton & Allison (1972)
HMM, Host-mediated assay, Salmonella typhimurium TA1530 in male Swiss–Webster mice	–		1.25, im or po	Simmon et al. (1979)
HMM, Host-mediated assay, Salmonella typhimurium TA1535 in male Swiss–Webster mice	–		103, im or po	Simmon et al. (1979)
HMM, Host-mediated assay, Salmonella typhimurium TA1538 in male Swiss–Webster mice	–		1.25, im or po	Simmon et al. (1979)
HMM, Host-mediated assay, Saccharomyces cerevisiae in mice	–		103, im or po	Simmon et al. (1979)
MVM, Micronucleus test, mouse bone marrow in vivo	–		116, po × 1	Ashby et al. (1990)
Beryllium oxide				
BSD, Bacillus subtilis (spores) rec assay, differential toxicity	–[h]	0	0.1	Kuroda et al. (1991)
SA0, Salmonella typhimurium TA100, reverse mutation	–[h]	–	0.08	Kuroda et al. (1991)
SA9, Salmonella typhimurium TA98, reverse mutation	–[h]	–	0.08	Kuroda et al. (1991)
DIA, DNA strand breaks, rat tracheal epithelial cells	+[i]	0	0.36	Steele et al. (1989)
DIA, DNA strand breaks, rat tracheal epithelial cells	?[j]	0	10	Steele et al. (1989)

Table 19 (contd)

Test system	Result		Dose[a] (LED/HID)	Reference
	Without exogenous metabolic system	With exogenous metabolic system		
Beryllium oxide (contd)				
SIC, Sister chromatid exchange, Chinese hamster V79 lung cells *in vitro*	−[g]	0	0.03	Kuroda *et al.* (1991)
TCL, Cell transformation, rat tracheal epithelial cells *in vitro*	+[i]	0	0.1	Steele *et al.* (1989)
TCL, Cell transformation, rat tracheal epithelial cells *in vitro*	?[j]	0	10	Steele *et al.* (1989)

+, considered to be positive; (+), considered to be weakly positive in an inadequate study; −, considered to be negative; ?, considered to be inconclusive (variable responses in several experiments within an adequate study); 0, not tested

[a]LED, lowest effective dose; HID, highest ineffective dose. In-vitro tests, μg/ml; in-vivo tests, mg/kg bw. Doses given as concentration of element, not concentration of compound; im, intramuscularly; po, orally; NR, not reported

[b]Precipitate

[c]Comutation with 9-aminoacridine (100 μmol/plate) (not on profile)

[d]Comutation with ultraviolet radiation (not on profile)

[e]Results from four independent laboratories

[f]Negative in two laboratories, inconsistently positive in two laboratories

[g]Enhancement of effect of X irradiation (not on profile)

[h]BeO unspecified

[i]Low-fired oxide

[j]High-fired oxide

***Not displayed on profiles

medium (Rossman *et al.*, 1987). [The Working Group noted that the lack of toxicity of beryllium compounds in many studies of bacteria suggests lack of uptake.] In mammalian cells, intracellular transfer is from lysozyme to nucleus (reviewed by Skilleter, 1984).

Beryllium chloride (1–10 mM) increased misincorporation of nucleoside triphosphates during polymerization of poly-d(A–T) by *Micrococcus luteus* DNA polymerase (Luke *et al.*, 1975). In a similar system, beryllium chloride reduced the fidelity of DNA synthesis *in vitro* in the presence of avian myeloblastosis virus DNA polymerase, a synthetic prime template and complementary and noncomplementary nucleoside triphosphates. This effect was observed at concentrations at which even incorporation of complementary triphosphates was inhibited and was ascribed to the noncovalent binding of ionic divalent beryllium to DNA polymerase rather than to DNA (Sirover & Loeb, 1976). [It is not clear that such effects can occur within the cell, where the concentrations of Be^{2+} would probably be much lower; e.g. chromosomal aberrations have been reported at an extracellular concentration of $< 5 \mu M$.] The binding of beryllium by purified DNA is very weak ($K_a = 7 \times 10^3$/mol) (Truhaut *et al.*, 1968). It was reported in an abstract that beryllium can induce DNA–protein complexes (Kubinski *et al.*, 1977). [The Working Group considered that any 'genotoxic' effects of Be^{2+} are probably not caused by direct damage to DNA.]

5. Summary of Data Reported and Evaluation

5.1 Exposure data

Beryllium is found at low concentrations in the Earth's crust. Since the early twentieth century, it has been produced and used in a variety of applications as the metal, in alloys and as its oxide.

Although only a relatively small number of workers worldwide are potentially exposed to high levels of beryllium, mainly in the refining and machining of the metal and in production of beryllium-containing products, a growing number of workers are potentially exposed to lower levels of beryllium in the aircraft, aerospace, electronics and nuclear industries. Although the range of industrial processes with potential occupational exposure to beryllium has expanded over the past two decades, exposures have generally decreased over the same period.

The most important source of exposure to beryllium in the general environment is the burning of coal.

5.2 Human carcinogenicity data

In an early series of cohort mortality studies of workers at two beryllium extraction, production and fabrication facilities in the USA, a consistent, marginally significant excess of deaths from lung cancer was observed. The excess increased with time since first exposure. In a more recent mortality analysis of some 9000 workers at seven beryllium plants in the USA, including the two plants studied previously, a small but significant excess in mortality from lung cancer was found in the total cohort. The risks for lung cancer were consistently higher in those plants in which there was also excess mortality from nonmalignant respiratory disease. Also, the risk for lung cancer increased with time since first exposure and was greater in workers first hired in the period when exposures to beryllium in the work place were relatively uncontrolled. Mortality from cancers at other sites was not increased. The association between lung cancer risk and exposure to beryllium was judged not to be confounded by smoking.

Follow-up of deaths among workers entered into the US Beryllium Case Registry (which registered cases of acute beryllium-related pneumonitis and chronic beryllium-related nonmalignant lung disease, including cases from the plants mentioned above) revealed excess mortality from lung cancer; the excess was greater in those who were entered into the Registry with acute beryllium pneumonitis. Potential confounding by smoking was addressed in several ways and did not appear to explain the increased risk for lung cancer. The results of the follow-up of the Case Registry subjects yielded a higher risk for lung cancer than had been found in the previous cohort mortality study of the seven production facilities.

In a nested case–control study of cancers of the central nervous system among workers at two nuclear facilities in the USA, an increasing risk of cancer of the central nervous system was suggested with longer duration of employment in jobs with more highly ranked exposure to beryllium.

Several aspects of the two most recent cohort studies support the conclusion that the work environment of workers involved in refining, machining and producing beryllium metal and alloys was causally associated with an increased risk of lung cancer: the large number of lung cancer cases, providing a stable estimate of the mortality ratio; the consistency of the lung cancer excess in most of the locations; the greater excess in workers hired before 1950, when exposures to beryllium in the work place were relatively uncontrolled and much higher than in subsequent decades; the highest risk for lung cancer being found in the plant from which the greatest proportion of cases of acute beryllium pneumonitis was provided to the Beryllium Case Registry; the increasing risks with increasing latency; the greater lung cancer risk observed in the Beryllium Case Registry cohort, the highest risk for lung cancer being observed among individuals diagnosed with acute beryllium-induced pneumonitis, who represent a group that had the most intense exposure to beryllium; and the highest risks for lung cancer occurring in the plants where the risk for pneumoconiosis and other respiratory diseases was highest. Aspects of the studies which limit their interpretation are: the absence of any individual measurements of exposures to beryllium, the relatively low excess risk for lung cancer and the absence of any mention of exposure of workers to other lung carcinogens in the work place, although there is no evidence that other lung carcinogens were present.

5.3 Animal carcinogenicity data

Beryl ore and bertrandite ore were tested for carcinogenicity in rats, hamsters and monkeys by inhalation exposure in three experiments in one study. Beryl ore was shown to produce malignant and benign lung tumours in rats. The experiments in hamsters and monkeys were inadequate for evaluation, as were all experiments with bertrandite ore.

In one study in rats by single intratracheal instillation, beryllium metal, passivated beryllium metal (99% beryllium, 0.26% chromium as chromate) and beryllium–aluminium alloy (62% beryllium) produced dose-related increases in the incidence of lung tumours, which were mostly adenocarcinomas and adenomas.

Various beryllium compounds were tested by inhalation in five studies in rats, rabbits and monkeys. In two studies in rats, beryllium sulfate tetrahydrate produced lung tumours, which were mostly adenocarcinomas. In one study, both beryllium oxide and beryllium chloride produced dose-related increases in the incidence of malignant epithelial lung tumours in rats. The studies in rabbits and monkeys were considered to be inadequate for evaluation. Beryllium hydroxide and low- and high-temperature-fired beryllium oxide were tested in rats by intratracheal instillation; beryllium hydroxide produced lung adenocarcinomas and adenomas in one study, and low-temperature-fired (below 900 °C) beryllium oxide produced malignant lung tumours in two studies.

Rabbits given intravenous injections of beryllium metal and various compounds of beryllium (zinc beryllium silicate, beryllium silicate, beryllium oxide and beryllium phosphate) developed osteosarcomas. Similar findings were obtained in rabbits treated by implantation or injection into the bone of beryllium oxide, zinc beryllium silicate and beryllium carbonate.

5.4 Other relevant data

Increased levels of beryllium have been found in the lungs of people exposed up to 20 years previously. In dogs and rats, the lung clearance of beryllium oxide calcined at high temperatures is slower than for that calcined at low temperatures. After inhalation, beryllium also accumulates in tracheobronchial lymph nodes. Gastrointestinal absorption of beryllium and beryllium compounds is very limited. Beryllium accumulates in bone and, to a lesser extent, in the liver. Absorbed beryllium is excreted mostly in the urine.

Beryllium may cause a fatal acute pneumonitis and, after long-term exposure, a chronic, non-caseating granulomatous pulmonary disease with a high rate of fatality; the pathogenesis of the latter disease involves cell-mediated immunological reactions. Susceptibility to chronic beryllium disease varies between individuals, and the disease may develop after low environmental exposures in some people. A similar disease is seen in exposed dogs, guinea-pigs and sensitized rats. Beryllium causes contact dermatitis, which is also associated with cell-mediated immunological reactions.

Beryllium sulfate did not induce micronuclei in the bone marrow of mice treated *in vivo*. Beryllium salts induced sister chromatid exchange and possibly chromosomal aberrations in mammalian cells *in vitro*. Beryllium sulfate induced morphological transformation in a number of different systems. In one report, beryllium chloride induced gene mutation in mammalian cells. In bacteria, beryllium chloride was comutagenic with 9-aminoacridine but not with ultraviolet radiation. Beryllium compounds are not mutagenic in most bacterial systems. In assays of differential toxicity, beryllium salts gave mixed results.

In cultured mammalian cells, low-temperature-fired beryllium oxide induced single-strand breaks in DNA and morphological transformation; an unspecified beryllium oxide did not induce sister chromatid exchange in mammalian cells or differential toxicity or mutation in bacteria.

5.5 Evaluation[1]

There is *sufficient evidence* in humans for the carcinogenicity of beryllium and beryllium compounds.

There is *sufficient evidence* in experimental animals for the carcinogenicity of beryllium and beryllium compounds.

Overall evaluation

Beryllium and beryllium compounds *are carcinogenic to humans (Group 1)*.

6. References

Agency for Toxic Substances and Disease Registry (1988) *Toxicological Profile for Beryllium* (ATSDR/TP-88/07; US NTIS PB89-148233), Atlanta, GA, US Public Health Service

Aldrich Chemical Co. (1992) *Aldrich Catalog/Handbook of Fine Chemicals 1992–1993*, Milwaukee, WI, pp. 142–143

Aldridge, W.N., Barnes, J.M. & Denz, F.A. (1950) Biochemical changes in acute beryllium poisoning. *Br. J. exp. Pathol.*, **31**, 473–484

Alfa Products (1990) *Alfa Catalog—Research Chemicals and Accessories*, Ward Hill, MA, pp. 56, 460

American Conference of Governmental Industrial Hygienists (1992) *1992–1993 Threshold Limit Values for Chemical Substances and Physical Agents and Biological Exposure Indices*, Cincinnati, OH, p. 13

Angerer, J. & Schaller, K.H., eds (1985) *Analysis of Hazardous Substances in Biological Materials*, Vol. 1, Weinheim, VCH Verlagsgesellschaft, pp. 57–65

Anon. (1992) Occupational exposure limits. *BIBRA Bull.*, **31**, 287

Apostoli, P., Porru, S. & Alessio, L. (1989a) Behaviour of urinary beryllium in general population and in subjects with low-level occupational exposure. *Med. Lav.*, **80**, 390–396

Apostoli, P., Porru, S., Minoia, C. & Alessio, L. (1989b) Beryllium. In: Alessio, L., Berlin, A., Boni, M. & Roi, R., eds, *Biological Indicators for the Assessment of Human Exposure to Industrial Chemicals* (EUR 12174 EN), Luxembourg, Commission of the European Communities, pp. 3–21

Araki, M., Okada, S. & Fujita, M. (1954) Beryllium. Experimental studies on beryllium-induced malignant tumours of rabbits (Jpn.). *Gann*, **45**, 449–451

Arbeidsinspectie [Labour Inspection] (1986) *De Nationale MAC-Lijst 1986* [National MAC List 1986], Voorburg, p. 8

Arbejdstilsynet [Labour Inspection] (1992) *Graensevaerdier for Stoffer og Materialer* [Limit Values for Compounds and Materials] (No. 3.1.0.2), Copenhagen, p. 52

Arbetarskyddsstyrelsens [National Board of Occupational Safety and Health] (1991) *Hygieniska Gränsvärden* [Hygienic Limit Values], Stockholm, p. 14

Arlauskas, A., Baker, R.S.U., Bonin, A.M., Tandon, R.K., Crisp, P.T. & Ellis, J. (1985) Mutagenicity of metal ions in bacteria. *Environ. Res.*, **36**, 379–388

---

[1]For definition of the italicized terms, see Preamble, pp. 26–30.

Asami, T. & Fukazawa, F. (1985) Beryllium contents of uncontaminated soil and sediments in Japan. *Soil Sci. Plant Nutr.*, **31**, 43–53

Ashby, J., Ishidate, M., Jr, Stoner, G.D., Morgan, M.A., Ratpan, F. & Callander, R.D. (1990) Studies on the genotoxicity of beryllium sulphate *in vitro* and *in vivo*. *Mutat. Res.*, **240**, 217–225

Atomergic Chemetals Corp. (undated) *High Purity Metals Brochure*, Farmingdale, NY

Ballance, J., Stonehouse, A.J., Sweeney, R. & Walsh, K. (1978) Beryllium and beryllium alloys. In: Mark, H.F., Othmer, D.F., Overberger, C.G., Seaborg, G.T. & Grayson, N., eds, *Kirk-Othmer Encyclopedia of Chemical Technology*, 3rd ed., Vol. 3, New York, John Wiley & Sons, pp. 803–823

Barlow, S. & Sullivan, F. (1982) *Reproductive Hazards of Industrial Chemicals. An Evaluation of Animal and Human Data*, London, Academic Press, pp. 119–125

Barna, B.P., Chiang, T., Pillarisetti, S.G. & Deodhar, S.D. (1981) Immunologic studies of experimental beryllium lung disease in the guinea pig. *Clin. Immunol. Immunopathol.*, **20**, 402–411

Barna, B.P., Deodhar, S.D., Chiang, T., Gautam, S. & Edinger, M. (1984) Experimental beryllium-induced lung disease. I. Differences in immunologic responses to beryllium compounds in strains 2 and 13 guinea pigs. *Int. Arch. Allergy appl. Immunol.*, **73**, 42–48

Barnes, J.M. (1950) Experimental production of malignant tumours by beryllium (Letter to the Editor). *Lancet*, **i**, 463

Barnes, J.M., Denz, F.A. & Sissons, H.A. (1950) Beryllium bone sarcomata in rabbits. *Br. J. Cancer*, **4**, 212–222

Baumgardt, B., Jackwerth, E., Otto, H. & Tölg, G. (1986) Trace analysis to determine heavy metal load in lung tissue. A contribution to substantiation of occupational hazards. *Int. Arch. occup. environ. Health*, **58**, 27–34

Bencko, V., Brezina, M., Benes, B. & Cikrt, M. (1979) Penetration of beryllium through the placenta and its distribution in the mouse. *J. Hyg. Epidemiol. Microbiol. Immunol.*, **23**, 361–367

Bencko, V., Vasil'eva, E.V. & Symon, K. (1980) Immunological aspects of exposure to emissions from burning coal of high beryllium content. *Environ. Res.*, **22**, 439–449

Berry, J.-P., Escaig, F. & Galle, P. (1987) Study of intracellular localization of beryllium by analytical ionic microscopy (Fr.). *C.R. Acad. Sci. Paris*, **304** (Sér. III), 239–243

Berry, J.-P., Mentre, P., Hallegot, P., Levi-Setti, R. & Galle, P. (1989) Cytochemical study of abnormal intranuclear structures rich in beryllium. *Biol. Cell*, **67**, 147–157

Boiana, J.M. (1980) *Technical Assistance Report: Walter Reed Army Medical Center, Washington, DC* (NIOSH Report No. TA-80-60-756), Cincinnati, OH, National Institute for Occupational Safety and Health

Bowen, H.J.M. (1966) *Trace Elements in Biochemistry*, London, Academic Press, pp. 150–176

Breslin, A.J. & Harris, W.B. (1959) Health protection in beryllium facilities. Summary of ten years of experience. *Arch. ind. Health*, **19**, 596–648

Brooks, A.L., Griffith, W.C., Johnson, N.F., Finch, G.L. & Cuddihy, R.G. (1989) The induction of chromosome damage in CHO cells by beryllium and radiation given alone and in combination. *Radiat. Res.*, **120**, 494–507

Brush Wellman (1992) *Material Safety Data Sheet—No. A111: AlBeMet*^{TM}, Cleveland, OH

Brush Wellman (undated) *BeO*, Cleveland, OH

Budavari, S. (1989) *The Merck Index*, 4th ed., Rahway, NJ, Merck & Co., pp. 181–183

Bussy, A.A.B. (1828) Pharmacy section: glucinium (Fr.). *J. Chim. méd. Pharm. Toxicol.*, **4**, 453–456

Carlier, M.-F., Didry, D., Melki, R., Chabre, M. & Pantaloni, D. (1988) Stabilization of microtubules by inorganic phosphate and its structural analogues, the fluoride complexes of aluminum and beryllium. *Biochemistry*, **27**, 3555–3559

Carlier, M.-F., Didry, D., Simon, C. & Pantaloni, D. (1989) Mechanism of GTP hydrolysis in tubulin polymerization: characterization of the kinetic intermediate microtubule-GDP-P_i using phosphate analogues. *Biochemistry*, **28**, 1783–1791

Caroli, S., Coni, E., Alimonti, A., Beccaloni, E., Sabbioni, E. & Pietra, R. (1988) Determination of trace elements in human lungs by ICP-AES (inductivity coupled plasma–atomic emission spectrometry) and NAA (neutron activation analysis). *Analysis*, **16**, 75–80

Carpenter, A.V., Flanders, W.D., Frome, E.L., Tankersley, W.G. & Fry, S.A. (1988) Chemical exposures and central nervous system cancers: a case–control study among workers at two nuclear facilities. *Am. J. ind. Med.*, **13**, 351–362

Casto, B.C., Meyers, J. & DiPaolo, J.A. (1979) Enhancement of viral transformation for evaluation of the carcinogenic or mutagenic potential of inorganic metal salts. *Cancer Res.*, **39**, 193–198

CERAC, Inc. (1991) *Advanced Specialty Inorganics*, Milwaukee, WI, pp. 71–72

Cherniack, M.G. & Kominsky, J.R. (1984) *Health Hazard Evaluation Report. Chemetco Incorporated, Alton, Illinois* (NIOSH Report No. 82-024-1428), Cincinatti, OH, National Institute for Occupational Safety and Health

Cholak, J., Schafer, L. & Yeager, D. (1967) Exposures to beryllium in a beryllium alloying plant. *Am. ind. Hyg. Assoc. J.*, **28**, 399–407

Clary, J.J., Bland, L.S. & Stokinger, H.E. (1975) The effect of reproduction and lactation on the onset of latent chronic beryllium disease. *Toxicol. appl. Pharmacol.*, **33**, 214–221

Cloudman, A.M., Vining, D., Barkulis, S. & Nickson, J.J. (1949) Bone changes observed following intravenous injections of beryllium (Abstract). *Am. J. Pathol.*, **25**, 810–811

Commission of the European Communities (1980) Council Directive of 17 December 1979 on the protection of groundwater against pollution caused by certain dangerous substances (80/68/EEC). *Off. J. Eur. Commun.*, **L20**, 43

Commission of the European Communities (1991a) Thirteenth Commission Directive of 12 March 1991 (91/814/EEC) on the approximation of the laws of the Member States relating to cosmetic products. *Off. J. Eur. Commun.*, **L91**, 59–62

Commission of the European Communities (1991b) Council Directive of 12 December 1991 on hazardous wastes (91/689/EEC). *Off. J. Eur. Commun.*, **L377**, 20

Commission of the European Communities (1991c) Amendment to the Council Directive 67/548/EEC of June 1967 on the approximation of the laws, regulations and administrative provisions relating to the classification, packaging and labelling of dangerous substances. *Off. J. Eur. Commun.*, **L180**, 79

Commission of the European Communities (1992) Fifteenth Commission Directive of 21 October 1992 (92/86/EEC) on the approximation of the laws of the Member States relating to cosmetic products. *Off. J. Eur. Commun.*, **L325**, 18–22

Cook, W.A. (1987) *Occupational Exposure Limits—Worldwide*, Akron, OH, American Industrial Hygiene Association, pp. 117, 129, 165

Crowley, J.F., Hamilton, J.G. & Scott, K.G. (1949) The metabolism of carrier-free radioberyllium in the rat. *J. biol. Chem.*, **177**, 975–984

Cullen, M.R., Cherniack, M.G. & Kominsky, J.R. (1986) Chronic beryllium disease in the United States. *Semin. respir. Med.*, **7**, 203–209

Cullen, M.R., Kominsky, J.R., Rossman, M.D., Cherniack, M.G., Rankin, J.A., Balmes, J.R., Kern, J.A., Daniele, R.P., Palmer, L., Naegel, G.P., McManus, K. & Cruz, R. (1987) Chronic beryllium disease in a precious metal refinery. Clinical epidemiologic and immunologic evidence for continuing risk from exposure to low level beryllium fume. *Am. Rev. respir. Dis.*, **135**, 201–208

Curtis, G.H. (1951) Cutaneous hypersensitivity due to beryllium. A study of thirteen cases. *Arch. Dermatol. Syphilol.*, **64**, 470–482

Dayan, A.D., Hertel, R.F., Heseltine, E., Kazantzis, G., Smith, E.M. & van der Venne, M.T., eds (1990) *Immunotoxicity of Metals and Immunotoxicology. Proceedings of an International Workshop*, New York, Plenum Press, p. 7

DeNardi, J.M., Van Ordstrand, H.S. & Curtis, G.H. (1952) Berylliosis. Summary and survey of all clinical types in ten year period. *Cleveland clin. Q.*, **19**, 171–193

Deodhar, S.D. & Barna, B.P. (1991) Immune mechanisms in beryllium lung disease. *Cleveland Clin. J. Med.*, **58**, 157–160

Deodhar, S.D., Barna, B. & Van Ordstrand, H.S. (1973) A study of the immunologic aspects of chronic berylliosis. *Chest*, **63**, 309–313

Deutsche Forschungsgemeinschaft (1992) *MAK- and BAT-Values 1992. Maximum Concentrations at the Workplace and Biological Tolerance Values for Working Materials* (Report No. 28), Weinheim, Verlagsgesellschaft, p. 21

D.F. Goldsmith Chemical & Metal Corp. (undated) *High Purity Elements; Fine Inorganic Chemicals; Precious Metals; Mercury*, Evanston, IL, p. 6

DiPaolo, J.A. & Casto, B.C. (1979) Quantitative studies of in vitro morphological transformation of Syrian hamster cells by inorganic metal salts. *Cancer Res.*, **39**, 1008–1013

Drury, J.S., Shriner, C.R., Lewis, E.G., Towill, L.E. & Hammons, A.S. (1978) *Reviews of the Environmental Effects of Pollutants: VI. Beryllium* (Report No. EPA-600/1-78-028), Cincinatti, OH, US Environmental Protection Agency

Dunkel, V.C., Pienta, R.J., Sivak, A. & Traul, K.A. (1981) Comparative neoplastic transformation responses of Balb/3T3 cells, Syrian hamster embryo cells, and Rauscher murine leukemia virus-infected Fischer 344 rat embryo cells to chemical carcinogens. *J. natl Cancer Inst.*, **67**, 1303–1315

Dunkel, V.C., Zeiger, E., Brusick, D., McCoy, E., McGregor, D., Mortelmans, K., Rosenkranz, H.S. & Simmon, V.F. (1984) Reproducibility of microbial mutagenicity assays: I. Tests with *Salmonella typhimurium* and *Escherichia coli* using a standardized protocol. *Environ. Mutag.*, **6** (Suppl. 2), 1–254

Dutra, F.R. & Largent, E.J. (1950) Osteosarcoma induced by beryllium oxide. *Am. J. Pathol.*, **26**, 197–209

Dutra, F.R., Largent, E.J. & Roth, J.L. (1951) Osteogenic sarcoma after inhalation of beryllium oxide. *Arch. Pathol.*, **51**, 473–479

Dvivedi, N. & Shen, G. (1983) Beryllium toxicity in the laboratory processing of dental alloy (Abstract No. 568). *J. dent. Res.*, **62**, 232

Dylevoi, M.V. (1990) Evaluation of the DNA-damaging action of the carcinogenic metal beryllium by means of bacterial repair test (Russ.). *Mikrobiol. Zh. (Kiev)*, **52**, 34–38

Eisenbud, M. (1984) Commentary and update: chemical pneumonia in workers extracting beryllium oxide. *Cleveland clin. Q.*, **51**, 441–447

Eisenbud, M. & Lisson, J. (1983) Epidemiological aspects of beryllium-induced nonmalignant lung disease: a 30-year update. *J. occup. Med.*, **25**, 196–202

Eller, P.M., ed. (1984) Method 7300. In: *NIOSH Manual of Analytical Methods*, 3rd Ed., Vol. 1 (DHHS (NIOSH) Publ. No. 84-100), Washington DC, US Government Printing Office, pp. 7300-1–7300-5

Eller, P.M., ed. (1987) Method 7102. In: *NIOSH Manual of Analytical Methods*, 3rd Ed., Suppl. 2 (DHHS (NIOSH) Publ. No. 84-100), Washington DC, US Government Printing Office, pp. 7102-1–7102-3

Epstein, P.E., Dauber, J.H., Rossman, M.D. & Daniele, R.P. (1982) Bronchoalveolar lavage in a patient with chronic berylliosis: evidence for hypersensitivity pneumonitis. *Ann. intern. Med.*, **97**, 213–216

Everest, D.A. (1973) Beryllium. In: Bailar, J.C., Jr, Emeléus, H.J., Nyholm, R. & Trotman-Dickenson, A.F., eds, *Comprehensive Inorganic Chemistry*, Vol. 1, Oxford, Pergamon Press, pp. 531–590

Feingold, L., Savitz, D.A. & John, E.M. (1992) Use of a job–exposure matrix to evaluate parental occupation and childhood cancer. *Cancer Causes Control*, **3**, 161–169

Feldman, I., Havill, J.R. & Neuman, W.F. (1953) The state of beryllium in blood plasma. *Arch. Biochem. Biophys.*, **46**, 443–453

Finch, G.L., Verburg, R.J., Mewhinney, J.A., Eidson, A.F. & Hoover, M.D. (1988) The effect of beryllium compound solubility on in vitro canine alveolar macrophage cytotoxicity. *Toxicol. Lett.*, **41**, 97–105

Finch, G.L., Mewhinney, J.A., Hoover, M.D., Eidson, A.F., Haley, P.J. & Bice, D.E. (1990) Clearance, translocation, and excretion of beryllium following acute inhalation of beryllium oxide by beagle dogs. *Fundam. appl. Toxicol.*, **15**, 231–241

Fluka Chemie AG (1993) *Fluka Chemika-BioChemika*, Buchs, p. 175

Fodor, I. (1977) Histogenesis of beryllium-induced bone tumours. *Acta morphol. acad. sci. hung.*, **25**, 99–105

Freiman, D.G. & Hardy, H.L. (1970) Beryllium disease. The relation of pulmonary pathology to clinical course and prognosis based on a study of 130 cases from the US Beryllium Case Registry. *Hum. Pathol.*, **1**, 25–44

Furchner, J.E., Richmond, C.R. & London, J.E. (1973) Comparative metabolism of radionuclides in mammals. VIII. Retention of beryllium in the mouse, rat, monkey and dog. *Health Phys.*, **24**, 293–300

Gardner, L.U. & Heslington, H.F. (1946) Osteosarcoma from intravenous beryllium compounds in rabbits (Abstract). *Fed. Proc.*, **5**, 221

Gilles, D. (1976) *Health Hazard Evaluation Determination. Hardric Laboratories, Waltham, Massachusetts* (NIOSH Report No. HEE-76-103-349), Cincinnati, OH, National Institute for Occupational Safety and Health

Gosink, T.A. (1976) Gas chromatographic analysis of beryllium in the marine system. Interference, efficiency, apparent biological discrimination and some results. *Marine Sci. Commun.*, **2**, 183–199

Grewal, D.S. & Kearns, F.X. (1977) A simple and rapid determination of small amounts of beryllium in urine by flameless atomic absorption. *At. Absorpt. Newsl.*, **16**, 131–132

Groth, D.H., Kommineni, C. & MacKay, G.R. (1980) Carcinogenicity of beryllium hydroxide and alloys. *Environ. Res.*, **21**, 63–84

Gunter, B.J. & Thoburn, T.W. (1986) *Health Hazard Evaluation Report. Rockwell International, Rocky Flats Plant, Golden, Colorado* (NIOSH Report No. 84-510-1691), Cincinnati, OH, National Institute for Occupational Safety and Health

Guyatt, B.L., Kay, H.D. & Branion, H.D. (1933) Beryllium 'rickets'. *J. Nutr.*, **6**, 313–324

Haley, P.J. (1991) Mechanisms of granulomatous lung disease from inhaled beryllium: the role of antigenicity in granuloma formation. *Toxicol. Pathol.*, **19**, 514–525

Haley, P.J., Finch, G.L., Mewhinney, J.A., Harmsen, A.G., Hahn, F.F., Hoover, M.D., Muggenburg, B.A. & Bice, D.E. (1989) A canine model of beryllium-induced granulomatous lung disease. *Lab. Invest.*, **61**, 219–227

Haley, P.J., Finch, G.L., Hoover, M.D. & Cuddihy, R.G. (1990) The acute toxicity of inhaled beryllium metal in rats. *Fundam. appl. Toxicol.*, **15**, 767-778

Hamel, E., Lin, C.M., Kenney, S. & Skehan, P. (1991) Highly variable effects of beryllium and beryllium fluoride on tubulin polymerization under different reaction conditions: comparison of assembly reactions dependent on microtubule-associated proteins, glycerol, dimethyl sulfoxide, and glutamate. *Arch. Biochem. Biophys.*, **286**, 57-69

Hamel, E., Lin, C.M., Kenney, S., Skehan, P. & Vaughns, J. (1992) Modulation of tubulin-nucleotide interactions by metal ions: comparison of beryllium with magnesium and initial studies with other cations. *Arch. Biochem. Biophys.*, **295**, 327-339

Hamilton, E.I. & Minsky, M.J. (1973) Abundance of the chemical elements in man's diet and possible relations with environmental factors. *Sci. total Environ.*, **1**, 375-394

Hanifin, J.M., Epstein, W.L. & Cline, M.J. (1970) In vitro studies of granulomatous hypersensitivity to beryllium. *J. invest. Dermatol.*, **55**, 284-288

Hardy, H.L. (1965) Beryllium poisoning. Lessons in control of man-made disease. *New Engl. J. Med.*, **273**, 1188-1199

Hardy, H.L. & Tabershaw, I.R. (1946) Delayed chemical pneumonitis occurring in workers exposed to beryllium compounds. *J. ind. Hyg. Toxicol.*, **28**, 197-211

Hardy, H.L. & Tepper, L.B. (1959) Beryllium disease. A review of current knowledge. *J. occup. Med.*, **1**, 219-224

Hardy, H.L., Rabe, E.W. & Lorch, S. (1967) United States Beryllium Case Registry (1952-1966). Review of its methods and utility. *J. occup. Med.*, **9**, 271-276

Henderson, W.R., Fukuyama, K., Epstein, W.L. & Spitler, L.E. (1972) In vitro demonstration of delayed hypersensitivity in patients with berylliosis. *J. invest. Dermatol.*, **58**, 5-8

Hinds, M.W., Kolonel, L.N. & Lee, J. (1985) Application of a job-exposure matrix to a case-control study of lung cancer. *J. natl Cancer Inst.*, **75**, 193-197

Hiruma, T. (1991) Rabbit osteosarcoma induced by hydroxypropylcellulose mixed beryllium oxide pellet—comparison between implantations into the bone marrow cavity and into fracture callus of the femur (Jpn.). *Nippon Seikeigeka Gakkai Zasshi* [*J. Jpn. Orthop. Assoc.*], **65**, 775-786

Hoagland, M.B., Grier, R.S. & Hood, M.B. (1950) Beryllium and growth. I. Beryllium-induced osteogenic sarcomata. *Cancer Res.*, **10**, 629-635

Hoar, S.K., Morrison, A.S., Cole, P. & Silverman, D.T. (1980) An occupation and exposure linkage system for the study of occupational carcinogenesis. *J. occup. Med.*, **22**, 722-726

Huang, H., Meyer, K.C., Kubai, L. & Auerbach, R. (1992) An immune model of beryllium-induced pulmonary granulomata in mice. Histopathology, immune reactivity and flow-cytometric analysis of bronchoalveolar lavage-derived cells. *Lab. Invest.*, **67**, 138-146

IARC (1972) *IARC Monographs on the Evaluation of Carcinogenic Risk of Chemicals to Man*, Vol. 1, *Some Inorganic Substances, Chlorinated Hydrocarbons, Aromatic Amines, N-Nitroso Compounds and Natural Products*, Lyon, pp. 17-28

IARC (1980) *IARC Monographs on the Evaluation of the Carcinogenic Risk of Chemicals to Humans*, Vol. 23, *Some Metals and Metallic Compounds*, Lyon, pp. 143-204

IARC (1987a) *IARC Monographs on the Evaluation of Carcinogenic Risks to Humans*, Suppl. 7, *Overall Evaluations of Carcinogenicity: An Updating of* IARC Monographs *Volumes 1 to 42*, Lyon, pp. 127-128

IARC (1987b) *IARC Monographs on the Evaluation of Carcinogenic Risks to Humans*, Suppl. 7, *Overall Evaluations of Carcinogenicity: An Updating of* IARC Monographs *Volumes 1 to 42*, Lyon, pp. 139-142

IARC (1987c) *IARC Monographs on the Evaluation of Carcinogenic Risks to Humans*, Suppl. 7, *Overall Evaluations of Carcinogenicity: An Updating of* IARC Monographs *Volumes 1 to 42*, Lyon, pp. 230–232

IARC (1987d) *IARC Monographs on the Evaluation of Carcinogenic Risks to Humans*, Suppl. 7, *Overall Evaluations of Carcinogenicity: An Updating of* IARC Monographs *Volumes 1 to 42*, Lyon, pp. 341–343

IARC (1990a) *IARC Monographs on the Evaluation of Carcinogenic Risks to Humans*, Vol. 49, *Chromium, Nickel and Welding*, Lyon, pp. 49–256

IARC (1990b) *IARC Monographs on the Evaluation of Carcinogenic Risks to Humans*, Vol. 49, *Chromium, Nickel and Welding*, Lyon, pp. 257–445

IARC (1991) *IARC Monographs on the Evaluation of Carcinogenic Risks to Humans*, Vol. 52, *Chlorinated Drinking-water; Chlorination By-products; Some Other Halogenated Compounds; Cobalt and Cobalt Compounds*, Lyon, pp. 363–472

Ikebe, K., Tanaka, R., Kuzuhara, Y., Suenaga, S. & Takabatake, E. (1986) Studies on the behavior of beryllium in environment. Behavior of beryllium and strontium in atmospheric air (Jpn.). *Eisei Kagaku*, **32**, 159–166

Infante, P.F., Wagoner, J.K. & Sprince, N.L. (1980) Mortality patterns from lung cancer and nonneoplastic respiratory disease among white males in the Beryllium Case Registry. *Environ. Res.*, **21**, 35–43

Institut National de Recherche et de Sécurité [National Institute of Research and Safety] (1990) *Valeurs Limites pour les Concentrations de Substances Dangereuses dans l'Air des Lieux de Travail* [Limit Values for Concentrations of Dangerous Substances in the Air of Work Places] (DN 1609-125-90), Paris, p. 572

International Labour Office (1991) *Occupational Exposure Limits for Airborne Toxic Substances: Values of Selected Countries* (Occupational Safety and Health Series No. 37), 3rd Ed., Geneva, pp. 46–47

Ishinishi, N., Mizunoe, M., Inamasu, T. & Hisanaga, A. (1980) Experimental study on carcinogenicity of beryllium oxide and arsenic trioxide to the lung of rats by an intratracheal instillation (Jpn.). *Fukuoka Igaku Zasshi*, **71**, 19–26

Izmerov, N.F., ed. (1985) *Beryllium* (Scientific Reviews of Soviet Literature on Toxicity and Hazards of Chemicals Series), Geneva, International Register of Potentially Toxic Chemicals, Moscow, Centre of International Projects

Janes, J.M., Higgins, G.M. & Herrick, J.F. (1954) Beryllium-induced osteogenic sarcoma in rabbits. *J. Bone Jt Surg.*, **36B**, 543–552

Jones Williams, W. (1977) Beryllium disease—pathology and diagnosis. *J. Soc. occup. Med.*, **27**, 93–96

Jones Williams, W., Fry, E. & James, E.M.V. (1972) The fine structure of beryllium granulomas. *Acta pathol. microbiol. scand., Sect. A.80*, **Suppl. 233**, 195–202

Kada, T., Hirano, K. & Shirasu, Y. (1980) Screening of environmental chemical mutagens by the rec-assay system with *Bacillus subtilis*. In: de Serres, F.J. & Hollaender, A., eds, *Chemical Mutagens. Principles and Methods for Their Detection*, Vol. 6, New York, Plenum, pp. 149–173

Kanarek, D.J., Wainer, R.A., Chamberlin, R.I., Weber, A.L. & Kazeni, H. (1973) Respiratory illness in a population exposed to beryllium. *Am. Rev. respir. Dis.*, **108**, 1295–1302

Karkinen-Jääskeläinen, M., Määttä, K., Pasila, M. & Saxén, L. (1982) Pulmonary berylliosis: report on a fatal case. *Br. J. Dis. Chest*, **76**, 290–297

Kawecki Berylco Industries (1968) *Product Specifications: Beryllium Chemical Compounds* (File 401 1-SP1), New York

KBAlloys (1985) *KBI® Aluminum Master Alloys: KBI® Aluminum Beryllium (MA-PD 6)*, Reading, PA

Kelly, P.J., Janes, J.M. & Peterson, L.F.A. (1961) The effect of beryllium on bone. A morphological study of the progressive changes observed in rabbit bone. *J. Bone Jt Surg.*, **43A**, 829–844

Kleinman, M.T., Rhodes, J.R., Guinn, V.P. & Thompson, R.J. (1989a) 822. General atomic absorption procedure for trace metals in airborne material collected on filters. In: Lodge, J.P., Jr, ed., *Methods of Air Sampling and Analysis*, 3rd Ed., Chelsea, MI, Lewis Publishers, pp. 608–618

Kleinman, M.T., Courtney, W.J., Guinn, V.P., Rains, T.C., Rhodes, J.R. & Thompson, R.J. (1989b) 822A. General method for preparation of tissue samples for analysis for trace metals. In: Lodge, J.P., Jr, ed., *Methods of Air Sampling and Analysis*, 3rd Ed., Chelsea, MI, Lewis Publishers, pp. 619–622

Klemperer, F.W., Martin, A.P. & Liddy, R.E. (1952) The fate of beryllium compounds in the rat. *Arch. Biochem. Biophys.*, **41**, 148–152

Kline, E.M., Inkley, S.R. & Pritchard, W.H. (1951) Five cases from the fluorescent lamp industry. Treatment of chronic beryllium poisoning with ACTH (adrenocorticotrophic hormone) and cortisone. *Arch. ind. Hyg. occup. Med.*, **3**, 549–564

Komitowski, D. (1968) Experimental beryllium-induced bone tumours as a model of osteogenic sarcoma (Pol.). *Chir. Narzad. Ruchu Ortop. Pols.*, **33**, 237–242

Komitowski, D. (1974) Beryllium-induced bone sarcomas (Ger.). *Verh. dtsch. Ges. Pathol.*, **58**, 438–440

Kramer, D.A. (1985a) Beryllium. In: *Minerals Yearbook 1984*, Vol. 1, *Metals and Minerals*, Washington DC, Bureau of Mines, US Department of the Interior, pp. 153–157

Kramer, D.A. (1985b) Beryllium. In: *Mineral Commodity Summaries 1985*, Washington DC, Bureau of Mines, US Department of the Interior, pp. 18–19

Kramer, D.A. (1987) Beryllium. In: *Mineral Commodity Summaries 1987*, Washington DC, Bureau of Mines, US Department of the Interior, pp. 20–21

Kramer, D.A. (1990) Beryllium. In: *Mineral Commodity Summaries 1990*, Washington DC, Bureau of Mines, US Department of the Interior, pp. 30–31

Kramer, D.A. (1991a) *Annual Report: Beryllium 1990*, Washington DC, Bureau of Mines, US Department of the Interior

Kramer, D.A. (1991b) Beryllium. In: *Mineral Commodity Summaries 1991*, Washington DC, Bureau of Mines, US Department of the Interior, pp. 24–25

Kramer, D.A. (1992a) *Annual Report: Beryllium 1991*, Washington DC, Bureau of Mines, US Department of the Interior

Kramer, D.A. (1992b) Beryllium. In: *Mineral Commodity Summaries 1992*, Washington DC, Bureau of Mines, US Department of the Interior, pp. 34–35

Kreiss, K., Newman, L.S., Mroz, M.M. & Campbell, P.A. (1989) Screening blood test identifies subclinical beryllium disease. *J. occup. Med.*, **31**, 603–608

Kriebel, D., Sprince, N.L., Eisen, E.A. & Greaves, I.A. (1988a) Pulmonary function in beryllium workers: assessment of exposure. *Br. J. ind. Med.*, **45**, 83–92

Kriebel, D., Brain, J.D., Sprince, N.L. & Kazemi, H. (1988b) The pulmonary toxicity of beryllium. *Am. Rev. respir. Dis.*, **137**, 464–473

Kubinski, H., Zeldin, P.E. & Morin, N.R. (1977) Survey of tumor-producing agents for their ability to induce macromolecular complexes (Abstract No. 61). *Proc. Am. Assoc. Cancer Res.*, **18**, 16

Kuroda, K., Endo, G., Okamoto, A., Yo, Y.S. & Horiguchi, S.-I. (1991) Genotoxicity of beryllium, gallium and antimony in short-term assays. *Mutat. Res.*, **264**, 163–170

Larramendy, M.L., Popescu, N.C. & DiPaolo, J.A. (1981) Induction by inorganic metal salts of sister chromatid exchanges and chromosome aberrations in human and Syrian hamster cell strains. *Environ. Mutag.*, 3, 597–606

Laskin, S., Turner, R.A.N. & Stokinger, H.E. (1950) An analysis of dust and fume hazards in a beryllium plant. In: Vorwald, A.J., ed., *Pneumoconiosis. Beryllium, Bauxite Fumes Compensation*, New York, Paul B. Hoeber, pp. 360–386

Levi-Setti, R., Berry, J.-P., Chabala, J.M. & Galle, P. (1988) Selective intracellular beryllium localization in rat tissue by mass-resolved ion microprobe imaging. *Biol. Cell.*, 63, 77–82

Lewis, F.A. (1980) *Health Hazard Evaluation Determination Report. Bertoia Studio, Bally, Pennsylvania* (NIOSH Report No. HE-79-78-655), Cincinnati, OH, National Institute for Occupational Safety and Health

Lewis, R.E. (1988) Aluminum alloys: beryllium as alloying element. In: Cahn, R.W., ed., *Encyclopedia of Materials Science and Engineering*, Suppl. vol. 1, Cambridge, MA, MIT Press, pp. 9–14

Lide, D.R., ed. (1991) *CRC Handbook of Chemistry and Physics*, 72nd Ed., Boca Raton, FL, CRC Press, pp. 4-43–4-44

Lieben, J., Dattoli, J.A. & Israel, H.L. (1964) Probable berylliosis from beryllium alloys. *Arch. environ. Health*, 9, 473–477

Litvinov, N.N., Kazenashev, V.F. & Bugryshev, P.F. (1983) Blastomogenic activities of various beryllium compounds (Russ.). *Eksp. Onkol.*, 5, 23–26

Litvinov, N.N., Popov, V.A., Vorozheikina, T.V., Kazenashev, V.F. & Bugryshev, P.F. (1984) Materials to specify MAC for beryllium in the work environment (Russ.). *Gig. Tr. prof. Sanit. Zabol.*, 1, 34–37

Livey, D.T. (1986) Beryllium oxide. In: Bever, M.B., ed., *Encyclopedia of Materials Science and Engineering*, Vol. 1, Cambridge, MA, MIT Press, pp. 297–298

Love, J.R. & Donohue, M.T. (1983) *Health Hazard Evaluation Report: International Brotherhood of Painters and Allied Trades, Electric Boat Division of General Dynamics Corporation, Groton, CI* (NIOSH Report No. HETA-78-135-1333), Cincinnati, OH, National Insitute for Occupational Safety and Health

Luke, M.Z., Hamilton, L. & Hollocher, T.C. (1975) Beryllium-induced misincorporation by a DNA polymerase: a possible factor in beryllium toxicity. *Biochem. biophys. Res. Commun.*, 62, 497–501

Mancuso, T.F. (1970) Relation of duration of employment and prior respiratory illness to respiratory cancer among beryllium workers. *Environ Res.*, 3, 251–275

Mancuso, T.F. (1979) Occupational lung cancer among beryllium workers. In: Lemen, R. & Dement, J., eds, *Dusts and Disease*, Park Forest, IL, Pathotox Publishers, pp. 463–471

Mancuso, T.F. (1980) Mortality study of beryllium industry workers' occupational lung cancer. *Environ. Res.*, 21, 48–55

Mancuso, T.F. & El-Attar, A.A. (1969) Epidemiological study of the beryllium industry. Cohort methodology and mortality studies. *J. occup. Med.*, 11, 422–434

Marcotte, J. & Witschi, H.P. (1972) Synthesis of RNA and nuclear proteins in early regenerating rat livers exposed to beryllium. *Res. Commun. chem. Pathol. Pharmacol.*, 3, 97–104

Marx, J.J., Jr & Burrell, R. (1973) Delayed hypersensitivity to beryllium compounds. *J. Immunol.*, 111, 590–598

Mathur, R., Sharma, S., Mathur, S. & Prakash, A.O. (1987) Effect of beryllium nitrate on early and late pregnancy in rats. *Bull. environ. Contam. Toxicol.*, 38, 73–77

Matsuura, K. (1974) Experimental studies on the production of osteosarcoma by beryllium compounds, and the effects of irradiation (Jpn.). *Jpn. J. Orthop. Assoc.*, 48, 403–418

Mazabraud, A. (1975) Experimental production of osteosarcomas in rabbits by single local injection of beryllium (Fr.). *Bull. Cancer*, **62**, 49–58

Measures, C.I. & Edmond, J.M. (1982) Beryllium in the water column of the central North Pacific. *Nature*, **297**, 51–53

Meehan, W.R. & Smythe, L.E. (1967) Occurrence of beryllium as a trace element in environmental materials. *Environ. Sci. Technol.*, **1**, 839–844

Mellor, J.W. (1946) *A Comprehensive Treatise on Inorganic and Theoretical Chemistry*, Vol. 4, London, Longmans, Green & Co., pp. 221–248

Merrill, J.R., Lyden, E.F.X, Honda, M. & Arnold, J.R. (1960) The sedimentary geochemistry of the beryllium isotopes. *Geochim. cosmochim. Acta*, **18**, 108–129

Minkwitz, R., Fröhlich, N. & Lehmann, E. (1983) *Untersuchungen von Schadstoffbelastungen an Arbeitsplätzen bei der Herstellung und Verarbeitung von Metallen: Beryllium, Cobalt und deren Legierungen* [Examination of Charges of Harmful Substances at Work Place during the Production and Processing of Metals: Beryllium, Cobalt and Their Alloys] (Forschungsbericht No. 367), Dortmund, Bundesanstalt für Arbeitsschutz

Minoia, C., Sabbioni, E., Apostoli, P., Pietra, R., Pozzoli, L., Gallorini, M., Nicolaou, G., Alessio, L. & Capodaglio, E. (1990) Trace element reference values in tissues from inhabitants of the European Community. I. A study of 46 elements in urine, blood and serum of Italian subjects. *Sci. total Environ.*, **95**, 89–105

Miyaki, M., Akamatsu, N., Ono, T. & Koyama, H. (1979) Mutagenicity of metal cations in cultured cells from Chinese hamster. *Mutat. Res.*, **68**, 259–263

Müller, J. (1979) Beryllium, cobalt, chromium and nickel in particulate matter of ambient air. In: *Proceedings of the International Conference on Heavy Metals in the Environment, London, September 1979*, Edinburgh, CEP Consultants Ltd, pp. 300–303

Mullen, A.L., Stanley, R.E., Lloyd, S.R. & Moghissi, A.A. (1972) Radioberyllium metabolism by the dairy cow. *Health Phys.*, **22**, 17–22

Nesnow, S., Triplett, L.L. & Slaga, T.J. (1985) Studies on the tumor initiating, tumor promoting, and tumor co-initiating properties of respiratory carcinogens. In: Mass, M.J., Kaufman, D.G., Siegfried, J.M., Steele, V.E. & Nesnow, S., eds, *Carcinogenesis*, Vol. 8, New York, Raven Press, pp. 257–277

Newland, L.W. (1984) Arsenic, beryllium, selenium and vanadium. In: Hutzinger, O., ed., *The Handbook of Environmental Chemistry*, Vol. 3, Part B, *Anthropogenic Compounds*, New York, Springer-Verlag, pp. 27–67

Newman, L.S. & Campbell, P.A. (1987) Mitogenic effect of beryllium sulfate on mouse B lymphocytes but not T lymphocytes *in vitro*. *Int. Arch. Allergy appl. Immunol.*, **84**, 223–227

Newman, L.S., Kreiss, K., King, T.E., Jr, Seay, S. & Campbell, P.A. (1989) Pathologic and immunologic alterations in early stages of beryllium disease. Re-examination of disease definition and natural history. *Am. Rev. respir. Dis.*, **139**, 1479–1486

Nishioka, H. (1975) Mutagenic activities of metal compounds in bacteria. *Mutat. Res.*, **31**, 185–189

Ogawa, H.I., Tsuruta, S., Niyitani, Y., Mino, H., Sakata, K. & Kato, Y. (1987) Mutagenicity of metal salts in combination with 9-aminoacridine in *Salmonella typhimurium*. *Jpn. J. Genet.*, **62**, 159–162

Parker, V.H. & Stevens, C. (1979) Binding of beryllium to nuclear acidic proteins. *Chem.-biol. Interactions*, **26**, 167–177

Paschal, D.C. & Bailey, G.G. (1986) Determination of beryllium in urine with electrothermal atomic absorption using the L'vov platform and matrix modification. *At. Spectrosc.*, **7**, 1–3

Paton, G.R. & Allison, A.C. (1972) Chromosome damage in human cell cultures induced by metal salts. *Mutat. Res.*, **16**, 332–336

Petkof, B. (1982) Beryllium. In: *Mineral Yearbook 1981*, Vol. 1, *Metals and Minerals*, Washington DC, Bureau of Mines, US Department of the Interior, pp. 137–140

Petzow, G., Fritz Aldinger, W.C., Jönsson, S. & Preuss, O.P. (1985) Beryllium and beryllium compounds. In: Gerhartz, W., Yamamoto, Y.S., Campbell, F.T., Pfefferkorn, R. & Rounsaville, J.F., eds, *Ullmann's Encyclopedia of Industrial Chemistry*, 5th ed., Vol. A4, Weinheim, VCH Verlagsgesellschaft, pp. 11–33

Pienta, R.J., Poiley, J.A. & Lebherz, W.B., III (1977) Morphological transformation of early passage golden Syrian hamster embryo cells derived from cryopreserved primary cultures as a reliable in vitro bioassay for identifying diverse carcinogens. *Int. J. Cancer*, **19**, 642–655

Powers, M.B. (1991) History of beryllium. In: Rossman, M.D., Preuss, O.P. & Powers, M.B., eds, *Beryllium. Biomedical and Environmental Aspects*, Baltimore, Williams & Wilkins, pp. 9–24

Preuss, O.P. (1988) Beryllium. In: Zenz, C., ed., *Occupational Medicine: Principles and Practical Applications*, Chicago, IL, Year Book Medical Publishers, pp. 517–525

Price, R.J. & Skilleter, D.N. (1985) Stimulatory and cytotoxic effects of beryllium on proliferation of mouse spleen lymphocytes in vitro. *Arch. Toxicol.*, **56**, 207–211

Reeves, A.L. (1986) Beryllium. In: Friberg, L., Nordberg, G.F. & Vouk, V.B., eds, *Handbook of the Toxicology of Metals*, Vol. 2, *Specific Metals*, 2nd Ed., Amsterdam, Elsevier, pp. 95–116

Reeves, A.L. (1989) Beryllium: toxicological research of the last decade. *J. Am. Coll. Toxicol.*, **8**, 1307–1313

Reeves, A.L. & Vorwald, A.J. (1961) The hormonal transport of beryllium. *J. occup. Med.*, **3**, 567–574

Reeves, A.L. & Vorwald, A.J. (1967) Beryllium carcinogenesis. II. Pulmonary deposition and clearance of inhaled beryllium sulfate in the rat. *Cancer Res.*, **27**, 446–451

Reeves, A.L., Deitch, D. & Vorwald, A.J. (1967) Beryllium carcinogenesis. I. Inhalation exposure of rats to beryllium sulfate aerosol. *Cancer Res.*, **27**, 439–445

Reichert, J.K. (1974) Beryllium: a toxic element in the human environment with special regard to its occurrence in water (Ger.). *Wasser*, **41**, 209–216

Rhoads, K. & Sanders, C.L. (1985) Lung clearance, translocation, and acute toxicity of arsenic, beryllium, cadmium, cobalt, lead, selenium, vanadium and ytterbium oxides following deposition in rat lung. *Environ. Res.*, **36**, 359–378

Rosenkranz, H.S. & Poirier, L.A. (1979) Evaluation of the mutagenicity and DNA-modifying activity of carcinogens and noncarcinogens in microbial systems. *J. natl Cancer Inst.*, **62**, 873–892

Rossman, T.G. & Molina, M. (1986) The genetic toxicology of metal compounds: II. Enhancement of ultraviolet light-induced mutagenesis in *Escherichia coli* WP2. *Environ. Mutag.*, **8**, 263–271

Rossman, T.G., Molina, M. & Meyer, L.W. (1984) The genetic toxicology of metal compounds: I. Induction of λ prophage in *E. coli* WP2$_s$(λ). *Environ. Mutag.*, **6**, 59–69

Rossman, T.G., Zelikoff, J.T., Agarwal, S. & Kneip, T.J. (1987) Genetic toxicology of metal compounds: an examination of appropriate cellular models. *Toxicol. environ. Chem.*, **14**, 251–262

Rossman, M.D., Kern, J.A., Elias, J.A., Cullen, M.R., Epstein, P.E., Preuss, O.P., Markham, T.N. & Daniele, R.P. (1988) Proliferative response of bronchoalveolar lymphocytes to beryllium. A test for chronic beryllium disease. *Ann. intern. Med.*, **108**, 687–693

Rössner, P. & Bencko, V. (1980) Beryllium toxicity testing in the suspension culture of mouse fibroblasts. *J. Hyg. Epidemiol. Microbiol. Immunol.*, **24**, 150–155

Safe Drinking Water Committee (1977) *Drinking Water and Health*, Washington DC, National Research Council, National Academy of Science, pp. 211, 231–232

Saltini, C., Winestock, K., Kirby, M., Pinkston, P. & Crystal, R.G. (1989) Maintenance of alveolitis in patients with chronic beryllium disease by beryllium-specific helper T cells. *New Engl. J. Med.*, **320**, 1103–1109

Sanders, C.L., Cannon, W.C., Powers, G.J., Adee, R.R. & Meier, D.M. (1975) Toxicology of high-fired beryllium oxide inhaled by rodents. I. Metabolism and early effects. *Arch. environ. Health*, **30**, 546–551

Saracci, R. (1985) Beryllium: epidemiological evidence. In: Wald, N.J. & Doll, R., eds, *Interpretation of Negative Epidemiological Evidence for Carcinogenicity* (IARC Scientific Publications No. 65), Lyon, IARC, pp. 203–219

Sauer, C. & Lieser, K.H. (1986) Determination of trace elements in raw water and in drinking-water (Ger.). *Wasser*, **66**, 277–284

Savitz, D.A., Whelan, E.A. & Kleckner, R.C. (1989) Effects of parents' occupational exposures on risk of stillbirth, preterm delivery, and small-for-gestational-age infants. *Am. J. Epidemiol.*, **129**, 1201–1218

Sax, N.I. & Lewis, R.J. (1987) *Hawley's Condensed Chemical Dictionary*, 11th ed., New York, Van Nostrand Reinhold, pp. 140–142

Schepers, G.W.H., Durkan, T.M., Delehant, A.B. & Creedon, F.T. (1957) The biological action of inhaled beryllium sulfate. A preliminary chronic toxicity study in rats. *Arch. ind. Health*, **15**, 32–58

Schroeder, H.A. & Mitchener, M. (1975) Life-term studies in rats: effects of aluminum, barium, beryllium and tungsten. *J. Nutr.*, **105**, 421–427

Schulert, A.R., Glasser, S.R., Stant, E.G., Jr, Brill, A.B., Koshakji, R.P. & Mansour, M.M. (1969) *Development of Placental Discrimination among Homologous Elements* (Atomic Energy Commission Symposium Series 17), pp. 145–152

Scott, J.K., Neuman, W.F. & Allen, R. (1950) The effect of added carrier on the distribution and excretion of soluble ^{7}Be. *J. biol. Chem.*, **182**, 291-298

Sendelbach, L.E., Witschi, H.P. & Tryka, A.F. (1986) Acute pulmonary toxicity of beryllium sulfate inhalation in rats and mice: cell kinetics and histopathology. *Toxicol. appl. Pharmacol.*, **85**, 248–256

Sendelbach, L.E., Tryka, A.F. & Witschi, H. (1989) Progressive lung injury over a one-year period after a single inhalation exposure to beryllium sulfate. *Am. Rev. respir. Dis.*, **139**, 1003–1009

Shacklette, H.T., Hamilton, J.L., Boerngen, J.G. & Bowles, J.M. (1971) *Elemental Composition of Surficial Materials in the Conterminous United States* (US Geological Survey, Professional Paper 574-D), Washington DC, US Government Printing Office

Simmon, V.F. (1979a) In vitro mutagenicity assays of chemical carcinogens and related compounds with *Salmonella typhimurium*. *J. natl Cancer Inst.*, **63**, 893–899

Simmon, V.F. (1979b) In vitro assays for recombinogenic activity of chemical carcinogens and related compounds with *Saccharomyces cerevisiae* D3. *J. natl Cancer Inst.*, **62**, 901–909

Simmon, V.F., Rosenkranz, H.S., Zeiger, E. & Poirier, L.A. (1979) Mutagenic activity of chemical carcinogens and related compounds in the intraperitoneal host-mediated assay. *J. natl Cancer Inst.*, **62**, 911-918

Sirover, M.A. & Loeb, L.A. (1976) Metal-induced infidelity during DNA synthesis. *Proc. natl Acad. Sci. USA*, **73**, 2331–2335

Sissons, H.A. (1950) Bone sarcomas produced experimentally in the rabbit, using compounds of beryllium. *Acta unio int. contra cancrum*, **7**, 171–172

Skilleter, D.N. (1984) Biochemical properties of beryllium potentially relevant to its carcinogenicity. *Toxicol. environ. Chem.*, **7**, 213–228

Skilleter, D.N. (1986) Selective cellular and molecular effects of beryllium on lymphocytes. *Toxicol. environ. Chem.*, **11**, 301–312

Skilleter, D.N. & Legg, R.F. (1989) Inhibition of epidermal growth factor-stimulated hepatocyte proliferation by the metallocarcinogen beryllium. *Biochem. Soc. Transact.*, **17**, 1040–1041

Skilleter, D.N. & Price, R.J. (1978) The uptake and subsequent loss of beryllium by rat liver parenchymal and non-parenchymal cells after the intravenous administration of particulate and soluble forms. *Chem.-biol. Interactions*, **20**, 383–396

Skilleter, D.N. & Price, R.J. (1984) Lymphocyte beryllium binding: relationship to development of delayed beryllium sensitivity. *Int. Arch. Allergy appl. Immunol.*, **73**, 181–183

Smugeresky, J.E. (1986) Beryllium and beryllium alloys. In: Bever, M.B., ed., *Encyclopedia of Materials Science and Engineering*, Vol. 1, Cambridge, MA, MIT Press, pp. 289–294

Sprince, N.L. & Kazemi, H. (1980) US Beryllium Case Registry through 1977. *Environ. Res.*, **21**, 44–47

Sprince, N.L. Kazemi, H. & Hardy, H.L. (1976) Current (1975) problem of differentiating between beryllium disease and sarcoidosis. *Ann. N.Y. Acad. Sci.*, **278**, 654–664

Sprince, N.L., Kanarek, D.J., Weber, A.L., Chamberlin, R.I. & Kazemi, H. (1978) Reversible respiratory disease in beryllium workers. *Am. Rev. respir. Dis.*, **117**, 1011–1017

Steele, V.E., Wilkinson, B.P., Arnold, J.T. & Kutzman, R.S. (1989) Study of beryllium oxide genotoxicity in cultured respiratory epithelial cells. *Inhal. Toxicol.*, **1**, 95–110

Steenland, K. & Ward, E. (1991) Lung cancer incidence among patients with beryllium disease: a cohort mortality study. *J. natl Cancer Inst.*, **83**, 1380–1385

Sterner, J.H. & Eisenbud, M. (1951) Epidemiology of beryllium intoxication. *Arch. ind. Hyg. occup. Med.*, **4**, 123–151

Stiefel, T., Schulze, K., Zorn, H. & Tölg, G. (1980) Toxicokinetic and toxicodynamic studies of beryllium. *Arch. Toxicol.*, **45**, 81–92

Stoeckle, J.D., Hardy, H.L. & Weber, A.L. (1969) Chronic beryllium disease. Long-term follow-up of sixty cases and selective review of the literature. *Am. J. Med.*, **46**, 545–561

Stonehouse, A.J. & Zenczak, S. (1991) Properties, production, processes, and applications. In: Rossman, M.D., Preuss, O.P. & Powers, M.B., eds, *Beryllium. Biomedical and Environmental Aspects*, Baltimore, Williams & Wilkins, pp. 27–55

Strem Chemicals (1992) *Catalog No. 14—Metals, Inorganics and Organometallics for Research*, Newburyport, MA, pp. 18–19

Sussmann, V.H., Lieben, J. & Cleland, J.G. (1959) An air pollution study of a community surrounding a beryllium plant. *Ind. Hyg. J.*, **20**, 504–508

Tapp, E. (1966) Beryllium induced sarcomas in the rabbit tibia. *Br. J. Cancer*, **20**, 778–783

Tapp, E. (1969) Osteogenic sarcoma in rabbits following subperiosteal implantation of beryllium. *Arch. Pathol.*, **88**, 89–95

Truhaut, R., Festy, B. & Le Talaer, J.-Y. (1968) Interaction of beryllium with DNA and its effect on some enzymatic systems (Fr.). *C.R. Acad. Sci. Paris Ser. D*, **266**, 1192–1195

Tso, W.-W. & Fung, W.-P. (1981) Mutagenicity of metallic cation. *Toxicol. Lett.*, **8**, 195–200

UNEP (1993) *IRPTC PC Data Base*, Geneva

US Environmental Protection Agency (1986a) Method 6010. Inductively coupled plasma atomic emission spectroscopy. In: *Test Methods for Evaluating Solid Waste—Physical/Chemical Methods*, 3rd Ed., Vol. 1A (US EPA No. SW-846), Washington DC, Office of Solid Waste and Emergency Response, pp. 6010-1–6010-17

US Environmental Protection Agency (1986b) Method 7090. Beryllium (atomic absorption, direct aspiration). In: *Test Methods for Evaluating Solid Waste—Physical/Chemical Methods*, 3rd Ed., Vol. 1A (US EPA No. SW-846), Washington DC, Office of Solid Waste and Emergency Response, pp. 7090-1–7090-3

US Environmental Protection Agency (1986c) Method 7091. Beryllium (atomic absorption, furnace technique). In: *Test Methods for Evaluating Solid Waste—Physical/Chemical Methods*, 3rd ed., Vol. 1A (US EPA No. SW-846), Washington DC, Office of Solid Waste and Emergency Response, pp. 7091-1–7091-3

US Environmental Protection Agency (1987) *Health Assessment Document for Beryllium* (EPA Report No. 600/8-84-026F), Research Triangle Park, NC, Office of Research and Development

US Environmental Protection Agency (1992) National emission standard for beryllium. *US Code fed. Regul.*, **Title 40**, Subpart C, Sections 61.30–61.44, pp. 23–26

US National Institute for Occupational Safety and Health (1972) *Criteria Document: Recommendations for an Occupational Exposure Standard for Beryllium* (NIOSH Report No. Tr-003-72; HSM 72-10268), Rockville, MD

US National Institute for Occupational Safety and Health (1990) *NIOSH Pocket Guide to Chemical Hazards* (DHHS (NIOSH) Publication No. 90-117), Cincinnati, OH, pp. 46–47

US National Library of Medicine (1992) *Hazardous Substances Data Bank* (HSDB), Bethesda, MD

US Occupational Safety and Health Administration (1989) Air contaminants—permissible exposure limits. *US Code fed. Regul.*, **Title 29**, Part 1910.1000, p. 599

Vacher, J. & Stoner, H.B. (1968) The transport of beryllium in rat blood. *Biochem. Pharmacol.*, **17**, 93–107

Vacher, J., Deraedt, R. & Benzoni, J. (1974) Role of the reticuloendothelial system in the production of α-macrofetoprotein in the rat following intravenous injection of beryllium and other particles. *Toxicol. appl. Pharmacol.*, **28**, 28–37

Vegni Talluri, M. & Guiggiani, V. (1967) Action of beryllium ions on primary cultures of swine cells. *Caryologia*, **20**, 355–367

Vorwald, A.J. (1967) The induction of experimental pulmonary cancer in the primate (Abstract I-07-e). In: Harris, R.J., ed., *Proceedings of the IX International Cancer Congress, Tokyo, 1966*, Berlin, Springer, p. 125

Votto, J.J., Barton, R.W., Gionfriddo, M.A., Cole, S.R., McCormick, J.R. & Thrall, R.S. (1987) A model for pulmonary granulomata induced by beryllium sulfate in the rat. *Sarcoidosis*, **4**, 71–76

Wagner, W.D., Groth, D.H., Holtz, J.L., Madden, G.E. & Stokinger, H.E. (1969) Comparative chronic inhalation toxicity of beryllium ores, bertrandite and beryl, with production of pulmonary tumors by beryl. *Toxicol. appl. Pharmacol.*, **15**, 10–29

Wagoner, J.K., Infante, P.F. & Bayliss, D.L. (1980) Beryllium: an etiologic agent in the induction of lung cancer, nonneoplastic respiratory disease and heart disease among industrially exposed workers. *Environ. Res.*, **21**, 15–34

Walsh, K. & Rees, G.H. (1978) Beryllium compounds. In: Kirk, R.E. & Othmer, D.F., eds, *Encyclopedia of Chemical Technology*, 3rd ed., Vol. 3, New York, John Wiley & Sons, pp. 824–829

Ward, E., Okun, A., Ruder, A., Fingerhut, M. & Steenland, K. (1992) A mortality study of workers at seven beryllium processing plants. *Am. J. ind. Med.*, **22**, 885–904

Weber, H.H. & Engelhardt, W.E. (1933) Apparatus for production of highly constant, low concentrations of dust and a method for microgravimetric analysis of dust. Application to the study of dusts from beryllium production (Ger.). *Zbl. Gewerbehyg.*, **10**, 41–47

WHO (1990) *Beryllium* (Environmental Health Criteria 106), Geneva

Williams, G.M., Laspia, M.F. & Dunkel, V.C. (1982) Reliability of the hepatocyte primary culture/DNA repair test in testing of coded carcinogens and noncarcinogens. *Mutat. Res.*, **97**, 359-370

Witschi, H.P. (1968) Inhibition of deoxyribonucleic acid synthesis in regenerating rat liver by beryllium. *Lab. Invest.*, **19**, 67-70

Witschi, H.P. (1970) Effects of beryllium on deoxyribonucleic acid-synthesizing enzymes in regenerating rat liver. *Biochem. J.*, **120**, 623-634

Witschi, H.P. & Aldridge, W.N. (1968) Uptake, distribution and binding of beryllium to organelles of the rat liver cell. *Biochem. J.*, **106**, 811-820

Wöhler, F. (1828) On beryllium and yttrium (Ger.). *Pogg. Ann.*, **13**, 577-582

Yamaguchi, S. (1963) Study of beryllium-induced osteogenic sarcoma (Jpn.). *Nagasaki Iggakai Zasshi*, **38**, 127-138

Zakour, R.A. & Glickman, B.W. (1984) Metal-induced mutagenesis in the *lacI* gene of *Escherichia coli*. *Mutat. Res.*, **126**, 9-18

Zielinski, J.F. (1961) Seven-year experience summaries of beryllium air pollution in a modern alloy foundry. In: *NIOSH Workshop on Beryllium*, Cincinatti, OH, Kettering Laboratory, University of Cincinnati, pp. 592-600

Zorn, H. & Diem, H. (1974) Importance of beryllium and its compounds in occupational medicine (Ger.). *Zbl. Arbeitsmed.*, **24**, 3-8

Zorn, H., Stiefel, T. & Diem, H. (1977) Importance of beryllium and its compounds in occupational medicine. Part 2 (Ger.). *Zbl. Arbeitsmed.*, **27**, 83-88

Zorn, H., Stiefel, T. & Porcher, H. (1986) Clinical and analytical follow-up of 25 persons exposed accidentally to beryllium. *Toxicol. environ. Chem.*, **12**, 163-171

Zorn, H.R., Stiefel, T.W., Breuers, J. & Schlegelmilch, R. (1988) Beryllium. In: Seiler, H.G. & Sigel, H., eds, *Handbook on Toxicity of Inorganic Compounds*, New York, Marcel Dekker, pp. 105-114

CADMIUM AND CADMIUM COMPOUNDS

Cadmium and cadmium compounds were considered by previous working groups, in 1972, 1975 and 1987 (IARC, 1973, 1976, 1987a). New data have since become available, and these are included in the present monograph and have been taken into consideration in the evaluation. The agents considered are metallic cadmium, cadmium alloys and some cadmium compounds.

1. Exposure Data

1.1 Chemical and physical data and analysis

1.1.1 *Synonyms, trade names and molecular formulae*

Synonyms, trade names and molecular formulae for cadmium, cadmium–copper alloy and some cadmium compounds are presented in Table 1. The cadmium compounds shown are those for which data on carcinogenicity or mutagenicity were available or which are commercially important compounds. It is not an exhaustive list and does not necessarily include all of the most commercially important cadmium-containing substances.

Table 1. Synonyms (Chemical Abstracts Service (CAS) names are in italics), trade names and atomic or molecular formulae of cadmium and cadmium compounds

Chemical name	CAS Reg. No.[a]	Synonyms and trade names	Formula
Cadmium	7440-43-9	Cadmium metal; CI 77180	Cd
Cadmium acetate	543-90-8 (24558-49-4; 29398-76-3)	*Acetic acid, cadmium salt*; bis(acetoxy)-cadmium; cadmium(II) acetate; cadmium diacetate; cadmium ethanoate; CI 77185	$Cd(CH_3COO)_2$
Cadmium carbonate	513-78-0 [93820-02-1]	*Carbonic acid, cadmium salt*; cadmium carbonate ($CdCO_3$); cadmium monocarbonate; chemcarb; kalcit; mikrokalcit; supermikrokalcit	$CdCO_3$
Cadmium chloride	10108-64-2	Cadmium dichloride; dichlorocadmium	$CdCl_2$
Cadmium hydroxide	21041-95-2 (1306-13-4; 13589-17-8)	*Cadmium hydroxide ($Cd(OH)_2$)*; cadmium dihydroxide	$Cd(OH)_2$
Cadmium nitrate	10325-94-7 (14177-24-3)	*Nitric acid, cadmium salt*; cadmium dinitrate; cadmium(II) nitrate; cadmium nitrate ($Cd(NO_3)_2$)	$Cd(NO_3)_2$
Cadmium stearate	2223-93-0	Alaixol II; cadmium distearate; cadmium octadecanoate; cadmium(II) stearate; octadecanoic acid; cadmium salt; SCD; stabilisator SCD; stabilizer SCD; stearic acid, cadmium salt	$Cd(C_{36}H_{72}O_4)$

Table 1 (contd)

Chemical name	CAS Reg. No.[a]	Synonyms and trade names	Formula
Cadmium sulfate	10124-36-4 (62642-07-3) [31119-53-6]	Cadmium monosulfate; cadmium sulfate; *sulfuric acid, cadmium salt (1:1)*	$CdSO_4$
Cadmium sulfide	1306-23-6 (106496-20-2)	Cadmium monosulfide; cadmium orange; cadmium yellow; CI 77199	CdS
Cadmium oxide	1306-19-0	Cadmium monoxide	CdO
Cadmium–copper alloy[b]	37364-06-0	*Copper base, Cu,Cd*	Cd.Cu
	12685-29-9 (52863-93-1)	*Cadmium nonbase, Cd,Cu*	Cd.Cu
	132295-56-8	*Copper alloy, base, Cu 99.75-100, Cd 0.05–0.15*; IMI 143; UNS C14300	Cd.Cu
	132295-57-9	*Copper alloy, base, Cu 99.60-100, Cd 0.1–0.3*; UNS C14310	Cd.Cu

[a]Replaced CAS Registry numbers are shown in parentheses; alternative CAS Registry numbers are shown in brackets.
[b]116 cadmium-copper alloys are registered with the Chemical Abstracts Service.

1.1.2 *Chemical and physical properties of the pure substances*

Selected chemical and physical properties of most of the cadmium and cadmium compounds covered in this monograph are presented in Table 2.

Cadmium (atomic number, 48; relative atomic mass, 112.41) is a metal, which belongs, together with zinc and mercury, to group IIB of the periodic table. The oxidation state of almost all cadmium compounds is +2, although a few compounds have been reported in which it is +1. There are eight naturally occurring isotopes (abundance is given in parentheses): 106 (1.22%), 108 (0.88%), 110 (12.39%), 111 (12.75%), 112 (24.07%), 113 (12.26%), 114 (28.86%) and 116 (7.58%). Although cadmium is slowly oxidized in moist air at ambient temperature, it forms a fume of brown-coloured cadmium oxide when heated in air. Other elements that react readily with cadmium metal upon heating include halogens, phosphorus, selenium, sulfur and tellurium (Hollander & Carapella, 1978; Schulte-Schrepping & Piscator, 1985).

There is no evidence that organocadmium compounds (in which the metal is bound covalently to carbon) occur in nature, although cadmium may bind to proteins and other organic molecules and form salts with organic acids (e.g. cadmium stearate) (WHO, 1992a).

Cadmium has a relatively high vapour pressure (0.001 mm Hg [0.133 Pa] at 218 °C; 1.0 mm Hg [133.3 Pa] at 392 °C; 100 mm Hg [13.3 kPa] at 611 °C). When reactive gases or vapours, such as oxygen, carbon dioxide, water vapour, sulfur dioxide, sulfur trioxide or hydrogen chloride, are present, cadmium vapour reacts to produce cadmium oxide, carbonate, hydroxide, sulfite, sulfate or chloride, respectively. These compounds may be formed in stacks and emitted into the environment (Schulte-Schrepping & Piscator, 1985; WHO, 1992a).

Table 2. Physical and chemical properties of cadmium and cadmium compounds

Chemical name	Relative atomic/molecular mass	Melting-point (°C)	Typical physical description	Density (g/cm^3)	Solubility
Cadmium metal	112.41	320.9	Silver–white, blue-tinged malleable metal	8.642	Soluble in ammonium nitrate, dilute nitric acid, hot sulfuric acid; insoluble in water
Cadmium acetate	230.50	256	Colourless crystal with slight acetic acid odour	2.341	Soluble in water, ethanol, methanol
Cadmium carbonate	172.42	321 (dec.)	White trigonal solid	4.26 (4 °C)	Practically insoluble in water (28 μg/L) and ammonia; soluble in dilute acids; insoluble in organic solvents
Cadmium chloride	183.32	568	Colourless to white, hygroscopic, rhombohedral or hexagonal crystals	4.047	Soluble in water (1400 g/L) and acetone; slightly soluble in methanol, ethanol; insoluble in diethyl ether
Cadmium hydroxide	146.43	130 (dec.)	White trigonal crystal or amorphous solid	4.79 (15 °C)	Almost insoluble in water (2.6 mg/L); soluble in dilute acids and ammonium salts; insoluble in alkaline solutions
Cadmium nitrate	236.43	350	Colourless solid	NR	Soluble in water (1 kg/L at 0 °C, 3.3 kg/L at 60 °C); soluble in diethyl ether, ethyl acetate, acetone, ethanol; very soluble in dilute acids
Cadmium sulfate	208.47	1000	Colourless to white orthorhombic crystals	4.691	Soluble in water (755 g/L); insoluble in acetone, ammonia, ethanol
Cadmium sulfide	144.47	1750 (at 100 atm [101 × 10^2 kPa])	Yellow–orange hexagonal (α) or cubic (β) dimorphic, semi-transparent crystals; yellow-brown powder	4.82 (α); 4.50 (β)	Soluble in concentrated or warm dilute mineral acids with evolution of hydrogen sulfide; very slightly soluble in ammonium hydroxide; almost insoluble in water (1.3 mg/L); forms a colloid in hot water
Cadmium oxide	128.41	> 1500	Dark-brown cubic crystals or amorphous powder	8.15 (crystal); 6.95 (amorphous)	Soluble in dilute acids and ammonium salts; almost insoluble in water (9.6 mg/L); insoluble in alkali

From Hollander & Carapella (1978); Parker (1978); Sax & Lewis (1987); Budavari (1989); Cadmium Association/Cadmium Council (1991); Lide (1991); WHO (1992a); Agency for Toxic Substances and Disease Registry (1989). NR, not reported; dec., decomposes

Some cadmium compounds, such as cadmium sulfide, carbonate and oxide, are practically insoluble in water. Few data are available, however, on the solubility of these compounds in biological fluids, e.g. in the gastrointestinal tract and lung. The water-insoluble compounds can be changed to water-soluble salts by acids or light and oxygen; e.g. aqueous suspensions of cadmium sulfide gradually photooxidize to soluble (ionic) cadmium. Cadmium sulfate, nitrate and halides are water-soluble (Ulicny, 1992; WHO, 1992a).

1.1.3 *Technical products and impurities*

Cadmium metal—produced in a wide range of forms and purities for various uses. Purities range from 99.0% (reagent grade) to 99.9999% (zone-refined), and forms include powder, foils, wires, ingots and others. Typical impurities (%, max.) include: Zn, 0.02–0.1; Cu, 0.0001–0.015; Pb, 0.0001–0.025; Fe, 0.0001–0.001; Bi, 0.0005; Sn, 0.01; Ag, 0.01; Sb, 0.001; and As, 0.003 (J.T. Baker, 1989; Alfa Products, 1990; Spectrum Chemical Mfg Corp., 1991; Aldrich Chemical Co., 1992; Strem Chemicals, 1992; Atomergic Chemetals Corp., undated; D.F. Goldsmith Chemical & Metal Corp., undated)

Cadmium acetate—reagent grade; 99.999% (Alfa Products, 1990)

Cadmium chloride—purities: 99.0– > 99.99%; American Chemical Society reagent grade, 95– > 99%; anhydrous, 99.99–99.999%; impurities (%): NO_3, 0.003; SO_4, 0.005–0.01; NH_4, 0.002–0.01; Cu, 0.001; Fe, 0.001; Pb, 0.005; and Zn, 0.1 (J.T. Baker, 1989; Alfa Products, 1990; CERAC, Inc., 1991; Spectrum Chemical Mfg Corp., 1991; Aldrich Chemical Co., 1992; Strem Chemicals, 1992)

Cadmium sulfate (as $3CdSO_4.8H_2O$)—purities: 98–99.999%; American Chemical Society reagent grade, 98–99.0%; impurities (%): Cl, 0.001; NO_3, 0.003; Cu, 0.002; Fe, 0.001; Pb, 0.003; Zn, 0.1; and As, 1–2 ppm (J.T. Baker, 1989; Alfa Products, 1990; Aldrich Chemical Co., 1992)

Cadmium sulfide—purities: > 98–99.999%; phosphor (luminescent) grade, 99.99–99.999% (Alfa Products, 1990; CERAC, Inc., 1991; Aldrich Chemical Co., 1992; Strem Chemicals, 1992; D.F. Goldsmith Chemical & Metal Corp., undated). Some of the trade names associated with cadmium sulfide include: Cadmium Golden; Cadmium Golden 366; Cadmium Lemon Yellow; Cadmium Lemon Yellow 527; Cadmium Orange; Cadmium Primrose 819; Cadmium Sulfide Yellow; Cadmium Yellow; Cadmium Yellow 000; Cadmium Yellow 892; Cadmium Yellow Conc. Deep; Cadmium Yellow Conc. Golden; Cadmium Yellow Conc. Lemon; Cadmium Yellow Conc. Primrose; Cadmium Yellow 10G Conc.; Cadmium Yellow OZ Dark; Cadmium Yellow Primrose 47-4100; Cadmopur Golden Yellow N; Cadmopur Yellow; Capsebon; C.P. Golden Yellow 55; Ferro Lemon Yellow; Ferro Orange Yellow; Ferro Yellow; GSK; PC 108; Primrose 1466.

Cadmium oxide—purities: 99.0–99.9999%; reagent grade, 99.0%; commercial grade, 99.7%; impurities (%): Cl, 0.002; NO_3, 0.01; SO_4, 0.20; Cu, 0.005; Fe, 0.002; and Pb, 0.01 (J.T. Baker, 1989; Alfa Products, 1990; CERAC, Inc., 1991; Aldrich Chemical Co., 1992; Strem Chemicals, 1992; D.F. Goldsmith Chemical & Metal Corp., undated).

Impurities that occur in cadmium compounds that have been the subjects of previous monographs are lead (IARC, 1987b) and arsenic (IARC, 1987c).

1.1.4 Analysis

Selected methods for the determination of cadmium and cadmium compounds in various media are presented in Table 3.

Table 3. Methods for the analysis of cadmium and cadmium compounds (as Cd)

Sample matrix	Sample preparation	Assay procedure	Limit of detection	Reference
Air	Collect on membrane filter; dissolve with nitric acid	FLAA	0.03 µg/m^3; 0.002 µg/ml	Kleinman et al. (1989a)
	Collect on cellulose ester membrane filter; add nitric and hydrochloric acids; heat, then cool	FLAA	0.05 µg/sample	Eller (1987)
	Collect on cellulose ester membrane filter; ash with nitric:perchloric acid solution (4:1); heat; repeat; heat to dryness; dilute with nitric:perchloric acid solution (4:1)	ICP	1 µg/sample	Eller (1984a)
Water, ground- and surface	Acidify with nitric and hydrochloric acids (Method 3005)	FLAA; ICP at 226.5 nm	0.005 mg/L; 4 µg/L	US Environmental Protection Agency (1986a,b) (Methods 6010 & 7130)
Aqueous samples, extracts, wastes	Acidify with nitric acid; heat and evaporate to low volume; cool; add nitric acid; reheat and reflux with hydrochloric acid (Method 3010)			
Oils, greases, waxes	Dissolve in xylene or methyl isobutyl ketone (Method 3040)			
Sediments, sludges, soils	Digest with nitric acid and hydrogen peroxide; reflux with hydrochloric acid (Method 3050)			
Aqueous samples, extracts, wastes	Acidify with nitric acid; evaporate to low volume; cool; add nitric acid; heat to complete digestion (Method 3020)	GFAA	0.1 µg/L	US Environmental Protection Agency (1986c) (Method 7131)
Sediments, sludges, soils	Digest with nitric acid and hydrogen peroxide; reflux with nitric acid (Method 3050)	GFAA	0.1 µg/L	US Environmental Protection Agency (1986c) (Method 7131)
Tissue samples	Ash in hot concentrated nitric acid	AA	0.0006 µg/ml	Kleinman et al. (1989b)
Urine	Adjust pH to 2.0 and add polydithiocarbamate resin; filter through cellulose ester membrane filter; ash in low-temperature oxygen plasma or with nitric:perchloric acid solution (4:1)	ICP	0.1 µg/sample	Eller (1984b)

Table 3 (contd)

Sample matrix	Sample preparation	Assay procedure	Limit of detection	Reference
Urine (contd)	Complex with hexamethylene ammonium/hexamethylene dithiocarbamate; extract with diisopropyl ketone/xylene	GFAA	0.2 µg/L	Angerer & Schaller (1988)
Blood	Solubilize with Triton-X-100; deproteinate with 1 M nitric acid (Recommended reference method of the Commission of Toxicology of IUPAC)	GFAA	0.2 µg/L	Stoeppler & Brandt (1980); Angerer & Schaller (1985)

Abbreviations: FLAA, flame atomic absorption spectrometry; ICP, inductively coupled argon plasma atomic emission spectrometry; GFAA, graphite furnace atomic absorption spectrometry; AA, atomic absorption spectrometry

The cadmium concentrations in environmental and biological specimens vary widely: only a few nanograms of cadmium may be present in specimens of air, water and biological fluids, whereas hundreds of micrograms or more may be present in kidney, sewage sludge and plastics. Different techniques are therefore required for sample collection and preparation and for analysis. Atomic absorption spectrometry, electrochemical methods such as anodic stripping voltammetry and pulse polarography, neutron activation, X-ray microanalysis and spark source emission spectroscopy are used for the determination of cadmium in various media.

In general, the techniques available for measuring cadmium in the environment and in biological materials cannot differentiate between different compounds. With special separation techniques, cadmium-containing proteins can be isolated and identified. In most studies to date, the concentration or amount of cadmium in water, air, soil, plants and other environmental or biological material has been determined as the element.

The most commonly used methods, atomic absorption spectrometry and polarography, were discussed in detail in WHO (1992b). Atomic absorption spectrometry is the most reliable and practicable method, especially for the biological monitoring of exposure to cadmium. The sensitivity of flame atomic absorption spectrometry is about 10 µg/L; with graphite furnace atomic absorption spectroscopy, cadmium concentrations of about 0.1 µg/L can be determined in urine and blood. Standardized methods for the determination of cadmium in blood and urine have been published (Stoeppler & Brandt, 1980; Angerer & Schaller, 1985, 1988).

The precision and accuracy of the results are strongly influenced by the pre-analytical phase, so that special care must be taken to avoid contamination during sampling, transport and storage of specimens, particularly liquid samples. Contamination of biological samples by sampling devices, containers and sample preparations has been reported (WHO, 1992b). It is strongly recommended that analysis of cadmium be accompanied by an adequate internal and external quality assurance programme. Quality control materials are available for daily use in intralaboratory control and in national and international intercomparison programmes for the determination of cadmium in blood and urine (Herber *et al.*, 1990a,b; Schaller *et al.*, 1991; Brown, 1992; WHO, 1992b).

A noninvasive technique for determination of cadmium in liver and kidney *in vivo* has been developed, which is based on the principle of neutron activation analysis and takes advantage of the very large cross-sectional area for capture of thermal neutrons of one of the naturally occurring stable isotopes of cadmium, ^{113}Cd (Ellis *et al.*, 1981; Roels *et al.*, 1981). The lowest detection limits for 'field work' techniques currently in use are about 1.5 mg/kg in liver and 2.2 mg/kg in kidney (Ellis *et al.*, 1981). An alternative method for determination of cadmium concentrations in kidney cortex *in vivo* involves X-ray-generated atomic fluorescence (Ahlgren & Mattsson, 1981; Christoffersson & Mattsson, 1983). Skerfving *et al.* (1987) found the limit of detection of this method to be 17 mg/kg in kidney cortex. The analytical validity of these in-vivo techniques has not been studied sufficiently (WHO, 1992b; see also section 4.1).

1.2 Production and use

1.2.1 *Production*

(a) *Cadmium metal*

Cadmium is often considered to be a metal of the twentieth century: Unlike some other heavy metals, such as lead and mercury which have been used since ancient times, cadmium has been refined and used only relatively recently, and over 65% of the cumulative world production has taken place in the last few decades. After its discovery by Strohmeyer in 1817 as an impurity in zinc carbonate, more than a century elapsed before the metal or its compounds were used to any significant extent, and only in the last 40–50 years have production and consumption risen (Hollander & Carapella, 1978; Schulte-Schrepping & Piscator, 1985). Cadmium is a relatively rare element and is not found in the pure state in nature. Cadmium minerals do not occur in concentrations or quantities sufficient to justify mining them in their own right, and cadmium is almost invariably recovered as a by-product from the processing of sulfide ores of zinc, lead (see IARC, 1987b) and copper (Cadmium Association/Cadmium Council, 1991; WHO, 1992b).

Because cadmium is primarily a by-product of zinc processing, the level of cadmium output has closely followed the pattern of zinc production, little being produced prior to the early 1920s. The subsequent rapid increase corresponded to the commercial development of cadmium electroplating. Worldwide production reached a plateau in the 1970s, but appeared to be increasing again in the 1980s (Table 4). Canada is the largest source of cadmium concentrate; other major suppliers are Australia, Europe, Japan, Mexico, Peru and the USA. Outside of the former USSR (for which only estimates of production are available), Japan is the largest producer of primary refined cadmium, as it treats concentrates from South America and Australia as well as from its own mines. Australia, Belgium, Canada, China, Germany, Italy, Mexico and the USA are also major producers of refined cadmium. An important source of cadmium is the recycling of secondary raw materials, including cadmium-containing products which have become unusable, such as nickel–cadmium batteries (for the monograph on nickel, see IARC, 1990a); cadmium-containing by-products, such as steel industry dust and electroplating sludges; and other types of materials the reprocessing of which has become economically feasible or required by law (Förstner, 1984; Cadmium Association/Cadmium Council, 1991; WHO, 1992b).

Table 4. World production of refined cadmium (tonnes)

Country or region	1980	1981	1982	1983	1984	1987	1988	1989	1990	1991
Algeria	60	65	65	50	50	102	55	46	65	65
Argentina	18	NR	21	19	20	46	46	54	48	50
Australia	1 012	1 031	1 010	1 100	1 200	944	855	696	638	800
Austria	36	55	48	46	45	26	26	49	44	22
Belgium	1 524	1 176	996	800	850	1 308	1 836	1 761	1 956	1 800
Brazil	41	45	73	189	180	214	161	197	200	200
Bulgaria	210	210	200	200	200	250	300	350	309	300
Canada	1 303	1 298	809	1 107	1 200	1 571	1 694	1 620	1 437	1 400
China	250	270	300	300	300	680	750	800	1 000	1 200
Democratic People's Republic of Korea	140	140	100	100	100	100	100	100	100	100
Finland	581	621	566	616	600	690	703	612	568	593
France	789	663	793	540	500	457	558	790	780	700
Germany	1 210	1 208	1 046	1 111	1 116	1 143	1 189	1 234	990	1 105
India	89	113	131	131	120	214	237	275	277	280
Italy	568	489	475	450	400	320	705	770	665	734
Japan	2 173	1 977	2 034	2 214	2 400	2 450	2 614	2 694	2 451	2 889
Mexico	778	590	607	642	650	935	1 117	976	882	900
Namibia	69	NR	110	25	25	51	106	88	75	75
Netherlands	455	518	497	521	525	517	563	505	590	549
Norway	130	117	104	117	110	147	169	206	286	236
Peru	172	307	421	451	460	351	303	352	265	350
Poland	698	580	570	570	570	620	642	485	373	350
Republic of Korea	365	300	320	320	300	NR	490	500	500	450
Romania	85	85	80	80	80	75	75	70	62	60
Spain	309	303	286	278	250	297	438	361	355	350
United Kingdom	375	278	354	340	340	498	399	395	438	449
USA	1 578	1 603	1 007	1 052	1 686	1 515	1 885	1 550	1 678	1 676
Former USSR	2 850	2 900	2 900	3 000	3 000	3 000	3 000	3 000	2 800	2 500
Former Yugoslavia	201	208	174	48	100	305	405	471	362	280
Zaire	168	230	281	308	310	299	281	224	213	120
Total[a]	18 238	17 381	16 378	16 725	17 687	19 169	21 761	21 325	20 493	20 673

From Plunkert (1985) for 1980–84; Llewellyn (1992) for 1987–91; some figures are estimates. NR, not reported
[a]Totals do not add up because they have been revised.

Figure 1 summarizes the individual steps in the process and their combination for the production of cadmium metal. The flue dust on which volatile cadmium collects when zinc, copper and lead ores are heated in air is the primary starting material for cadmium recovery and refining. This dust must usually be recirculated in order to obtain high concentrations of cadmium. If the primary flue dust is reduced in a rotary oven, lead and zinc remain, while the cadmium is volatilized and enriched in the secondary flue dust (Schulte-Schrepping & Piscator, 1985).

Fig. 1. Processes for the production of cadmium metal

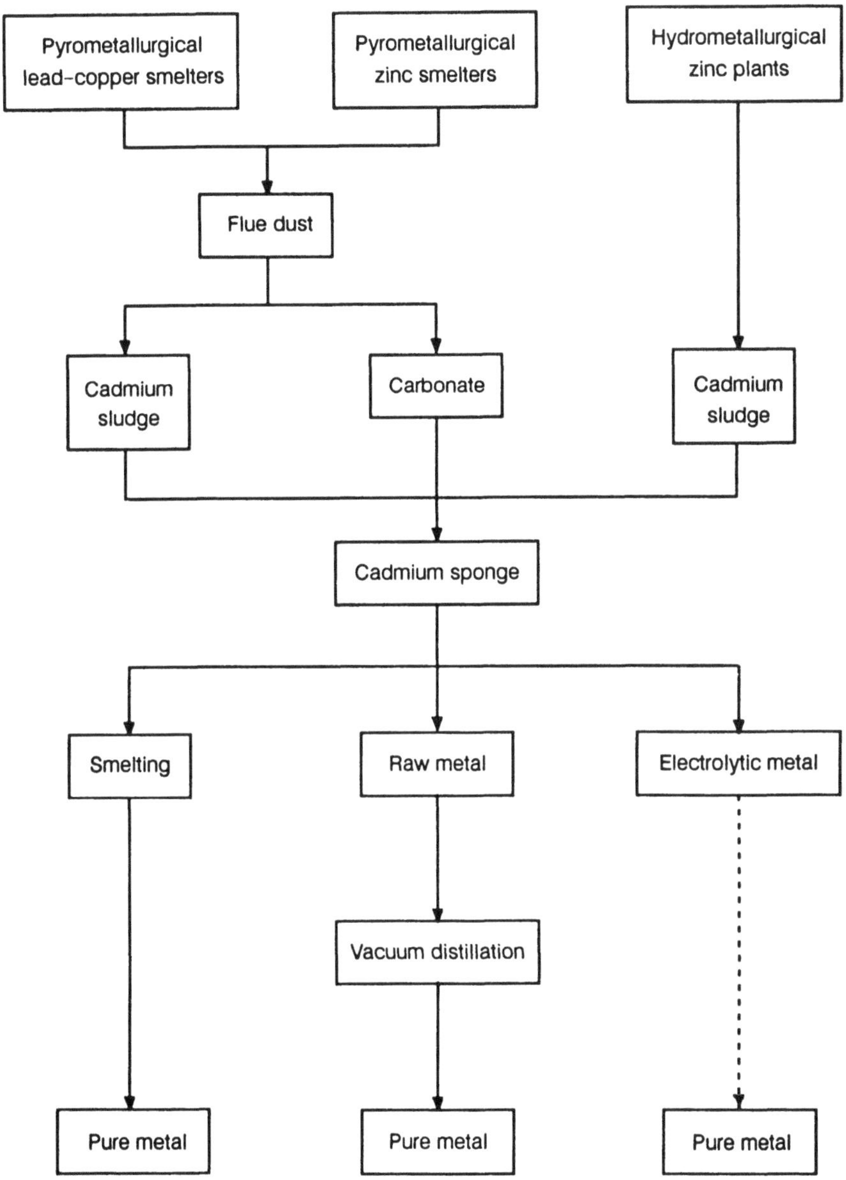

From Schulte-Schrepping & Piscator (1985)

Zinc metal can be produced by either pyrometallurgical or electrolytic processes, and cadmium is recovered and refined at a number of stages. In one type of pyrometallurgical process, complex lead–zinc ores are refined by the Imperial smelting process. When the concentrate is roasted at 700–1200 °C in sintering furnaces, cadmium-containing flue dust and fume are produced. This is leached in a sulfuric acid solution, and the cadmium is subsequently precipitated as cadmium carbonate, which is dried and refined by distillation to cadmium metal. The cadmium in secondary raw materials, after enrichment in a special furnace, can be added to the concentrate and processed at the same time (Schulte-Schrepping & Piscator, 1985; Cadmium Association/Cadmium Council, 1991).

In hydrometallurgical zinc refining, cadmium-containing zinc concentrate is leached with sulfuric acid, and cadmium is removed from the solution together with copper by reduction with zinc dust, to give a metallic sludge. These cadmium sludges are the most important starting materials for cadmium refining today (Schulte-Schrepping & Piscator, 1985).

In electrolytic processes, the zinc concentrate is also roasted under oxidizing conditions to remove the sulfur, usually in fluidized bed roasters which produce a fine calcine suitable for acid leaching. The calcine is dissolved in sulfuric acid in a leaching plant, then neutralized to precipitate any iron. The bulk of the cadmium is precipitated from the sulfate solution during the second zinc dust stage and the remainder in the third stage. The cadmium precipitate is filtered and forms a cake containing about 25% cadmium, 50% zinc and small amounts of copper and lead; the cake is redissolved in sulfuric acid. A reasonably pure cadmium sponge is produced after two additional acid solution/zinc dust precipitation stages. The sponge is again dissolved in sulfuric acid, and the solution is passed into electrolytic cells where the cadmium is deposited on cathodes. The cathodes are then removed and stripped, and the cadmium is melted and cast into required shapes; it is typically 99.99% pure (Cadmium Association/Cadmium Council, 1991).

(b) Cadmium alloys

Cadmium can be combined with a number of other nonferrous metals to form alloys with useful commercial properties. Typically, metallic cadmium is added to the molten metal(s) with which it is to be alloyed and, after thorough mixing, the resultant alloy is cast into the desired form (ingot, wire, rod). Depending on the alloy and its application, the cadmium content ranges from < 0.1 to 15%. To facilitate mixing, a master alloy containing much higher levels of cadmium may be prepared first and added to the molten alloying metal (Hollander & Carapella, 1978; Holden, 1982).

(c) Cadmium acetate

Cadmium acetate is produced by the reaction of acetic acid with cadmium metal or oxide, or by treating cadmium nitrate with acetic anhydride. The dihydrate is obtained by dissolving cadmium metal or oxide in acetic acid, followed by crystallization. Calcination of the dihydrate can be controlled to yield cadmium acetate monohydrate and the anhydrous acetate (Parker, 1978; Budavari, 1989).

(d) Cadmium chloride

Cadmium chloride is produced by reacting molten cadmium with chlorine gas at 600 °C or by dissolving cadmium metal or the oxide, carbonate, sulfide or hydroxide in hydrochloric acid (see IARC, 1992), and subsequently vaporizing the solution to produce a hydrated crystal. In order to prepare the anhydrous salt, the hydrate is refluxed with thionyl chloride or calcined in a hydrogen chloride atmosphere. It may also be obtained by the addition of dry cadmium acetate to a mixture of glacial acetic acid and acetyl chloride or by distillation from a mixture of cadmium nitrate tetrahydrate in hot concentrated hydrochloric acid (Parker, 1978; Schulte-Schrepping & Piscator, 1985; Sax & Lewis, 1987).

(e) Cadmium hydroxide

Cadmium hydroxide has been prepared by the addition of a solution of cadmium nitrate to boiling sodium or potassium hydroxide (Parker, 1978). It has also been produced by the action of sodium hydroxide on a cadmium salt solution (Sax & Lewis, 1987).

(f) Cadmium nitrate

Cadmium nitrate has been produced by the action of nitric acid on cadmium metal or cadmium oxide, hydroxide or carbonate (Parker, 1978; Schulte-Schrepping & Piscator, 1985; Sax & Lewis, 1987).

(g) Cadmium oxide

Cadmium oxide is produced by the reaction of cadmium metal vapour with air. Pure cadmium metal is melted in a cast-iron or steel kettle and pumped to a heated chamber, where it is vaporized. The vapour is conducted to a reactor, and air is blown through, oxidizing the cadmium and carrying the reaction product into a 'baghouse'. Finer or coarser particles are produced, depending on the ratio of air to cadmium vapour. Cadmium oxide can also be obtained by thermal decomposition of cadmium nitrate or carbonate or by oxidation of molten cadmium by an oxidizing agent (Parker, 1978; Schulte-Schrepping & Piscator, 1985). Cadmium oxide is generated as either a dust or fume, depending on how it is produced.

(h) Cadmium stearate

Cadmium stearate, one of the cadmium alkanoate salts used as polyvinyl chloride stabilizers, is prepared by the addition of sodium stearate to a solution of cadmium chloride. The cadmium salt precipitates from solution and is filtered, washed and dried. Other salts (laurate, myristate, palmitate) are prepared in analogous reactions (Parker, 1978).

(i) Cadmium sulfate

The principal cadmium sulfates are $CdSO_4$, $CdSO_4.H_2O$ [13477-20-8] and $3CdSO_4.8H_2O$ [7790-84-3]. They are crystallized from cadmium sulfate solutions or can be precipitated by addition of ethanol. Anhydrous cadmium sulfate is prepared by oxidation of the sulfide or sulfite at elevated temperatures, or by the action of dimethyl sulfate on finely powdered cadmium nitrate, halides, oxide or carbonate. Solutions are prepared by dissolving cadmium metal, oxide, sulfide, hydroxide or carbonate in sulfuric acid. Anhydrous cadmium sulfate is also produced by melting cadmium with ammonium or sodium peroxodisulfate. Cadmium sulfate monohydrate, which is the form usually marketed, is produced by evaporating a cadmium sulfate solution above 41.5 °C (Parker, 1978; Schulte-Schrepping & Piscator, 1985).

(j) *Cadmium sulfide*

Cadmium sulfide can be prepared by the reaction between hydrogen sulfide and cadmium vapour at 800 °C, or by heating a mixture of cadmium or cadmium oxide with sulfur. Usually, the sulfides are precipitated from aqueous solutions of cadmium salts by adding hydrogen sulfide or a soluble sulfide such as sodium sulfide. Cadmium sulfide can also be prepared by passing hydrogen sulfide gas into a solution of a cadmium salt acidified with hydrochloric acid; the precipitate is filtered and dried. It also occurs naturally as the mineral greenockite. The dimorphic sulfide, CdS, is the most widely used cadmium compound. The β form can be transformed to the α form by heating at 750 °C in a sulfur atmosphere. Both forms can be prepared in colours ranging from lemon-yellow through orange and red, depending on the method of preparation and particle size (Parker, 1978; Sax & Lewis, 1987).

1.2.2 *Use*

Typical use patterns for cadmium and its compounds and alloys in several industrialized countries are presented in Table 5.

Table 5. Patterns of use of cadmium in several industrialized countries (%)

Use category	1970[a]	1973[a]	1976[a]	1979[a]	1982[a]	1990[b]
Coating and plating	37	30	36.5	34	29	8
Batteries	8	15	21.5	23	28.5	55
Pigments	24	30	25	27	24	20
Stabilizers for PVC	23	17	12	12	12	10
Alloys and other uses	8	8	5	4	6.5	7

[a]From Schulte-Schrepping & Piscator (1985); figures are based on totals of published statistics for Germany, Japan, the United Kingdom and the USA.
[b]From Cadmium Association/Cadmium Council (1991); figures are for Belgium, France, Germany, Japan, the United Kingdom and the USA.

(a) *Cadmium*

Cadmium has a limited number of principal applications, but within the range the metal, its alloys and compounds are used in a large variety of consumer and industrial materials. The principal applications of cadmium fall into five categories: active electrode material in nickel–cadmium batteries; pigments used mainly in plastics, ceramics and glasses; to stabilize polyvinyl chloride (PVC) against heat and light; engineering coatings on steel and some nonferrous metals; and as a component of various specialized alloys. Detailed statistics on use are available for only a limited number of countries, but these indicate that the pattern of use varies considerably from country to country (Cadmium Association/Cadmium Council, 1991; WHO, 1992a).

Japan is by far the largest user of cadmium, followed by the USA, Belgium, the United Kingdom, France and Germany. Worldwide consumption of cadmium for all uses in 1990 was estimated to have been 18 500 tonnes. The cadmium compounds of greatest commercial importance are cadmium oxide and cadmium sulfide; other important compounds are the hydroxide, chloride, nitrate, sulfate and stearate (adapted from Cadmium Association/Cadmium Council, 1991).

Examination of the reported trends in cadmium consumption over the last 25 years reveals considerable change in the relative importance of the major applications. The use of cadmium for engineering coatings and electroplating represents the most striking decrease; in 1960, this sector accounted for over half the cadmium consumed worldwide, but in 1985 its share was less than 25%. The decline is usually linked to the widespread introduction of progressively more stringent limits on effluents from plating works and, more recently, to the introduction of restrictions on certain cadmium products in some European countries. In contrast, the use of cadmium in batteries has shown considerable growth in recent years, from only 8% of the total market in 1970 to 37% by 1985. The use of cadmium in batteries is particularly important in Japan, where it represented over 75% of total consumption in 1985 (WHO, 1992b).

Of the remaining applications of cadmium, pigments and stabilizers are the most important, accounting for 22 and 12%, respectively, of total world consumption in 1985. The share of the market represented by cadmium pigments remained relatively stable between 1970 and 1985, but use of the metal in stabilizers during the period showed a considerable decline, largely as a result of economic factors. The use of cadmium as a constituent of alloys is relatively small and has also declined in importance in recent years: it accounted for about 4% of total cadmium use in 1985 (WHO, 1992b).

(b) *Cadmium alloys* (from Cadmium Association/Cadmium Council, 1991, unless otherwise specified)

Cadmium forms many binary and more complex alloys, which have useful properties for many commercial applications. Most commercial alloys containing cadmium fall into two major groups, where:

(i) the presence of cadmium improves some feature of the alloy. Small amounts of cadmium can improve hardness and wear resistance, mechanical strength, fatigue strength, castability and electrochemical properties. Cadmium is added principally to alloys based on copper, tin, lead and zinc, although several others benefit from its presence.

(ii) lower melting-points are obtained. Such alloys range from low-melting-point eutectic ('fusible') alloys to high-melting-point non-eutectic alloys used in metal joining.

Cadmium–copper alloys, which have almost twice the mechanical strength and wear resistance of pure copper yet still retain 90% of its conductivity, contain 0.8–1.2% cadmium. The major uses of such alloys are in telephone wires, wiring for railway overhead electrification, conductors for flexible telephone cords, special cables for military and aerospace uses and electrical components such as contact strips and electric blanket and heating-pad elements (Ricksecker, 1979).

Zinc alloys containing 0.1% cadmium improve the mechanical properties of rolled, drawn or extruded zinc. Zinc alloys containing cadmium in the range of 0.025 to 0.15% are used in anodes to protect structural steelwork immersed in seawater against corrosion.

Lead alloys with up to 0.075% cadmium are sometimes used as sheaths for cables subject to cyclic stress.

Tin-based white metal-bearing alloys with up to 1% cadmium have adequate tensile and fatigue strength for use in marine engines and gearboxes.

Precious metal alloys for jewellery incorporate cadmium for improved hardness and strength. Levels of up to 5% cadmium in gold–silver–copper alloys make Greek gold, a greenish-tinged gold.

Silver electric contacts incorporating 10–15% cadmium or cadmium oxide are useful in many heavy duty electrical applications, such as relays, switches and thermostats.

A *tin–lead–bismuth–cadmium alloy*, which melts at 70 °C, is more commonly known as Woods metal and is used in the bonding of metallized ceramic and glass components to metal frames and chassis, where higher soldering temperatures are not possible. The presence of Woods metal in water sprinkler valves automatically activates the water supply when the local temperature exceeds 70 °C, when it melts.

Cadmium alloyed with silver, zinc or tin makes excellent solders, with tensile strengths two to three times greater than most common solders in the same temperature range. Cadmium is an important component in quaternary alloys with silver, copper and zinc in the lower temperature range of brazing alloys.

The low melting-points and rapid fusing or solidifying characteristics of *low-temperature fusible alloys* containing cadmium lead to a variety of uses. Heat-sensitive fusible links in fire safety devices or kilns and ovens can activate control mechanisms when they melt at specific temperatures. The alloys are used to mount glass lenses firmly during grinding operations.

(c) *Cadmium acetate*

Cadmium acetate is the starting material for cadmium halides and is a colourant in glass, ceramics (iridescent glazes) and textiles. It is also used in electroplating baths, as a laboratory reagent and in the separation of mercaptans from crude oils and gasolines (Greene, 1974; Parker, 1978; Sax & Lewis, 1987).

(d) *Cadmium chloride*

Cadmium chloride is used in electroplating. The significance of cadmium chloride as a commercial product is declining; however, it occurs as an intermediate in the production of cadmium-containing stabilizers and pigments, which are often obtained from cadmium chloride solutions, themselves obtained from cadmium metal, oxide, hydroxide or carbonate. It is also used in the preparation of cadmium sulfide, in analytical chemistry, in photography, in dyeing and calico printing, in the manufacture of special mirrors and of cadmium yellow, in the vacuum tube industry and as a lubricant (Schulte-Schrepping & Piscator, 1985; Sax & Lewis, 1987; Budavari, 1989).

(e) *Cadmium hydroxide*

Cadmium hydroxide is a component of cadmium–nickel and silver–cadmium batteries. It often replaces the oxide as the starting material for other cadmium compounds (Parker, 1978; Schulte-Schrepping & Piscator, 1985; Cadmium Association/Cadmium Council, 1991).

(f) *Cadmium nitrate*

Cadmium nitrate is the preferred starting material for cadmium hydroxide; it is also used in photographic emulsions (Budavari, 1989; Parker, 1978) and in colouring glass and porcelain (Schulte-Schrepping & Piscator, 1985; Sax & Lewis, 1987).

(g) *Cadmium stearate*

Cadmium stearate is commonly used in combination with other salts to retard the degradation processes which occur in PVC and related polymers on exposure to heat and ultraviolet light (sunlight). The stabilizers consist of mixtures of barium, lead and organic cadmium salts, usually cadmium stearate or cadmium laurate, which are incorporated into the PVC before processing and which arrest any degradation reactions as soon as they occur. They ensure that PVC develops good initial colour and clarity and allow high processing temperatures to be employed; they also ensure longer service life.

Barium–cadmium stabilizers typically contain 1–15% cadmium and usually constitute about 0.5–2.5% of the final PVC compound. They are incorporated into PVC used, for example, in rigid profiles for window and door frames, water and drain pipes, hoses and electrical insulation (Parker, 1978; Cadmium Association/Cadmium Council, 1991).

(h) *Cadmium sulfate*

Cadmium sulfate is used in electroplating and as a starting material for pigments, stabilizers and other cadmium compounds that can be precipitated from aqueous solution. It is also used to produce fluorescent materials, in analytical chemistry and as a nematocide. Cadmium sulfate solution is a component of Weston cells (portable standards for electromagnetic frequency) (Schulte-Schrepping & Piscator, 1985; Sax & Lewis, 1987; Budavari, 1989).

(i) *Cadmium sulfide*

The main use of cadmium sulfide is for pigments. Pure yellow cadmium sulfides are formulated with red cadmium selenides in varying proportions to make chemically pure toners ranging from yellows and oranges with a low selenium content to reds and maroons with a high selenium content. Cadmium colourants are used in special paints (especially artists' colours, such as cadmium yellow), for colouring textiles, paper, rubber, plastics, glasses and ceramic glazes and in fireworks. Red and yellow cadmium sulfide–zinc sulfide fluorescent and phosphorescent pigments are also produced. Cadmium sulfide is used in the conversion of solar energy to electrical power. Its photoconductive and electroluminescent properties have been applied not only in photocells but also in a wide variety of phosphors, light amplifiers, radiation detectors, thin film transistors and diodes, electron beam-pumped lasers and household smoke detectors (Parker, 1978; Sax & Lewis, 1987; Budavari, 1989).

(j) Cadmium oxide

The main use of cadmium oxide is in the manufacture of nickel–cadmium batteries. In the first step in the preparation of negative electrodes (paste preparation), cadmium oxide is hydrated to form a paste of cadmium hydroxide. The dried paste is then mixed with graphite, iron oxide and paraffin, milled and finally compacted between rollers (Malcolm, 1983; Adams, 1992).

Cadmium oxide is used as a starting material for PVC heat stabilizers and for other inorganic cadmium compounds. It is also used as a catalyst in oxidation–reduction reactions, dehydrogenation, cleavage, polymerization, the production of saturated alcohols, hydrogenation of unsaturated fatty acids and as a mixed catalyst component to produce methanol from carbon monoxide and water. Further uses are in resistant enamels, metal coatings for plastics, heat-resistant plastics and selenium ruby glass. Cadmium oxide combined with an alkali-metal cyanide is the salt mixture used in baths for cadmium electroplating. High-purity cadmium oxide is used as a second depolarizer (in addition to silver oxide) in silver–zinc storage batteries. It is temperature resistant and, together with silver, useful in heavy-duty electrical contacts. In veterinary medicine, it has been used as a nematocide, vermicide and ascaricide in swine (Parker, 1978; Schulte-Schrepping & Piscator, 1985; Sax & Lewis, 1987; Budavari, 1989; Cadmium Association/Cadmium Council, 1991).

Other cadmium compounds used industrially include: cadmium cyanide (electroplating), cadmium carbonate (starting material for pigments), cadmium arsenides (electronic devices), cadmium selenide (photocells, luminous paints, colourant in glass), cadmium telluride (photocells, infra-red optics) and cadmium tungstate (X-ray screens, phosphors) (Parker, 1978; Schulte-Schrepping & Piscator, 1985).

1.3 Occurrence

1.3.1 *Natural occurrence*

Cadmium is widely but sparsely distributed over the Earth's surface; it is found most commonly as the mineral greenockite (cadmium sulfide) and in weathered ores such as otavite (cadmium carbonate). Other minerals that contain cadmium are hawleyite (cadmium sulfide), xanthocroite (cadmium sulfide hydrate), cadmoselite (cadmium selenide) and monteponite (cadmium oxide). It occurs in nature associated mainly with zinc but also with lead or copper; in minerals and ores, cadmium and zinc are present typically in a ratio of 1:100 to 1:1000 (Fairbridge, 1974; Alessio *et al.*, 1983; Förstner, 1984).

Cadmium is a relatively rare element, comprising about 0.1–0.5 mg/kg of the Earth's crust; however, higher concentrations (15 mg/kg) are present in some sedimentary rocks. Trace quantities of cadmium can also be found in fossil fuels and oils (Bowen, 1966; WHO, 1992a,b).

1.3.2 *Occupational exposure*

Workers may be exposed to cadmium and cadmium compounds in a variety of occupational settings (Table 6). The major sources of such exposure are smelting and refining of zinc, lead and copper ores, electroplating, manufacture of cadmium alloys and of pigments and plastic stabilizers, production of nickel–cadmium batteries and welding.

Table 6. Occupations in which there is potential exposure to cadmium and cadmium compounds

Alloy production[a]
Battery production[a]
Brazing
Coating
Diamond cutting
Dry colour formulation
Electroplating
Electrical contacts production
Enamelling
Engraving
Glasswork
Laser cutting
Metallizing
Paint production and use
Pesticide production and use
Phosphorus production
Pigment production and use[a]
Plastics production[a]
Plating
Printing
Semiconductor and superconductor production
Sensors production
Smelting and refining[a]
Solar cells production
Soldering
Stabilizer production
Textile printing
Thin film production
Transistors production
Welding[a]

[a]Activities in which risk is highest because atmospheric concentrations of cadmium can be high and because the number of workers employed is relevant (modified from Odone *et al.*, 1983)

It has been estimated that about 510 000 workers in the USA are exposed to cadmium (Thun *et al.*, 1991). In 1987, an estimated 210 000 workers were exposed to concentrations equal to or greater than 1 $\mu g/m^3$; 65% were exposed to concentrations of 1–39 $\mu g/m^3$, 21% to 40–99 $\mu g/m^3$ and 14% to concentrations greater than 100 $\mu g/m^3$ (US National Toxicology Program, 1991). Airborne concentrations of cadmium found in occupational settings vary considerably according to the type of industry and to specific working conditions. Cadmium oxide fumes are generated at high temperatures (US Occupational Safety and Health Administration, 1992) and can be absorbed very efficiently through the lung, while deposition and absorption of dust of different cadmium compounds depends on particle size (Alessio *et al.*, 1983; Thun *et al.*, 1991). Improvements in occupational hygiene have led to a progressive reduction in the concentrations of cadmium in occupational environments, and 5–20 µg/m^3 can now be achieved (Hassler et al., 1983; Friberg et al., 1986a; US Occupational Safety and Health Administration, 1992).

Data on exposure to cadmium and cadmium compounds and the results of biological monitoring in different occupational situations are summarized below. Occupational exposure to cadmium can be assessed both by ambient air monitoring ('external dose') and by biological monitoring ('internal dose'). Individual external doses can be measured only by personal sampling of ambient air; individual uptake is estimated by biological monitoring of cadmium in blood and urine (Alessio et al., 1983; Ghezzi et al., 1985; see also section 4.1).

(a) Cadmium production and refining

Smith et al. (1980) made a detailed assessment of exposures to cadmium in a production facility in the USA where cadmium metal had been refined and cadmium compounds, such as cadmium oxide and yellow cadmium pigment, had been produced since 1925. An epidemiological study carried out at the plant (Thun et al., 1985) is described on pp. 152–153. Exposure to cadmium oxide dusts occurred during sampling, loading and transport of dust between the roasting, mixing and calcining operations and during loading of purified oxide. Exposure to cadmium oxide fume occurred in roaster, calcining, retort and foundry operations. Exposure to cadmium sulfate mist occurred during solution and tankhouse operations. The concentrations of cadmium differed substantially between the departments and with time. The highest exposures (1500 µg/m^3) were estimated to have occurred in the mixing and retort areas prior to 1950 and in the calcining area prior to 1960. Estimates of exposures by inhalation, based on historical data derived from area monitoring and adjusted to reflect actual exposures of workers wearing respirators, were 200–1500 µg/m^3 before 1950 and 40–600 µg/m^3 during 1965–76. In 1946, an average concentration of 18 900 µg/m^3 was reported during grinding of cadmium sulfide and 31 300 µg/m^3 in the cadmium sulfide packaging room (Princi, 1947); cadmium concentrations in the solution room were approximately 3000 µg/m^3 before 1955, 1500 µg/m^3 in 1955–64 and 150 µg/m^3 subsequently (Thun et al., 1985; Commission of the European Communities, 1991a,b).

At a zinc–lead–cadmium smelter in the United Kingdom, mean airborne cadmium concentrations were 80 µg/m^3 in the cadmium plant and 200 µg/m^3 in the sintering plant before 1970, whereas a mean level of 15 µg/m^3 was measured in each department in 1977. These assessments were considered to be accurate within a factor of 2–5. Urinary cadmium concentrations ranged from a geometric mean of 2.5 nmol/mmol creatinine [2.5 µg/g creatinine] for workers in the sinter area to 6.3 nmol/mmol creatinine (6.3 µg/g creatinine) for workers in the cadmium plant. [Some of the workers were exposed to cadmium sulfate and cadmium sulfide, but cadmium oxide is the compound to which they were most likely to have been exposed predominantly.] Copper and, from time to time, arsenic had also been refined in the plant (Kazantzis & Armstrong, 1983; Ades & Kazantzis, 1988). Epidemiological studies at the smelter are described on pp. 154–156.

Concentrations of cadmium were measured in the blood and urine of workers employed at two cadmium-producing factories and at a nickel–cadmium battery plant in Belgium. The cadmium content of the airborne respirable dust was usually below 90 µg/m^3. In 96 workers without kidney damage, the mean urinary concentration of cadmium was 16.3 ± 1.7

(SE) μg/g creatinine and that in blood was 21.4 ± 1.9 μg/L. In 25 workers with kidney lesions, the levels were 48.2 ± 8.5 μg/g creatinine and 38.8 ± 7.7 μg/L, respectively (Lauwerys *et al.*, 1976).

Airborne cadmium concentrations of 2500–6500 μg/m^3 in the crushing and roasting area, 10 800–23 300 μg/m^3 in the dry smelting area, 10–160 μg/m^3 in the cadmium melting area and 2800–4700 μg/m^3 in the ingot making area were measured in 1988 at a Chinese plant which employed about 10 000 workers; 358 were employed in those areas (Nomiyama *et al.*, 1992).

As part of an epidemiological study of Chinese smelter workers (see p. 156), Ding *et al.* (1987) reported a mean air concentration of 186 μg/m^3 in the cadmium shop, where workers were exposed to cadmium oxide, and 14 μg/m^3 in the sintering shop. The concentrations in the cadmium shop were reported to have been much higher (535 μg/m^3) prior to 1980.

(b) *Cadmium–copper and silver–cadmium alloy production*

In two plants for the production of cadmium–copper alloys in the United Kingdom, mean exposure concentrations of cadmium oxide as cadmium were 38–106 μg/m^3 in 1953 in one factory (Bonnell *et al.*, 1959) and 13–89 μg/m^3 in the rocker furnace area in the other factory (King, 1955). Concentrations of cadmium oxide were reported to have been at least 1000 μg/m^3 prior to 1953, up to 150 μg/m^3 between 1953 and 1957 and approximately 50 μg/m^3 subsequently (Holden, 1980a,b). Similar levels (mean, 130 μg/m^3) were reported in the 1960s at a Japanese silver–cadmium alloy factory (Tsuchiya, 1967).

In an Italian cadmium alloy plant in 1982, mean concentrations of 67 μg/m^3 and 28 μg/m^3 were detected using personal samplers in two foundries in the same factory; during alloy processing, 3 μg/m^3 were measured. Atmospheric concentrations of cadmium of up to 1500 μg/m^3 were measured with area samplers in 1975 (Ghezzi *et al.*, 1985).

As part of an epidemiological study of copper–cadmium alloy workers in Sweden (see pp. 151–152), the concentration of cadmium in cadmium oxide fumes was reported to be 100–400 μg/m^3 during the 1960s and 50 μg/m^3 during the 1970s (Kjellström *et al.*, 1979).

(c) *Battery manufacture*

Although the oxide is the form of cadmium used as the raw material in the manufacture of nickel–cadmium batteries, it is converted to cadmium hydroxide during the process. No information was available in the studies described below about which species of cadmium workers were actually exposed to. Exposures to nickel during the manufacture of nickel–cadmium batteries were described in a previous monograph (IARC, 1990a).

In a nickel–cadmium battery factory in Singapore, atmospheric, urinary and blood concentrations of cadmium were measured. The highest geometric mean atmospheric concentration (870 μg/m^3) was detected during spot welding; measurements during the period 1973–80 showed levels of 31–2900 μg/m^3. The geometric mean concentration of cadmium in blood was 75.2 μg/L for 41 women and 40.4 μg/L for six men; the geometric means in urine were 66.0 and 22.9 μg/g creatinine, respectively. The highest concentrations were detected in the subgroup of spot welders (Chan *et al.*, 1982).

The average concentrations of cadmium in a battery factory in the United Kingdom in 1957 were 500 μg/m^3 in the plate-making department and 100 μg/m^3 in the assembly department (Adams *et al.*, 1969). In a nickel–cadmium battery factory in the United Kingdom, in which an epidemiological stdy was conducted (see pp. 149–150), the air concentration of cadmium in plate-making and assembly shops was 600–2800 µg/m^3 in 1949. After installation of local exhaust ventilation in 1950, concentrations were reduced to less than 500 µg/m^3 in most parts of the factory. After further improvements in the ventilation systems and the building of new departments in 1975, the levels were below 50 µg/m^3 (Sorahan & Waterhouse, 1983).

In a Swedish nickel–cadmium battery factory, where a series of epidemiological studies were carried out (see pp. 150–151), the concentration of cadmium was about 1000 µg/m^3 before 1947 but decreased gradually thereafter, to about 300 µg/m^3 in 1947–62 and 50 µg/m^3 in 1962–74. After 1975, 20 µg/m^3 was seldom exceeded (Adamsson, 1979; Elinder *et al.*, 1985). In 1977 in the same factory, the arithmetic mean concentration of cadmium in workroom air, based on 181 observations, was 7.6 µg/m^3; the arithmetic mean concentration in samples from 18 workers was 14.1 µg/L in blood and 4.9 µg/g creatinine in urine (Hassler *et al.*, 1983).

(d) Polyvinyl chloride compounding

A study was carried out in eight PVC production factories in Singapore where cadmium compounds were used as thermal stabilizers in liquid form or as cadmium stearate powder. A geometric mean concentration of 100 µg/m^3 cadmium was measured in the mixing area of one plant, where maintenance and work practices were poor; and < 10 µg/m^3 in the other seven plants. Geometric mean concentrations in samples from 53 male workers were 0.78 ± 2.9 µg/g creatinine in urine and 2.25 ± 2.51 µg/L in blood (Chan *et al.*, 1982).

(e) Pigment manufacture

Concentrations of cadmium in respirable dust were measured in 1976 and 1977 in a small Australian plant producing cadmium selenosulfide and cadmium sulfide pigments; exposure to cadmium carbonate also occurred. All time-weighted average exposures in the furnace, crushing–cleaning and general duties areas were greater than 1000 µg/m^3 in 1977; about 50% of the dust particles were in the respirable range. Biological monitoring of nine workers was begun in 1976: concentrations of < 0.5–32 µg/L were found for urinary cadmium and 6–54 µg/L for blood cadmium (De Silva & Donnan, 1981).

In a Japanese factory for the manufacture of cadmium pigments, cadmium sulfide and cadmium selenide, the arithmetic mean atmospheric concentrations of cadmium in seven areas of the plant in 1986 ranged from 3 to 350 µg/m^3; the highest values were found in the canning area. The geometric mean urinary cadmium concentrations in nine subjects who worked in the canning area were 1.7 (0.5–5.8) µg/g creatinine in April 1986 and 2.3 (1.3–4.1) µg/g creatinine in September 1986 (Kawada *et al.*, 1989).

(f) Soldering

One limited investigation in the United Kingdom indicated air concentrations of cadmium in excess of 50 µg/m^3 in five firms involved in the small specialized trade for both the manufacture and repair of metal frames (jigs), which entails soldering with cadmium-containing electrodes in small workrooms without exhaust ventilation. All 32 workers with more than five years of exposure and 11 of 21 with fewer than five years of exposure had 'raised' blood and urinary concentrations of cadmium; 30 had urinary cadmium concentrations in excess of 10 nmol/mmol (μg/g) creatinine (Smith *et al.*, 1986).

(g) *Other*

A biological monitoring programme was conducted between 1980 and 1989, involving 919 workers employed in 16 different cadmium-processing industries in The Netherlands. The main industrial processes included in the survey were metal recycling, alloy production, enamelling, printing, production of coloured plastics, stabilizers, paints and pigments, electroplating and manufacture of cathode-ray tubes. The cadmium compounds to which workers were exposed included the oxide, chloride, carbonate, laurate, cyanide, sulfate and phosphate. Urinary cadmium concentrations ranged from 0 to 60.4 μg/g creatinine and those in blood from 0 to 48.4 μg/L. The highest concentrations were measured in workers using silver–cadmium solder (Zwennis & Franssen, 1992).

1.3.3 *Air*

Most of the cadmium that occurs in air is associated with particulate matter in the respirable range. Cadmium oxide is presumed to constitute a large proportion of airborne cadmium, but, in principle, other cadmium salts, such as cadmium chloride, used as stabilizers and pigments in plastics, could enter the environment, especially during incineration. Atmospheric emissions of cadmium from man-made sources exceed those of natural origin by one order of magnitude (UNEP, 1984, 1992). Traditional municipal solid-waste incinerators may make a significant contribution to the concentration of cadmium in ambient air and to its deposition rates. The rates of emission of cadmium from incinerators in Europe, Canada and the USA ranged from 20 to 2000 μg/m^3 from the stacks of traditional incinerators and from 10 to 40 μg/m^3 from advanced incinerators. Such emissions could result in deposition rates of 1–40 and 0.02–0.8 μg/m^2 per day, respectively (WHO, 1988). Cadmium sulfate also occurs in atmospheric emissions from thermal processes involving cadmium (IARC, 1976; Friberg *et al.*, 1985, 1986b).

Estimated emissions of cadmium to the atmosphere from natural and human sources are shown in Table 7. In both the European Economic Community and worldwide, 10–15% of total airborne emissions arise from natural processes, volcanic action being one of the major sources (WHO, 1992a,b). Mean global emission rates were estimated in 1983 to be 1000 tonnes cadmium per year from natural sources and 7570 tonnes from human sources (Nriagu & Pacyna, 1988).

In many countries, cadmium concentrations in the atmosphere are monitored regularly. In European countries, average values were 0.001–0.005 μg/m^3 in rural areas, 0.005–0.015 in urban areas and up to 0.05 μg/m^3 in industrialized areas. Concentrations of 0.003–0.023 μg/m^3 were found in urban areas of the USA, and 0.003–0.0063 μg/m^3 cadmium have been measured in urban areas in Japan (Friberg *et al.*, 1974, 1985, 1986b; WHO, 1992b). Higher concentrations of cadmium have been detected in areas close to atmospheric sources of the metal, such as cadmium-related industries. The nonferrous metal industry accounts for the largest fraction of cadmium emitted (Nriagu & Pacyna, 1988). Fluctuations in the data occur as a result of changing emission characteristics and weather conditions (WHO, 1992b).

Table 7. Estimated atmospheric emissions of cadmium (tonnes/year) from natural and human sources

Source	European Economic Community	Worldwide
Natural source	20	800
Nonferrous metal production		
Mining	NR	0.6–3
Zinc and cadmium	20	920–4600
Copper	6	1700–3400
Lead	7	39–195
Secondary production	NR	2.3–3.6
Iron and steel production	34	28–284
Fossil fuel combustion		
Coal	6	176–882
Oil	0.5	41–246
Refuse incineration	31	56–1400
Sewage sludge incineration	2	3–36
Phosphate fertilizer manufacture	NR	68–274
Cement manufacture	NR	8.9–534
Wood combustion	NR	60–180
Total	130	3900–12 800

Modified from WHO (1992a,b). NR, not reported

In Sweden, weekly mean levels of 0.3 μg/m^3 were recorded 500 m from a factory where cadmium–copper alloys were used. In Japan, a mean level of 0.2 μg/m^3 was recorded 400 m from a zinc smelter (Friberg et al., 1971). In Colorado (USA), the mean annual airborne concentration of cadmium in an area about 1 km from a zinc smelter was 0.023 μg/m^3 (Wysowski et al., 1978).

1.3.4 Water

Cadmium enters the aquatic environment from numerous diffuse and point sources and by different routes. At the global level, the smelting of nonferrous metal ores has been estimated to be the largest human source of cadmium released into the aquatic environment (Nriagu & Pacyna, 1988). The cadmium content of ore bodies, mine management policies and climatic and geographical conditions all influence the quantities of cadmium released from individual sites. Contamination can arise from entry into aquifers of mine drainage water, wastewater, overflow from tailing ponds and rainwater run-off from mine areas (WHO, 1992a).

Other human sources are spent solutions from plating operations and phosphate fertilizers, which are known to contain cadmium: cadmium constitutes up to 255 mg/kg of phosphorus pentoxide in West Africa and up to 35 mg/kg in the USA (WHO, 1992a,b). Atmospheric fall-out of cadmium to water courses and marine waters represents the major worldwide source of cadmium in the environment (Nriagu & Pacyna, 1988). Acidification of soils and lakes may result in mobilization of the metal from soils and sediments toward surface and groundwaters (Impens *et al.*, 1989; WHO, 1992b). Other point sources are mining residue dumps, solid-waste deposits and wastewater of both municipal and industrial origin (Muntau & Baudo, 1992). Cadmium salts such as cadmium carbonate, cadmium chloride and cadmium sulfate may also contaminate surface waters as a result of run-off from industrial processes (IARC, 1976). In polluted rivers, high concentrations can be found in bottom sediments (Muntau & Baudo, 1992).

The concentration of cadmium dissolved in surface waters of the open ocean is less than 0.005 µg/L (WHO, 1992b). Ice samples from the Arctic contained an average of 5 ng/kg, while those from the Antarctic contained 0.3 ng/kg (Wolff & Peel, 1985).

The concentration of cadmium in drinking-water is generally less than 1 µg/L, but it may increase up to 10 µg/L as a result of industrial discharge and leaching from metal or plastic pipes (Friberg *et al.*, 1971).

1.3.5 *Soil and plants*

The sources of cadmium in soil are nonferrous metal mines and smelters, agricultural application of phosphate fertilizers, use of batteries, PVC stabilizers, pigments and alloys, sewage-sludge landfill, sewage-sludge and solid-waste incineration, and application of municipal sewage sludge to agricultural soil (UNEP, 1984, 1992; WHO, 1992a,b). The concentration of cadmium in soil can vary widely. In non-polluted areas, concentrations are usually below 1 mg/kg (Friberg *et al.*, 1971, 1974), whereas in polluted areas levels of up to 800 mg/kg have been detected (Friberg *et al.*, 1985; 1986b; WHO, 1992b). With increasing acidification of soils due to acid rain and the use of fertilizers (and sewage sludge), increased uptake of cadmium from soil may occur (UNEP, 1984; 1992; WHO, 1992b).

Plants may be contaminated with cadmium *via* two routes: (i) soil–plant transfer, due to absorption of mobile forms of cadmium by the roots: increased soil content of cadmium results in increased plant uptake of the metal; the long-term availability of cadmium to plants is uncertain; (ii) air–plant transfer, due to deposition of cadmium particles and to precipitation of soluble forms on the epigeal parts of plants (Impens *et al.*, 1989). Cadmium residues in plants are normally less than 1 mg/kg (Friberg *et al.*, 1986a); however, plants growing in soil contaminated with cadmium may contain significantly higher levels (UNEP, 1984, 1992; WHO, 1992b).

1.3.6 *Cigarette smoke*

Tobacco plants naturally accumulate relatively high concentrations of cadmium in the leaves. The cadmium content of cigarette tobacco is generally 1–2 µg per cigarette, although the concentrations differ among regions. A smoker who smokes 20 cigarettes per day has an estimated daily uptake of 2–4 µg and accumulates 0.5 mg cadmium in one year (Lewis *et al.*, 1972; UNEP, 1984; Friberg *et al.*, 1985; IARC, 1986a; UNEP, 1992; WHO, 1992b).

1.3.7 *Food*

Food is the main source of cadmium for non-occupationally exposed people, although uptake (gastrointestinal absorption) from food is generally much less efficient than from water or air, as cadmium binds to food constituents. Cadmium is present in most foods, and an extremely wide range of concentrations in foodstuffs has been reported from different countries (Friberg et al., 1986a,b; WHO, 1992b). While average dietary concentrations are usually below the provisional tolerable weekly intake of 7 µg/kg bw proposed by FAO/WHO (1989), they are exceeded in some population groups (UNEP, 1984, 1992).

Meat, eggs, fish and milk products generally contain little cadmium—less than 0.01 µg/g wet weight—whereas internal organs, especially liver and kidney, may contain much more: concentrations of up to 1 µg/g wet weight have been reported in animal organs. Even higher concentrations have been detected in oysters (up to 8 µg/g) and salmon flesh (3 µg/g) (Friberg et al., 1974); internal organs of fish and shellfish may also contain high amounts of the metal (Banat et al., 1972; WHO, 1992b).

In general, vegetable products contain more cadmium than animal products. Two important dietary staples, rice and wheat, accumulate high amounts of the metal, depending on the season (Nordberg & Nordberg, 1988). In unpolluted areas, concentrations of 0.01–0.1 µg/g have been reported in rice and wheat, whereas in Japan and some other Asian countries the cadmium content may be higher (Friberg et al., 1985; Watanabe et al., 1989; Rivai et al., 1990). An analysis of the cadmium content of 207 samples of common rice and glutinous rice collected in various areas of Asia showed no difference; the geometric mean cadmium concentration was about 20 ng/g dry wt (range, 0.8–259.3) (Watanabe et al., 1989).

The average daily intake of cadmium varies among countries, and large individual variations occur. In unpolluted areas, intake is estimated to be 10–60 µg/day; values tend to be lower in Europe and North America than in Japan. In areas of Japan that are considered to be unpolluted, average daily intakes are generally 15–50 µg, whereas in polluted areas values as high as 500 µg have been reported (Friberg et al., 1974; Kowal et al., 1979; Friberg et al., 1985; Watanabe et al., 1985; Louekari et al., 1991; Watanabe et al., 1992; WHO, 1992b).

1.3.8 Animal tissues (some of which may be used as food)

High levels of cadmium have been found particularly in seabirds and sea mammals; much of the cadmium occurs in the kidney and liver. Typical concentrations are in the range 0.1–2 mg/kg wet weight in liver and 1–10 mg/kg wet weight in kidney (Elinder, 1992; WHO, 1992b).

Long-lived terrestrial mammals, such as horses and moose, can also have remarkable burdens of cadmium in liver and kidney; concentrations of up to 200 mg/kg have been reported in kidney cortex samples of old horses (Elinder, 1992; WHO, 1992a). In small mammals living in polluted areas, cadmium also accumulates in the liver and kidney: concentrations ranged from 1.5 to 280 mg/kg dry weight in liver and from 7.4 to 193 mg/kg in kidney. In animals from unpolluted sites, concentrations in liver ranged from 0.5 to 25 mg/kg and those in kidney from 1.5 to 26 mg/kg (WHO, 1992a).

1.3.9 Human tissues and secretions

Cadmium accumulates in the body. The total body burden of non-occupationally exposed adult subjects has been estimated to range from 9.5 to 40 mg in the USA and Europe. The International Register of Potentially Toxic Chemicals (UNEP, 1984, 1992) considered that the body burden of a proportion of the population is already approaching the critical value of 10–15 μg, which is the amount that must be retained daily to result in impaired kidney function after 50 years. Cadmium deposition increases with age and is greater in smokers then nonsmokers (Alessio et al., 1983). Concentrations of 1–3 mg/kg wet weight have been detected in liver and 15–50 mg/kg in kidney cortex. Concentrations are usually higher in the Japanese; average concentrations in kidney cortex ranging from about 50 to 100 mg/kg were detected in people 50 years of age (Friberg et al., 1985).

After long-term exposure to low levels, 40–80% of the retained cadmium (mainly bound to metallothionein) was found in liver and kidneys and about one-third in kidneys alone. Concentrations of 100–450 mg/kg wet weight were measured in kidney cortex of cadmium-exposed subjects who showed no renal changes or only slight changes in tubular function. The lungs of non-occupationally exposed subjects contained about 2% of the cadmium body burden (Alessio et al., 1983; WHO, 1992b). In unselected autopsies in Germany, the mean concentrations of cadmium in lungs were found to be 1.48 ± 1.22 μg/g dry weight in the age group 20–45, 1.73 ± 1.42 μg/g in the age group 45–65 and 1.18 ± 1.27 μg/g for people aged > 65 (Kollmeier et al., 1990). Placentas from nonsmokers contained 13.7 ± 6.4 ng/g cadmium, and those from smokers contained 18.1 ± 7.3 ng/g (Kuhnert et al., 1982).

Concentrations of cadmium in urine and blood of subjects non-occupationally exposed to the metal have been reported in only a few studies, most of which were not designed for the definition of reference values but involved control groups for toxicological and epidemiological investigations (Alessio et al., 1992). Mean urinary cadmium concentrations measured in several countries in Europe, Japan and the USA ranged from about 0.4 to 4 μg/L. Urinary cadmium concentrations are significantly higher in smokers than in nonsmokers; on a group basis, they increase with age in nonsmokers. Mean blood concentrations ranged from about 0.2 to 4 μg/L; they were significantly higher in smokers and were influenced by age (Kowal et al., 1979; Bruaux et al., 1983; Elinder et al., 1983; Friberg et al., 1985; Watanabe et al., 1985; Abe et al., 1986; Pocock et al., 1988; Alessio et al., 1990; Buchet et al., 1990; Alessio et al., 1992; Kawada et al., 1992).

1.4 Regulations and guidelines

Occupational exposure limits and guidelines, whether legally binding or not, established in different parts of the world are given in Table 8. Separate engineering control air limits for cadmium in selected industries in the USA are shown in Table 9. WHO (1980, 1987, 1988) estimated the hazards to human health of lifetime exposure to different levels of cadmium in air and concluded that the concentration of cadmium in respirable dust should be well below 20 μg/m^3, and short-term exposures to cadmium oxide fumes and respirable dust should not exceed 250 μg/m^3.

In Sweden, an 8-h time-weighted average concentration of 0.01 mg/m^3 became applicable for respirable dust of cadmium and cadmium compounds in new and renovated plants as of 1 July 1991 (UNEP, 1993).

The American Conference of Governmental Industrial Hygienists (1992) adopted a biological exposure index of 10 μg/g creatinine for cadmium in urine and 10 μg/L for cadmium in blood. They have also proposed a reduction in these values to 5 μg/g creatinine in urine and 5 μg/L in blood, in agreement with the health-based biological limits recommended by WHO (1980).

Table 8. Occupational exposure limits and guidelines for cadmium and cadmium compounds

Country or region	Year valid	Concentration (mg/m³)	Substances affected	Interpretation[a]
Argentina	1991	0.05	Cadmium and cadmium salts (as Cd)	TWA, potential carcinogen
Australia	1990	0.05	Cadmium, cadmium compounds (as Cd), cadmium oxide, fumes	TWA, probable human carcinogen
Austria	1982	0.05	Cadmium dusts and salts (as Cd)	TWA
Belgium	1990	0.05	Cadmium, cadmium compounds (as Cd), cadmium oxide	TWA
		0.05	Cadmium oxide, fumes	Ceiling
Bulgaria	1984	0.1	Cadmium oxide, fumes (as Cd)	TWA
China	1979	0.1	Cadmium oxide, fumes (as Cd)	TWA
Denmark	1990	0.01	Cadmium, cadmium oxide, fumes	TWA
		0.01	Inorganic cadmium compounds (as Cd)	TWA, suspected carcinogen
Finland	1990	0.02	Cadmium, cadmium compounds (as Cd)	TWA, suspected of having carcinogenic potential
		0.01	Cadmium oxide, fumes	TWA, suspected of having carcinogenic potential
		0	Cadmium (respirable dust), cadmium chloride, inorganic cadmium compounds (as Cd), inorganic cadmium compounds (respirable dust) (as Cd)	Suspected of having carcinogenic potential
France	1990	0.05	Cadmium oxide	TWA
		0.05	Cadmium oxide, fumes	STEL
		0	Cadmium chloride	Suspected carcinogen
Germany	1992	0	Cadmium, cadmium compounds (as Cd), cadmium oxide, cadmium chloride, cadmium sulfate, cadmium sulfide	A2
Hungary	1983	0.05	Cadmium oxide, fumes (as Cd)	TWA
		0.1	Cadmium oxide, fumes (as Cd)	STEL (twice during one work shift)
Indonesia	1978	0.2	Cadmium dusts and salts (as Cd)	TWA
		0.2	Cadmium oxide, fumes (as Cd)	Ceiling
Italy	1978	0.05	Cadmium dusts and salts (as Cd)	TWA
		0.01	Cadmium oxide, fumes (as Cd)	TWA
Japan	1990	0.05	Cadmium, cadmium compounds (as Cd)	TWA

Table 8 (contd)

Country or region	Year valid	Concentration (mg/m³)	Substances affected	Interpretation[a]
Mexico	1984	0.05	Cadmium dusts and salts (as Cd); cadmium oxide, fumes (as Cd); cadmium oxide, production (as Cd)	TWA
		0.2	Cadmium dusts and salts (as Cd); cadmium oxide, fumes (as Cd); cadmium oxide, production (as Cd)	STEL (15 min four times a day)
Netherlands	1986	0.02	Cadmium and cadmium compounds (as Cd)	TWA, suspected carcinogen
Poland	1984	0.05	Cadmium oxide, fumes (as Cd)	TWA
Romania	1975	0.1	Cadmium oxide, fumes (as Cd)	TWA
		0.2	Cadmium oxide, fumes (as Cd)	STEL
Sweden	1991	0.05	Cadmium (total dust), inorganic cadmium compounds (as Cd) (total dust)	TWA, suspected of having carcinogenic potential
		0.02	Cadmium (respirable dust), inorganic cadmium compounds (respirable dust)	TWA, suspected of having carcinogenic potential
Switzerland	1984	0.05	Cadmium dusts and salts (as Cd), cadmium chloride	TWA
		0.05	Cadmium oxide, fumes (as Cd)	Ceiling
Taiwan	1981	0.1	Cadmium dusts and salts (as Cd)	TWA
United Kingdom[b]	1992	0.05	Cadmium and cadmium compounds (dusts and fumes) (as Cd) (except cadmium oxide fumes and cadmium sulfide pigments), cadmium oxide fumes (as Cd)	TWA, MEL
		0.05	Cadmium oxide fumes (as Cd)	STEL, MEL (10 min)
		0.04	Cadmium sulfide pigments (respirable dust) (as Cd)	TWA
USA				
OSHA	1992	0.005	Cadmium	TWA, PEL
		0.015–0.050	Cadmium	SECAL (see Table 9)
ACGIH[c]	1992	0.05	Cadmium dusts and salts (as Cd), cadmium oxide production	TWA, TLV
		0.05	Cadmium oxide fumes (as Cd)	Ceiling

Table 8 (contd)

Country or region	Year valid	Concentration (mg/m^3)	Substances affected	Interpretation[a]
Venezuela	1978	0.05	Cadmium dusts and salts (as Cd)	TWA
		0.15	Cadmium dusts and salts (as Cd), cadmium compounds (as Cd)	Ceiling
		0.05	Cadmium oxide, fumes (as Cd)	Ceiling

From Arbeidsinspectie (1986); Cook (1987); International Labour Office (1991); American Conference of Governmental Industrial Hygienists (ACGIH) (1992); Deutsche Forschungsgemeinschaft (1992); Health and Safety Executive (1992); US Occupational Safety and Health Administration (OSHA) (1992); UNEP (1993)

[a]The concentrations given may or may not have regulatory or legal status in the various countries; for interpretation of the values, the original references or other authoritative sources should be consulted. TWA, time-weighted average; STEL, short-term exposure limit; MEL, maximal exposure limit; PEL, permissible exposure limit; SECAL, separate engineering control air limit; TLV, threshold limit value; A2, compounds which in the Commission's opinion have proven so far to be unmistakably carcinogenic in animal experimentation only; namely under conditions which are comparable to those for possible exposure of a human being at the work place, or from which such comparability can be deduced.

[b]New maximal exposure limits have been proposed, to take effect from 1 January 1994: 0.04 mg/m^3 for cadmium sulfide and its pigments, and 0.025 mg/m^3 for cadmium and other cadmium compounds (Anon., 1992).

[c]A change has been proposed in the 'adopted' values: to 0.01 mg/m^3 for total dust or particulates of cadmium and cadmium compounds, and 0.002 mg/m^3 for the respirable fraction of dust (respirable particulate mass), considered to be suspected human carcinogens.

Table 9. Separate engineering control air limits (SECALs) for cadmium processes in selected US industries

Industry	Process	SECAL (mg/m^3)
Nickel–cadmium battery	Plate-making, plate preparation	0.050
	All other processes	0.015
Zinc and cadmium refining[a]	Cadmium refining, casting, melting, oxide production, sinter plant	0.050
Pigment manufacture	Calcining, crushing, milling, blending	0.050
	All other processes	0.015
Stabilizer manufacture[a]	Cadmium oxide charging, crushing, drying, blending	0.050
Lead smelting[a]	Sinter plant, blast furnace, baghouse, yard area	0.050
Plating[a]	Mechanical plating	0.015

From US Occupational Safety and Health Administration (1992)

[a]Processes used in these industries that are not specified in the table must achieve the permissible exposure limit by using engineering controls and changing work practices. Industries that are not listed must meet the permissible exposure limit of 0.005 mg/m^3 (see Table 8).

In Sweden, cadmium workers are required to undergo a medical examination twice a year. Workers who have blood cadmium concentrations exceeding 150 nmol/L (16.5 µg/L) are removed from exposure and are not allowed to return until the concentration is below 100 nmol (11 µg/L) (Arbetarskyddsstyrelsens, 1989).

The guideline for all forms of cadmium in drinking-water recommended by WHO (1984, 1992c) is 3 µg/L. The maximal level of cadmium in drinking-water and the permissible level in bottled water in the USA is 10 µg/L (US Environmental Protection Agency, 1991; US Food and Drug Administration, 1992).

The Joint FAO/WHO Expert Committee of Food Additives (WHO, 1989) proposed a provisional tolerable weekly intake for cadmium of 7 µg/kg body weight. The provisional guidelines set by the Japanese Ministry of Health and Welfare are 0.4 mg/kg in rice and up to 10 µg/L in drinking-water (Förstner, 1984).

Cadmium and cadmium compounds are not permitted in cosmetic products in the countries of the European Economic Community (Commission of the European Communities, 1990, 1991c). A Directive has been adopted aimed at restricting the manufacture and use of certain cadmium-bearing pigments, stabilizers and plating and the discharge of cadmium into the environment (Commission of the European Communities, 1983, 1991d,e; Shagarofsky-Tummers, 1992). In Sweden, cadmium is not allowed for use as a pigment, for surface coatings or as a stabilizer (Svensk Författningssamling, 1979, 1980).

The International Register of Potentially Toxic Chemicals of UNEP included cadmium together with lead and mercury in its listing of environmentally dangerous chemical substances and processes of global significance (UNEP, 1984, 1992).

2. Studies of Cancer in Humans

The occupations covered in the studies reviewed below involve recovery of cadmium from zinc refining, manufacture of cadmium oxide, alloys and pigment and production of nickel–cadmium batteries. The Working Group did not review studies of other occupations, such as electroplating, welding (see IARC, 1990b), painting (see IARC, 1989) and glass-making (see p. 347), in which exposure to cadmium occurs, but which involve lower or more sporadic exposures. The use of cadmium was noted to be increasing in the production of nickel–cadmium batteries (US Occupational Safety and Health Administration, 1992) but decreasing in other applications. In general, the maximal concentrations of cadmium in work-place air decreased by up to 100 times since the 1940s in the work sites studied. Given the long latency of cancer, the health effects noted among long-term workers may reflect former rather than current conditions of exposure.

The Working Group considered other occupational respiratory carcinogens, such as nickel (see IARC, 1990a) in nickel–cadmium battery plants and arsenic (see IARC, 1987c) in localized areas of metallurgical plants, that might introduce a spurious association between exposure to cadmium and lung cancer. Potential confounding by occupational exposures to other substances was not considered in the studies of prostatic cancer.

2.1 Descriptive studies

Shigematsu *et al.* (1982) assessed mortality in four pairs of populations in cadmium-polluted and unpolluted areas of four prefectures of Japan during 1948–77, when exposure to cadmium in the polluted areas occurred through ingestion of cadmium-contaminated rice. Average concentrations ranged from 0.2 to 0.7 ppm in the polluted area and from 0.02 to 0.1 ppm in the unpolluted areas. No difference was seen between the two areas in the rate of mortality from cancers at all sites or from cancers of the stomach or liver. The rate of mortality from prostatic cancer was significantly higher (standardized mortality ratio [SMR], 1.66) in the polluted than in the unpolluted area of one prefecture, as was the incidence of hyperplasia of the prostate. Figures for respiratory cancer were not reported.

Bako *et al.* (1982) studied age-adjusted incidence rates for prostatic cancer in various census divisions of Alberta, Canada, in relation to the occurrence of cadmium in the environment, i.e. in samples of flowing fresh water, municipal waste water, soil, and wheat and barley stems. Significantly high and low incidence rates were seen: the city with high incidence, 53.2 cases per 100 000 population, had consistently higher cadmium concentrations in the samples taken (0.006 ppm in waste water, 0.27 in soil, 0.004 in flowing water); and the city with the lowest incidence, 10.6 cases per 100 000 population, had consistently low concentrations (< 0.001, 0.19 and 0.001 ppm, respectively). Other environmental parameters also differed.

Campbell *et al.* (1990) reported analyses of a comprehensive cross-sectional survey of possible risk factors for primary liver cancer in 48 counties in China. County mortality rates were correlated positively with mean daily cadmium intake (0–90 µg/day) from foods of plant origin, as estimated by dietary surveys.

2.2 Cohort studies (see Tables 10 and 11, pp. 157 *et seq.*)

The relation between exposure to cadmium and cancers of the lung and prostate has been studied in six occupational cohorts in Europe and the USA, most of which covered overlapping populations, and in one in China. The cohorts are generally small, particularly when restricted to long-term, highly exposed workers with prolonged follow-up. Recent studies have expanded the number of subjects by including many short-term, minimally exposed or recently hired workers, so that the need for subanalyses by dose and latency is increased. In order to facilitate interpretation, the studies are grouped according to plant; the published data on cancer of the lung are summarized in Table 10 and those for prostatic cancer in Table 11.

2.2.1 *Nickel–cadmium battery manufacture, United Kingdom*

Workers from two nickel–cadmium battery plants in the United Kingdom, one of which operated from 1923 to 1947 and the other from 1937 to the present, were the subject of a series of studies. The plants were amalgamated in 1947. The concentrations of cadmium in cadmium oxide (hydroxide) dust in high-exposure jobs (plate-making and assembly shops) were 0.6–2.8 mg/m^3 [236 mg/m^3 in the negative active material department where cadmium oxide is prepared (Potts, 1965)] in 1949, $\leq$ 0.5 mg/m^3 between 1950 (when extensive local exhaust ventilation was installed) and 1967 (when a new plate-making department was built), < 0.2 mg/m^3 from 1968 to 1975 and < 0.05 mg cadmium/m^3 after 1975 (Sorahan & Waterhouse, 1983). [The Working Group noted that the process was probably similar to those in the Swedish study described below, where exposure to nickel hydroxide dust was reported to be higher than that to cadmium oxide.]

Potts (1965) identified three deaths from cancer of the prostate and one from lung cancer out of eight deaths among 74 men who had been exposed to cadmium oxide dust in the plant for at least 10 years before 1965. No referent rates were used to compute the expected number of fatal cancers. [The Working Group had no information on the completeness of ascertainment and whether, therefore, the 74 men were representative of the exposed population.]

Kipling and Waterhouse (1967) assembled a cohort of 248 men with at least one year of exposure to cadmium oxide at the same plants, including the 74 men reported by Potts (1965). [The Working Group had no published information on exposure levels in these jobs; however, in subsequent studies of the same plants, these job titles were classified as involving high exposure.] They compared cancer incidence rates through 1966 with regional rates from the local cancer registry. One new case of prostatic cancer was detected. This case, combined with the three deaths reported by Potts (1965), exceeded the 0.58 expected (standardized incidence ratio [SIR], 6.90 [95% confidence interval (CI), 1.86–17.66]). The incidence of lung cancer was not significantly elevated (5 observed, 4.4 expected; SIR, 1.14 [95% CI, 0.37–2.65]). [The Working Group noted that there was no analysis of incidence by latency or duration of exposure.]

Sorahan and Waterhouse (1983) enlarged the cohort to include 3025 people (2559 men) first employed at the plants between 1923 and 1975 for a minimum of one month. An initial study of mortality from prostatic cancer reported eight deaths between January 1946 and

January 1981, whereas 6.6 were expected on the basis of mortality rates in the general population of England and Wales (relative risk [RR], 1.21 [95% CI, 0.52–2.39]). In a later study, Sorahan and Waterhouse (1985) identified 15 incident cases of prostatic cancer entered into the Birmingham Regional Cancer Registry between 1950 and 1980; comparison with the 11.0 cases expected from regional rates gave an RR of 1.36 [95% CI, 0.76–2.25]. Eight of the cases occurred in a subgroup of 458 workers who had been employed for at least one year in jobs entailing high exposure to cadmium oxide dust (8 observed, 1.99 expected; RR, 4.02 [95% CI, 1.73–7.92]). Four of the eight cases were additional to those reported by Kipling and Waterhouse (1967); this number was greater than that expected but not significant (4 observed, 1.78 expected; RR, 2.25 [95% CI, 0.60–5.75]).

Sorahan (1987) examined lung cancer mortality between 1946 and 1984 in the same workforce of 3025 workers. Overall, 110 deaths from lung cancer were observed, while 84.5 were expected (RR, 1.30 [95% CI, 1.07–1.57]). The RRs for lung cancer in high-exposure jobs were slightly greater (1.3–1.5) than that for workers with no or minimal exposure but did not increase with years of employment in high-exposure jobs (Table 10). [The Working Group noted that the analysis did not incorporate exposure measurements, nor was the intensity of exposure considered simultaneously with duration. Tobacco smoking was controlled for indirectly in internal dose–response comparisons. Exposure to nickel hydroxide could not be controlled for, since few workers were exposed to cadmium in the absence of nickel.]

2.2.2 *Nickel–cadmium battery manufacture, Sweden*

Concentrations of cadmium in air containing cadmium oxide dust at a single nickel–cadmium battery plant in Sweden, where a series of studies was done, averaged about 1 mg/m^3 before 1947, 0.3 mg/m^3 between 1947 and 1962, 0.05 mg/m^3 between 1962 and 1974 and 0.02 mg/m^3 after 1975 (Elinder *et al.*, 1985). Exposures to nickel hydroxide dust were reported to have been 2–10 times higher than those to cadmium oxide, although no measurements were reported (Kjellström *et al.*, 1977).

Kjellström *et al.* (1979) studied 228 men who had been employed at the plant for five or more years between 1940 and 1959, who were followed up from 1959 to 1975. Incident cancers among the workers were identified from the Swedish National Cancer Registry, which started in 1959, and were compared with national rates of incidence. The numbers of new cases were as follows: lung, 2 observed, 1.35 expected (RR, 1.48 [95% CI, 0.17–5.35]), prostate, 2 observed, 1.2 expected (RR, 1.67 [95% CI, 0.19–6.02]) and nasopharynx, 2 observed, 0.20 expected (RR, 10.0 [95% CI, 1.23–36.1]). [The Working Group noted that cancers of the nasal cavity and sinuses and not nasopharyngeal cancers are associated with exposure to nickel, and that only cases of cancers that occurred after 1959 were included.]

Andersson *et al.* (1984) and Elinder *et al.* (1985) extended the cohort to include 522 male workers who had been exposed to cadmium for at least one year between 1940 and 1980, and who were still alive in 1951; follow-up was from 1951 to 1983. In that period, there were eight deaths from lung cancer (6.01 expected; RR, 1.33 [95% CI, 0.57–2.62]), four from prostatic cancer (3.70 expected; RR, 1.08 [95% CI, 0.29–2.77]) and one from cancer of the nasopharynx (expected near 0). Seven of the eight cases of lung cancer occurred among workers with five or more years of exposure and 20 years' latency (7 observed, 4.0 expected;

RR, 1.75 [95% CI, 0.70–3.61]). [The Working Group noted that the small number of cases precluded a dose–response analysis.]

2.2.3 *Copper–cadmium alloy plants, United Kingdom*

Holden (1980a,b) described cadmium exposures at two plants, in rural and urban locations in the United Kingdom, where copper–cadmium alloy was produced from 1922 to 1966 and from 1925 to the present, respectively. The numbers of workers in each plant were not given; a total of 347 workers at the two plants had been employed for at least one year. Exposure to cadmium fume at the urban plant exceeded 1 mg/m^3 before 1953, with a peak of 3.6 mg/m^3, was < 0.15 mg/m^3 from 1953 to 1957 and was < 0.05 mg/m^3 thereafter. Although air concentrations at the rural plant were not described, proteinuria was common in workers at both plants before 1950, indicating high exposures to cadmium (Holden, 1980b).

Mortality from respiratory cancer, followed from 1921 to 1978, was higher among urban cadmium workers [number not given] than in the general population of England and Wales (8 observed, 4.50 expected; RR, 1.78 [95% CI, 0.77–3.50]) but was significantly lower among the rural workers [number not given] (2 observed, 7.85 expected; RR, 0.25 [95% CI, 0.03–0.92]). One death from prostatic cancer was observed in the combined workforce (1.58 expected; RR, 0.63 [95% CI, 0.01–3.52]). In the same study, 624 'vicinity' workers from the urban plant, who produced arsenical copper and other alloys in the same workshop, were followed up. Their mean cadmium exposures were low (≤ 0.07 mg/m^3; King, 1955), but their arsenic exposures were high [figures not given]. These workers had significantly higher mortality rates from both respiratory (36 observed, 26.08 expected; RR, 1.38 [95% CI, 0.97–1.91]) and prostatic cancer (8 observed, 3.0 expected; RR, 2.67 [95% CI, 1.15–5.26]) than the general population of England and Wales (Holden, 1980a,b). [The Working Group noted that no regional comparison was made, and it is unclear whether the general population is comparable with the rural population with respect to smoking. It is unlikely, however, that urban–rural differences would completely explain the low risk for lung cancer in the rural workers.]

Kazantzis *et al.* (1989) reported briefly the results of a nested case–control study of cancer of the lung in the same copper–cadmium alloy cohort described above. Long-term employees were reported also to have been exposed to arsenic in the production of arsenical copper. An analysis in which 50 lung cancer deaths were compared with 158 controls matched on age and year at hire showed a stronger association between lung cancer and exposure to arsenic (odds ratio, 2.15; 90% CI, 1.22–3.79) than with exposure to cadmium (odds ratio, 1.27; 90% CI, 0.61–2.51). [The Working Group found the report difficult to interpret with respect to cadmium, because it lacks information on exposure classification and no statement is made about control for urban *versus* rural location or simultaneous control of exposure to cadmium and arsenic in the analysis.]

2.2.4 *Copper–cadmium alloy plants, Sweden*

Kjellström *et al.* (1979) investigated the incidence of prostatic cancer among 94 workers employed for five or more years between 1940 and 1978 at a cadmium–copper alloy plant in

Sweden. Production of the alloy was begun in the 1930s. The levels of cadmium oxide fume in air were 0.1–0.4 mg/m^3 in the 1960s and about 0.05 mg/m^3 in the 1970s. Mortality from prostatic cancer between 1940 and 1975 was above that expected from national rates (4 observed, 2.69 expected; RR, 1.49 [95% CI, 0.40–3.81]). A reference group of 328 workers not exposed to cadmium had lower mortality from prostatic cancer than expected (4 observed, 6.42 expected; RR, 0.62 [95% CI, 0.17–1.60]).

2.2.5 *Cadmium recovery plant in the USA*

Several mortality studies have been conducted at a US plant where cadmium oxide, sulfide and metal were made from cadmium oxide dust recovered from the waste of nonferrous smelters since 1926 (especially zinc smelters). Estimated average air concentrations of cadmium in dust and fumes in high-exposure departments were 1.16 mg/m^3 before 1950, 0.50 mg/m^3 in 1950–59, 0.34 mg/m^3 in 1960–64 and 0.26 mg/m^3 in 1965–76 (Smith *et al.*, 1980). As extensive measurements had been made throughout the plant since 1943, mortality could be analysed by both intensity and duration of exposure to cadmium. Other metals, such as lead, arsenic, indium and thallium, had been produced intermittently in localized areas of the plant, and the facility had been an arsenic smelter in 1918–25 and a lead smelter from 1886 to 1918. Some contamination of incoming feed material with arsenic persisted after 1926: The proportion of arsenic in feedstock was ≥ 50% before 1926, about 7% in 1926–27, 1.5–5.6% in 1928–33, 1.9–3.7% in 1934–40 and 1.0–2.0% after 1940 (Thun *et al.*, 1985, 1986). In 1973, arsenic was present at 0.3–1.1 μg/m^3 in the pre-melt department and 1.4 μg/m^3 in the retort department; the respective values for cadmium were 74.8–90.3 and 1105 μg/m^3. Bulk samples of preprocessed ore contained 70% cadmium, 6.0% zinc, 4.3% lead and 0.3% arsenic; after initial roasting, bulk samples contained 42.2% cadmium, 3.53% zinc, no lead and 0.02% arsenic. Additional refining steps reduced the levels of impurities further, so that exposure of workers to trace metals other than cadmium was considered to be insignificant (Lemen *et al.*, 1976).

Lemen *et al.* (1976) studied 292 white male hourly workers exposed for two or more years between 1940 and 1969 and followed from 1940 through to 1973. There were four deaths from cancer of the prostate (1.15 expected; RR, 3.48; [95% CI, 0.94–8.91]). Mortality from this cancer was significantly increased in workers with ≥ 20 years latency (4 observed, 0.88 expected [RR, 4.55; 95% CI, 1.22–11.64]). The number of deaths from respiratory cancer also exceeded that expected (12 observed, 5.11 expected; RR, 2.35 [95% CI, 1.21–4.10]). [The Working Group noted that the association with lung cancer was not examined in relation to cumulative exposure to cadmium or exposure to other work-related exposures, including arsenic.]

Thun *et al.* (1985) expanded the cohort to a total of 602 white men who had been employed in cadmium production between 1940 and 1969 for at least six months. Estimates of exposure based on air measurements over time were combined with work exposure categories to estimate cumulative exposures to cadmium. No additional death from prostatic cancer had occurred during the extended follow-up from 1974 to 1978. As the cohort was limited to cadmium production workers, one of the four prostatic cancer deaths observed by Lemen *et al.* (1976) was excluded from the analysis. The remaining three deaths from prostatic cancer occurred among workers with two or more years of employment and 20 or more years of latency (3 observed, 1.41 expected; RR, 2.13; 95% CI, 0.44–6.22). [The Working Group noted that increased screening for prostatic cancer could result in early detection and therefore greater survival, thus biasing the results of mortality studies of this cancer.]

Lung cancer mortality was examined first through 1978 (Thun *et al.*, 1985) and later through 1984 (Stayner *et al.*, 1992). All analyses of lung cancer mortality in relation to exposure to cadmium were restricted to 576 men who were first employed after 1 January 1926, when the plant ceased arsenic smelting, although (as noted above) some arsenic remained in the material being processed, decreasing with time. Death rates from lung cancer in the overall cohort through 1984 were slightly greater than those expected from US white male rates (24 observed, 16.07 expected; RR, 1.49 [95% CI, 0.96–2.22]), and the RR increased with estimated cumulative exposure to cadmium: 0.34, 1.63, 2.17 and 2.72 in workers with cumulative exposures of ≤ 584, 585–1460, 1461–2920 and > 2920 mg/m^3-days (Table 10). The mortality rates for lung cancer among the workers were compared with Colorado State rates for white men for the follow-up period through 1978. The RRs were higher for this follow-up period when compared with local rather than national rates: The RR in the most highly exposed group was 3.87 when compared to State rates (7 observed, 1.81 expected [95% CI, 1.55–7.97]) and 2.80 when national rates were used for comparison (Thun *et al.*, 1986).

Several authors have examined whether exposure to cigarette smoking or arsenic could account for the excess mortality from lung cancer at the US plant. Nearly half of the cadmium workers were men of Mexican–American descent, who in the 1980s smoked fewer cigarettes per day on average and had less than half the incidence of lung cancer of other US white males (US National Cancer Institute, 1986). Lower rates from lung cancer among Mexican–Americans as compared with other whites were also reported in earlier years in Denver, where the plant is located: The RR was about 0.3 in 1969–71 and 0.7 in 1979–81, when men with Latino surnames were compared with other whites (Savitz, 1986). Stayner *et al.* (1992) showed that the excess mortality from lung cancer at the US plant is confined to non-Mexican–American cadmium workers when compared to US white males (21 observed, 9.95 expected; RR, 2.11 [95% CI, 1.31–3.23]), and no excess was seen in Mexican–American workers (3 observed, 6.12 expected; RR, 0.49 [95% CI, 0.10–1.43]). Comparisons with the US population, however, result in overestimates of the expected number of deaths among Mexican–Americans and underestimates of the effect of occupation. The tobacco smoking habits of the non-Mexican–American workers were similar to those of all US white males, yet 11 excess deaths from lung cancer were observed (RR, 2.11; $p < 0.01$) (US Occupational Safety and Health Administration, 1992). [The Working Group noted that confounding by cigarette smoking is unlikely to explain a dose–response relationship and strength of association of this magnitude in an occupational cohort study (Axelson, 1978; Siemiatycki *et al.*, 1988).]

A second extraneous factor that could contribute to mortality from lung cancer at the US plant is arsenic. Three studies were designed to isolate the effect of cadmium from that of arsenic in the cohort by using year of hire before or after 1940 as a proxy for exposure to arsenic. These analyses are based on identical exposure data and overlapping study populations.

Lamm et al. (1992) performed a nested case–control analysis in which 25 cases of fatal lung cancer diagnosed through 1982 were each matched with three controls on year of hire; no association was found between exposure to cadmium and risk for lung cancer. The mean cumulative exposure of the cases (9.24 mg/m^3-year) was not different from that of the controls (mean, 9.29 mg/m^3-year). [The Working Group found the results difficult to interpret, in that exposure data identical to those for the full cohort were used and therefore the same results as in the full cohort should have been obtained. One possible explanation is that matching was done on year of hire, but no matched analysis was done, thereby potentially biasing the results.]

In further analyses, Stayner et al. (1992) categorized the 576 cadmium workers employed after January 1926 into pre-1940 and post-1940 and included this variable in Poisson and proportional hazards analyses of lung cancer rates. Dose–response relationships between exposure to cadmium remained significant in nearly all multivariate analyses after controlling for age, Mexican–American ethnicity (a proxy for lighter tobacco use) and period of hire.

As noted by Doll (1992), part of the explanation for the differences between the results of Lamm et al. (1992) and Stayner et al. (1992) could be that the two studies had only 21 cases in common. Lamm's series also included four cases hired before 1926, which were excluded by Stayner et al. Three cases included by Stayner et al. died of lung cancer between 1982 and 1984 and were therefore not reported by Lamm et al. [The Working Group noted that the methodological differences between the studies of Lamm et al. and Stayner et al. may account for the contradictory results reported.]

In a subsequent analysis, Stayner et al. (1993) conducted a nested case–control analysis using approximately 50 controls per case. The odds ratio increased with increasing cumulative exposure to cadmium, as in the full cohort. They also presented an odds ratio analysis of workers hired after 1940, when arsenic exposures were low. For non-Mexican–Americans, the odds ratio was 0.32 [95% CI, 0.0–1.78] at < 584 mg/m^3-days, 2.81 [1.02–6.10] at 585–1460 mg/m^3-days and 4.70 [1.51–10.97] at 1461–2920 mg/m^3-days. No lung cancer death was observed in the highest exposure category (> 2920 mg/m^3-days), but only 0.6 were expected. [The Working Group noted that the dose–response pattern was stronger in workers hired after 1940, indicating that the result was not likely to be due to exposure to arsenic.]

Thun et al. (1986) addressed the question of the extent to which exposure to arsenic could be held responsible for the excess of lung cancer observed in the cohort. They estimated average cumulative exposure to arsenic in relation to a potency estimate for exposure to arsenic and lung cancer used by the US Occupational Safety and Health Administration and concluded that 0.77 lung cancer deaths could be attributed to arsenic. In a more detailed analysis, the US Occupational Safety and Health Administration (1992) estimated that exposure to arsenic would have resulted in 0.52–0.97 lung cancer deaths in the cohort.

2.2.6 Cadmium processing plants in the United Kingdom

Armstrong and Kazantzis (1983) and Kazantzis et al. (1988) studied mortality among workers at 17 plants in the United Kingdom where cadmium is produced or used, including primary production, copper–cadmium alloy production, silver–cadmium alloy production, pigments and oxide production and stabilizer production. The cohort comprised 6958 men born before 1940 and employed for more than one year on or near a cadmium process between 1942 and 1970. The plants at which nickel–cadmium batteries and copper–cadmium alloys were produced and which were described by Sorahan (1987) and Holden (1980b) were excluded. Jobs were assessed for each relevant year as involving high, medium or low exposure to cadmium on the basis of discussions with hygienists and others with knowledge of past working procedures, taking into account available results of biological or environmental monitoring. The years at risk of the study population were divided on the basis of these categories and recorded job histories into three groups; 'ever high' (minimum one year), 'ever medium' (minimum one year) and 'always low'. A total of 198 workers (3%; Kazantzis *et al.*, 1992) were classified as having had 'ever high' exposure, 17% were considered to have had 'ever medium' exposure, and the exposures of 80% were classified as 'always low' (Armstrong & Kazantzis, 1983). Kazantzis *et al.* (1992) stated that in these epidemiological studies consideration should be given to concomitant exposure to other potential carcinogens, in particular to arsenic, but also to beryllium (see p. 41), nickel (see IARC, 1990a), chromium (see IARC, 1990c) and emissions from a variety of heated mineral oils (see IARC, 1987d) in the various plants.

Kazantzis *et al.* (1988) described mortality from 1943 to 1984 in this cohort, and Kazantzis and Blanks (1992) and Kazantzis *et al.* (1992) extended follow-up through 1989 for 6910 workers. No increased risk for death from prostatic cancer was observed in the overall cohort (37 observed, 49.5 expected; RR, 0.75; 95% CI, 0.53–1.03). One death from prostatic cancer was seen in the 'ever high' exposure group (1.0 expected; RR, 0.97), but none was observed in the 'ever medium' group (6.2 expected; RR, 0; 95% CI, 0–0.59). Mortality from lung cancer was significantly increased in the overall cohort (339 observed, 304.1 expected; RR, 1.12; 95% CI, 1.00–1.24), with some evidence of a trend across exposure categories; these do not, however, attain significance (low: 270 observed, 249.9 expected; RR, 1.08; 95% CI, 0.96–1.22; medium: 55 observed, 45.6 expected; RR, 1.21; 95% CI, 0.91–1.57; high: 14 observed, 8.6 expected; RR, 1.62; 95% CI, 0.89–2.73). With regard to duration of exposure, mortality from lung cancer was significantly raised for men employed for 20–29 years in the cohort as a whole (65 observed, 49.6 expected; RR, 1.31; 95% CI, 1.01–1.67) and in the low-exposure category (54 observed, 38.4 expected; RR, 1.41; 95% CI, 1.06–1.84). In the 'ever high' exposure category, mortality from lung cancer was significantly increased among men first employed between 1930 and 1939 (4 observed, 1.0 expected; RR, 3.81; 95% CI, 1.03–9.76). There is suggestive evidence of a relationship with both intensity of exposure and duration of employment for workers employed before 1940, but no such pattern was seen for workers who started work after 1950. A significantly increased risk was observed for stomach cancer in the cohort as a whole (106 observed, 85.3 expected; RR, 1.24; 95% CI, 1.02–1.50), but this was not related to intensity of exposure, with 91 of the deaths occurring in the low-exposure group (71.4 expected; RR, 1.28; 95% CI 1.03–1.57). As in the earlier studies of this cohort, an increased risk significantly related to intensity of exposure was observed only for bronchitis.

Ades and Kazantzis (1988) reported separately on the experience of 4393 men who had been employed for at least one year at a lead–zinc smelter that comprised 64% of the entire

United Kingdom cadmium cohort and at which no exposure was classified as 'ever high'. There was excess mortality from lung cancer overall when compared with regional rates (182 observed, 146.2 expected; RR, 1.25; 95% CI, 1.07–1.44) and when updated by Kazantzis *et al.* (1992): 237 observed, 194.3 expected; RR, 1.22, 95% CI, 1.02–1.39. A significant trend in SMR was seen with increasing duration of employment. A nested case–control analysis and matched logistic regression were used to compare 174 fatal cases of lung cancer with 2717 controls matched to the cases on year of birth, date of starting work (within three years) and length of follow-up (at least 10 years). The odds ratio for lung cancer increased by 1.23 fold per mg/m^3-years of exposure to cadmium, but the trend was not significant. The trend in RR was significant for exposure to arsenic and lead. Only 21 (12%) cases had ever worked in the two departments (sinter and cadmium plant) where exposures to cadmium generally exceeded 0.010 mg/m^3.

2.2.7 *Smelter in China*

Cancer mortality among male workers employed for at least one year in a smelter in China was followed from 1972 to 1985 and compared with rates for the city in which the smelter was located (Ding *et al.*, 1987). When the plant was divided into five areas, industrial hygiene sampling indicated that exposures to cadmium were highest in the cadmium shop and the sintering shop, with mean air concentrations of 0.186 and 0.014 mg/m^3, respectively. The levels in the cadmium shop were reported to have been much higher prior to 1980 (0.535 mg/m^3). Exposure to arsenic was also reported to have occurred in the sintering area (0.196 mg/m^3 As_2O_3). One case of lung cancer (0.15 expected, SMR, 6.65) and two of liver cancer (0.11 expected, SMR, 17.9) were observed among cadmium shop workers. Four lung cancers (0.24 expected, SMR, 16.8; $p < 0.05$), one stomach cancer (0.31, SMR, 3.18) and three liver cancers (0.18 expected, SMR, 17.0) were observed among sintering shop workers. The men who died of cancer were reported to have had 10–30 years of exposure. Mortality from lung cancer was also increased in the other three areas. The authors stated that there was no obvious association with smoking. [The Working Group noted that the numbers of workers employed were not given.]

2.3 Case–control studies

Abd Elghany *et al.* (1990) conducted a population-based case–control study of exposure to cadmium based on 358 cases of prostatic cancer newly diagnosed in 1984–85 and 679 controls in four urban Utah (USA) counties. Analyses were also conducted for the subgroup of cases classified as aggressive tumours, in order to differentiate more clearly the cases from the controls (which may have included some latent prostatic tumours). In general, there was little evidence of an increased risk for prostatic cancer associated with occupations with potential exposure to cadmium (odds ratio, 0.9; 95% CI, 0.7–1.2), with cigarette smoking (odds ratio, 1.1; 95% CI, 0.8–1.4) or with diet (odds ratio, 1.4; 95% CI, 1.0–2.1). A composite measure of potentially high exposure to cadmium from any source was not associated with prostatic cancer in general (odds ratio, 1.0; 95% CI, 0.7–1.3) but was associated with aggressive tumours (odds ratio, 1.7; 95% CI, 1.0–3.1).

A hypothesis-generating case–control study of 20 cancer sites was conducted in the Montréal (Canada) metropolitan area (Siemiatycki, 1991) and is described in detail in the

Table 10. Cohort studies of lung cancer in workers exposed to cadmium

Type of plant, country (reference)	Population (duration of exposure)	Lung cancers (obs/exp)	Exposure level	Cadmium levels Years	Estimated levels (mg/m³)		Relative risk (95% CI[a])	Comment
Nickel–cadmium battery (cadmium oxide)								
United Kingdom								
Potts (1965)	74 men (≥ 10 years)	1/NR	Overall				Cannot be calculated	Mortality through 1965 No referent group
Kipling & Waterhouse (1967)	248 men (≥ 1 year)	5/4.40	Overall	1949	0.6–2.8		1.14 [0.37–2.65] (Sorahan & Waterhouse, 1983)	Incidence through 1966 at same plant as Potts (1965)
Sorahan (1987)	3025 men and women (≥ 1 month)	110/84.5	Overall None[b] < 2 years 2– 5– ≥ 15	1950–67 1968–75 > 1975	< 0.5 < 0.2 < 0.05		1.30 [1.07–1.57] 1.0 1.4 1.3 1.3 1.5 (Sorahan & Waterhouse (1983)	Mortality 1946–84 Dose-response based on years employed in high-exposure jobs. Trend not significant
Sweden								
Kjellström et al. (1979)	228 men (≥ 5 years)	2/1.35	Overall	< 1947	1		1.48 [0.17–5.35] (Elinder et al. 1985)	Incidence 1959–75
Elinder et al. (1985)	522 men (> 1 year)	8/6.01	Overall > 5 years and ≥ 20 years latency	1947–62 1962–74 > 1975	0.3 0.05 0.02		1.33 [0.57–2.62] 1.75 [0.70–3.61] (Elinder et al., 1985)	Mortality 1940–80 at same plant
Copper–cadmium alloy								
United Kingdom								
Holden (1980a)	Urban ≥ 1 year Rural ≥ 1 year 624 vicinity ≥ 1 year	8/4.50 2/7.85 36/26.08	Overall Overall Overall	< 1953 1953–57 > 1957	1 < 0.15 < 0.05		1.78 [0.77–3.50] 0.26 [0.03–0.92] 1.38 [0.97–1.91]	Mortality, number of workers not stated Expected deaths based on national rates Vicinity workers also exposed to arsenic
Cadmium recovery								
USA								
Lemen et al. (1976)	292 men (≥ 2 years)	12/5.11					2.35 [1.21–4.10] (Smith et al., 1980)	Mortality 1940–73
Stayner et al. (1992)	579 men (≥ 6 months)	24/16.07	Overall ≤ 584[c] 585–1460 1461–2920 > 2920	< 1950 1950–59 1960–64 1965–76	(personal) 1.16 0.50 0.34 0.26	(ambient) 1–45 0.1–20 0.4–0.5 0.05–0.6	1.49 [0.95–2.21] 0.34 1.63 2.17 2.72	Mortality 1940–84 Excludes workers hired before 1 January 1926 Test for trend significant

Table 10 (contd)

Type of plant, country (reference)	Population (duration of exposure)	Lung cancers (obs/exp)	Exposure level	Cadmium levels		Relative risk (95% CI[a])		Comment
				Years	Estimated levels (mg/m³)			

Cadmium recovery (contd)

						Odds ratio		
						Non-Mexican-American (no.)	Mexican-American (no.)	
USA (contd) Stayner et al. (1993)	Subgroup of cohort of Stayner et al. (1992) hired after 1940			< 584 584–1460 1461–2920 > 2920		0.32 (1) 2.81 (6) 4.70 (5) 0 (0.6 exp.)	0.42 (1) 0 (0 exp.) 0.82 (1) 2.46 (2)	

Cadmium processing

| United Kingdom Kazantzis et al. (1992); Kazantzis & Blanks (1992) | 6910 men > 1 year | 339/304.1 270 55 14 | Overall Always low Ever medium Ever high | | | 1.12 (1.00–1.24) 1.08 (0.96–1.22) 1.21 (0.91–1.57) 1.62 (0.89–2.73) | | Mortality 1943–89; 17 plants; 3% of workers had ever high exposure. |

NR, not reported
[a]Approximate 95% confidence intervals calculated by the Working Group are given in square brackets.
[b]Referent group includes jobs with no or 'minimal' exposure to cadmium.
[c]Units are mg/m³-days

Table 11. Cohort studies of prostatic cancer in cadmium workers

Type of plant, country (reference)	Population (duration of exposure)	Prostatic cancers (obs/exp)	Exposure level	Relative risk (95% CI[a])	Comment
Nickel–cadmium battery (cadmium oxide)					
United Kingdom					
Potts (1965)	74 men (≥10 years)	3/NR	Overall	Cannot be calculated	Mortality through 1965. No referent group
Kipling & Waterhouse (1967)	248 men (≥1 year)	4/0.58	Overall	6.90 [1.86–17.66]	Incidence through 1966 includes three deaths from Potts (1965).
Sorahan & Waterhouse (1983)	2559 men (≥1 month)	8/6.6	Overall	1.21 [0.52–2.39]	Mortality 1946–80
Sorahan & Waterhouse (1985)	2559 men (≥1 month)	15/11.02	Overall >1 year and high	1.36 [0.76–2.25] 4.02 [1.73–7.92]	Incidence 1950–80 including 4 cases from Kipling & Waterhouse (1967)
Sweden					
Kjellström et al. (1979)	228 men (≥5 years)	2/1.2	Overall	1.67 [0.19–6.02]	Incidence 1959–75
Elinder et al. (1985)	522 men (>1 year)	4/3.70	Overall >5 years and ≥20 years' latency	1.08 [0.29–2.77] 1.48 [0.40–3.79]	Mortality 1951–83
Copper–cadmium alloy					
United Kingdom					
Holden (1980a)	347 male cadmium workers (≥1 year)	1/1.58	Exposed	0.63 [0.01–3.52]	Mortality
	624 vicinity workers (≥1 year)	8/3.0	Less exposed	2.67 [1.15–5.26]	

Table 11 (contd)

Type of plant, country (reference)	Population (duration of exposure)	Lung cancers (obs/exp)	Exposure level	Relative risk (95% CI[a])	Comment
Copper–cadmium alloy (contd)					
Sweden					
Kjellström et al. (1979)	94 men (≥ 5 years)	4/2.69	Exposed	1.49 [0.40–3.81]	Mortality 1940–75. Data described as preliminary
	328 controls	4/6.42	Unexposed	0.62 [0.17–1.60]	
Cadmium recovery					
USA					
Lemen et al. (1976)	292 men (≥ 2 years)	4/1.15	Overall ≥ 20 years' latency	3.48 [0.94–8.91] [4.55 (1.22–11.64)]	Mortality 1940–73
Thun et al. (1985)	602 men (≥ 6 months)	3/1.41	≥ 2 years' employment and ≥ 20 years' latency	2.13 (0.44–6.22)	Mortality 1940–78
Cadmium processing					
United Kingdom					
Kazantzis et al. (1992); Kazantzis & Blanks (1992)	6910 men (> 1 year)	37/49.3 36 0 1	Overall Always low Ever medium Ever high	0.75 (0.53–1.03) 0.85 (0.60–1.18) 0 (0.0–0.59) 0.97 (0.01–5.40)	Mortality 1943–89 Regional adjustment

NR, not reported
[a]Approximate 95% confidence intervals calculated by the Working Group are given in square brackets.

monograph on exposures in the glass manufacturing industry (p. 347). The prevalence of exposure to cadmium compounds was 1%. Bladder was the only cancer site to be associated with exposure to cadmium compounds (six exposed cases; odds ratio, 1.6; 90% CI, 0.7–3.8). When the analysis was restricted to substantial exposure, only four cases of bladder cancer had been exposed (odds ratio, 4.9; 90% CI, 1.2–19.6). No association was found with cancers of the lung or prostate.

3. Studies of Cancer in Experimental Animals

The carcinogenic and toxicological effects of cadmium have been reviewed (Oberdörster, 1986; Peters *et al.*, 1986; Kazantzis, 1987; Oberdörster, 1989; Waalkes & Oberdörster, 1990; Heinrich, 1992; Nordberg *et al.*, 1992; Waalkes *et al.*, 1992a).

3.1 Oral administration

3.1.1 *Mouse*

A group of 48 male and 39 female weanling Swiss mice (Charles River strain) received 5 ppm [5 mg/L] cadmium as **cadmium acetate** in the drinking-water for life. A group of 44 male and 60 female control mice were given 'metal-free' drinking-water. Body weight was generally similar in treated and control animals. Cadmium treatment did not result in an increased incidence of any type of tumour, and the incidence of lung tumours in treated males was reduced compared to controls (0/48 *versus* 8/44; $p < 0.01$, χ^2 test); no such effect was observed in females (5/39 *vs* 9/60) (Schroeder *et al.*, 1964). [The Working Group considered that the single exposure level used was too low for an evaluation of carcinogenicity.]

Groups of 50 eight-week-old male specified pathogen-free (SPF) Swiss mice were administered 0.44, 0.88 or 1.75 mg/kg bw cadmium as **cadmium sulfate** (3 $CdSO_4.8H_2O$) in distilled-water by gavage once a week for 18 months, at which time the experiment was terminated. A control group of 150 male mice received distilled-water alone. No difference in survival or weight gain was observed between cadmium-treated mice and controls. Among the mice surviving after 18 months of treatment, groups of 20 animals were selected at random from the high-dose group and from the control group for histological analysis of selected tissues, including urogenital tract, stomach, lung, liver and kidney, while only macroscopically abnormal tissues were examined from other animals. Tumour incidence was no different in treated and control animals. Special attention was paid to the prostate, but no neoplastic or preneoplastic lesion was observed in this organ (Levy *et al.*, 1975). [The Working Group noted the low dose levels used and the limited histopathological examination in terms of numbers of animals and tissues.]

3.1.2 *Rat*

Groups of 69 male and 58 female weanling Long–Evans rats received 0 or 5 ppm [5 mg/L] cadmium as **cadmium acetate** in the drinking-water until death. Body weights and survival did not differ significantly among treated and control groups; about 50% of test and control animals survived more than 24 months. Histopathology was performed on gross lesions. Tumour incidences in various organs in the 48 treated male and 36 treated female rats examined were similar to those in the 35 male and 35 female controls examined (Schroeder *et al.*, 1965). [The Working Group noted that the single exposure level used was too low for an evaluation of carcinogenicity.]

A group of 47 weanling Long–Evans rats [sex distribution unspecified] received 5 ppm [mg/L] cadmium as **cadmium acetate** in the drinking-water for life. A control group of 34 rats received drinking-water alone. Growth rate and survival were similar. Only macroscopically visible tumours were sectioned for histological analysis. Tumour incidence (as analysed by χ^2) in the cadmium-treated animals was similar to that in the control group (Schroeder *et al.*, 1963; Kanisawa & Schroeder, 1969). [The Working Group noted the single, low exposure level, the lack of sex-specific data and that histopathology was performed only on macroscopic lesions.]

Three groups of 30 male SPF CB hooded rats, 12 weeks of age, received weekly gastric instillations of 0.09, 0.18 and 0.35 mg/kg bw cadmium as **cadmium sulfate** ($3CdSO_4.8H_2O$) dissolved in sterile distilled-water for 104 weeks, at which time surviving animals were killed. A control group of 90 rats received weekly gastric instillations of sterile distilled-water. Histopathological examination was performed on all animals. There was no difference in body weights or survival. Tumour incidence was similar in cadmium-exposed animals and controls (Levy & Clack, 1975). [The Working Group noted the low doses used and that the spontaneous incidence of interstitial-cell tumours of the testis (seen in 75% of animals) may have obscured any cadmium-induced effects within that tissue.]

Groups of 50 male and 50 female Wistar (W74) rats, four to five weeks of age, were fed diets containing 1, 3, 10 or 50 ppm (mg/kg diet) Cd^{2+} as **cadmium chloride** ($CdCl_2.H_2O$) for a period of 104 weeks. Control groups of 100 rats of each sex were used. Survival was not affected by cadmium treatment, and body weights were significantly reduced only in high-dose males [exact extent or time point not given]. Histological examination was performed on all animals, and tumour incidence data were tested by the Fisher exact test. The incidences of testicular and prostatic tumours and of other tumour types were similar in treated groups and controls (Löser, 1980a).

Groups of 30 male Wistar (TNO/W74) rats, 13–16 weeks old, received a single intragastric dose of 50 mg/kg bw or 10 weekly doses of 5 mg/kg bw cadmium as **cadmium chloride** ($CdCl_2.H_2O$) in distilled-water. Two groups of 10 controls received vehicle only. Five animals in each group of treated animals and two or three animals of each group of control animals were killed at 12 and 18 months, and the remaining animals were killed at 133 weeks. Survival was similar in all groups. Following the single administration of 50 mg/kg bw, growth was slightly retarded [data not shown, extent or time point not given]. Testis, epididymis, seminal vesicles, prostates and gross lesions were examined histologically. Rats treated with cadmium did not have an increased incidence of testicular tumours or of tumours at other sites (Bomhard *et al.*, 1987). [The Working Group noted the short duration of exposure.]

In a study on the effect of chronic dietary deficiency of zinc on the carcinogenicity of orally administered cadmium, groups of 28 male Wistar (WF/NCr) rats, eight weeks of age, were fed diets containing either adequate zinc (60 ppm [60 mg/kg diet]) or a zinc concentration (7 ppm [7 mg/kg diet]) that produced a significant reduction (40%) in serum zinc in the absence of overt toxicity. Starting two weeks later, these diets were fed together with cadmium at 0, 25, 50, 100 or 200 (maximum-tolerated dose) ppm [mg/kg diet] as **cadmium chloride** hemipentahydrate, for 77 weeks, at which time the study was terminated. Histological examination was performed on all animals and lesions. Zinc deficiency alone did not affect food consumption, weight gain or survival; cadmium did not affect survival or food consumption, and body weight was consistently reduced only at the highest doses (100 and 200 mg/kg diet), by 10% and 12–17%, respectively. At the two highest doses of cadmium, rats fed zinc-deficient diets had a significantly increased food consumption when compared with zinc-deficient controls. The combined incidence of prostatic proliferative lesions (hyperplasia and adenoma), but not those of the lesions separately, was significantly ($p < 0.05$; Fisher exact test) greater in rats given zinc-adequate diets containing 50 ppm cadmium (5/22; 22.7%) than in controls (1/28; 3.6%), and in rats receiving zinc-deficient diets (4/26; 15.4%) than in controls (0/26). At higher doses of cadmium (100 and 200 ppm), an increased incidence of prostatic atrophy was observed in the rats receiving zinc-deficient diets, which may have been responsible for the lower incidence of prostatic lesions seen in rats fed zinc-deficient diets. Cadmium treatment resulted in a dose-related (Cochran–Armitage trend tests) increase in the incidence of leukaemia in rats fed zinc-deficient diets throughout the dose range and in rats fed zinc-adequate diets receiving up to and including 100 ppm. The highest incidence of leukaemia occurred in rats receiving 200 ppm cadmium and the zinc-deficient diet (7/25; 28%), when compared with controls (2.27; 7.4%). Exposure to cadmium at a concentration of 200 ppm in conjunction with the zinc-adequate diet also induced a significant increase in testicular interstitial-cell tumours (6/27, 22.2% compared with controls, 1/28, 3.6%) (Waalkes & Rehm, 1992).

3.2 Inhalation exposure[1]

3.2.1 *Mouse*

Groups of 48 female Han:NMRI mice [age unspecified] were exposed to cadmium at 30 or 90 µg/m^3 as **cadmium chloride**, 30 or 90 µg/m^3 as **cadmium sulfate**, 90, 270 or 1000 µg/m^3 as **cadmium sulfide**, 10, 30, 90 or 270 µg/m^3 as **cadmium oxide dust** or 10, 30 or 90 µg/m^3 as **cadmium oxide fume**. The mass median aerodynamic diameter of all compounds was 0.2–0.6 µm [geometric standard deviation, 1.6]. For each treated group, a control group of 48 animals receiving filtered air was available. Exposure was for 19 or 8 h per day for five days a week, and the exposure time ranged from six to 69 weeks; exposure was terminated in some groups when the mortality rats started to increase. The duration of the study was 71–107 weeks; controls were followed for about 106 weeks. Histological examination was performed on all animals. Survival was reduced in 12 of the 19 experimental groups; survival was similar to that of controls in groups exposed to 90 or 270 µg/m^3 as cadmium sulfide, to 10, 30 or 90 µg/m^3 as cadmium oxide fume and to 10 or 270 µg/m^3 as cadmium oxide dust. The incidence of lung tumours was significantly increased in the groups receiving 30 and 90 µg/m^3

---

[1]The Working Group was aware of a study by inhalation in progress in rats and mice (Ghess et al., 1992).

as cadmium oxide fumes and 10 µg/m³ as cadmium oxide dust, but not in the group given 270 µg/m³ as cadmium oxide (see Table 12). In six other groups receiving cadmium oxide dust at various concentrations, survival was significantly decreased, but the probability of dying with a lung tumour was greater than in the controls (by life-table analysis) (Heinrich *et al.*, 1989; Heinrich, 1992). [The Working Group noted the variable spontaneous lung tumour rate and that the histopathological types of tumours were not reported.]

3.2.2 *Rat*

Four groups of 40 male SPF Wistar (TNO/W75) rats, six weeks old, were exposed to 12.5, 25 or 50 µg/m³ cadmium as **cadmium chloride** aerosol (mass median aerodynamic diameter, 0.55 µm; geometric standard deviation, 1.8) for 23 h a day on seven days a week for 18 months. Animals were observed for an additional 13 months, at which time the experiment was ended. A group of 41 rats exposed to filtered air served as controls. Histological examination was performed on all animals. Body weights and survival were not affected by cadmium treatment. A dose-related increase in the incidence of malignant pulmonary tumours (mostly adenocarcinomas) was observed in cadmium chloride-treated rats (12.5 µg/m³, 6/39 [15%]; 25 µg/m³, 20/38 [53%]; 50 µg/m³, 25/35 [71%]) compared with controls (0/38). Multiple pulmonary tumours were observed frequently; several tumours showed metastases or were regionally invasive. The incidence of adenomatous hyperplasia was also increased by cadmium treatment (Takenaka *et al.*, 1983).

Groups of 20–40 male and 20 female Wistar (BOR-WISW) [formerly called TNO/W75] SPF rats, nine weeks of age, were exposed to aerosols of **cadmium chloride, cadmium sulfate, cadmium sulfide, cadmium oxide dust** or **cadmium oxide fume** (for all compounds, mass median aerodynamic diameter, 0.2–0.5 µm; geometric standard deviation, 1.6) for up to 18 months and observed for up to an additional 13 months (see Table 13). Two additional groups received both zinc oxide dust and cadmium oxide dust at two different levels. Exposure was generally for 22 h a day for seven days a week, although some groups received continuous exposure for 6 months or discontinuous exposure for 40 h per week for 6 months. Inhalation and observation periods were terminated when mortality reached ≥ 25% or ≥ 75%, respectively, or at 31 months. Histological examination was performed on all rats. Mortality rates were generally greater in rats treated with the high dose of cadmium [body weights not given]. Generally, all forms of cadmium appeared to increase the incidence of primary pulmonary tumours over that in controls [statistical analysis not performed], to a maximum of 90% (cadmium sulfate in females) compared to 0 in controls; in general, no male:female difference was observed. Except in males exposed to 90 µg/m³ cadmium oxide and 900 µg/m³ zinc oxide, zinc oxide reduced the carcinogenicity of cadmium oxide at that dose. The tumours observed were mostly adenomas and adenocarcinomas, but a few rats had bronchioloalveolar adenomas and squamous-cell carcinomas (Glaser *et al.*, 1990). [The Working Group noted that the groups exposed to cadmium oxide fume had significantly lower lung tumour incidences than the groups exposed to the other cadmium compounds ($p < 0.0001$; likelihood ratio by χ^2 test). Animals exposed to cadmium oxide fume, however, had only about half the cadmium content in their lungs as animals exposed to the same concentration of the other cadmium compounds over the same period, which was attributed

Table 12. Percentages of animals bearing lung tumours among mice exposed to cadmium with no reduction in mean survival time

Cadmium compound	Concentration ($\mu g/m^3$ Cd)	Exposure time (weeks)		50% survival (weeks)		Experimental time (weeks)	% Tumour-bearing animals	
		h/day	Weeks	Treated	Controls		Treated	Controls
Cadmium sulfide	90	19	64	76	70	98	21.1	14.6
	270	8	26	78	80	101	25	36.9
Cadmium oxide fume	10	19	55	75	71	98	20.9	20.0
	30	19	50	68	71	93	29.6*	20.0
	90	8	64	74	70	105	34.0*	14.6
Cadmium oxide dust	10	19	64	76	70	105	26.1*	14.6
	270	8	59	66	89	107	25.5	27.7

Modified from Heinrich (1992)
*$p < 0.05$ (χ^2 test)

Table 13. Lung tumour incidence in animals with long-term exposure to cadmium by inhalation

Group	Cadmium aerosol (µg/m³)	Duration (months)[a] Exposure	Study	Animals bearing primary lung tumours/animals examined
Males				
Control	0	0	31	0/40
Cadmium chloride	30	18	30	15/20
	90	6	30	11/20
Cadmium sulfate	90	14	31	11/20
Cadmium sulfide	90	18	30	17/20
	270	16	30	14/20
	810	7	30	11/20
	2430	4	30	7/16
	270[b]	6	27	3/20
Cadmium oxide dust	30	18	31	28/39
	90	7	31	12/39
	90[b]	6	31	4/20
	30[c]	18	29	25/38
Cadmium oxide fume	10	18	31	0/40
	30	18	31	8/38
Cadmium oxide/zinc oxide	30/300	18	31	0/20
	90/900	18	31	8/20
Females				
Control	0	0	31	0/20
Cadmium chloride	30	18	31	13/18
	90	6	29	3/18
Cadmium sulfate	90	18	29	18/20
Cadmium sulfide	90	18	31	15/20
	270	16	30	16/19
	810	10	29	13/20
	2430	3	31	6/19
	270[b]	6	29	3/20
Cadmium oxide dust	30	18	31	15/20
	90	11	31	14/19
	90[b]	6	31	3/20
Cadmium oxide/zinc oxide	30/300	18	31	0/20
	90/900	18	31	7/20

Modified from Glaser et al. (1990)

[a]Exposure was stopped when 25% mortality had occurred, and the study was terminated when 75% of the animals had died.
[b]Discontinuous exposure for 40 h per week
[c]Rats maintained on a zinc-deficient (24 ppm) diet

to a lower pulmonary deposition (Oberdörster & Cox, 1990) of the chain-like electric arc-generated fume particles. The Working Group was also aware of the fact that the generation of cadmium sulfide aerosols in this study from an aqueous suspension had resulted in the generation of a cadmium sulfate:cadmium sulfide mixture (50:50), due to photo-oxidation of cadmium sulfide, which may have confounded the number of tumours induced by cadmium sulfide (Glaser et al., 1992; König et al., 1992; Oberdörster & Cherian, 1992)].

3.2.3 Hamster

Groups of 24 male and 24 female Syrian golden [Hoe:SYHK] hamsters [age unspecified] were exposed to cadmium at 30 or 90 µg/m³ as **cadmium chloride**, 30 or 90 µg/m³ as **cadmium sulfate**, 90, 270 or 1000 µg/m³ as **cadmium sulfide**, 10, 30, 90 or 270 µg/m³ as **cadmium oxide dust** or 10, 30 or 90 µg/m³ as **cadmium oxide fume** (mass median aerodynamic diameter, 0.2–0.6 µm [geometric standard deviation, 1.6]) for 19 or 8 h per day on five days a week; the exposure time ranged from 13 to 65 weeks and the total experimental time from 60 to 113 weeks. Control groups received filtered air. Exposure was terminated earlier when mortality started to increase; the experimental time was 61–87 weeks for exposed females and 60–113 weeks for males, as increased mortality occurred earlier in females than in males. Survival was reduced in 12 of the 19 groups of exposed male hamsters, but none showed an increased incidence of lung tumours. Histological examination was performed on all animals. In only six of the exposed groups (males and females combined) was there one or, in one case, two animals with a papilloma or a polypoid adenoma of the trachea; one papilloma was also found in the control group (Heinrich et al., 1989; Heinrich, 1992). [The Working Group noted the limited reporting of the data on tumours and the insensitivity of the hamster to induction of tumours of the lung in studies by long-term inhalation.]

3.3 Intratracheal administration

Rat: Groups of male Fischer 344 rats received either a single intratracheal instillation of 25 µg **cadmium oxide** (median diameter, 0.5 µm) suspended in saline at 70 days of age (48 rats), one instillation at both 70 and 100 days of age (total dose, 50 µg/rat; 46 rats) or one instillation at 70, 100 and 130 days of age (total dose, 75 µg/rat; 50 rats) and were compared with 46 rats receiving intratracheal instillations of saline only. [The dose of 25 µg/rat was approximately 75% of the single intratracheal LD_{50}.] Animals were observed for up to 880 days, and all were examined histologically. Cadmium treatment did not affect survival [body weights not given]. Two pulmonary adenocarcinomas were seen in rats given 50 µg (nonsignificant; χ^2) but none in other groups. Increased incidences of mammary gland fibroadenomas were reported in all groups receiving cadmium oxide: 25 µg/rat, 7/44 (16%); 50 µg/rat, 5/41 (12%); 75 µg/rat, 11/48 (23%); controls, 3/45 (7%). No other significant difference in tumour incidence was seen (Sanders & Mahaffey, 1984). [The Working Group noted that the mammary tumours that occurred in treated groups had to be pooled in order to reach statistical significance.]

Groups of about 40 female Wistar (WU/Kiβlegg) rats, 11 weeks of age, received 20 weekly intratracheal instillations in saline of 1 or 3 µg or 15 weekly instillations of 9 µg cadmium as **cadmium chloride** hydrate (purity, 99%) or **cadmium oxide** [purity not given] (total doses, 20, 60 or 135 µg/rat for both compounds) or 10 weekly instillations of 63, 250 or 1000 µg cadmium as **cadmium sulfide** (> 99.9% pure; total doses, 630, 2500 or 10 000 µg/rat) and were observed for up to 124 weeks. Concurrent controls received saline only. [Body weights were not given.] Only the lungs and trachea were examined histologically. Cadmium chloride induced moderate, dose-related increases in the incidence of lung tumours: controls, 0/40; 20 µg/rat, 0/38; 60 µg/rat, 3/40 (7.5%); 135 µg/rat, 2/36 (5.6%) [$p < 0.01$; trend test]. Cadmium oxide also induced some lung tumours: 20 µg/rat, 2/37 (5.4%); 60 µg/rat, 2/40 (5.0%); 135 µg/rat, 0/39 (not significant). Cadmium sulfide induced a dose-related increase in the incidence of lung tumours: 2/39 (5.1%) at 630 µg/rat, 8/36 (22.2%) at 2500 µg/rat and 7/36 (19.4%) at 10 000 µg/rat [$p < 0.005$; trend test]. The authors reported that mortality was increased at the highest dose. The lung tumours induced were primarily adenocarcinomas, although a few adenomas and squamous-cell carcinomas were also observed (Pott *et al.*, 1987). [The Working Group noted that the cadmium sulfide particles had been administered in an aqueous suspension, which may have resulted in photo-oxidation of some fraction of the cadmium sulfide to cadmium sulfate; however, even under the assumption of worst-case conditions—24-h exposure of cadmium sulfide suspension to light—the amount of cadmium sulfate should not have exceeded 3% of the total cadmium in the middle dose (Oberdörster & Cherian, 1992). Therefore, photo-decomposition of cadmium sulfide to cadmium sulfate could not have accounted for the carcinogenic response observed.]

3.4 Subcutaneous and/or intramuscular administration

3.4.1 *Mouse*

In a study to examine the effect of zinc on the carcinogenicity of cadmium, a group of 26 male Charles River mice, eight weeks of age, received a single subcutaneous injection of 0.03 mmol/kg bw (5.5 mg/kg bw) **cadmium chloride** [vehicle unspecified] in the interscapular region and were observed for 14 months. Control groups consisted of 25 untreated mice and 25 mice that received a single subcutaneous injection of 0.03 mmol/kg bw cadmium chloride and three concurrent subcutaneous injections of 1.0 mmol/kg zinc acetate (total dose, 3.0 mmol/kg; 550 mg/kg bw) at three different sites over a period of 25 h before and after the cadmium injection. No injection-site tumour was reported. Only testes were examined histologically [weight gains and survival not reported]. Of the mice that received cadmium alone, 77% (20/26) had interstitial-cell tumours of the testis; none occurred in cadmium–zinc treated animals or in untreated controls. Zinc also prevented the induction by cadmium of non-neoplastic lesions of the testes in almost all of the animals (Gunn *et al.*, 1961, 1963).

A group of 20 male CB mice, six to seven weeks of age, received 11 weekly subcutaneous injections of 0.05 mg **cadmium sulfate** tetrahydrate in 0.2 ml sterile distilled-water into the right flank (total dose of cadmium, 0.22 mg). A group of 20 untreated animals served as controls [body weights not reported]. Only gross and testicular lesions were taken for histological analysis. None of the cadmium-treated mice developed tumours at the site of injection, and the incidence of tumours at other sites did not exceed control rates [statistical analysis not given]; however, non-neoplastic changes typical of cadmium treatment, such as testicular degeneration and interstitial-cell hyperplasia, were observed in 6/16 [17 in table] animals that survived for eight months or more and in none of 15 control mice surviving at least to the same time point. [The Working Group noted the short duration of the study.] In a separate study, 10 six-week-old male CB mice received three weekly subcutaneous injections of 5 mg cadmium sulfate-precipitated rat ferritin into the right flank, followed six weeks later by 12 weekly injections of 0.5 mg of the same preparation (total dose, 0.36 mg cadmium). No tumour was observed at the site of injection during the following 20 months (Haddow *et al.*, 1964; Roe *et al.*, 1964).

3.4.2 *Rat*

The earliest suspicion that cadmium might be carcinogenic came from a brief report by Haddow *et al.* (1961), who detected malignant tumours at the injection site (subcutaneous or intramuscular) of ferritin prepared from rat liver by cadmium precipitation in 8/20 male rats [strain unspecified]. Additionally, 10/20 of these rats had interstitial-cell tumours of the testes.

Groups of 10 female hooded rats, two to three months old, received a single intramuscular injection of 14 or 28 mg **cadmium metal** powder (dimensions: 1.7 μm diameter for spheres, 85 μm × 50 μm for ellipsoids and rods and 220 μm × 50 μm × 50 μm for other shapes) suspended in 0.4 ml fowl serum into the thigh muscle. The total duration of the study was 84 weeks. [Weight gain was not determined and necropsy protocol was not stated.] Two of the rats receiving 28 mg cadmium powder were killed within two week of injection in order to study acute local reactions. Malignant tumours developed at the site of injection in 9/10 rats given 14 mg and in 6/8 rats given 28 mg cadmium powder. Most of the tumours were rhabdomyosarcomas; some fibrosarcomas were seen which metastasized to lymph nodes (Heath *et al.*, 1962; Heath & Daniel, 1964). [The Working Group noted that, while the authors stated that zinc or tungsten metal powders did not induce local sarcomas at the injection site, no details were reported.]

A group of 25 male Wistar rats, 12 weeks of age, received a single subcutaneous injection of 0.03 mmol/kg bw [5.5 mg/kg bw] **cadmium chloride** [vehicle unspecified] in the interscapular region and were observed for 11 months. Control groups consisted of 20 untreated rats and 17 rats that received a single subcutaneous injection of 0.03 mmol/kg bw cadmium chloride and three concurrent subcutaneous injections of 1.0 mmol/kg zinc acetate (total dose, 3.0 mmol/kg; 550 mg/kg bw) in the lumbosacral area over a period of 25 h before and after the cadmium injection. Only testes were examined histologically. [Weight gains and survival were not stated.] Of the rats that received cadmium alone, 17/25 (68%) had interstitial-cell tumours of the testes; 2/17 occurred in cadmium–zinc treated animals, and 0/20 occurred in controls (Gunn *et al.*, 1961, 1963, 1965).

Ten six-month-old female Wistar CB rats received subcutaneous injections of 25 mg **cadmium sulfide** (diameter, 0.5 μm; equivalent to 20 mg cadmium) suspended in 0.25 ml saline into both sides of the dorsal midline. Ten three-month-old rats received subcutaneous injections of 0.25 ml saline and served as controls. [Body weights and necropsy protocol were not stated.] Over the following 12 months, 6/10 treated rats and none of the controls developed fibrosarcomas (Kazantzis, 1963). In a further study, 15 male and 15 female Wistar CB rats, nine months of age, received subcutaneous injections of 25 mg cadmium sulfide suspended in 0.25 ml saline into both sides of the dorsal midline. Of the 26 rats that survived for more than six months, six developed sarcomas at the site of injection. In a separate experiment, seven male and seven female rats, eight months old, were given a single intramuscular injection of 50 mg cadmium sulfide suspended in 0.5 ml saline into the thigh. [Body weights and necropsy protocol not stated.] Four animals died during the first nine months after injection. Sarcomas at the site of injection developed in 6/14 rats over a 17-month period. In a further study, 10 three-month-old female rats received subcutaneous injections of 25 mg cadmium oxide suspended in 0.25 ml saline into both sides of the dorsal midline; 8/10 developed fibrosarcomas at the site of injection within one year (Kazantzis & Hanbury, 1966).

A group of 22 four-month-old male Wistar rats received single subcutaneous injections of 0.03 mmol/kg bw [5.5 mg/kg bw] **cadmium chloride** (equivalent to 1.35 mg cadmium [vehicle not stated]) into the interscapular region and were observed for 10 months. Only testes and subcutaneous tumours at the site of injection were examined histologically. Sarcomas developed at the site of injection in 9/22 rats, while 21/22 rats developed interstitial-cell tumours of the testis. A group of 17 rats received the same treatment with cadmium chloride and subcutaneous injections of 1 mmol/kg bw (183.5 mg/kg bw) zinc acetate in the lumbosacral area; the zinc acetate treatment resulted in lower incidences of sarcomas at the site of injection (2/17) and of testicular tumours (3/17) than those induced by cadmium. No interstitial-cell tumour of the testis developed in 18 untreated controls (Gunn *et al.*, 1964).

A group of 20 male CB rats, three weeks of age, received an initial subcutaneous injection of 20 mg **cadmium sulfate**-precipitated rat liver ferritin [vehicle unspecified] into the right flank followed by another injection of 20 mg 46 days later and then 2 mg once a week for eight weeks, all in approximately the same area. A group of 16 untreated rats served as controls. Only gross lesions were taken for histological examination. Of the cadmium–ferritin-treated rats, 7/20 (35%) developed injection-site sarcomas and 11/15 (73%) examined developed interstitial-cell tumours of the testis over the total observation period of 28 months. No such lesion was observed in 15 control rats that survived to a similar time (Haddow *et al.*, 1964; Roe *et al.*, 1964). In a subsequent study, no tumour at the site of injection and no testicular tumour was induced in CB Wistar rats by cadmium-free ferritin (Roe *et al.*, 1968). A separate group of 20 male CB rats, six to seven weeks old, received 10 weekly subcutaneous injections into the right flank of 0.5 mg cadmium sulfate tetrahydrate in 0.1 ml sterile distilled-water. By 20 months, 14/20 rats had developed sarcomas at the site of injection (Haddow *et al.*, 1964), while 10/18 examined had developed interstitial-cell tumours of the testis (Roe *et al.*, 1964).

A group of 49 male Wistar rats, four months of age, received a single injection of 1.8 mg cadmium as **cadmium chloride** [vehicle unspecified] either subcutaneously into the interscapular region (23 rats) or intramuscularly into the thigh (26 rats) and were observed for 14 months. No concurrent controls were available [body weights and necropsy protocol not given]. More sarcomas occurred at the site of injection when cadmium was injected subcutaneously (10/23; 43.5%) than intramuscularly (3/26; 11.5%) (Gunn *et al.*, 1967).

Six male Sprague–Dawley rats, three months of age, received a single subcutaneous injection of 10 mg/kg **cadmium chloride** [site and vehicle unspecified] and were observed for a further 13 months. A group of 16 untreated rats of the same age served as controls. All six cadmium-treated rats developed interstitial-cell tumours of the testis. Baseline urinary testosterone concentrations in cadmium-treated rats bearing tumours were 26–29% those of control animals (Favino et al., 1968). [The Working Group noted the limited reporting of the study.]

Eighty 12-week-old male Wistar rats received a a single subcutaneous injection of 0.03 mmol/kg bw [5.5 mg/kg bw] **cadmium chloride** as the dihydrate (3.4 mg/kg bw cadmium) dissolved in sterile distilled-water into the hip area and were observed for up to two years. Twenty untreated rats served as controls. Animals were examined grossly and histologically [body weights not stated]. Dermal atrophy, ulcerative necrosis, acute and chronic inflammation, fibrosis and mineralization were observed at the site of injection during the two months following administration of cadmium. Of the rats that survived to seven months (the time of appearance of the first sarcoma at the site of injection), 6/45 had local spindle-cell sarcomas after 18 months (Knorre, 1970a,b). In a second experiment with 104 male rats treated by the same schedule, interstitial-cell tumours of the testis were found by 698 days in 10/25 rats still alive at 355 days (when the first tumour of the testis appeared) (Knorre, 1971). One sarcoma at the site of injection metastasized to the peritoneum [possibly invasion], and several others metastasized to regional lymph nodes (Knorre, 1970a). A single cadmium-induced histologically confirmed testicular interstitial-cell tumour metastasized to the colon and liver [a rare event]. No interstitial-cell tumour of the testis was seen in 32 control animals (Knorre, 1971).

A group of 15 male Wistar rats weighing 100–300 g received single subcutaneous injections [site unspecified] of 0.02–0.03 mmol/kg bw [3.7–5.5 mg/kg bw] **cadmium chloride** and were observed for 11 months. Interstitial-cell tumours of the testis developed in 13/13 rats still alive at 11 months, and two rats developed pleomorphic sarcomas at the site of injection (Lucis et al., 1972).

Three groups of 25 male SPF CB hooded rats, 12 weeks of age, received weekly subcutaneous injections of 0.05, 0.1 or 0.2 mg **cadmium sulfate** (3 $CdSO_4.8 H_2O$; 0.02–0.09 mg Cd) dissolved in sterile distilled-water into alternate flanks over a period of two years. The control group consisted of 75 animals that received weekly injections of distilled-water alone. Extensive macroscopic and microscopic examinations were performed, with special attention to the genital gland complex. Body weights were suppressed ($p < 0.001$) [test unspecified; data not shown; extent not stated] in the high-dose group after two years. Sarcomas at the site of injection were found in 1/25 rats given the low dose, 1/25 given the medium dose and 4/25 given the high dose. No neoplastic change was seen in any other tissue, including the prostate. All groups, including controls, had high incidences of testicular interstitial-cell tumours (67–77%) [which may have obscured any effect of cadmium on that tissue]. The concentration of cadmium in the kidney in the highest dose group was about 500 µg/g tissue [analysed polarographically after dithizone extraction] (Levy et al., 1973).

Twenty male Fischer 344 rats, four to five weeks old, received a single subcutaneous injection of 0.03 mmol/kg bw **cadmium chloride** [5.5 mg/kg bw], and 10 control rats received subcutaneous injections of saline [body weight, survival data and necropsy protocol not given]. Interstitial-cell tumours of the testis (11 bilateral) developed in 16/20 treated rats over the one-year observation period, while none developed in control rats (Reddy et al.,

1973). [The Working Group noted that the Fischer 344 strain generally has a > 80% spontaneous incidence of interstitial-cell tumours of the testis by two years of age.]

In a 110-week study to examine the potential effects of calcium and magnesium salts on the carcinogenicity of cadmium, groups of 25 male Wistar rats weighing 120–150 g were kept for two weeks and then given subcutaneous injections of 0.02 or 0.04 mmol/kg bw [3.67 or 7.34 mg/kg bw] **cadmium chloride** hemipentahydrate into the nape of the neck. Rats received either no further treatment or treatment with calcium acetate or magnesium acetate, either in the diet (3%) two weeks prior and two weeks after cadmium chloride treatment or by three separate subcutaneous injections (calcium acetate, 0.16 mmol/kg bw [25.3 mg/kg bw]; magnesium acetate, 4.0 mmol/kg bw [570 mg/kg bw]) in the same area as the cadmium chloride 24 h before, at the same time as and 24 h after cadmium chloride injection. Control rats received saline injections instead of cadmium chloride. All animals were examined histologically. The highest dose of cadmium chloride caused slight weight suppression but only up to 12 weeks after injection. Survival was not affected by any of the treatments. Tumours at the site of injection (predominantly fibrosarcomas) occurred to a similar extent (approximately 33% of rats at risk) in all groups receiving cadmium chloride, regardless of the dose or of other treatments, with the exception of injected magnesium acetate which significantly reduced (to 0; $p < 0.02$; χ^2) the response to cadmium at the injection site. Both levels of cadmium chloride increased the incidence of testicular interstitial-cell tumours (approximately 85%) over that in controls (30%); the increase was generally unchanged by other treatments, with the exception of dietary calcium acetate, which resulted in a lower incidence than in animals receiving cadmium chloride alone, but only at the high dose. When all groups receiving cadmium chloride were considered together, a significantly ($p < 0.02$) higher incidence of pancreatic islet-cell tumours (mainly adenomas) occurred (22/258 rats; 8.5%) when compared with rats not receiving cadmium chloride (3/137; 2.2%) (Poirier et al., 1983).

Groups of 30 male Wistar Crl:(WI)BR rats, six weeks of age, received a single subcutaneous injection of 1.0, 2.5, 5.0, 10.0, 20.0 or 40.0 μmol/kg bw [0.18–7.3 mg/kg bw] **cadmium chloride** dissolved in saline into the dorsal thoracic midline area and were observed for two years. Other groups received either four separate subcutaneous injections of 5 μmol/kg cadmium chloride on days 0, 2, 4 and 7 or a subcutaneous injection of 5 μmol/kg [0.9 mg/kg] cadmium chloride followed two days later by a dose of 10 or 20 [1.8 or 3.6] μmol/kg bw. A group of 45 controls received subcutaneous injections of saline alone. All animals were examined histologically. Cadmium chloride did not modify survival in any group. The highest dose (40 μmol/kg) reduced body weight by about 5–10%. The incidences of sarcomas at the site of injection were found to depend on accumulated dosage at the site and approached 45% incidence at the highest dose of cadmium. The incidences of testicular tumours (mostly interstitial-cell tumours) were correlated with the extent of testicular degeneration induced by cadmium and showed a positive dose-dependence with single doses of cadmium: 83% at 40 μmol/kg and 72% at 20 μmol/kg, as compared with 18% in controls ($p \leq 0.05$; Cochran–Armitage test). The 5-μmol/kg and 20-μmol/kg doses did not increase the incidence of testicular tumours. Prostatic tumour incidence was significantly elevated at the 2.5 μmol/kg dose (8/26; 31%; $p \leq 0.05$, Fisher exact test) compared with controls (5/44; 11%), and a positive dose–effect relationship was seen between 0 and 2.5 μmol/kg in both tumour incidence and multiplicity ($p \leq 0.05$; Cochran–Armitage test). A reduction to the control level in the tumour response of the prostate to higher doses of cadmium (≥ 5.0 μmol/kg) was attributed by the authors to testicular degeneration and consequent loss of androgenic support. Cadmium chloride suppressed the induction of tumours of the pancreas (both islet-cell and acinar-cell) from 60% in controls to 20% in animals receiving 40 μmol/kg cadmium, with a negative dose dependence ($p \leq 0.05$, Cochran–Armitage test) (Waalkes et al., 1988a).

Groups of 30 male Wistar Crl:(WI)BR rats, six weeks of age, received a single subcutaneous injection of 30 μmol/kg bw (5.5 mg/kg bw) **cadmium chloride** dissolved in saline into the dorsal thoracic midline area and three subcutaneous injections of 0.1, 0.3 or 1.0 mmol/kg [18.4, 55.1 or 183.5 mg/kg bw] zinc acetate in saline into the right, left and midline lumbosacrum 6 h before, at the same time as and 18 h after the cadmium treatment. Animals were observed for up to two years. Two other groups of 30 rats received either 30 μmol/kg cadmium chloride intramuscularly plus 1.0 mmol/kg zinc subcutaneously into the right, left and midline lumbosacrum 4 h before, at the same time as and 18 h after the cadmium treatment or 30 μmol/kg cadmium chloride subcutaneously and, starting two weeks previously, 100 ppm [100 mg/L] zinc as zinc acetate in the drinking-water for the duration of the study. A control group of 84 rats received saline injections and tap water. All animals were examined histologically. The treatments did not modify survival in any group. Injection-site sarcomas occurred in 12/30 rats given only the subcutaneous injection of cadmium, and the incidence was significantly ($p \leq 0.05$; Fisher exact test) reduced by the highest subcutaneous dose of zinc (6/29) and by administration of zinc in the drinking-water (1/30). Intramuscular injection of cadmium produced sarcomas at the site of injection in 3/29 rats given cadmium alone and in 1/29 rats also given zinc subcutaneously. Testicular tumours (mostly interstitial-cell tumours) were observed in 22/30 (73%) rats given only the subcutaneous injection of cadmium chloride and in 3/28 (11%) rats receiving both cadmium chloride subcutaneously and three subcutaneous doses of 1 mmol/kg zinc; 9/83 (11%) were observed in saline control rats. The incidence of testicular tumours overall showed a negative dependence on the subcutaneous dose of zinc ($p \leq 0.05$; Cochran–Armitage test), although zinc in the drinking-water had no effect on induction by subcutaneous cadmium chloride (25/30 rats, 83%). Subcutaneous administration of cadmium caused extensive testicular degeneration, which was prevented in a dose-related fashion by subcutaneous zinc. Intramuscular administration of cadmium did not increase the incidence of tumours of the testis. Prostatic adenoma incidence was elevated in the groups receiving cadmium subcutaneously and the high dose of zinc (8/27; 30%; $p \leq 0.05$, Fisher exact test), intramuscular cadmium (11/26; 42%; $p \leq 0.05$) or intramuscular cadmium and subcutaneous zinc (7/28; 25%; $p \leq 0.05$), compared with controls (8/83; 10%). The tumour response of the prostate to cadmium in animals given the highest dose of zinc was attributed by the authors to prevention of cadmium-induced testicular degeneration and consequent loss of androgenic support (Waalkes et al., 1989).

A group of 70 male Fischer F344/NCr rats, eight weeks old, received a single subcutanous injection of 30.0 μmol/kg bw [5.5 mg/kg bw] **cadmium chloride** hemipentahydrate dissolved in saline into the dorsal thoracic midline area and were observed for 90 weeks. Fifty control animals received a single subcutaneous injection of saline only. In the

33 animals still alive at the time of appearance of the first tumour (32 weeks), cadmium chloride reduced survival but not body weight. Cadmium chloride induced sarcomas (primarily fibrosarcomas) at the site of injection in 21/32 rats (1/50 in controls). The incidence of testicular interstitial-cell tumours was 97% in cadmium chloride-treated rats and 84% in controls. The incidence of large granular lymphocytic leukaemia (2/31) was reduced ($p = 0.028$) by cadmium chloride from that in controls (12/47) (Waalkes *et al.*, 1991a).

Groups of 28 male Wistar Hsd:(WI)BR rats, eight weeks of age, were fed diets either adequate in zinc (60 ppm [60 mg/kg diet]) or marginally zinc-deficient (7 ppm [7 mg/kg diet]), as defined by significant reductions (40%) in serum zinc in the absence of overt weight suppression. The diets were given for two weeks prior to a single subcutaneous injection of 0, 5.0, 10.0 or 30.0 μmol/kg bw (0.92–5.5 mg/kg bw) **cadmium chloride** hemipentahydrate dissolved in saline into the dorsal thoracic midline area. Animals were observed for the next 92 weeks. All animals were examined histologically. Zinc deficiency alone did not affect food consumption, weight gain or survival. Cadmium chloride affected weight gain only at the highest dose (30 μmol/kg), at which body weight was reduced approximately 15%, only for the first 10 weeks after injection; thereafter, weights were not different from those of controls. Survival was reduced in rats fed zinc-adequate diets and given the highest dose of cadmium chloride ($p \leq 0.05$). Injection-site sarcomas occurred in 7/25 rats receiving 30 μmol cadmium chloride and zinc-deficient diets ($p < 0.05$), in 3/24 rats given 30 μmol cadmium chloride and zinc-adequate diets and in 0/49 controls. Dietary zinc level did not affect the incidence of cadmium-induced interstitial-cell tumours of the testis, and a dose–response relationship in tumour incidence occurred with cadmium up to a maximum incidence of approximately 70% (control, < 10%) at both levels of dietary zinc. Rats receiving zinc-deficient diets showed an increased multiplicity of testicular interstitial-cell tumours (Waalkes *et al.*, 1991b).

3.5 Other routes of administration

3.5.1 *Mouse*

In a screening study based on the accelerated induction of lung adenomas in a strain highly susceptible to development of this neoplasm, groups of 20 male and female strain A/Strong mice, six to eight weeks old, received thrice weekly intraperitoneal injections of **cadmium acetate** in saline for a total of 23 injections, while controls received a total of 24 injections of saline alone. The total doses of cadmium acetate were designed to be 7, 14 and 28 mg/kg bw. All mice given 28 mg/kg bw died prior to completion of the study (30 weeks). Lung adenomas occurred in 6/14 (43%) animals given 7 mg/kg bw and in 3/10 (30%) animals given 14 mg/kg bw, compared with 37% of controls. The average number of lung tumours per mouse was unaltered by treatment ($p > 0.05$; Student's *t* test) (Stoner *et al.*, 1976).

3.5.2 *Rat*

A group of 207 male Wistar rats, six weeks of age, received injections of 0.15 ml of a 1-mol [*sic*] solution of **cadmium chloride** [16.86 mg/rat; 241 mg/kg bw] in saline directly into the prostate. A further group of 50 rats received one to five subcutaneous injections of 0.05 ml of the 1-mol solution of cadmium chloride [5.62–28.1 mg/rat; 80–401 mg/kg bw] in saline [site unspecified]. Concurrent controls were not included [body weights, survival, necropsy protocol and observation time not specified]. Prostatic tumours, generally carcinomas, developed in 17/207 (8.2%) rats given injections directly into the prostate. In the animals given cadmium chloride subcutaneously, a possible early adenocarcinoma of the prostate was observed (Scott & Aughey, 1978). [The Working Group noted that the absence of concurrent controls makes these data difficult to interpret.]

A group of 125 inbred male rats of the Okamoto-toki strain, 12 months of age, were anaesthetized and injected with 0.44 mg cadmium (1.2 mg/kg bw) as **cadmium chloride** in saline into the right lobe of the ventral prostate. Twenty saline-injected rats of the same age served as controls. Animals were observed for 270 days after cadmium chloride injection [body weights and survival not given]. Lesions of the prostate were classified as hyperplasia, atypical hyperplasia, carcinoma *in situ* (Hoffmann *et al.*, 1985a) [modified to atypical hyperplasia with severe dysplasia by Hoffmann *et al.*, 1985b] and invasive carcinoma. The first case of invasive prostatic carcinoma was detected 56 days after treatment, and a total of five cases occurred in 100 rats examined in this group. Other prostatic changes induced by cadmium chloride treatment included 'carcinoma *in situ*' in 11 rats (Hoffmann *et al.*, 1985a), atypical hyperplasia in 29 rats and simple hyperplasia in 38. Of the 20 controls examined, five had simple hyperplasia and one had atypical hyperplasia (Hoffmann *et al.*, 1985a,b). [The Working Group noted the small number of controls and the short obervation period.]

Female Wistar WU/Kißlegg rats [number not given], 12 weeks of age, each received a single intraperitoneal injection of 50 mg cadmium as **cadmium sulfide** (81 rats examined) or two weekly intraperitoneal injections of 0.125 mg cadmium as **cadmium oxide** (47 rats examined) dissolved in saline. Animals were observed for up to 123 weeks. No concurrent controls were reported. Only gross lesions of the peritoneal cavity were examined histologically. Three of the rats given cadmium oxide and 54/81 given cadmium sulfide had peritoneal cavity tumours, described as sarcomas, mesotheliomas and carcinomas of the abdominal cavity [no further details reported]. In the 204 rats injected with saline alone (combined controls), five intraperitoneal tumours (one carcinoma, one mesothelioma and three sarcomas) were observed (Pott *et al.*, 1987).

Groups of male Okamoto-aoki rats, 12 months of age, were injected twice with 2.25 mg/kg bw (10 rats) or three times with 3.35 mg/kg bw (20 rats) **cadmium chloride** [time course and vehicle unspecified] into the right lobe of the ventral prostate. No concurrent controls were used. Animals were killed after 170 or 240 days, respectively. Prostatic carcinomas occurred in 2/8 rats receiving the lower dose of cadmium and in 9/15 rats given the higher dose (Hoffmann *et al.*, 1988). [The Working Group noted that the absence of a control group makes this study difficult to interpret.]

3.6 Administration with known carcinogens

3.6.1 *Mouse*

Groups of 25 three-week-old female Swiss mice received 5, 10 or 50 ppm [mg/L] cadmium as **cadmium chloride** in deionized water or drinking-water alone (controls) for

15 weeks. After three weeks of exposure, all mice received an intraperitoneal injection of 1.5 mg/g bw [1.5 g/kg bw] urethane in saline. At the end of the 15-week exposure period, all mice were killed. Treatment did not affect average body weight gain or water consumption. Only lungs were examined histologically. Cadmium did not modify the size or number of pulmonary adenomas induced by urethane per animal (Blakley, 1986).

A group of 100 female hybrid CBA × C57Bl/6 mice, weighing 10–12 g, received 0.01 mg/L **cadmium chloride** together with 10 ppm [mg/L] N-nitrosodimethylamine (NDMA) in the drinking-water *ad libitum* for nine months, at which time the experiment was terminated. A positive control group of 50 mice received NDMA alone. The total dose of cadmium chloride received from drinking-water was stated to be 0.007 mg. Survival was similar in both groups [body weights not given]. All animals were examined histologically. Treatment with cadmium chloride plus NDMA significantly increased ($p \leq 0.05$, χ^2) the proportion of animals with tumours of any type (95.3%) over that of mice given NDMA alone (80.0%) among animals that survived to the time of appearance of the first tumour. The tumours were primarily pulmonary adenomas, renal adenomas and hepatic haemangiomas and haemangioendotheliomas (Litvinov *et al.*, 1986). [The Working Group noted the high incidence of tumours in the group given NDMA alone and the absence of a concurrent untreated control group and of a group receiving cadmium chloride alone.]

In a study of promotion, groups of 50 male B6C3F1 mice, five weeks of age, were given a single intraperitoneal injection of 90 mg/kg bw N-nitrosodiethylamine (NDEA) in tricaprylin or vehicle alone followed two weeks later by administration of 0, 500 or 1000 ppm [mg/L] **cadmium chloride** hemipentahydrate in drinking-water. Groups of 10 mice were killed at 16, 24 and 36 weeks, and the remainder were killed at 52 weeks. Cadmium chloride markedly suppressed body weight gain in the group given 1000 mg/L. All animals were examined histologically. Cadmium chloride was not associated with an increased incidence of tumours, regardless of NDEA treatment, and animals treated with cadmium chloride had a dose-related reduction in NDEA-induced pulmonary adenomas of alveolar-cell origin and liver tumours (typically basophilic adenomas) (Waalkes *et al.*, 1991c).

In a study of initiation, groups of male B6C3F1 mice, five weeks of age, were given a single subcutaneous injection of vehicle (30 mice) or cadmium at 20.0 (30 mice) or 22.5 (60 mice) μmol/kg bw (2.25 or 2.53 mg/kg bw) as **cadmium chloride** hemipentahydrate in saline, followed two weeks later by administration of water or 500 ppm [mg/L] sodium barbital in the drinking-water (540 mice in all). Both doses of cadmium chloride caused focal hepatocellular necrosis; the 20.0 μmol/kg dose caused 8% (5/60) mortality and 22.5 μmol/kg caused 39% (47/120) mortality within the first two days (all treated groups combined). Final body weights were similar in animals that survived the acute toxicity. Groups of 10 mice were killed 40 weeks after cadmium injection, and the remainder were killed at 92 weeks. Histological examination was performed, with special emphasis on liver lesions. Cadmium chloride treatment was not associated with increases in the incidence of any tumours; it reduced ($p \leq 0.05$) liver tumour incidence and the numbers of tumours/liver, but not tumour size (Waalkes *et al.*, 1991c).

3.6.2 Rat

Groups of 15 male Fischer 344 rats, seven weeks old, were administered 500 mg/L N-nitrosoethyl-N-hydroxyethylamine in drinking-water for two weeks followed by 100 mg/L **cadmium chloride** hemipentahydrate for 25 weeks. Cadmium chloride did not affect body weight or survival. Only kidneys and liver were examined histologically. Cadmium chloride did not increase the kidney tumour incidence significantly but it significantly ($p \leq 0.05$; Student's t test) increased the mean number of renal dysplastic foci/cm^2 of tissue (0.69 ± 0.32) in comparison with nitrosamine-treated controls (0.23 ± 0.28) (Kurokawa et al., 1985, 1989). [The Working Group noted the short duration of the study.]

Groups of 40 male Wistar (Sim:Wistar) rats, nine weeks of age, were treated with estimated daily dietary doses of 50 mg/kg of diet [ppm] cyproterone acetate for three weeks followed by three daily subcutaneous injections of 25 mg testosterone propionate and then a single intravenous injection of 50 mg/kg bw N-methyl-N-nitrosourea (MNU). One group then received 100 ppm (100 mg/L) **cadmium chloride** in the drinking-water, and another received standard drinking-water and served as controls. Survival and body weight were not affected by cadmium, and the mean survival time was 58 weeks. All animals were examined histologically. One intraductal carcinoma of the prostate occurred in a cadmium-treated rat, but none occurred in controls. The incidences of tumours at other sites were not affected by cadmium (Nakao, 1986). [The Working Group noted the short duration of the study, the minimal effect of MNU alone and the absence of concurrent untreated controls or controls receiving cadmium chloride alone.]

Groups of 20 male Wistar rats [age at onset unspecified] were given 100 ppm [mg/L] N-methyl-N'-nitro-N-nitrosoguanidine in their drinking-water and fed a diet supplemented with 10% sodium chloride for eight weeks to initiate stomach tumour formation. **Cadmium chloride** was then given in the drinking-water at a concentration of 100 ppm [mg/L] for the following 32 weeks. A group of 28 rats received the nitrosamine then distilled drinking-water and served as controls. Cadmium chloride did not modify the incidence of gastroduodenal tumours or preneoplastic lesions (Kurokawa et al., 1989).

Groups of 20 male Fischer 344 rats [age at onset unspecified] were given 50 ppm [mg/L] NDEA in the drinking-water for four weeks followed by 100 ppm [mg/L] **cadmium chloride** in the drinking-water for the following 30 weeks. Controls received NDEA followed by drinking-water. Cadmium chloride significantly ($p < 0.01$) reduced the incidence of hepatocellular carcinomas induced by NDEA (Kurokawa et al., 1989).

Groups of 42–58 female hooded rats, 10–12 weeks of age, were given one treatment of either crocidolite alone (1.82 mg/rat suspended in Tyrode's solution by intratracheal instillation), crocidolite plus cadmium (0.18 mg cadmium/rat as powdered **cadmium metal** suspended in Tyrode's solution by intratracheal instillation), crocidolite plus cadmium plus N-nitrosoheptamethyleneimine (NHMI; 1 mg/rat dissolved in saline given subcutaneously into the dorsal thoracic area six weeks after intratracheal instillation of crocidolite and cadmium for 12 weeks) or NHMI alone. Survival was similar in all the cadmium-treated groups. The overall lung tumour incidence in animals receiving crocidolite, cadmium and NHMI (14/45) was significantly ($p \leq 0.05$) higher than that in groups receiving NHMI alone (10/58), crocidolite and cadmium (2/51) or crocidolite and NMHI (7/42). The tumours were primarily squamous-cell carcinomas (Harrison & Heath, 1986). [The Working Group noted that concurrent untreated controls and groups treated with cadmium metal only were not available.]

Groups of male Wistar Cr1:[WI]BR rats, 22 weeks old, were given a single intraperitoneal injection of 18 mg/kg bw NDMA followed 4 h and four days later by intramuscular injections of **cadmium chloride** into the thigh (total doses of cadmium, 1.5 mg/kg bw [20 rats] or 3.0 mg/kg bw [30 rats]) or no further treatment (20 rats). Two other groups of 20 rats were given cadmium alone, and a group of five untreated rats served as controls. The animals were observed for 52 weeks. Cadmium chloride alone was not acutely lethal; NDMA alone caused 5% mortality, low-dose cadmium plus NDMA induced 10% mortality and high-dose cadmium plus NDMA induced 30% mortality. All treatments markedly reduced body weight [extent not stated] within one week of exposure, but by the end of the experiment the weights were similar to those of untreated controls. Only rats surviving to week 30 were included in the tumour analysis. Cadmium chloride increased ($p \leq 0.05$, Fisher exact test) the incidence of renal tumours induced by NDMA (NDMA alone, 2/18 rats examined; NDMA plus low-dose cadmium chloride, 10/18; NDMA plus high-dose cadmium chloride, 11/21) but did not induce significant numbers when given alone (low-dose, 1/20; high-dose, 0/20). Cadmium chloride also increased the incidence of hepatocellular adenoma (NDMA alone, 1/18; NDMA plus pooled cadmium chloride groups, 9/39). In a second experiment, 30 rats (same strain, six weeks old) were given intramuscular injections of cadmium as cadmium chloride at a dose of 1 mg/kg bw into the thigh on days 0, 4, 5 and 6 and of 2 mg/kg bw on day 12; one day later, the animals received an intraperitoneal injection of 18 mg/kg bw NDMA. Further groups received NDMA alone (20 rats), cadmium chloride alone (20 rats) or remained untreated (four rats). Survival and body weights were similar in all groups. Cadmium chloride increased ($p \leq 0.05$, Fisher exact test) the incidence of NDMA-induced renal tumours (NDMA alone, 2/19; NDMA plus cadmium chloride, 15/26) but did not induce any renal tumours when given alone (0/20). The incidences of hepatocellular adenomas were: NDMA alone, 3/19; NDMA plus cadmium chloride, 0/26; cadmium chloride alone, 1/20 (Wade *et al.*, 1987).

4. Other Relevant Data

The extensive literature on cadmium has been reviewed (Friberg *et al.*, 1985, 1986b; Nordberg & Nordberg, 1988; Nordberg *et al.*, 1992; US Occupational Safety and Health Administration, 1992; WHO, 1992b). The following summary comprises illustrative studies only.

4.1 Absorption, distribution, metabolism and excretion

4.1.1 *Humans*

Cadmium may enter the body by ingestion, inhalation and, to a very limited extent, by passage through the skin, but few studies have examined fractional absorption of cadmium in humans. In one study, rice was cultured in a nutrient solution containing cadmium-115 [compound unspecified] and then cooked and administered to a healthy male subject. Whole-body counting for three days and counting in faeces and urine suggested that 5% of the cadmium had been absorbed. When cadmium-115 was administered in an acid solution [presumably on an empty stomach], the absorption was almost 30% (Yamagata *et al.*, 1975). In another study, faecal elimination of cadmium-115 was detected up to 20–30 days after oral intake of the tracer as the chloride, probably reflecting sloughing of mucosal cells containing cadmium; the remaining whole-body retention averaged 4.6% (McLellan *et al.*, 1978). A higher absorption rate has been seen in women, in whom fractional absorption of ^{115}Cd-cadmium chloride was correlated inversely with serum ferritin concentration (Flanagan *et al.*, 1978).

The extent of deposition in the lungs depends on particle size and shape, ventilatory parameters and airway geometry. The fact that smokers have higher cadmium levels in the body shows that cadmium is absorbed in the lungs (see section 1.3.9). In a study of autopsy specimens, lower pulmonary concentrations of cadmium were observed in ex-smokers than in smokers. A half-time for pulmonary cadmium of 9.4 years was calculated from these data (Paäkkö *et al.*, 1989).

Low excretion rates of cadmium lead to efficient retention in the body. Analysis of cadmium in autopsied organs shows that most of the body burden is retained in the kidneys and liver. The biological half-time in kidneys was estimated to be 12–20 years (Elinder *et al.*, 1976; Tsuchiya *et al.*, 1976; Kjellström & Nordberg, 1978; Roels *et al.*, 1981; WHO, 1992b) and that in the liver somewhat shorter (Tsuchiya *et al.*, 1976; Kjellström & Nordberg, 1978). Neutron activation analysis has been used to determine cadmium concentrations in liver and kidney of cadmium-exposed workers *in vivo*. In workers without kidney dysfunction, the cadmium concentrations in the two organs correlated well, and both correlated well with urinary cadmium excretion (Roels *et al.*, 1981). As also reflected in other studies (Lauwerys *et al.*, 1980), urinary cadmium excretion can be regarded as a measure of the body burden of this metal in individuals with normal kidney function. In 64 active and retired smelter workers without kidney dysfunction, urinary excretion of metallothionein also correlated well with the cadmium burdens of liver and kidneys (Shaikh *et al.*, 1990). In workers with cadmium-induced kidney dysfunction, urinary cadmium excretion is higher, and kidney burdens tend to decrease relative to the concentrations in the liver (Roels *et al.*, 1981).

The concentration of cadmium in the blood depends mainly on recent absorption of the metal and tends to stabilize within a few months after a change in exposure (Lauwerys *et al.*, 1980). The concentrations of cadmium in blood were measured over more than 10 years in five workers in a copper–cadmium alloy factory who had had high exposures to cadmium in the past. The data fitted a two-compartment model, with a first mean half-time of 75–128 days and a second of 7.4–16 years. Two workers with proteinuria had shorter half-times than workers without kidney dysfunction (Järup *et al.*, 1983).

Urinary excretion of absorbed cadmium is the major route of elimination, but it is also excreted in the bile (Friberg *et al.*, 1986b). In an autopsy study of deceased smelter workers, increased lung concentrations of cadmium were found. High concentrations were related particularly to tobacco smoking (Gerhardsson *et al.*, 1986).

Cadmium concentrations in the prostate (50–500 ng/g wet weight) were < 1% of those found in the kidneys (8000–39 000 ng/g wet weight) in five men aged 61–76 years, but within the prostate the concentrations varied considerably, with the highest concentrations at the base (Lindegaard et al., 1990).

A placental barrier seems to exist: at delivery, cadmium concentrations in umbilical cord blood were about half of those occurring in maternal blood, and cadmium concentrations in human placenta reached a level about 10-fold higher than that seen in maternal blood (Hubermont et al., 1978). Placental transfer was also demonstrated in more recent studies (Kuhnert et al., 1982, 1987).

4.1.2 Experimental systems

In mice given ordinary food pellets, average fractional absorption of a single dose of cadmium chloride was 0.2% of non-toxic doses; five to eight times higher absorption rates were recorded in mice on a semisynthetic diet resembling human food (Andersen et al., 1992).

In a study of male Wistar rats exposed by inhalation to cadmium aerosols (see pp. 164, 166–167), the cadmium concentrations in lung tissue homogenate and lung cytosol supernatant were about twice as high for cadmium oxide as for cadmium chloride, both at the end of the 30-day exposure period and two months later. Exposure to a cadmium sulfide aerosol (a combination of sulfide and sulfate) at a 10-fold higher level (1 mg/m^3) resulted in cytosol cadmium concentrations similar to those caused by administration of cadmium oxide at 0.1 mg/m^3. The amount of absorbed cadmium that was retained in the liver and kidneys was higher if delivered as cadmium oxide than if given as cadmium chloride at the same concentration (Glaser et al., 1986).

In a study of Long–Evans and Fischer 344 rats exposed to aerosols of cadmium chloride, oxide dust and sulfide dust, pulmonary retention of cadmium chloride and sulfide (half-time, 85 days and 11–76 days, respectively) was similar, whereas that of cadmium oxide dust was somewhat longer (half-time, 217 days). In contrast, there was no transfer to the kidney or liver of cadmium administered as cadmium sulfide, but the levels in faeces were high. Monkeys (Macaca fascicularis) did not accumulate cadmium in the kidney after inhaling cadmium sulfide dust but did so after inhaling cadmium oxide (Oberdörster & Cox, 1989).

A low-molecular-weight protein, metallothionein, occurs mainly in liver and kidney and binds cadmium. Its synthesis is induced by cadmium and other divalent metals. Metallothionein-bound cadmium released from the liver is cleared by glomerular filtration and taken up by the renal tubules (Nordberg et al., 1971; Nordberg, 1972). Metallothionein production in the intestinal mucosa was induced by oral administration of zinc to Wistar rats. Subsequent oral administration of cadmium increased the retention of cadmium in the kidneys but decreased retention in the liver in comparison with non-pretreated rats (Min et al., 1991). Induced mallothionein production was not detectable in rat ventral prostate, and cadmium in these cells seems to bind to other (non-inducible) proteins. In male Wistar rats, subcutaneous injection of cadmium stimulated expression of the metallothionein-I gene in the liver and the dorsal prostate, while gene expression in the ventral prostate remained unchanged (Waalkes et al., 1992a,b).

Zinc deficiency may affect tissue deposition of cadmium. In male Wistar rats given a diet low in zinc (7 ppm) for nine weeks with different levels of cadmium for the last six weeks, retention of cadmium was enhanced in liver, kidney and testis, with concomitant, marked reductions in renal and testicular zinc concentrations. Zinc deficiency also decreased cadmium-induced metallothionein retention in the kidneys (Waalkes, 1986). After acute exposure to cadmium, low doses, which probably become bound to metallothionein, are retained mainly in the kidneys, while higher doses show a retention pattern that probably reflects saturation of metallothionein binding (Lehman & Klaassen, 1986).

Metallothionein-bound cadmium-109 given orally to male C57Bl/6J mice initially showed the same fractional absorption as cadmium chloride, but the relative retention in the kidney was greater (Cherian et al., 1978). Kidney retention of cadmium-109 in male CF-1 mice was similar after oral intake of metallothionein-bound cadmium generated in different ways; heat-treatment of the material did not affect the retention pattern (Maitani et al., 1984).

The reported half-times of cadmium in the body vary from weeks to two years (or as long as half the lifespan of the animal); the biological half-time of cadmium in the kidney and whole body decreases when renal tubular dysfunction has developed (WHO, 1992b).

After inhaling cadmium chloride aerosols at a concentration of 100 $\mu g/m^3$ for four weeks, male Fischer 344 rats showed no significant increase in the concentration of metallothionein in lung tissue; the concentration was increased in female BALB/c mice treated similarly. Metallothionein concentrations were higher, however, in lung cells obtained by bronchoalveolar lavage from the exposed rats than in those from the mice (Oberdörster et al., 1993).

The rate of cadmium uptake in Chinese hamster V79 variant cells resistant to cadmium was about 10–15% of that seen in the parental line; however, metallothionein induction and the rate of glutathione synthesis after depletion were similar in the two cell types. Depletion of glutathione enhanced the sensitivity of wild-type cells to cadmium ion but had no effect on the resistant variant. Inhibition of protein synthesis by cycloheximide did not affect cadmium uptake, but blocking of sulfhydryl groups with N-ethylmaleimide suppressed cadmium uptake (Ochi, 1991).

Cadmium has been observed to cross the hamster placenta on day 8 but not on day 9 of gestation (Dencker, 1975). No cadmium was seen in rat fetuses after their dams had received an injection of a sub-embryolethal dose of cadmium chloride (40 μmol [7.3 mg]/kg) on day 12 of gestation (Saltzman et al., 1989). Concentrations in rat fetuses after injection of a teratogenic dose of cadmium (1.25 mg/kg) to the dam on day 12 of gestation have been reported to be 1% of those in the placenta (Webb & Samarawickrama, 1981). Christley and Webster (1983) reported similar percentages of embryonic cadmium uptake when mice were injected with cadmium at 0.66, 40 or 2400 μg/kg as cadmium chloride on gestation day 9.

4.2 Toxic effects

4.2.1 Humans

A worker who inhaled high concentrations of cadmium fumes died five days later. Both lungs showed acute pneumonitis (Lucas et al., 1980).

Long-term exposure to cadmium may result in kidney disease. Twenty-three workers with cadmium-induced kidney dysfunction were examined at various times after their removal from exposure. Over a five-year period, a significant increase was noted in the concentrations of β_2-microglobulin and creatinine in serum, indicating considerable progression in kidney dysfunction despite cessation of exposure (Roels *at al.*, 1989). Similar progression was observed in a population residing in a cadmium-polluted community (Kido *et al.*, 1988). Cadmium-induced kidney dysfunction may, however, be reversible, depending on the severity of the damage (Kasuya *et al.*, 1986; Saito, 1987; WHO, 1992b). In Japan, ingestion of cadmium-contaminated rice resulted in a disease (*itai-itai* or 'ouch-ouch' disease) characterized by kidney damage (mainly in proximal tubuli but also in other parts of the nephron) and osteomalacia, which mainly affected women who had given birth to many children (Shigematsu *et al.*, 1982; Williams *et al.*, 1983; Kasuya *et al.*, 1992).

Ten patients with cadmium-induced kidney dysfunction had decreased serum concentrations of 24,25-dihydroxyvitamin D; the five patients with the most severe kidney dysfunction also had decreased concentrations of 1α,25-dihydroxyvitamin D, while serum 25-hydroxyvitamin D levels were similar to those seen in five controls (Nogawa *et al.*, 1990).

A group of 101 men who had worked for at least one year at a copper–cadmium alloy manufacturing company were examined for respiratory symptoms by questionnaire, lung function testing and chest X-ray and were compared with a control group matched for age, sex and employment status; the two groups contained a similar proportion of smokers. Individual exposure to cadmium was estimated from data on cumulative exposure or from activation analysis of liver cadmium concentrations *in vivo*. The forced expiratory volume in 1 sec (FEV_1) and carbon monoxide transfer (diffusion capacity) were significantly decreased in the cadmium-exposed workers; more frequent radiographic signs of emphysema were also recorded. The difference from the controls in carbon monoxide transfer coefficient increased linearly with increasing cumulative exposure; exposure of 2000 µg/m³-years resulted in a decrement of 0.05–0.3 mmol/min × kPa × L (Davison *et al.*, 1988).

In a study of men employed in two Belgian zinc–cadmium plants, the concentration of cadmium in the liver increased with years of past exposure (range, 3–40 years). The concentration of cadmium in the renal cortex increased up to a level of about 250 ppm after 10–15 years of exposure and decreased with longer duration of exposure. Most of the men with more than 20 years' mean exposure, but none of the men with fewer than 10 years' mean exposure, had signs of renal dysfunction. These findings were interpreted as evidence of accumulation of cadmium in the liver and kidneys up to the onset of renal dysfunction, which is followed by a progressive loss of the cadmium in the kidneys (Roels *et al.*, 1981). Ellis *et al.* (1985), in a study of workers occupationally exposed to cadmium, reported that cumulative exposure concentrations higher than 400–500 µg/m³-years (corresponding to about 40 ppm [mg/kg] in the liver) were associated with renal abnormalities.

Workers in the cadmium recovery plant studied by Thun *et al.* (1985) (described in detail on pp. 136 and 152–153) had slightly elevated mortality from nonmalignant respiratory disease (SMR, 1.54; 95% CI, 0.88–2.51). In the study of cadmium-exposed workers in 17 plants in the United Kingdom (Kazantzis & Blanks, 1992; see pp. 154–156), the rate of mortality from bronchitis was significantly increased in the cohort as a whole (SMR, 1.20; 95% CI, 1.03–1.39) and in the highly exposed group (SMR, 3.16; 1.68–5.40). In the whole cohort, the SMR for emphysema was elevated (1.37; 95% CI, 0.84–2.12), but that for nephritis and nephrosis was not (0.77; 95% CI, 0.45–1.23). Increased mortality from nephritis and nephrosis was, however, reported among workers in a Swedish nickel-cadmium battery plant (SMR, 3.00; not significant) (Elinder et al., 1985; see pp. 150–151).

Possible excess mortality due to diabetes and 'neuralgia' [not defined] was seen over periods of 6–30 years in Japanese communities with significant cadmium pollution (Shigematsu et al., 1982). In another study, mortality was recorded for an average of 6.3 years for 185 Japanese individuals over 50 years of age who had increased excretion of retinol-binding protein, indicating kidney dysfunction due to environmental cadmium pollution. The mortality rate was compared with that of a group of 2229 individuals who had no sign of proteinuria. Of the 76 deaths that occurred in the group with kidney dysfunction, five were due to respiratory disease (as compared to 1.30 expected), four in men to nephritis and renal insufficiency (0.14 expected) and three in women to diabetes (0.50 expected). These excesses were significant (Nakagawa et al., 1987).

In 12 women with *itai-itai* disease, immunoglobulin serum concentrations were normal and lymphocyte transformation and phytohaemagglutinin cytotoxicity responses *in vitro* were similar to those in a control group (Williams et al., 1983).

4.2.2 *Experimental systems*

Acute exposure of rodents to cadmium produces hepatotoxicity (Dudley et al., 1982), while chronic administration causes kidney damage. Cadmium-induced kidney dysfunction produced in experimental animals is very similar to the low-molecular proteinuria seen in cadmium workers. Histopathological examination of kidneys from horses and sea birds exposed environmentally to cadmium showed changes indicative of chronic interstitial nephritis (WHO, 1992a). In experimental animals, acute renal toxicity can be prevented by pretreatment with small doses of the metal (Nordberg et al., 1975). After repeated exposures resulting in cadmium concentrations in the kidney cortex greater than about 200 mg/kg, rats tend to develop proteinuria (WHO, 1992b); subsequently, no further accumulation of cadmium occurs in the kidneys, presumably because of the increased urinary excretion of cadmium that occurs with the induced proteinuria (Axelsson & Piscator, 1966). Interspecies differences in the critical concentrations of cadmium in the kidney have been reported (Nomiyama & Nomiyama, 1984; WHO, 1992b).

Injection into male Wistar rats of metallothionein with the same amount of bound cadmium but different amounts of bound zinc showed that renal toxicity decreased with increasing amounts of zinc (Kojima et al., 1991).

Inbred strains of mice show different susceptibility to cadmium-induced hepatotoxicity: C3H/He mice are sensitive, while DBA/2 mice are resistant; however, hepatic concentrations of metallothionein isoforms were similar in the two strains after injection of cadmium chloride. Susceptibiity is therefore not mediated by metallothionein (Kershaw & Klaassen, 1991).

In a carcinogenicity study (described in detail on pp. 164, 166–167), exposure (22 h per day for 6–18 months) to different cadmium compounds by inhalation increased mortality in Wistar rats in a dose-related fashion, mainly from pulmonary toxicity (Glaser et al., 1990).

Alveolar hyperplasia and interstitial fibrosis were recorded in mice and golden hamsters exposed by inhalation to similar aerosols (Heinrich et al., 1989; see pp. 163–164, 167). The earliest effect of cadmium chloride and cadmium oxide aerosols seems to be type I cell necrosis, which is followed by an increase in the number of macrophages and proliferation of type II cells. Cadmium sulfide appears to be much less toxic (Oberdörster, 1989). Dose-dependent increases in the volume density of hyperplastic areas occurred in male hamsters exposed to cadmium oxide. The volume density of hyperplastic areas was also increased in males exposed to 90 $\mu g/m^3$ cadmium sulfide and in females exposed to 30 $\mu g/m^3$ cadmium sulfate (Aufderheide et al., 1990).

Many studies have been carried out to elucidate the pathogenesis of *itai-itai* disease. In female rhesus monkeys given a diet low in vitamin D, calcium (0.3%), phosphorus (0.3%) and protein (14%) with a cadmium content of 3 mg/kg (as cadmium chloride) during the first 12 months, followed by 30 mg/kg, osteomalacia developed at 12 months and proteinuria was detected at 36 months (Kimura et al., 1988). When cadmium is included in hydroxyapatite, the main calcium-containing mineral in bone, the solubility of the crystal is considerably decreased (Christoffersen et al., 1988).

In female B6C3F1 mice given water containing 0, 10, 50 or 250 ppm (mg/L) cadmium chloride for 90 days, T- and B-lymphocyte proliferation was significantly reduced. Increased susceptibility to herpes 2 virus was also recorded (Thomas et al., 1985). In SPF female rats of the Brown–Norway and Lewis strains given subcutaneous injections of 0.8 mg/kg bw cadmium chloride five times a week for 15 days, the amount of cadmium that reached the thymus was similar; however, only Brown–Norway rats had a significant decrease in S-phase thymocytes and increases in the number of thymus cells in G_2 phase and in mitosis (Morselt et al., 1988).

At concentrations below 10 μmol/L [1 mg/L], cadmium selectively inhibited concanavalin A-induced T-cell proliferation but not bacterial lipopolysaccharide-induced B-cell proliferation of spleen cells from male BALB/c mice. The effect could be prevented by adding 30 μmol zinc to the culture medium, but the intracellular cadmium concentration and the cadmium-induced metallothionein level were not affected (Otsuka & Ohsawa, 1991).

Natural killer cell-mediated cytotoxicity and antibody-dependent cellular cytotoxicity of human peripheral blood lymphocytes *in vitro* were inhibited by cadmium concentrations of 1 μM [0.1 mg/L] and above. The inhibition of natural killer activity could be prevented partially by adding calcium or zinc to the culture medium, zinc being most effective (Cifone et al., 1991).

4.3 Reproductive and developmental effects

In a review of occupational exposures and defects of the central nervous system, Roeleveld et al. (1990) noted that cadmium could induce malformations of the brain in experimental animals but that no data were available on the effects of prenatal or postnatal exposure to cadmium in humans.

4.3.1 *Humans*

In a study of 77 pregnant smokers and 125 nonsmokers who delivered infants in Cleveland Metropolitan General Hospital (USA), samples of blood were obtained from the mothers within 1 h of delivery and from the umbilical cord immediately after delivery;

placental samples were obtained immediately after delivery. Cadmium concentrations were determined in maternal whole blood, placenta and placental, maternal and cord-vein plasma; zinc was determined in maternal and cord-vein red blood cells. Smoking status was confirmed by measuring plasma thiocyanate. The potential confounding variables that were taken into account in the analysis included maternal age, gravidity, parity, gestational age, sex of offspring, race, maternal red blood cell count, maternal haemoglobin concentration, haematocrit and cord-vein haemoglobin concentration. The birth weights of the infants of smokers were significantly reduced (3143 g *versus* 3534 g), and maternal whole blood cadmium and thiocyanate concentrations were negatively related to birth weight. After the confounding variables had been controlled for, thiocyanate concentration explained 5.8% of the birth weight variance among the infants of smokers, maternal whole blood cadmium concentration explained 8.5%, and cord-vein red blood cell zinc concentration explained 1.7%. All of variables together explained more than 30% of the variance in birth weight (Kuhnert *et al.*, 1987). [The Working Group noted that it was not clear whether the differences in birth weight could be fully explained by differences in smoking, since smoking increases blood cadmium levels, and thiocyanate measurements are only qualitative measures of smoking.]

The relationship between placental cadmium concentration and the birth weight of the children of a population of nonsmoking women living near a lead smelter in former Yugoslavia was compared with that in a neighbouring town. There were 106 placentas from the smelter region and 55 from the control region. The analysis was adjusted for ethnicity, gender of children, maternal age, height, parity and education, mid-pregnancy blood lead levels and alcohol consumption. The average placental cadmium concentrations were 0.73 nmol [82 ng]/g dry weight in the exposed area and 0.50 nmol [56 ng]/g in the control area. There was no association between placental cadmium levels and either birth weight or gestational age (Loiacono *et al.*, 1992).

4.3.2 *Experimental systems*

The effects of cadmium and cadmium compounds on reproduction in experimental systems have been reviewed (Barlow & Sullivan, 1982; Carmichael *et al.*, 1982; Parízek, 1983; Shepard, 1992).

Haemorrhagic necrosis of the ovaries was observed in Cr:RGH hamsters, in one strain of mice (DBA), but not in three others, and in immature Fischer 344/NCr and WF/NCr rats injected with 47.5 μmol/kg [8.7 mg/kg] cadmium chloride (Rehm & Waalkes, 1988). A single intraperitoneal injection of 2 mg/kg cadmium chloride to (101 × C3H)F_1 or (SEC × C57Bl)F_1 × X^{Gsy} female mice had no dominant lethal or other effect on fertility, except that it induced superovulation (Suter, 1975).

Dietary exposure to up to 10 (Lorke, 1978) or 68.8 ppm (Zenick *et al.*, 1982) cadmium chloride did not affect reproductive performance in male rats. Injection of cadmium chloride to adult male rats induced an acute vascular response in the testis, leading to oedema and, ultimately, necrosis of the seminiferous epithelium (Parízek, 1960). Vas deferens sperm concentration, release of human chorionic gonadotropin-stimulated testosterone 14 days after exposure and testicular weight 60 days after exposure were found to be the most sensitive of a variety of reproductive parameters in exposed male rats. Younger (30- or

50-day-old) male rats were less sensitive than older (70-day-old) rats to the effects of cadmium (Laskey *et al.*, 1984, 1986). Rat Sertoli cells in culture were at least four times more sensitive to cadmium than interstitial (primarily Leydig) cells, suggesting a direct action of cadmium on cells in the seminiferous epithelium (Clough *et al.*, 1990). Laskey and Phelps (1991) also showed a direct effect on rat Leydig cell function following exposure *in vitro* to cadmium chloride.

Metallothionein was not induced by cadmium in rat, mouse or monkey testis or in hamster ovary (Ohta *et al.*, 1988; Waalkes & Perantoni, 1988; Waalkes *et al.*, 1988b,c,d), which may determine the susceptibility of these organs to cadmium (Waalkes & Goering, 1990). In contrast, Abel *et al.* (1991) demonstrated a cadmium-induced increase in metallothionein concentration in a murine Leydig cell line and in purified rat Leydig cells.

Female mice received cadmium in their diet for six consecutive 42-day rounds of pregnancy and lactation. Litter size at birth and pup growth were reduced at 50 but not at 25 ppm [mg/kg] (Whelton *et al.*, 1988). When male and female rats were gavaged with up to 10 mg/kg bw cadmium chloride per day for six weeks prior to mating and females during pregnancy, the high dose reduced the incidence of copulation and of pregnant females and the numbers of implants and live fetuses. Fetuses of dams given the high dose were anaemic. No effect on male fertility was reported (Sutou *et al.*, 1980a,b).

In multigeneration studies in rats in which cadmium was incorporated into the diet, offspring body weight was reduced at 100 ppm [mg/kg] (Lorke, 1978; Löser, 1980b) and the number of litters per female was reduced in a group receiving a diet containing 6.9 μg/kg bw more than the control levels of 4.4 μg/kg bw (Wills *et al.*, 1981). In a multigeneration study in which rats received up to 5 ppm (mg/L) cadmium in the drinking-water, reductions in male body weights (day 130), liver weights (1 ppm, days 50 and 130), epididymal sperm content (5 ppm, day 130), serum progesterone in term F_1 females (5 ppm), kidney weights in F_1 neonates (5 ppm) and F_2 litter weights [no data presented] were reported. A significant decrease in the incidence of preimplantation death was observed in the F_1 females given 5.0 ppm (Laskey *et al.*, 1980). Exposure of rats by inhalation to 100 μg/m^3 cadmium chloride (as an aerosol) for three generations increased lung weight in males and females of all three generations, increased leukocyte counts in males of the first two generations and in females of all three generations, increased proteinuria in males of the first and third generations and decreased body weight in males of the second and third generations and in females of the third generation. No effect on reproduction was reported (Weischer & Greve, 1979).

Pre- and postimplantation mouse and rat embryos cultured *in vitro* were severely affected by the presence of microgram per millilitre concentrations of cadmium chloride or sulfate (Schmid *et al.*, 1983; Warner *et al.*, 1984; Yu *et al.*, 1985; Abraham *et al.*, 1986; Yu & Chan, 1987; Naruse & Hayashi, 1989; Müller *et al.*, 1990).

Danielsson and Dencker (1984) found decreased vitamin B_{12} transport to the fetuses of mice within 1 h of injection of an embryolethal dose of cadmium chloride (4 mg/kg bw) on gestation day 16; lower doses did not affect fetal development, but vitamin B_{12} transport was reduced within 24 h of exposure to doses as low as 0.5 mg/kg. Transport of α-aminobutyric acid and deoxyglucose across the placenta were largely unaffected by the treatment. A teratogenic dose of cadmium (1.25 mg/kg bw) reduced thymidine incorporation into embryonic DNA at 4 h and leucine incorporation into embryonic protein at 20 h (Webb &

Samarawickrama, 1981). Injection of rats on gestation day 12 or 18 with 40 μM/kg [7.3 mg/kg] cadmium chloride reduced blood flow from the uterus to the chorioallantoic placenta beginning some time between 12 and 16 h after exposure (Levin & Miller, 1981; Levin et al., 1987; Saltzman et al., 1989).

Lobes of placentas from normal-term deliveries of nonsmoking women were dually perfused *in vitro* with cadmium at 0, 10, 20 or 100 nmol/ml [0–11 μg/ml] for up to 12 h. The synthesis and release of human chorionic gonadotropin was decreased by all concentrations of cadmium, beginning at 4 h, and necrosis of the fetal vasculature was seen 5–8 h after perfusion with the high dose. Zinc transfer to the fetal circuit was decreased by addition of 10 nmol/ml cadmium to the maternal perfusate (Wier et al., 1990).

Exposure of QS/CH mice to 40 ppm (mg/L) cadmium in the drinking-water throughout gestation resulted in reduced maternal water intake and fetal growth retardation during gestation; the newborn mice were severely anaemic. Fetal body weights were reduced by concentrations of 10 ppm and above (Webster, 1978). No effect on fetal viability, weight or morphology was reported in a study in which albino rats received 100 ppm (mg/L) cadmium as cadmium acetate in the drinking-water throughout gestation (Saxena et al., 1986). Fetal growth retardation was observed in the offspring of Sprague–Dawley rats receiving 50 or 100 ppm (mg/L) cadmium as cadmium chloride in the drinking-water from day 6 to 20 of pregnancy; no effect was seen with 5 ppm. The higher doses also reduced the average daily body weight gain of dams; after adjustment for maternal weight at day 20, fetal weight deficit was seen only at 50 ppm. No gross defect was noted (Sorell & Graziano, 1990). Exposure of Wistar rats by inhalation to 0.2–0.6 mg/m^3 cadmium (median aerodynamic diameter, 0.6 μm) throughout gestation decreased maternal weight gain and increased lung weight. The fetuses of dam given the high dose were retarded in growth, and both high- and low-dose groups had nonsignificant decreases in haematocrit (Prigge, 1978). No effect on fetal development was reported following dietary exposure of Long–Evans rats to up to 100 ppm (mg/kg in diet) on days 6–15 of gestation (Machemer & Lorke, 1981). Exposure of rats during gestation by oral gavage to doses of 40 mg/kg bw per day and above was severely toxic to the dams; doses as low as 2 mg/kg per day had some maternal effects (Machemer & Lorke, 1981; Barański et al., 1982). Reductions in fetal body weight were seen in Wistar rats with doses as low as 8 mg/kg per day (Barański et al., 1982) and in Long–Evans rats at 30 mg/kg per day (Machemer & Lorke, 1981). Fetal hydropericardium was seen with 4 mg/kg per day and above (Barański et al., 1982), and at 30 mg/kg per day a variety of fetal defects (e.g. dysplasia of the facial bones and of the rear limbs, oedema, cleft palate) were observed in rats (Machemer & Lorke, 1981).

Parenteral administration of < 10 mg/kg of cadmium salts on single days during pregnancy induced a wide range of malformations (e.g. craniofacial, eyes, limbs) in hamsters (Gale, 1979), mice (Layton & Layton, 1979; Webster & Messerle, 1980; Murdoch & Cowen, 1981; Messerle & Webster, 1982; Feuston & Scott, 1985; Naruse & Hayashi, 1989; De et al., 1990; Padmanabhan & Hameed, 1990) and rats (Parzyck et al., 1978; Samarawickrama & Webb, 1979, 1981; Holt & Webb, 1987). Direct injection of cadmium into rat fetuses late in gestation resulted in lower fetal mortality than was expected from the body burden (Levin & Miller, 1980). Daston and coworkers (Daston & Grabowski, 1979; Daston, 1981a,b, 1982) demonstrated selective retardation in morphological and biochemical maturation of fetal rat lung at doses of cadmium chloride as low as 2 mg/kg per day injected intraperitoneally on days 12–15 of gestation. Respiratory distress was seen in the offspring at birth.

The postnatal consequences of exposure to cadmium *in utero* have been studied by several investigators. Barański *et al.* (1983) reported no effect on postnatal growth of rats following exposure of dams to up to 4 mg/kg per day by oral gavage beginning five weeks prior to and during gestation, but they observed reduced exploratory locomotor activity in females at two months of age after exposure of dams to doses as low as 0.04 mg/kg per day. Ali *et al.* (1986) followed the offspring of rats that had received cadmium in the drinking-water (4.2 or 8.4 µg/ml) during gestation and found impaired postnatal growth, delayed development of cliff avoidance and swimming behaviour, elevated locomotor activity on postnatal days 14 and 21 and reduced locomotor activity on postnatal day 60. Lehotzky *et al.* (1990) injected rats subcutaneously with cadmium chloride at 0.2, 0.62 or 2 mg/kg bw per day on days 7–15 of gestation and found reduced litter size at birth but no effect on growth. Horizontal motor activity was decreased on day 38, among offspring of dams given 0.62 or 2 mg/kg and in all groups on day 90. Saillenfait *et al.* (1991) examined renal function in the offspring of rats exposed to up to 2.5 mg/kg bw cadmium chloride by intraperitoneal injection on days 8, 10, 12 and 14 of gestation. Indications of compromised renal function were observed in offspring of each sex on postnatal day 3 and in male offspring on postnatal day 49 but not on postnatal day 12.

4.4 Genetic and related effects (see also Table 14, pp. 195 *et seq.* and Appendices 1 and 2)

4.4.1 *Humans*

The genetic effects of cadmium and cadmium compounds in exposed humans have been reviewed (Vainio & Sorsa, 1981; Fleig *et al.*, 1983; Bernard & Lauwerys, 1986).

(*a*) *Itai-itai* patients

Twelve female *itai-itai* patients had markedly higher incidences of chromosomal aberrations of all types in peripheral blood lymphocytes than a group of nine age-matched control subjects (six females and three males [no further detail provided]). The patients were women aged 52–72 years who had been living in cadmium-polluted areas of Japan for more than 30 years and had been exposed to cadmium in the diet (water, rice, fish). Eight of the patients were sampled two to three times at three-month intervals. All types of chromatid and chromosomal aberrations were observed in the exposed women; the mean frequency of cells with any abnormality was 26.7% (range, 8.9–51.2%) in the exposed and 2.6 (range, 1.5–3.8%) in controls. The incidence of aneuploidy was four times or more that of the control group [smoking habits were not described] (Shiraishi, 1975).

In contrast, Bui *et al.* (1975) found no significant difference in the frequencies of cells with structural aberrations in cultures from blood of four female *itai-itai* patients and from four controls (three females, one male) living in an area of Japan known not to be cadmium-polluted; both had high frequencies of structural aberrations: 6.6 and 6.0%, respectively. The average age of the patients was 65 and that of controls, 75 years; blood cadmium levels ranged from 16 to 29 ng/g whole blood in exposed and 4.4–6.1 ng/g in controls. The samples were assayed in Sweden 96 h after sampling. The subjects were not suffering from viral diseases and had not been exposed to X-rays or cytostatic drugs. [The Working Group noted the long delay between sampling and culturing. Two of six samples were haemolysed and therefore discarded.]

(b) *Environmental and dietary exposure*

Nogawa et al. (1986) examined the frequency of sister chromatid exchange in peripheral lymphocytes from two groups of Japanese men and women. Group 1 (eight men and 16 women) lived in the cadmium-polluted Kakehashi river basin in Ishikawa Prefecture and had been diagnosed as having cadmium-induced renal damage. The comparison group 2 (two men and four women) came from Uchinada-machi, which was not contaminated by cadmium. The mean age was 76.6 years in group 1 and 68.3 years in group 2. The men, but not the women, in both groups had smoked tobacco. None of the subjects had used any known clastogenic drug or had undergone radiotherapy, and none had clinical evidence of viral infection at the time of examination. The mean cadmium concentrations in whole blood from men and women were 9.6 ± 5.8 (μg/L) in group 1 and not detectable in group 2; the mean concentrations in urine were 9.1 μg/g creatinine in group 1 and 2.7 μg/g creatinine in group 2. No difference was seen between the groups in the number of sister chromatid exchanges per cell: group 1, 8.0 ± 0.94; group 2, 9.0 ± 3.13.

Tang et al. (1990) investigated the frequency of chromosomal aberrations in a cadmium-polluted region of China. Twenty-one men (urinary cadmium concentration, 3.32 ± 1.46 μg/L) and 19 women (urinary cadmium, 3.83 ± 1.82 μg/L) living at Suichang in Zhejiang Province (soil cadmium, 1.103 ppm) for 11–62 years were compared with nine men (urinary cadmium, 2.34 ± 1.59 μg/L) and two women (urinary cadmium, 1.85 ± 0.65 μg/L) from an unpolluted region in the same general area (soil cadmium, 0.20 ppm). None of the subjects had been exposed to chromosome damaging drugs or radiotherapy and did not have viral infections. The frequency of abnormal cells, including structural aberrations, aneuploidy and endoreduplication, was not significantly different in the exposed group (5.80 ± 3.44) than in the controls (2.80 ± 1.99). (Statistical analysis using transformed data gave $p < 0.01$.) More individuals in the cadmium-polluted group (63.5%) had a high aberration prevalence (> 5%) than in controls (18.2%), and more severe structural aberrations, such as dicentrics, translocations and multiradials, were observed in the exposed group. A significant dose–effect relationship between urinary cadmium content and chromosomal aberration frequency was observed (linear regression equation given). Most men in the region were smokers, while none of the women smoked; no effect of smoking was observed.

(c) *Occupational exposure*

Deknudt and Léonard (1975) examined chromosomal aberrations in peripheral lymphocytes from three groups of workers in a cadmium plant: group 1, 23 cadmium workers with an average exposure of 12 years; group 2, 12 rolling-mill workers with an average exposure of 11 years; group 3, 12 controls (administrative department in the same plant). The materials to which exposure was considered to be relevant were: group 1, lead (60% w/w) and cadmium (10% w/w) in the absence of zinc; and group 2, mostly zinc but also low levels of lead (max. 4% w/w) and cadmium (max. 1% w/w). Both lead and cadmium concentrations in blood were measured in groups 1 and 2 at the time of sampling for cytogenetic analysis; the mean concentrations (in µg/L) were: group 1—lead, 446 ± 122.9; cadmium, 31.7 ± 33.11; group 2—lead, 208 ± 44.3; cadmium, 6.3 ± 5.51. Much of the variation in the concentration of cadmium of group 1 was due to a single individual who had 179 µg/L blood. [The Working Group noted that neither lead nor cadmium concentrations were measured in the blood of controls.] The proportions of cells (per 100 examined) with structural abnormalities were: group 1, 2.00; group 2, 3.96; and group 3, 3.04. The numbers of chromatid exchanges and chromosomal translocations, rings or dicentrics per 100 cells were: group 1, 0.89; group 2, 0.54; and group 3, 0.13. The exposed groups thus showed no increase in total aberrations but had a significantly increased frequency of more severe aberrations; however, the individual with a very high blood cadmium level had no aberration or gap. Seven workers in group 1 who had previously been employed in coal mines for 2.5–13 years had a mean rate of severe aberrations of [1.36/100 cells], compared with [0.69/100 cells] in the remainder of the group. [This effect was, however, due almost entirely to the rate of a single individual.] [The Working Group noted the absence of any record of other relevant exposures, such as tobacco smoking, viruses, X-rays and medicaments.]

Bui *et al.* (1975) examined chromosomal aberrations in peripheral lymphocytes from five men who had been employed in the electrode department of an alkaline battery factory for 5–24 years. The average cadmium concentration in the general air of the department during 1969–72 was 35 µg/m^3, and about twice this value was estimated in personal air samples. The control group consisted of three male office workers of about the same age as the exposed workers and from the same factory. Cadmium concentrations were measured in urine and blood [but it is not clear whether this was done at the same time as blood sampling for chromosomal analysis]. The subjects were not known to be suffering from viral disease and had not been exposed to X-rays or known clastogenic drugs. The mean cadmium concentrations in whole blood were 37.7 ± 15.5 ng/g in the exposed and 2.3 ± 0.9 ng/g in the controls; the concentrations in urine were 11.5 ± 11.5 µg/g creatinine in exposed and 2.5 ± 1.3 µg/g creatinine in controls. Lymphocytes were examined after culture times of both 48 h and 72 h: At neither time was there an increase in the frequency of cells with either structural chromosomal aberrations or numerical changes in the exposed group when compared with the control group.

Chromosomal aberrations were studied in peripheral lymphocytes from 24 male workers at a zinc smelting plant who had spent 3–6.5 years in zinc electrolysis, where they were exposed to fumes and dust containing zinc, lead and cadmium (Bauchinger *et al.*, 1976). The exposed workers had a mean lead blood concentration of 192.9 ± 66.2 µg/L and a cadmium concentration of 3.95 ± 2.68 µg/L but had no clinical sign of metal toxicity and had had no previous exposure to cytostatic drugs or X-irradiation. Fifteen (11 men, 4 women) unexposed healthy members of the general population not exposed to these metals were used as controls; the blood levels of lead and cadmium in this group were not measured but were assumed to be the average for industrial workers—120–130 µg/L lead and 1.5 µg/L cadmium. The numbers of cells with structural aberrations was significantly increased in the exposed group ($p < 0.001$, Mann–Whitney rank test). The percentages of cells with structural aberrations were 1.35 ± 0.99 (0.018 ± 0.015 assigned breaks/cell) for exposed workers and 0.47 ± 0.92 (0.0053 ± 0.011 assigned breaks/cell) for the controls.

No significant difference in chromosomal or chromatid aberration frequency was observed between 40 workers in a cadmium pigment plant (blood cadmium, 19.5 µg/L; range, < 2–140 µg/L) and 13 administrative and laboratory personnel at the same plant, used as controls (blood cadmium, < 2–29 µg/L), although four cells (out of 3740) with chromatid interchanges were observed in the exposed group only. No correlation was found between extent of damage and exposure levels or duration [data not shown]. Exposures ranged from six weeks to 34 years, and workers had not previously been exposed to chromosome damaging drugs or radiation (O'Riordan et al., 1978).

Fleig et al. (1983) also found no significant difference in the incidence of chromosomal aberrations (chromosome and chromatid type) in 14 workers exposed to cadmium-containing dusts for 6–25 years in cadmium pigment and stabilizer production plants (1.5% of cells with structural aberrations) when compared with 14 age-matched office workers (1.3% of cells with structural aberrations). The concentrations of cadmium in the blood of the workers (14–38 µg/L) were measured three years before the study; the levels for controls were not stated. The exposed workers had not been exposed to chromosome damaging drugs or radiotherapy.

Dziekanowska (1981) reported small increases in the incidence of chromosomal aberrations (8.91 ± 4.99), especially structural rearrangements (dicentrics, translocations), and disturbance of spiralization in 11 cadmium-exposed workers compared with 32 healthy non-smelter controls (6.66 ± 2.38). No difference was found in the frequency of sister chromatid exchange (cadmium-exposed group, 15.14 ± 4.7; controls, 16.9 ± 5.82). [The Working Group noted the high control value for sister chromatid exchange. It is not clear whether smoking habits were considered.]

The rates of abnormal metaphases (excluding gaps) were significantly higher in peripheral blood lymphocytes of a group of 40 male workers (10 nonsmokers, 24 smokers, 6 ex-smokers) exposed to fumes and dusts in the production of cadmium, zinc, copper and silver alloys in a single factory (2.6%) than in controls matched for age and smoking habits (1.7%, $p < 0.05$), whereas the total rates of abnormal metaphases did not differ between the two groups. Chromosome-type aberrations accounted for most of the observed increase. The mean cadmium concentration in blood, measured at the time of cytogenetic assay, was 5.10 ± 5.15 µg/L (range, 0.3–28.3), and the urinary concentration was 10.63 ± 7.99 µg/L (range, 1.5–31.6) in workers; levels for controls were not stated. When a cumulative exposure index was calculated for each subject (mean yearly atmospheric cadmium concentration × years of exposure), only high-intensity, long-term exposure was associated with a significant increase in the frequency of chromosome-type aberrations: Six of seven complex aberrations (dicentrics and rings) observed were found in the eight subjects of this group. The workers had not been exposed to radiation therapy, treatment with cytotoxic drugs, recent viral diseases or occupational exposure to known clastogens (Forni et al., 1990). [The Working Group noted that neither the exposure levels nor the blood and urine concentrations of other metals were measured.]

4.4.2 Experimental systems

The genetic effects of cadmium compounds in experimental systems have been reviewed (Degraeve, 1981; Hansen & Stern, 1984; Sunderman, 1984; Baker, 1985; IARC, 1987b;

Swierenga *et al.*, 1987), as have the mechanistic aspects of the effects (Léonard, 1988; Magos, 1991; Snow, 1992; Rossman *et al.*, 1992).

Most experimental systems have been used to study cadmium chloride. Some data are also available on cadmium acetate, cadmium oxide, cadmium sulfate, cadmium nitrate and cadmium sulfide, and the genetic and related effects of those compounds are listed separately in Table 14. The results are summarized here according to the solubility of the compounds in water, before they are added to biological media. Thus, cadmium sulfide, oxide and carbonate are very poorly soluble, while all of the other cadmium compounds are water-soluble at all concentrations tested. Water solubility does not, however, necessarily reflect solubility *in vivo*.

(a) *Cadmium compounds readily soluble in water (acetate, chloride, nitrate, sulfate)*

Cadmium chloride induced DNA strand breaks but not prophage in bacteria. Both cadmium chloride and cadmium sulfate, but not cadmium nitrate, induced differential toxicity in *Bacillus subtilis* and *Escherichia coli* strains. The compounds did not induce bacterial mutation reliably; precipitation in the bacterial media may have affected bioavailability. A few positive responses were reported with cadmium chloride and sulfate tested in *Salmonella typhimurium* strains (particularly TA102) and with cadmium nitrate in *E. coli* DG1153.

Cadmium chloride and cadmium sulfate induced gene conversion in *Saccharomyces cerevisiae*, but cadmium chloride did not induce reverse mutation in *S. cerevisiae* or aneuploidy in either *S. cerevisiae* or *Aspergillus nidulans*.

Cadmium chloride induced micronuclei in *Vicia faba* and water hyacinth and aneuploidy in Chinese spring wheat.

Cadmium chloride and cadmium nitrate did not induce mutation in *Drosophila melanogaster*, and cadmium chloride did not induce aneuploidy in one study but did in another, more sensitive assay.

Cadmium acetate and cadmium chloride induced DNA strand breaks in several cultured, non-human mammalian cell lines. Cadmium sulfate induced DNA strand breaks in primary cultures of rat hepatocytes, and cadmium chloride and cadmium nitrate induced unscheduled DNA synthesis in the same type of cell. Cadmium chloride did not induce DNA strand breaks in primary cultures of rat Leydig cells, which are an important target *in vivo* (see section 4.2).

Cadmium chloride and cadmium sulfate are mutagenic to cultured, non-human mammalian cells. The mutagenic activity of the chloride salt has been demonstrated at the *hprt* locus in Chinese hamster V79 cells and at the *tk* locus in mouse lymphoma L5178Y cells.

In non-human mammalian cells *in vitro*, cadmium chloride induced a dose-dependent increase in sister chromatid exchange frequency in one study but not in two others, in which only single doses were used; in one of the two studies, neither cadmium acetate nor cadmium nitrate induced sister chromatid exchange. A much higher degree of reproducibility has been observed in the induction of chromosomal aberrations by cadmium chloride and cadmium sulfate and in the induction of cell transformation by cadmium acetate and cadmium chloride. The chloride also induced aneuploidy in some cultured cells.

In cultured human cells, cadmium acetate and cadmium chloride induced DNA strand breaks, but cadmium chloride did not induce chromosomal aberrations. Cadmium acetate was reported to have induced aberrations in one study at very high doses. In the only pertinent study in which a human cell line was used, cadmium chloride induced aneuploidy, as demonstrated by the presence of centromeres in micronuclei. Cadmium chloride, but not cadmium sulfate, induced sister chromatid exchange in human lymphocytes.

Conflicting results have been reported for the genetic effects of cadmium chloride in mice: micronuclei and chromosomal aberrations have been observed in bone-marrow cells in several studies but not in others. Cadmium chloride did not induce aneuploidy in bone-marrow cells or spermatocytes of mice treated *in vivo*, but it induced aneuploidy in oocytes of Syrian hamsters and, in two of three studies, of mice. Cadmium chloride did not induce dominant lethal mutation in male rodents in five of six studies with mice or in a single study with rats and did not induce germ-line cell translocations in mice, either cytologically or in breeding experiments. Cadmium chloride induced morphologically abnormal sperm in mice in three of four studies. The discrepancies in the results of the different studies do not appear to be due to dose levels or frequency or route of treatment.

(b) *Cadmium compounds sparingly soluble in water*

Cadmium oxide [particle size not given] did not induce mutation in *S. typhimurium*, and cadmium carbonate [particle size not given] did not induce micronuclei in cells of *Vicia faba*.

Only cadmium sulfide, which exists in crystalline and amorphous forms, has been tested in cultured mammalian cells. Crystalline cadmium sulfide induced DNA strand breaks [particle size not given] and cell transformation [particle size, 0.64 μm], whereas amorphous cadmium sulfide [particle size, 0.64 μm] did not induce cell transformation. Cadmium sulfide [form unspecified] induced chromosomal aberrations in cultured human lymphocytes.

Considerations with regard to genotoxic mechanisms

As metal ions may be precipitated as their insoluble phosphates by *ortho*-phosphate ions in normal bacteriological culture medium and may not be detected as mutagens, modified media were used in some studies (e.g. Pagano & Zeiger, 1992). Ochi *et al.* (1984) reported a higher chromosomal aberration incidence after treatment in saline than in serum-containing medium, and that a post-treatment recovery period of Chinese hamster cells, which allows DNA synthesis to resume, was needed for efficient detection of cadmium-induced chromosomal aberrations.

Cadmium compounds are very toxic *in vitro*. In a screening study for cytotoxicity in BALB/c 3T3 cells, cadmium ranked second only to methylmercury in toxic potency (Borenfreund & Babich, 1987). Prostatic fibroblasts were more sensitive to cadmium toxicity than prostatic epithelial cells from the same species (Terracio & Nachtigal, 1986).

It was reported in many studies that exposure to cadmium induced DNA strand breaks (see Table 14). Ochi and Ohsawa (1983) reported single-strand breaks and, possibly, DNA–protein cross-links in Chinese hamster cells. *In vitro*, cadmium–metallothionein, but not cadmium alone, caused DNA strand breaks (Müller *et al.*, 1991). [The Working Group noted that the significance of this observation for the cell is questionable, since zinc pretreatment (which causes induction of metallothionein) resulted in a reduction of cadmium toxicity and DNA strand breaks (Coogan et al., 1992).]

The frequencies of cadmium-induced DNA strand breaks and chromosomal aberrations are reduced in cells treated with antioxidants, suggesting a relationship between single-strand breaks and active oxygen species. Various scavengers of active oxygen species were assayed for their ability to block chromosomal aberrations induced by cadmium chloride; no effect was seen with superoxide dismutase or dimethylfuran (a scavenger of singlet oxygen), but catalase blocked the induction of aberrations in a dose-dependent manner. D-Mannitol, a scavenger of hydroxyl radicals, also blocked aberration induction, as did the antioxidant butylated hydroxytoluene (a diffusible radical scavenger) (see IARC, 1986b). These results suggest that cadmium chloride is genotoxic by producing hydrogen peroxide, which can form hydroxyl radicals in the presence of iron or copper ions (Rossman et al., 1992). Cadmium chloride treatment also reduced the cellular glutathione level (Ochi et al., 1983; Ochi & Ohsawa, 1985; Ochi et al., 1987; Snyder, 1988). Selenium may also inhibit the clastogenic effects of cadmium in mouse bone marrow, but the interaction, if confirmed, appears to be complex (Mukherjee et al., 1988a). [The Working Group considered this an interesting observation, which could contribute to an understanding of the difficulty in reproducing the genetic effects of cadmium compounds *in vivo*, since selenium levels in rodent diets differ with time and place.]

Various studies have shown that cadmium compounds synergistically increase the effects of other chemicals. For example, cadmium increased the induction of micronuclei by NDMA in mice (Watanabe et al., 1982), enhanced ultraviolet-induced mutagenesis in V79 Chinese hamster cells (Hartwig & Beyersmann, 1989), but not in *E. coli* (Rossman & Molina, 1986), enhanced meiotic nondisjunction induced by γ-irradiation in *Drosophila* oocytes (Kogan et al., 1978) and enhanced benzo[a]pyrene-induced transformation of Syrian hamster embryo cells (Rivedal & Sanner, 1981). Inhibition of DNA repair by cadmium has been suggested as a mechanism for these interactions (e.g. Zasukhina & Sinelschikova, 1976). Cadmium inhibits human DNA polymerase β (a polymerase implicated in DNA replication) (Popenoe & Schmaeler, 1979) and O^6-methylguanine-DNA methyl transferase (Bhattacharyya et al., 1988). Other effects on DNA repair have been reviewed (Rossman et al., 1992).

Cadmium ion induces a number of genes in animal cells. Doses of 5–10 μM [917–1834 μg] cadmium chloride induced transient accumulation of c-*jun* and c-*myc* mRNA 2–4 h after treatment of L6J1 rat myoblasts (Jin & Ringertz, 1990). Cadmium chloride inhibited differentiation of *Drosophila* embryonic cultures, while inducing the entire set of heat-shock proteins (Bournias-Vardiabasis et al., 1990). It also induced haem oxygenase in human skin fibroblasts (Keyse & Tyrrell, 1989) and rat small intestinal epithelium (Rosenberg & Kappas, 1991) and metallothionein in Leydig cells (Abel et al., 1991). The induction of hepatocytic transdifferentiation by cadmium in rat pancreas (Konishi et al., 1990) and characteristics of the granulocyte phenotype in promyelocytic leukaemic cells (Richards et al., 1988) also suggest that it can modify gene expression.

Various researchers have reported that cadmium affects the spindle apparatus (possibly through interactions with thiol compounds, which have a high affinity for cadmium ion [$pK_d \sim 17$] [Verbost et al., 1989]). Kogan et al. (1978) and Ramel and Magnusson (1979)

Table 14. Genetic and related effects of cadmium and cadmium compounds

Test system	Result		Dose[a] (LED/HID)	Reference
	Without exogenous metabolic system	With exogenous metabolic system		
Itai-itai patients				
CLH, Chromosomal aberrations, human lymphocytes *in vivo*	–		0.029 (blood, max.) 0.031 (per g urinary creatinine, max.)	Bui *et al.* (1975)
CLH, Chromosomal aberrations, human lymphocytes *in vivo*	+		NR	Shiraishi (1975)
AVH, Aneuploidy, human lymphocytes *in vivo*	+		NR	Shiraishi (1975)
Environmental/dietary exposure				
SLH, Sister chromatid exchange, human lymphocytes *in vivo*	–		0.01 (blood) 0.01 (per g urinary creatinine)	Nogawa *et al.* (1986)
SLH, Chromosomal aberrations, human lymphocytes *in vivo*	+		NR 0.003 (urine, men) 0.004 (urine, women)	Tang *et al.* (1990)
Occupational exposure				
SLH, Sister chromatid exchange, human lymphocytes *in vivo*	–		NR	Dziekanowska (1981)
CLH, Chromosomal aberrations, human lymphocytes *in vivo*	?[b]		0.032 (blood)	Deknudt & Léonard (1975)
CLH, Chromosomal aberrations, human lymphocytes *in vivo*	–		0.061 (blood) 0.031 (per g urinary creatinine, max.)	Bui *et al.* (1975)
CLH, Chromosomal aberrations, human lymphocytes *in vivo*	(+)[b]		0.004 (blood)	Bauchinger *et al.* (1976)
CLH, Chromosomal aberrations, human lymphocytes *in vivo*	–		0.020 (blood)	O'Riordan *et al.* (1978)
CLH, Chromosomal aberrations, human lymphocytes *in vivo*	(+)		NR	Dziekanowska (1980)
CLH, Chromosomal aberrations, human lymphocytes *in vivo*	–		0.038 (blood)	Fleig *et al.* (1983)
CLH, Chromosomal aberrations, human lymphocytes *in vivo*	+		0.0003–0.0283 (blood) 0.0015–0.0316 (urine)	Forni *et al.* (1990)

Table 14 (contd)

Test system	Result		Dose[a] (LED/HID)	Reference
	Without exogenous metabolic system	With exogenous metabolic system		
Cadmium acetate				
DIA, DNA strand breaks, cross-links, hamster fibroblasts in vitro	+	0	0.11	Casto (1983)
SIC, Sister chromatid exchange, Chinese hamster DON cells in vitro	–	0	0.13	Ohno et al. (1982)
TCS, Cell transformation, Syrian hamster embryo cells, clonal assay in vitro	+	0	0.04	DiPaolo & Casto (1979)
TCS, Cell transformation, Syrian hamster embryo cells, clonal assay in vitro	(+)	0	0.21	Rivedal & Sanner (1981)
T7S, Cell transformation, SA7/Syrian hamster embryo cells in vitro	+	0	0.11	Casto et al. (1979)
DIH, DNA strand breaks, cross-links, human cells in vitro	+	0	21	Casto (1983)
CHL, Chromosomal aberrations, human lymphocytes in vitro	(+)	0	11.2	Gasiorek & Bauchinger (1981)
Cadmium chloride				
PRB, λ Prophage induction/SOS/strand breaks/cross-links	–	0	7.2	Rossman et al. (1984)
ECB, Escherichia coli, DNA strand breaks	+	0	0.34	Mitra & Bernstein (1978)
BSD, Bacillus subtilis rec strains, differential toxicity	+	0	280	Nishioka (1975)
BSD, Bacillus subtilis rec strains, differential toxicity	+	0	28	Kanematsu et al. (1980)
ERD, Escherichia coli differential toxicity	+	+	60	De Flora et al. (1984a)
SAF, Salmonella typhimurium TA1537, forward mutation to 8-azaguanine resistance	+	0	56	Mandel & Ryser (1984)
SA0, Salmonella typhimurium TA100, reverse mutation	–	–	150	Bruce & Heddle (1979)
SA0, Salmonella typhimurium TA100, reverse mutation	–	0	1120	Tso & Fung (1981)
SA0, Salmonella typhimurium TA100, reverse mutation	–	0	56	Mandel & Ryser (1984)

Table 14 (contd)

Test system	Result		Dose[a] (LED/HID)	Reference
	Without exogenous metabolic system	With exogenous metabolic system		

Cadmium chloride (contd)

Test system	Without	With	Dose	Reference
SA0, *Salmonella typhimurium* TA100, reverse mutation	–	–	610	Mortelmans et al. (1986)
SA0, *Salmonella typhimurium* TA100, reverse mutation	–	–	NR	De Flora et al. (1984a)
SA2, *Salmonella typhimurium* TA102, reverse mutation	(+)	(+)	8	De Flora et al. (1984b)
SA5, *Salmonella typhimurium* TA1535, reverse mutation	+	0	56	Mandel & Ryser (1984)
SA5, *Salmonella typhimurium* TA1535, reverse mutation	–	–	610	Mortelmans et al. (1986)
SA5, *Salmonella typhimurium* TA1535, reverse mutation	–	–	NR	De Flora et al. (1984a)
SA7, *Salmonella typhimurium* TA1537, reverse mutation	–	–	150	Bruce & Heddle (1979)
SA7, *Salmonella typhimurium* TA1537, reverse mutation	+	0	56	Mandel & Ryser (1984)
SA7, *Salmonella typhimurium* TA1537, reverse mutation	–	–	610	Mortelmans et al. (1986)
SA7, *Salmonella typhimurium* TA1537, reverse mutation	–	–	NR	De Flora et al. (1984a)
SA7, *Salmonella typhimurium* TA1538, reverse mutation	–	–	NR	De Flora et al. (1984a)
SA8, *Salmonella typhimurium* TA98, reverse mutation	–	–	150	Bruce & Heddle (1979)
SA9, *Salmonella typhimurium* TA98, reverse mutation	–	–	610	Mortelmans et al. (1986)
SA9, *Salmonella typhimurium* TA98, reverse mutation	–	–	NR	De Flora et al. (1984a)
SA9, *Salmonella typhimurium* TA97, reverse mutation	–	–	NR	De Flora et al. (1984b)
SAS, *Salmonella typhimurium* TA1975, reverse mutation	(+)	–	56	Mandel & Ryser (1984)
SAS, *Salmonella typhimurium* TA97, reverse mutation	–[c]	0	22.4	Pagano & Zeiger (1992)
SCG, *Saccharomyces cerevisiae*, gene conversion	+	0	11.2	Fukunaga et al. (1982)
SCG, *Saccharomyces cerevisiae*, gene conversion	+	0	61	Schiestl et al. (1989)
SCR, *Saccharomyces cerevisiae*, reverse mutation	–	0	34	Fukunaga et al. (1982)
SCN, *Saccharomyces cerevisiae*, aneuploidy	–	0	50	Whittaker et al. (1989)
SCN, *Saccharomyces cerevisiae*, aneuploidy	–	0	9	Albertini (1990)
ANN, *Aspergillus nidulans*, aneuploidy	–	0	610	Crebelli et al. (1991)
PLI, *Vicia faba*, micronuclei	+	0	45	De Marco et al. (1988)

Table 14 (contd)

Test system	Result		Dose[a] (LED/HID)	Reference
	Without exogenous metabolic system	With exogenous metabolic system		
Cadmium chloride (contd)				
PLI, Water hyacinth root tips, micronuclei	+	0	0.006	Rosas et al. (1984)
PLN, Chinese spring wheat, aneuploidy	+	0	0.61	Sandhu et al. (1991)
DMM, Drosophila melanogaster, somatic mutation or recombination	–		240	Rasmuson (1985)
DMX, Drosophila melanogaster, sex-linked recessive lethal mutations	–		30	Inoue & Watanabe (1978)
DMX, Drosophila melanogaster, sex-linked recessive lethal mutations	–		112	Kogan et al. (1978)
DMX, Drosophila melanogaster, sex-linked recessive lethal mutations	–		30	Chung & Kim (1982)
DMN, Drosophila melanogaster, aneuploidy	–		38	Ramel & Magnusson (1979)
DMN, Drosophila melanogaster, aneuploidy	+		12	Osgood et al. (1991)
DIA, DNA strand breaks, Chinese hamster ovary cells in vitro	+	0	11	Robison et al. (1982)
DIA, DNA strand breaks, Chinese hamster ovary cells in vitro	–	0	112	Hamilton-Koch et al. (1986)
DIA, DNA strand breaks, cross-links, Chinese hamster V79 cells in vitro	+	0	2.24	Ochi & Ohsawa (1983)
DIA, DNA strand breaks, TRL-1215 rat liver cells in vitro	+	0	56	Coogan et al. (1992)
DIA, DNA strand breaks, rat primary Leydig cells in vitro	–	0	45	Koizumi et al. (1992)
G9H, Gene mutation, Chinese hamster lung V79 cells, hprt locus, in vitro	+	0	0.11	Ochi & Ohsawa (1983)
G9H, Gene mutation, Chinese hamster lung V79 cells, hprt locus, in vitro	(+)	0	0.22	Hartwig & Beyersmann (1989)
G9H, Gene mutation, Chinese hamster lung V79 cells, hprt locus, in vitro	+	0	0.001	Kanematsu et al. (1990)

Table 14 (contd)

Test system	Result		Dose[a] (LED/HID)	Reference
	Without exogenous metabolic system	With exogenous metabolic system		
Cadmium chloride (contd)				
GST, Gene mutation, mouse lymphoma L5178Y cells, tk locus, in vitro	(+)	0	0.07	Amacher & Paillet (1980)
GST, Gene mutation, mouse lymphoma L5178Y cells, tk locus, in vitro	+	0	0.09	McGregor et al. (1988)
SIC, Sister chromatid exchange, Chinese hamster ovary cells in vitro	–	0	0.045	Deaven & Campbell (1980)
SIC, Sister chromatid exchange, Don Chinese hamster cells in vitro	–	0	0.11	Ohno et al. (1982)
SIC, Sister chromatid exchange, Chinese hamster ovary cells in vitro	+	0	0.001	Howard et al. (1991)
MIA, Micronucleus test (aneuploidy), Chinese hamster lung Cl-1 cells	+	0	1.22	Antoccia et al. (1991)
CIC, Chromosomal aberrations, Chinese hamster V79 cells in vitro	+	0	0.11	Deaven & Campbell (1980)
CIC, Chromosomal aberrations and polyploidy, Chinese hamster V79 cells in vitro	+	0	0.11	Ochi et al. (1984)
CIC, Chromosomal aberrations, Chinese hamster V79 cells in vitro	+	0	1.12	Ochi & Ohsawa (1985)
CIC, Chromosomal aberrations, Chinese hamster ovary cells in vitro	+	0	0.06	Lakkad et al. (1986)
CIC, Chromosomal aberrations, Chinese hamster ovary cells in vitro	+	0	0.01	Howard et al. (1991)
CIT, Chromosomal aberrations, mouse mammary carcinoma cells in vitro	–	0	3.58	Umeda & Nishimura (1979)
TBM, Cell transformation, BALB/c 3T3 mouse cells in vitro	+	0	0.17	Saffiotti & Bertolero (1989)

Table 14 (contd)

Cadmium chloride (contd)

Test system	Result		Dose[a] (LED/HID)	Reference
	Without exogenous metabolic system	With exogenous metabolic system		
TCL, Cell transformation, rat ventral prostate cells *in vitro*	+	0	0.003 × 7 days	Terracio & Nachtigal (1986)
TCL, Cell transformation, Indian muntjac skin fibroblasts *in vitro*	+	0	0.56 × 20 months	Chibber & Ord (1990)
T7S, Cell transformation, SA7/Syrian hamster embryo cells *in vitro*	+	0	0.22	Casto *et al.* (1979)
DIH, DNA strand breaks, human lymphocytes *in vitro*	+	0	2.8	Zasukhina & Sinelschikova (1976)
DIH, DNA strand breaks, human lymphocytes *in vitro*	–	0	5.6	McLean *et al.* (1982)
DIH, DNA strand breaks, human diploid (HSBP) fibroblasts *in vitro*	+	0	14	Hamilton-Koch *et al.* (1986)
DIH, DNA strand breaks, human diploid (HSBP) fibroblasts *in vitro*	+	0	14	Snyder (1988)
MIH, Micronuclei (aneuploidy), human LEO fibroblasts *in vitro*	+	0	0.03	Bonatti *et al.* (1992)
SHL, Sister chromatid exchange, human lymphocytes *in vitro*	+	0	0.56	Han *et al.* (1992)
CHL, Chromosomal aberrations, human lymphocytes *in vitro*	–	0	5.6	Deknudt & Deminatti (1978)
SVA, Sister chromatid exchange, mouse bone-marrow cells *in vivo*	+	0	0.51, ip × 1	Mukherjee *et al.* (1988b)
SVA, Sister chromatid exchange, pregnant mouse bone-marrow cells *in vivo*	–	0	7, sc × 1	Nayak *et al.* (1989)
SVA, Sister chromatid exchange, mouse fetal liver and lung cells *in vivo*	–	0	7, transplacentally × 1	Nayak *et al.* (1989)
MVM, Micronuclei, mice *in vivo*	–	0	9.15, ip	Bruce & Heddle (1979)
MVM, Micronuclei, mice *in vivo*	–	0	50, in drinking-water × 7 days	Watanabe *et al.* (1982)

CADMIUM AND CADMIUM COMPOUNDS

Table 14 (contd)

Test system	Result		Dose (LED/HID)	Reference
	Without exogenous metabolic system	With exogenous metabolic system		
Cadmium chloride (contd)				
MVM, Micronuclei, mice in vivo	+	0	0.92, ip × 1	Kozachenko et al. (1987)
MVM, Micronuclei, mice in vivo	(+)	0	4.12, ip × 1	Mukherjee et al. (1988b)
MVM, Micronuclei, mice in vivo	–	0	0.06, po × 2	Volkova & Karplyuk (1990)
MVM, Micronuclei, mice in vivo	–	0	6.10, ip × 1	Adler et al. (1991)
MVM, Micronuclei, mice in vivo	+	0	0.43, ip × 1	Han et al. (1992)
CBA, Chromosomal aberrations, mouse bone-marrow cells in vivo	–	0	44, in diet × 1 month	Deknudt & Gerber (1979)
CBA, Chromosomal aberrations, mouse bone-marrow cells in vivo	+	0	0.26, ip × 1	Mukherjee et al. (1988b)
CBA, Chromosomal aberrations, mouse bone-marrow cells in vivo	+		1.07, po × 7–21 days	Mukherjee et al. (1988a)
CBA, Chromosomal aberrations, mouse bone-marrow cells in vivo	–		30.5, ip × 1	Chopikashvili et al. (1989)
CBA, Chromosomal aberrations, mouse bone-marrow cells in vivo	+		0.43, ip × 1	Han et al. (1992)
CGC, Chromosomal aberrations, mouse spermatocytes in vivo	–		1.83, ip × 1	Gilliavod & Léonard (1975)
DLM, Dominant lethal mutation, mice in vivo	–		4.3, ip × 1	Epstein et al. (1972)
DLM, Dominant lethal mutation, mice in vivo	–		1.07, ip × 1	Gilliavod & Léonard (1975)
DLM, Dominant lethal mutation, mice in vivo	–		1.22, ip × 1	Suter (1975)
DLM, Dominant lethal mutation, mice in vivo	–		2.44, ip × 1	Ramaiya & Pomerantseva (1977)
DLM, Dominant lethal mutation, mice in vivo	–		2.44 ip × 1	Pomerantseva et al. (1980)
DLM, Dominant lethal mutation, mice in vivo	(+)		1.83, po × 5 days	Bleyl & Lewerenz (1980)

Table 14 (contd)

Test system	Result		Dose[a] (LED/HID)	Reference
	Without exogenous metabolic system	With exogenous metabolic system		
Cadmium chloride (contd)				
DLR, Dominant lethal mutation, rats in vivo	–		6.10, po × 6 weeks	Sutou et al. (1980b)
MHT, Heritable translocation, mice in vivo	–		1.07, ip × 1	Gilliavod & Léonard (1975)
AVA, Aneuploidy, mouse oocytes in vivo	(+)		3.66, sc × 1	Shimada et al. (1976)
AVA, Aneuploidy, mouse oocytes in vivo	(+)		3.66, sc × 1	Watanabe et al. (1977)
AVA, Aneuploidy, mouse oocytes in vivo	–		3.66, ip × 1	Mailhes et al. (1988)
AVA, Aneuploidy, Syrian hamster oocytes in vivo	+		0.61, sc × 1	Watanabe et al. (1979)
AVA, Aneuploidy, mouse spermatocytes in vivo	(+)		3.66, ip × 1	Miller & Adler (1992)
SPM, Sperm morphology, mice in vivo	+		2.44, ip × 1	Pomerantseva et al. (1980)
SPM, Sperm morphology, mice in vivo	–		9, ip, × 5	Bruce & Heddle (1979)
SPM, Sperm morphology, mice in vivo	+		0.51, ip × 5	Mukherjee et al. (1988b)
SPM, Sperm morphology, mice in vivo	+		0.37, ip × 1	Han et al. (1992)
***, Inhibition of DNA synthesis, mouse testis in vivo	+		10, ip × 1	Friedman & Staub (1976)
***, Decreased chromosome length, human lymphocytes in vitro	+	0	1.12, 4 h	Andersen et al. (1983)
***, Stimulation of DNA synthesis in mouse liver and other organs in vivo	+		1, ip × 1	Hellman (1986)
Cadmium nitrate				
BSD, Bacillus subtilis rec strains, differential toxicity	–	0	280	Nishioka (1975)
BSD, Bacillus subtilis rec strains, differential toxicity	+	0	28	Kanematsu et al. (1980)
SA0, Salmonella typhimurium TA100, reverse mutation	–	0	NR	Arlauskas et al. (1985)
SA5, Salmonella typhimurium TA1535, reverse mutation	–	0	NR	Arlauskas et al. (1985)

Table 14 (contd)

Test system	Result		Dose[a] (LED/HID)	Reference
	Without exogenous metabolic system	With exogenous metabolic system		
Cadmium nitrate (contd)				
SA7, *Salmonella typhimurium* TA1537, reverse mutation	–	0	NR	Arlauskas *et al.* (1985)
SA8, *Salmonella typhimurium* TA1538, reverse mutation	–	0	NR	Arlauskas *et al.* (1985)
SA9, *Salmonella typhimurium* TA98, reverse mutation	–	0	NR	Arlauskas *et al.* (1985)
ECR, *Escherichia coli* DG1153, reverse mutation	–[d]	0	NR	Arlauskas *et al.* (1985)
SIC, Sister chromatid exchange, Chinese hamster DON cells *in vitro*	–	0	0.18	Ohno *et al.* (1982)
DMM, *Drosophila melanogaster*, somatic mutation or recombination	–		132	Rasmuson (1985)
Cadmium sulfate				
ERD, *Escherichia coli* differential toxicity	+	+	67	De Flora *et al.* (1984a)
BSD, *Bacillus subtilis* rec strains, differential toxicity	+	0	28	Kanematsu *et al.* (1980)
SAS, *Salmonella typhimurium* TA97, reverse mutation	–	–	NR	De Flora *et al.* (1984a)
SA8, *Salmonella typhimurium* TA98, reverse mutation	–	–	NR	De Flora *et al.* (1984a)
SA0, *Salmonella typhimurium* TA100, reverse mutation	–	–	NR	De Flora *et al.* (1984a)
SA2, *Salmonella typhimurium* TA102, reverse mutation	(+)	(+)	7	De Flora *et al.* (1984b)
SA2, *Salmonella typhimurium* TA102, reverse mutation	–	0	0.03	Marzin & Phi (1985)
SA5, *Salmonella typhimurium* TA1535, reverse mutation	–	–	NR	De Flora *et al.* (1984a)
SA7, *Salmonella typhimurium* TA1537, reverse mutation	–	–	NR	De Flora *et al.* (1984a)
SA8, *Salmonella typhimurium* TA1538, reverse mutation	–	–	NR	De Flora *et al.* (1984a)
SCG, *Saccharomyces cerevisiae*, gene conversion	+	0	54	Schiestl *et al.* (1989)
DIA, DNA strand breaks, rat hepatocytes *in vitro*	+	0	3.36	Sina *et al.* (1983)
GST, Gene mutation, mouse lymphoma L5178Y cells, *tk* locus *in vitro*	+	0	0.08	Oberly *et al.* (1982)
CIC, Chromosomal aberrations, Chinese hamster fibroblasts *in vitro*	+	0	11.2	Röhr & Bauchinger (1976)

Table 14 (contd)

Test system	Result		Dose[a] (LED/HID)	Reference
	Without exogenous metabolic system	With exogenous metabolic system		
Cadmium sulfate (contd)				
CIC, Chromosomal aberrations, Chinese hamster ovary cells in vitro	+	0	0.11	Armstrong et al. (1992)
CIC, Chromosomal aberrations, Chinese hamster ovary cells in vitro	+	0	0.22	Bean et al. (1992)
SHL, Sister chromatid exchange, human lymphocytes in vitro	–	0	0.69	Bassendowska-Karska & Zawadzka-Kos (1987)
HMA, Chromosomal aberrations, mouse ascites tumour cells in vivo	–		0.02, parenterally × 1	Bishun & Pentecost (1981)
Cadmium sulfide				
DIA, DNA strand breaks, Chinese hamster ovary cells in vitro[e]	+	0	8 × 24 h	Robison et al. (1982)
TCS, Cell transformation, Syrian hamster embryo cells, clonal assay in vitro[e]	+	0	0.78	Costa et al. (1982)
TCS, Cell transformation, Syrian hamster embryo cells, clonal assay in vitro[f]	–	0	3.90	Costa et al. (1982)
CHL, Chromosomal aberrations, human lymphocytes in vitro (unspecified)	+	0	0.05 × 4 h	Shiraishi et al. (1972)
Cadmium oxide				
SA0, Salmonella typhimurium TA100, reverse mutation	–	0	1466	Mortelmans et al. (1986)
SA5, Salmonella typhimurium TA1535, reverse mutation	–	0	147	Mortelmans et al. (1986)
SA7, Salmonella typhimurium TA1537, reverse mutation	–	0	147	Mortelmans et al. (1986)

Table 14 (contd)

Test system	Result Without exogenous metabolic system	Result With exogenous metabolic system	Dose[a] (LED/HID)	Reference
Cadmium oxide (contd)				
SA9, *Salmonella typhimurium* TA98, reverse mutation	–	0	1466	Mortelmans *et al.* (1986)
Cadmium carbonate				
PLI, *Vicia faba*, micronuclei	–[g]	0	0	De Marco *et al.* (1988)

+, considered to be positive; (+), considered to be weakly positive in an inadequate study; –, considered to be negative; ?, considered to be inconclusive (variable responses in several experiments within an adequate study); 0, not tested

[a]LED, lowest effective dose; HID, highest ineffective dose. In-vitro tests, μg/ml; in-vivo tests, mg/kg bw. Doses given as concentration of element, not concentration of compound. ip, intraperitoneally; sc, subcutaneously; po, orally, by gavage; NR, not reported
[b]Exposed to lead and cadmium
[c]Positive at 12.5–25 μM in distilled deionized water
[d]Positive in fluctuation assay for *E. coli* DG1153 at 0.67 μg/ml
[e]Crystalline cadmium sulfide
[f]Amorphous cadmium sulfide
[g]Induced by 8×10^{-4} M in the presence of equimolar nitrilotriacetic acid 3Na salt
***Not displayed on profiles

reported non-disjunction of meiotic chromosomes in *D. melanogaster* after exposure to cadmium, suggesting damage to the mitotic apparatus. Lakkad *et al.* (1986) observed chromosomal damage after exposure of Chinese hamster ovary cells to very low concentrations of cadmium *in vitro*, which included micronuclei, lagging chromosomes, chromatid bridges and multinucleated cells, suggesting spindle damage. A project for the validation of tests for aneuploidy coordinated by the Commission of the European Communities included cadmium chloride among 10 known or presumed spindle poisons: Cadmium-induced spindle disturbances and aneuploidy were observed in test systems ranging from yeast to human cells and in mice *in vivo* (Table 14). Cadmium chloride also inhibited the assembly of purified *Drosophila* microtubules *in vitro* (Sehgal *et al.*, 1990).

The ionic charge and radius of Cd^{2+} are comparable to those of Ca^{2+} (Chao *et al.*, 1984). Thus, Cd^{2+} could conceivably replace Ca^{2+} at cellular Ca^{2+} binding sites and lead to disturbances in cellular calcium homeostasis. Verbost *et al.* (1989) observed inhibition of Ca^{2+}-ATPase-mediated Ca^{2+} extrusion in erythrocyte ghosts by Cd^{2+} at nanomolar concentrations, with involvement of thiol groups. [The Working Group noted that this effect occurred at very low concentrations and could have many consequences for cellular metabolism.]

5. Summary of Data Reported and Evaluation

5.1 Exposure data

Cadmium is found at low concentrations in the Earth's crust, mainly as the sulfide in zinc-containing mineral deposits. Since the early twentieth century, it has been produced and used in a variety of applications in alloys and in compounds. Among the important compounds of cadmium are cadmium oxide (used in batteries, as an intermediate and catalyst and in electroplating), cadmium sulfide (used as a pigment), cadmium sulfate (used as an intermediate and in electroplating) and cadmium stearate (used as a plastics stabilizer).

Occupational exposure to cadmium and cadmium compounds occurs mainly in the form of airborne dust and fume. Occupations in which the highest potential exposures occur include cadmium production and refining, nickel–cadmium battery manufacture, cadmium pigment manufacture and formulation, cadmium alloy production, mechanical plating, zinc smelting, soldering and polyvinylchloride compounding. Although levels vary widely among the different industries, occupational exposures generally have decreased in the last two decades.

Urinary and blood cadmium concentrations are generally much lower in non-occupationally exposed people, for whom the most important sources of exposure are cigarette smoking and, especially in polluted areas, eating certain foods (e.g. rice). Acidification of cadmium-containing soils and sediments may increase the concentrations of cadmium in surface waters and crops.

5.2 Human carcinogenicity data

Following a report of the occurrence of prostatic cancers in a small group of workers employed before 1965 in a plant manufacturing nickel–cadmium batteries in the United

Kingdom, a series of cohort analyses were undertaken, which did not confirm the excess among the remaining workers; however, an increase in mortality rates from lung cancer was detected. A small cohort working in the same industry was studied in Sweden: no excess of prostatic cancer was detected, but a nonsignificant increase in mortality from lung cancer was found among workers who had the longest duration of employment and latency.

Two small copper–cadmium alloy plants were studied in the United Kingdom. The rate of mortality from lung cancer was increased in one of them but decreased in the other. A case–control analysis of lung cancer did not show any association with exposure to cadmium. No increase in mortality from prostatic cancer was found in these two plants, while in a similar plant in Sweden a nonsignificant excess was detected.

Excess mortality from lung cancer was reported among workers employed in a US cadmium recovery plant, and a dose–response relationship was demonstrated between estimated cumulative exposure to cadmium and lung cancer risk. The latter was unlikely to be due to confounding by cigarette smoking and persisted among workers employed after 1940, when little arsenic was present in feedstock. Excess mortality from prostatic cancer was found initially, but the relative risk diminished and became nonsignificant with further follow-up.

In a large cohort of workers from 17 cadmium processing plants in the United Kingdom, decreased mortality from prostatic cancer was observed, while that from lung cancer was increased in the overall cohort and there were suggested trends with duration of employment and with intensity of exposure. The increase in lung cancer risk was stronger in the small proportion of workers with high cadmium exposure. Confounding by concomitant exposure to other cancer determinants, including arsenic, was not controlled for. Excess mortality from stomach cancer, which was not related to intensity of cadmium exposure, was also reported among these workers.

A number of early studies reported an increased risk for prostatic cancer among cadmium workers, but the results of later studies were not consistent. Early and recent studies provide consistent evidence that the risk for lung cancer is increased among workers exposed to cadmium.

Constraints that influence the assessment of both lung and prostatic cancer risk are that the number of long-term, highly exposed workers is small, the historical data on exposure to cadmium are limited, particularly for the non-US plants, and the ability to define and examine a gradient of cumulative exposure varies across studies. Additionally, for cohort studies, prostatic cancer poses special difficulties in that it is subject to the possibility of detection bias. Confounding by cigarette smoking in relation to lung cancer was addressed directly only in the study from the USA, but some other studies provided analyses based on internal comparisons, which are not likely to be affected by this problem. Control of the confounding effect of co-exposure to other metals, particularly arsenic and nickel, was limited; however, the analyses in which an attempt was made to distinguish US cadmium-exposed workers with different levels of exposure to arsenic indicated that the increase in lung cancer risk was unlikely to be explained by exposure to arsenic.

5.3 Animal carcinogenicity data

Cadmium chloride, cadmium sulfate and cadmium acetate have been tested by oral administration in several studies in mice and rats. Most of the studies were inadequate for an evaluation of carcinogenicity. Two adequate studies on cadmium chloride in rats are available. In one study with controlled dietary zinc levels in male rats, cadmium chloride produced dose-related increases in the incidences of leukaemia, interstitial-cell tumours of the testis and proliferative lesions of the prostate. In another study on cadmium chloride in rats, in which zinc levels in diet were not controlled, no increase in tumour incidence was seen.

In two inhalation studies in rats, malignant lung tumours were produced by cadmium chloride, cadmium sulfide/sulfate, cadmium sulfate and cadmium oxide fume and dust at low levels of exposure for short durations. In one study in rats by intratracheal instillation, malignant pulmonary tumours were produced by cadmium sulfide and cadmium chloride, but not by cadmium oxide. In one inhalation study in mice of cadmium chloride, cadmium sulfide/sulfate, cadmium sulfate and cadmium oxide fume and dust, some groups exposed to cadmium oxide fume or dust had increased incidences of lung tumours. In one inhalation study in hamsters of cadmium chloride, cadmium sulfide/sulfate, cadmium sulfate and cadmium oxide fume and dust, no increase in the incidence of lung tumours was found.

In several studies, single or multiple subcutaneous injections of cadmium chloride, cadmium sulfide, cadmium sulfate and cadmium oxide and of cadmium-containing rat liver ferritin caused local sarcomas in rats. Mice appear to be generally less susceptible than rats to induction of local tumours by cadmium compounds. Cadmium powder, cadmium chloride and cadmium sulfide produced local sarcomas in rats following intramuscular administration. In a single study by intraperitoneal injection in rats, cadmium sulfide induced malignant tumours within the peritoneal cavity. Cadmium chloride in mice and rats and cadmium sulfate and cadmium-precipitated rat liver ferritin in rats produced testicular interstitial tumours after subcutaneous administration. Dietary zinc deficiency enhanced the multiplicity of cadmium-induced interstitial-cell tumours of the testis and increased the incidence of local tumours at the site of subcutaneous cadmium injections. Subcutaneous injection of cadmium chloride to rats produced tumours of the prostate but only at doses below the level that induced cadmium-induced testicular degeneration or when such degeneration was prevented by concurrent exposure to zinc. Intramuscular administration of cadmium chloride also induced prostatic tumours in rats. Subcutaneous administration of cadmium chloride increased the incidence of pancreatic tumours in rats in one study and decreased the incidence in another.

In limited studies in rats, injection of cadmium chloride into the prostate produced malignant prostatic tumours.

Administration of excess zinc by inhalation, parenteral and oral routes has been shown to reduce the carcinogenic potential of cadmium after exposure systemically or by inhalation. When combined with known carcinogens, cadmium enhanced, suppressed or had no effect on tumour incidence, depending on a complex set of circumstances including, at least in part, the dose, time sequence of administration, site of tumour and route of administration.

5.4 Other relevant data

Cadmium enters the body mainly by inhalation and by ingestion. Fractional intestinal absorption is influenced by dietary factors and increases with dietary cadmium concentration. Pulmonary fractional absorption depends partly on the solubility *in vivo* of the compound. Cadmium induces synthesis of metallothionein, a low-molecular-weight protein that binds cadmium primarily in the liver and kidney. Metallothionein production can also be induced by e.g. zinc. When metallothionein-bound cadmium is released into the blood, it is filtered through the glomeruli and then reabsorbed in the proximal tubules. In certain mammalian tissues, such as rat ventral prostate, hamster ovary and rat, mouse and monkey testis, the concentrations of metallothionein are low and its synthesis is not induced by exposure to cadmium. Most of the body burden of cadmium is retained in the kidneys and the liver. The half-life of cadmium in human kidneys is probably 10–20 years. Cadmium concentrations in whole blood are affected by both recent exposure and body burden. Excretion occurs mainly *via* the urine. Urinary excretion of cadmium by individuals without renal dysfunction primarily reflects the amount of cadmium retained in the kidneys.

The target organs for cadmium toxicity depend on the type of exposure. Inhalation of cadmium can lead to chronic obstructive airway disease. Following long-term exposure, renal tubular and glomerular dysfunction can develop. Renal function can deteriorate further, even after cessation of exposure to cadmium. Cadmium can suppress cell-mediated immune responses *in vitro*.

Parenteral administration of cadmium salts produces adverse effects on the testes, ovaries, placenta and embryo in experimental animals; many of these effects have been shown to be preventable by administration of zinc compounds. Administration of cadmium at doses that affect placental morphology or function induces fetal anaemia, growth retardation, teratogenicity and embryonic and fetal death in experimental animals. Reproductive and developmental toxicity have been reported following exposure to cadmium compounds by oral and inhalation routes, but the effects are generally much less severe than after parenteral administration.

In three of five studies, the frequencies of chromosomal aberration were increased in peripheral blood lymphocytes of workers exposed to cadmium in the metal industry, where they were usually also exposed to other metals. No effect of cadmium was observed in a limited study of workers from a Swedish alkaline battery factory. In two studies of cadmium pigment plant workers, no increase in the frequency of chromosomal aberrations was observed. No increase in the frequency of sister chromatid exchange was seen in one study of workers exposed to cadmium.

In one of two limited studies of *itai-itai* patients, increased frequency and severity of chromosomal aberrations were observed. In one study, no increase in sister chromatid exchange frequency was observed in people living in a cadmium-polluted region of Japan. In a study of subjects living in a cadmium-polluted region of China, there were small but significant increases in chromosomal aberration frequency. A significant dose–effect relationship between urinary levels of cadmium and chromosomal aberration frequency was also observed, and more severe aberration types were observed in individuals with high urinary levels of cadmium.

In those studies in which significant responses were observed, the chromosomal aberrations tended to occur in the more heavily exposed groups and were of more complex types.

Chromosomal aberrations and aneuploidy were observed in animals exposed to cadmium chloride *in vivo*. Dominant lethal mutations were generally not induced in mice.

Cadmium chloride damages DNA of human cells *in vitro*. In the few studies available, chromosomal aberrations were observed in human cells treated with cadmium sulfide but not in those treated with cadmium chloride. Indications of aneuploidy were observed in human fibroblasts after treatment with cadmium chloride.

Studies using cultured animal cells show that exposure to cadmium compounds damages genetic material. DNA strand breaks, mutations, chromosomal damage and cell transformation have been observed *in vitro*. Cadmium compounds inhibit the repair of DNA damaged by other agents, thereby enhancing their genotoxicity.

Mutations have generally not been observed in *Drosophila* or bacteria; however, a weak response was observed in some studies in bacteria and there is evidence for cadmium-induced DNA damage in bacteria.

5.5 Evaluation[1]

There is *sufficient evidence* in humans for the carcinogenicity of cadmium and cadmium compounds.

There is *sufficient evidence* in experimental animals for the carcinogenicity of cadmium compounds.

There is *limited evidence* in experimental animals for the carcinogenicity of cadmium metal.

In making the overall evaluation, the Working Group took into consideration the evidence that ionic cadmium causes genotoxic effects in a variety of types of eukaryotic cells, including human cells.

Overall evaluation

Cadmium and cadmium compounds *are carcinogenic to humans (Group 1)*.

6. References

Abd Elghany, N., Schumacher, M.C., Slattery, M.L., West, D.W. & Lee, J.S. (1990) Occupation, cadmium exposure, and prostate cancer. *Epidemiology*, 1, 107–115

Abe, H., Watanabe, T. & Ikeda, M. (1986) Cadmium levels in the urine of female farmers in non-polluted areas in Japan. *J. Toxicol. environ. Health*, 18, 357–367

---

[1]For definition of the italicized terms, see Preamble, pp. 26–30.

Abel, J., de Ruiter, N. & Kühn-Velten, W.N. (1991) Comparative study on metallothionein induction in whole testicular tissue and isolated Leydig cells. *Arch. Toxicol.*, **65**, 228–234

Abraham, R., Charles, A.K., Mankes, R., LeFevre, R., Renak, V. & Ashok, L. (1986) In vitro effects of cadmium chloride on preimplantation rat embryos. *Ecotoxicol. environ. Saf.*, **12**, 213–219

Adams, R.G. (1992) Manufacturing process, resultant risk profiles and their control in the production of nickel–cadmium (alkaline) batteries. *Occup. Med.*, **42**, 101–106

Adams, R.G., Harrison, J.F. & Scott, P. (1969) The development of cadmium-induced proteinuria, impaired renal function, and osteomalacia in alkaline battery workers. *Q. J. Med. New Ser.*, **38**, 425–443

Adamsson, E. (1979) Long-term sampling of airborne cadmium dust in an alkaline battery factory. *Scand. J. Work Environ. Health*, **5**, 178–187

Ades, A.E. & Kazantzis, G. (1988) Lung cancer in a non-ferrous smelter: the role of cadmium. *Br. J. ind. Med.*, **45**, 435–442

Adler, I.-D., Kliesch, U., van Hummelen, P. & Kirsch-Volders, M. (1991) Mouse micronucleus tests with known and suspect spindle poisons: results from two laboratories. *Mutagenesis*, **6**, 47–53

Agency for Toxic Substances and Disease Registry (1989) *Toxicological Profile for Cadmium* (ATSDR/TP-88/08; US NTIS PB89-194476), Atlanta, GA, US Public Health Service

Ahlgren, L. & Mattsson, S. (1981) Cadmium in man measured *in vivo* by X-ray fluorescence analysis. *Phys. Med. Biol.*, **26**, 19–26

Albertini, S. (1990) Analysis of nine known or suspected spindle poisons for mitotic chromosome malsegregation using *Saccharomyces cerevisiae* D61.M. *Mutagenesis*, **5**, 453–459

Aldrich Chemical Co. (1992) *Aldrich Catalog/Handbook of Fine Chemicals 1992–1993*, Milwaukee, WI, pp. 241–243

Alessio, L., Odone, P., Bertelli, G. & Foà, V. (1983) Cadmium. In: Alessio, L., Berlin, A., Roi, R. & Boni, M., eds, *Human Biological Monitoring of Industrial Chemical Series* (EUR 8476 EN), Luxembourg, Commission of the European Communities, pp. 23–44

Alessio, L., Apostoli, P. & Ferioli, A. (1990) Identification of reference values for metals in general population groups. The example of cadmium. *Toxicol. environ. Chem.*, **27**, 39–48

Alessio, L., Apostoli, P., Duca, P.G. & Braga, M. (1992) Definition of reference values for Cd-B and Cd-U: methodological aspects and preliminary results. In: Nordberg, G.F., Herber, R.F.M. & Alessio, L., eds, *Cadmium in the Human Environment: Toxicity and Carcinogenicity* (IARC Scientific Publications No. 118), Lyon, IARC, pp. 93–99

Alfa Products (1990) *Alfa Catalog—Research Chemicals and Accessories*, Ward Hill, MA, pp. 78–81, 466–468

Ali, M.M., Murthy, R.C. & Chandra, S.V. (1986) Developmental and long-term neurobehavioral toxicity of low level in-utero cadmium exposure in rats. *Neurobehav. Toxicol. Teratol.*, **8**, 463–468

Amacher, D.E. & Paillet, S.C. (1980) Induction of trifluorothymidine-resistant mutants by metal ions in L5178Y/TK$^{+/-}$ cells. *Mutat. Res.*, **78**, 279–288

American Conference of Governmental Industrial Hygienists (1992) *1992–1993 Threshold Limit Values for Chemical Substances and Physical Agents and Biological Exposure Indices*, Cincinnati, OH, pp. 14, 39, 63, 69

Andersen, O., Rønne, M. & Nordberg, G.F. (1983) Effects of inorganic metal salts on chromosome length in human lymphocytes. *Hereditas*, **98**, 65–70

Andersen, O., Nielsen, J.B. & Nordberg, G.F. (1992) Factors affecting the intestinal uptake of cadmium from the diet. In: Nordberg, G.F., Herber, R.F.M. & Alessio, L., eds, *Cadmium in the Human Environment: Toxicity and Carcinogenicity* (IARC Scientific Publications No. 118), Lyon, IARC, pp. 173-187

Andersson, K., Elinder, C.-G., Hogstedt, C., Kjellström, T. & Spång, G. (1984) Mortality among cadmium and nickel-exposed workers in a Swedish battery factory. *Toxicol. environ. Chem.*, **9**, 53-62

Angerer, J. & Schaller, K.H., eds (1985) *Analyses of Hazardous Substances in Biological Materials*, Vol. 1, Weinheim, VCH Verlagsgesellschaft mbH, pp. 79-92

Angerer, J. & Schaller, K.H., eds (1988) *Analysis of Hazardous Substances in Biological Materials. Methods for Biological Monitoring*, Vol. 2, Weinheim, VCH Verlagsgesellschaft mbH, pp. 85-94

Anon. (1992) Occupational exposure limits. *BIBRA Bull.*, **31**, 287

Antoccia, A., Degrassi, F., Battistoni, A., Ciliutti, P. & Tanzarella, C. (1991) In vitro micronucleus test with kinetochore staining: evaluation of test performance. *Mutagenesis*, **6**, 319-324

Arbeidsinspectie [Labour Inspection] (1986) *De Nationale MAC-Lijst 1986* [National MAC List 1986], Voorburg, p. 9

Arbetarskyddsstyrelsens [National Board of Occupational Safety and Health] (1989) *Arbetarskyddsstyrelsens kungörelse om ändring i styrelsens kungörelse (AFS 1988:7) med föreskrifter om kadmium* [Notification by the National Board of Occupational Safety and Health of change in the notification of the Board (AFS 1988:7) with directives for cadmium and general advice of the Board on application of the directive] (AFS 1989:3), Stockholm

Arlauskas, A., Baker, R.S.U., Bonin, A.M., Tandon, R.K., Crisp, P.T. & Ellis, J. (1985) Mutagenicity of metal ions in bacteria. *Environ. Res.*, **36**, 379-388

Armstrong, B.G. & Kazantzis, G. (1983) The mortality of cadmium workers. *Lancet*, **i**, 1425-1427

Armstrong, M.J., Bean, C.L. & Galloway, S.M. (1992) A quantitative assessment of the cytotoxicity associated with chromosomal aberration detection in Chinese hamster ovary cells. *Mutat. Res.*, **265**, 45-60

Atomergic Chemetals Corp. (undated) *High Purity Metals Brochure*, Farmingdale, NY

Aufderheide, M., Mohr, U., Thiedemann, K.-U. & Heinrich, U. (1990) Quantification of hyperplastic areas in hamster lungs after chronic inhalation of different cadmium compounds. *Toxicol. environ. Chem.*, **27**, 173-180

Axelson, O. (1978) Aspects on confounding in occupational health epidemiology (Letter to the Editor). *Scand. J. Work Environ. Health*, **4**, 85-89

Axelsson, B. & Piscator, M. (1966) Renal damage after prolonged exposure to cadmium. An experimental study. *Arch. environ. Health*, **12**, 360-373

Baker, R.S.U. (1985) Evaluation of metals in in vitro assays, interpretation of data and possible mechanisms of action. In: Merian, E., ed., *Carcinogenic and Mutagenic Metal Compounds*, New York, Gordon & Breach, pp. 185-206

Bako, G., Smith, E.S.O., Hanson, J. & Dewar, R. (1982) The geographical distribution of high cadmium concentrations in the environment and prostate cancer in Alberta. *Can. J. Public Health*, **73**, 92-94

Banat, K., Förstner, U. & Müller, G. (1972) Heavy metals in sediments of the Danube, Rhine, Ems, Weser and Elbe in the Democratic Republic of Germany (Ger.). *Naturwissenschaften*, **59**, 525-528

Barański, B., Stetkiewicz, I., Trzcinka-Ochocka, M., Sitarek, K. & Szymczak, W. (1982) Teratogenicity, fetal toxicity and tissue concentration of cadmium administered to female rats during organogenesis. *J. appl. Toxicol.*, **2**, 255-259

Barański, B., Stetkiewicz, I., Sitarek, K. & Szymczak, W. (1983) Effects of oral, subchronic cadmium administration on fertility, prenatal and postnatal progeny developments in rats. *Arch. Toxicol.*, **54**, 297–302

Barlow, S.M. & Sullivan, F.M. (1982) *Reproductive Hazards of Industrial Chemicals. An Evaluation of Animal and Human Data*, London, Academic Press, pp. 136–177

Bassendowska-Karska, E. & Zawadzka-Kos, M. (1987) Cadmium sulfate does not induce sister chromatid exchanges in human lymphocytes *in vitro. Toxicol. Lett.*, **37**, 173–175

Bauchinger, M., Schmid, E., Einbrodt, H.J. & Dresp, J. (1976) Chromosome aberrations in lymphocytes after occupational exposure to lead and cadmium. *Mutat. Res.*, **40**, 57–62

Bean, C.L., Armstrong, M.J. & Galloway, S.M. (1992) Effect of sampling time on chromosome aberration yield for 7 chemicals in Chinese hamster ovary cells. *Mutat. Res.*, **265**, 31–44

Bernard, A. & Lauwerys, R. (1986) Cadmium in human population. *Experientia*, **50** (Suppl.), 114–123

Bhattacharyya, D., Boulden, A.M., Foote, R.S. & Mitra, S. (1988) Effects of polyvalent metal ions on the reactivity of human O^6-methylguanine-DNA methyltransferase. *Carcinogenesis*, **9**, 683–685

Bishun, N. & Pentecost, M. (1981) Cytogenetic effects of lead and cadmium compounds on ascitic tumour cells in the mouse. *Microbios Lett.*, **17**, 29–32

Blakley, B.R. (1986) The effect of cadmium on chemical- and viral-induced tumor production in mice. *J. appl. Toxicol.*, **6**, 425–429

Bleyl, D.W.R. & Lewerenz, H.J. (1980) Dominant lethal test in mice with repeated oral applications of cadmium chloride (Ger.). *Arch. exp. vet. Med.*, **34**, 399–404

Bomhard, E., Vogel, O. & Löser, E. (1987) Chronic effects of single and multiple oral and subcutaneous cadmium administrations on the testes of Wistar rats. *Cancer Lett.*, **36**, 307–315

Bonatti, S., Cavalieri, Z., Viaggi, S. & Abbondandolo, A. (1992) The analysis of 10 potential spindle poisons for their ability to induce CREST-positive micronuclei in human diploid fibroblasts. *Mutagenesis*, **7**, 111–114

Bonnell, J.A., Kazantzis, G. & King, E. (1959) A follow-up study of men exposed to cadmium oxide fume. *Br. J. ind. Med.*, **16**, 135–147

Borenfreund, E. & Babich, H. (1987) In vitro cytotoxicity of heavy metals, acrylamide, and organotin salts to neural cells and fibroblasts. *Cell Biol. Toxicol.*, **3**, 63–73

Bournias-Vardiabasis, N., Buzin, C. & Flores, J. (1990) Differential expression of heat shock proteins in *Drosophila* embryonic cells following metal ion exposure. *Exp. Cell Res.*, **189**, 177–182

Bowen, H.J.M. (1966) *Trace Elements in Biochemistry*, London, Academic Press

Brown, S.S. (1992) Quantitative analyses of cadmium: quality assured? In: Nordberg, G.F., Herber, R.F.M. & Alessio, L., *Cadmium in the Human Environment: Toxicity and Carcinogenicity* (IARC Scientific Publications No. 118), Lyon, IARC, pp. 73–81

Bruaux, P., Claeys-Thoreau, F., Ducoffre, G., Lafontaine, A., Grech, A. & Vassallo, A. (1983) Exposure to lead and cadmium of the general population of Malta. *Int. Arch. occup. environ. Health*, **53**, 119–125

Bruce, W.R. & Heddle, J.A. (1979) The mutagenic activity of 61 agents as determined by the micronucleus, *Salmonella*, and sperm abnormality assays. *Can. J. Genet. Cytol.*, **21**, 319–334

Buchet, J.P., Lauwerys, R., Roels, H., Bernard, A., Bruaux, P., Claeys, F., Ducoffre, G., De Plaen, P., Staessen, J., Amery, A., Lijnen, P., Thijs, L., Rondia, D., Sartor, F., Saint Remy, A. & Nick, L. (1990) Renal effects of cadmium body burden of the general population. *Lancet*, **336**, 699–702

Budavari, S., ed. (1989) *The Merck Index*, 11th ed., Rahway, NJ, Merck & Co., pp. 245–247

Bui, T.-H., Lindsten, J. & Nordberg, G.F. (1975) Chromosome analysis of lymphocytes from cadmium workers and itai-itai patients. *Environ. Res.*, **9**, 187–195

Cadmium Association/Cadmium Council (1991) *Technical Notes on Cadmium: Cadmium Production, Properties and Uses*, London/Greenwich, CT

Campbell, T.C., Chen, J., Liu, C., Li, J. & Parpia, B. (1990) Nonassociation of aflatoxin with primary liver cancer in a cross-sectional ecological survey in the People's Republic of China. *Cancer Res.*, **50**, 6882–6893

Carmichael, N.G., Backhouse, B.L., Winder, C. & Lewis, P.D. (1982) Teratogenicity, toxicity and perinatal effects of cadmium. *Hum. Toxicol.*, **1**, 159–186

Casto, B.C. (1983) Comparison of the sensitivity of rodent and human cells to chemical carcinogens using viral transformation, DNA damage, and cytotoxicity assays. *Basic Life Sci.*, **24**, 429–449

Casto, B.C., Meyers, J. & DiPaolo, J.A. (1979) Enhancement of viral transformation for evaluation of the carcinogenic or mutagenic potential of inorganic metal salts. *Cancer Res.*, **39**, 193–198

CERAC, Inc. (1991) *Advanced Specialty Inorganics*, Milwaukee, WI, pp. 78–80

Chan, O.Y., Tan, K.T., Kwok, S.F. & Chio, L.F. (1982) Study on workers exposed to cadmium in alkaline storage battery manufacturing and PVC compounding. *Ann. Acad. Med.*, **11**, 122–130

Chao, S.-H., Suzuki, Y., Zysk, J.R. & Cheung, W.Y. (1984) Activation of calmodulin by various metal cations as a function of ionic radius. *Mol. Pharmacol.*, **26**, 75–82

Cherian, M.G., Goyer, R.A. & Valberg, L.S. (1978) Gastrointestinal absorption and organ distribution of oral cadmium chloride and cadmium-metallothionein in mice. *J. Toxicol. environ. Health*, **4**, 861–868

Chibber, R. & Ord, M. (1990) Cadmium-induced multistep transformation of cultured Indian muntjac skin fibroblasts. *Biol. Metals*, **3**, 213–221

Chopikashvili, L.V., Bobyleva, L.A. & Zolotareva, G.N. (1989) Genotoxic effects of heavy metals and their salts in an experiment on *Drosophila* and mammals (Russ.). *Tsitol. Genet.*, **23**, 35–38

Christley, J. & Webster, W.S. (1983) Cadmium uptake and distribution in mouse embryos following maternal exposure during the organogenic period: a scintillation and autoradiographic study. *Teratology*, **27**, 305–312

Christoffersson, J.O. & Mattsson, S. (1983) Polarised x-rays in XRF-analysis for improved in vivo detectability of cadmium in man. *Phys. Med. Biol.*, **28**, 1135–1144

Christoffersen, J., Christoffersen, M.R., Larsen, R., Rostrup, E., Tingsgaard, P., Andersen, O. & Grandjean, P. (1988) Interaction of cadmium ions with calcium hydroxyapatite crystals: a possible mechanism contributing to the pathogenesis of cadmium-induced diseases. *Calcif. Tissue Int.*, **42**, 331–339

Chung, Y.J. & Kim, S.H. (1982) The effects of heavy metal compounds on mutagenicity of *Drosophila melanogaster* (Korean). *J. Korean Res. Inst. Better Living*, **29**, 55–61

Cifone, M.G., Napolitano, T., Festuccia, C., Cantalini, M.G., De Nuntiis, G., Santoni, G., Marinelli, G. & Santoni, A. (1991) Effects of cadmium on cytotoxic functions of human natural killer cells. *Toxicol. in vitro*, **5**, 525–528

Clough, S.R., Welsh, M.J., Payne, A.H., Brown, C.D. & Brabec, M.J. (1990) Primary rat Sertoli and interstitial cells exhibit a different response to cadmium. *Cell Biol. Toxicol.*, **6**, 63–79

Commission of the European Communities (1983) Council Directive of 26 September 1983 on limit values and quality objectives for cadmium discharges (83/513/EEC). *Off. J. Eur. Comm.*, **L291**, 1–8

Commission of the European Communities (1990) Proposal for a Council Directive on the approximation of the laws of the Member States relating to cosmetic products. *Off. J. Eur. Comm.*, **C322**, 29–77

Commission of the European Communities (1991a) Cadmium sulphide. In: Berlin, A., Draper, M.H., Duffus, J.H. & van der Venne, M.T., eds, *The Toxicology of Chemicals*, Series One, *Carcinogenicity. Summary Reviews of the Scientific Evidence*, Vol. III (EUR13765 EN), Luxembourg, pp. 75–81

Commission of the European Communities (1991b) Cadmium sulphate. In: Berlin, A., Draper, M.H., Duffus, J.H. & van der Venne, M.T., eds, *The Toxicology of Chemicals*, Series One, *Carcinogenicity. Summary Reviews of the Scientific Evidence*, Vol. III (EUR13765 EN), Luxembourg, pp. 67–74

Commission of the European Communities (1991c) Thirteenth Commission Directive of 12 March 1991 adapting to technical progress Annexes II, III, IV, V, VI and VII to Council Directive 76/768/EEC on the approximation of the laws of the Member States relating to cosmetic products (91/184/EEC). *Off J. Eur. Commun.*, **L91**, 59–62

Commission of the European Communities (1991d) Council Directive of 18 June 1991 amending for the 10th time Directive 76/769/EEC on the approximation of the laws, regulations and administrative provisions of the Member States relating to restrictions on the marketing and use of certain dangerous substances and preparations (91/338/EEC). *Off J. Eur. Commun.*, **L186**, 59–63

Commission of the European Communities (1991e) Council Directive of 23 December 1991 standardizing and rationalizing reports on the implementation of certain Directives relating to the environment (91/692/EEC). *Off J. Eur. Commun.*, **L377**, 48–54

Coogan, T.P., Bare, R.M. & Waalkes, M.P. (1992) Cadmium-induced DNA strand damage in cultured liver cells: reduction in cadmium genotoxicity following zinc pretreatment. *Toxicol. appl. Pharmacol.*, **113**, 227–233

Cook, W.A., ed. (1987) *Occupational Exposure Limits—Worldwide*, Akron, OH, American Industrial Hygiene Association, pp. 118, 131, 168

Costa, M., Heck, J.D. & Robison, S.H. (1982) Selective phagocytosis of crystalline metal sulfide particles and DNA strand breaks as a mechanism for the induction of cellular transformation. *Cancer Res.*, **42**, 2757–2763

Crebelli, R., Conti, G., Conti, L. & Carere, A. (1991) In vitro studies with nine known or suspected spindle poisons: results in tests for chromosome malsegregation in *Aspergillus nidulans*. *Mutagenesis*, **6**, 131–136

Danielsson, B.R.G. & Dencker, L. (1984) Effects of cadmium on the placental uptake and transport to the fetus of nutrients. *Biol. Res. Pregn.*, **5**, 93–101

Daston, G.P. (1981a) Toxicity of minimal amounts of cadmium to the developing rat lung and pulmonary surfactant. *Toxicol. Lett.*, **9**, 125–130

Daston, G.P. (1981b) Effects of cadmium on the prenatal ultrastructural maturation of rat alveolar epithelium. *Teratology*, **23**, 75–84

Daston, G.P. (1982) Fetal zinc deficiency as a mechanism for cadmium induced toxicity to the developing rat lung and pulmonary surfactant. *Toxicology*, **24**, 55–63

Daston, G.P. & Grabowski, C.T. (1979) Toxic effects of cadmium on the developing rat lung. I. Altered pulmonary surfactant and the induction of respiratory distress syndrome. *J. Toxicol. environ. Health*, **5**, 973–983

Davison, A.G., Newman Taylor, A.J., Darbyshire, J., Chettle, D.R., Guthrie, C.J.G., O'Malley, D., Mason, H.J., Fayers, P.M., Venables, K.M., Pickering, C.A.C., Franklin, D., Scott, M.C., Holden, H. & Wright, A.L. (1988) Cadmium fume inhalation and emphysema. *Lancet*, **i**, 663–667

De, S.K., Dey, S.K. & Andrews, G.K. (1990) Cadmium teratogenicity and its relationship with metallothionein gene expression in midgestation mouse embryos. *Toxicology*, **64**, 89–104

Deaven, L.L. & Campbell, E.W. (1980) Factors affecting the induction of chromosomal aberrations by cadmium in Chinese hamster cells. *Cytogenet. Cell Genet.*, **26**, 251–260

De Flora, S., Zanacchi, P., Camoirano, A., Bennicelli, C. & Badolati, G.S. (1984a) Genotoxic activity and potency of 135 compounds in the Ames reversion test and in a bacterial DNA-repair test. *Mutat. Res.*, **133**, 161–198

De Flora, S., Camoirano, A., Zanacchi, P. & Bennicelli, C. (1984b) Mutagenicity testing with TA97 and TA102 of 30 DNA-damaging compounds, negative with other *Salmonella* strains. *Mutat. Res.*, **134**, 159–165

Degraeve, N. (1981) Carcinogenic, teratogenic and mutagenic effects of cadmium. *Mutat. Res.*, **86**, 115–135

Deknudt, G. & Deminatti, M. (1978) Chromosome studies in human lymphocytes after in vitro exposure to metal salts. *Toxicology*, **10**, 67–75

Deknudt, G. & Gerber, G.B. (1979) Chromosomal aberrations in bone-marrow cells of mice given a normal or a calcium-deficient diet supplemented with various heavy metals. *Mutat. Res.*, **68**, 163–168

Deknudt, G. & Léonard, A. (1975) Cytogenetic investigations on leucocytes of workers from a cadmium plant. *Environ. Physiol. Biochem.*, **5**, 319–327

De Marco, A., Paglialunga, S., Rizzoni, M., Testa, A. & Trinca, S. (1988) Induction of micronuclei in *Vicia faba* root tips treated with heavy metals (cadmium and chromium) in the presence of NTA. *Mutat. Res.*, **206**, 311–315

Dencker, L. (1975) Possible mechanisms of cadmium fetotoxicity in golden hamsters and mice: uptake by the embryo, placenta and ovary. *J. Reprod. Fertil.*, **44**, 461–471

De Silva, P.E. & Donnan, M.B. (1981) Chronic cadmium poisoning in a pigment manufacturing plant. *Br. J. ind. Med.*, **38**, 76–86

Deutsche Forschungsgemeinschaft (1992) *MAK- and BAT-Values 1992. Maximum Concentrations at the Workplace and Biological Tolerance Values for Working Materials* (Report No. 28), Weinheim, VCH Verlagsgesellschaft, p. 24

D.F. Goldsmith Chemical & Metal Corp. (undated) *High Purity Elements; Fine Inorganic Chemicals; Precious Metals; Mercury*, Evanston, IL, p. 7

Ding, G.Y., Sun, G.F., Fen, Z.L., Li, L.-X. & Li, C.Y. (1987) Epidemiologic research of cancer in exposed cadmium, lead, and arsenic workers (Chin.). *J. Chin. med. Univ.*, **16**, 368–371

DiPaolo, J.A. & Casto, B.C. (1979) Quantitative studies of in vitro morphological transformation of Syrian hamster cells by inorganic metal salts. *Cancer Res.*, **39**, 1008–1013

Doll, R. (1992) Is cadmium a human carcinogen? *Ann. Epidemiol.*, **2**, 336–337

Dudley, R.E., Svoboda, D.J. & Klaassen, C.D. (1982) Acute exposure to cadmium causes severe liver injury in rats. *Toxicol. appl. Pharmacol.*, **65**, 302–313

Dziekanowska, D. (1981) Studies on mutagenic effect of environmental factors in heavy metal plants (Pol.). *Pat. Pol.*, **32**, 263–268

Elinder, C.-G. (1992) Cadmium as an environmental hazard. In: Nordberg, G.F., Herber, R.F.M. & Alessio, L., eds, *Cadmium in the Human Environment: Toxicity and Carcinogenicity* (IARC Scientific Publications No. 118), Lyon, IARC, pp. 123–132

Elinder, C.-G., Kjellström, T., Friberg, L., Lind, B. & Linnman, L. (1976) Cadmium in kidney cortex, liver, and pancreas from Swedish autopsies. Estimation of biological half time in kidney cortex, considering calorie intake and smoking habits. *Arch. environ. Health*, **31**, 292–302

Elinder, C.-G., Friberg, L., Lind, B. & Jawaid, M. (1983) Lead and cadmium levels in blood samples from the general population of Sweden. *Environ. Res.*, 30, 233-253

Elinder, C.-G., Kjellström, T., Hogstedt, C., Andersson, K. & Spång, G. (1985) Cancer mortality of cadmium workers. *Br. J. ind. Med.*, 42, 651-655

Eller, P.M., ed. (1984a) Method 7300. In: *NIOSH Manual of Analytical Methods*, Vol. 1, 3rd Ed. (DHHS (NIOSH) Publ. No. 84-100), Washington DC, US Government Printing Office, pp. 7300-1–7300-5

Eller, P.M., ed. (1984b) Method 8310. In: *NIOSH Manual of Analytical Methods*, Vol. 2, 3rd Ed. (DHHS (NIOSH) Publ. No. 84-100), Washington DC, US Government Printing Office, pp. 8310-1–8310-6

Eller, P.M., ed. (1987) Method 7048. In: *NIOSH Manual of Analytical Methods*, Suppl. 2, 3rd Ed. (DHHS (NIOSH) Publ. No. 84-100), Washington DC, US Government Printing Office, pp. 7048-1–7048-3

Ellis, K.J., Morgan, W.D., Zanzi, I., Yasumura, S., Vartsky, D. & Cohn, S.H. (1981) Critical concentrations of cadmium in human renal cortex: dose-effect studies in cadmium smelter workers. *J. Toxicol. environ. Health*, 7, 691-703

Ellis, K.J., Cohn, S.H. & Smith, T.J. (1985) Cadmium inhalation exposure estimates: their significance with respect to kidney and liver cadmium burden. *J. Toxicol. environ. Health*, 15, 173-187

Epstein, S.S., Arnold, E., Andrea, J., Bass, W. & Bishop, Y. (1972) Detection of chemical mutagens by the dominant lethal assay in the mouse. *Toxicol. appl. Pharmacol.*, 23, 288-325

Fairbridge, R.W. (1974) *The Encyclopedia of Geochemistry and Environmental Sciences*, Vol. IVA, *Encyclopedia of Earth Science Series*, New York, Van Nostrand Reinhold, pp. 99-100

FAO/WHO (1989) *Evaluation of Certain Food Additives and Contaminants. 33rd Report of the Joint FAO/WHO Expert Committee on Food Additives* (Technical Report Series 776), Geneva, pp. 28-31

Favino, A., Cavalleri, A., Nazari, G. & Tilli, M. (1968) Testosterone excretion in cadmium chloride induced testicular tumours in rats. *Med. Lav.*, 59, 36-40

Feuston, M.H. & Scott, W.J., Jr (1985) Cadmium-induced forelimb ectrodactyly: a proposed mechanism of teratogenesis. *Teratology*, 32, 407-419

Flanagan, P.R., McLellan, J.S., Haist, J., Cherian, M.G., Chamberlain, M.J. & Valberg, L.S. (1978) Increased dietary cadmium absorption in mice and human subjects with iron deficiency. *Gastroenterology*, 74, 841-846

Fleig, I., Rieth, H., Stocker, W.G. & Thiess, A.M. (1983) Chromosome investigations of workers exposed to cadmium in the manufacturing of cadmium stabilizers and pigments. *Ecotoxicol. environ. Saf.*, 7, 106-110

Forni, A., Toffoletto, F., Ortisi, E. & Alessio, L. (1990) Occupational exposure to cadmium: cytogenetic findings in relation to exposure levels. In: Seemayer, N.H. & Hadnagy, W., eds, *Environmental Hygiene II*, Berlin, Springer-Verlag, pp. 161-164

Förstner, U. (1984) Cadmium. In: Hutzingter, O., ed., *The Handbook of Environmental Chemistry*, Vol. 3, Part A, *Anthropogenic Compounds*, New York, Springer-Verlag, pp. 59-107

Friberg, L., Piscator, M. & Nordberg, G. (1971) *Cadmium in the Environment*, Cleveland, OH, CRC Press, pp. 19-26

Friberg, L., Piscator, M., Nordberg, G. & Kjellström, T., eds (1974) *Cadmium in the Environment*, 2nd Ed., Cleveland, OH, CRC Press

Friberg, L., Elinder, C.G., Kjellström, T. & Nordberg, G.F., eds (1985) *Cadmium and Health: A Toxicological and Epidemiological Appraisal*, Vol. I, *Exposure, Dose and Metabolism*, Cleveland, OH, CRC Press

Friberg, L., Kjellström, T. & Nordberg, G.F. (1986a) Cadmium. In: Friberg, L., Nordberg, G.F. & Vouk, V., eds, *Handbook on the Toxicology of Metals*, Vol. II, *Specific Metals*, 2nd Ed., Amsterdam, Elsevier, pp.130–184

Friberg, L., Elinder, C.-G., Kjellström, T. & Nordberg, G.F. (1986b) *Cadmium and Health: A Toxicological and Epidemiological Appraisal*, Vol. II, *Effects and Response*, Boca Raton, FL, CRC Press

Friedman, M.A. & Staub, J. (1976) Inhibition of mouse testicular DNA synthesis by mutagens and carcinogens as a potential simple mammalian assay for mutagenesis. *Mutat. Res.*, 37, 67–76

Fukunaga, M., Kurachi, Y. & Mizuguchi, Y. (1982) Action of some metal ions on yeast chromosomes. *Chem. pharm. Bull.*, 30, 3017–3019

Gale, T.F. (1979) Toxic effects of cadmium and amaranth on the developing hamster embryo. *Bull. environ. Contam. Toxicol.*, 22, 175–181

Gasiorek, K. & Bauchinger, M. (1981) Chromosome changes in human lymphocytes after separate and combined treatment with divalent salts of lead, cadmium, and zinc. *Environ. Mutag.*, 3, 513–518

Gerhardsson, L., Brune, D., Nordberg, G.F. & Wester, P.O. (1986) Distribution of cadmium, lead and zinc in lung, liver and kidney in long-term exposed smelter workers. *Sci. total Environ.*, 50, 65–85

Ghess, M.-J., Wilbourn, J.D. & Vainio, H. (1992) *Directory of Agents Being Tested for Carcinogenicity* (No. 15), Lyon, IARC, p. 172

Ghezzi, I., Toffoletto, F., Sesana, G., Fagioli, M.G., Micheli, A., Di Silvestro, P., Zocchetti, C. & Alessio, L. (1985) Behaviour of biological indicators of cadmium in relation to occupational exposure. *Int. Arch. occup. environ. Health*, 55, 133–140

Gilliavod, N. & Léonard, A. (1975) Mutagenicity tests with cadmium in the mouse. *Toxicology*, 5, 43–47

Glaser, U., Klöppel, H. & Hochrainer, D. (1986) Bioavailability indicators of inhaled cadmium compounds. *Ecotoxicol. environ. Saf.*, 11, 261–271

Glaser, U., Hochrainer, D., Otto, F.J. & Oldiges, H. (1990) Carcinogenicity and toxicity of four cadmium compounds inhaled by rats. *Toxicol. environ. Chem.*, 27, 153–162

Glaser, U., Oldiges, H., Stoeppler, M. & Oberdörster, G. (1992) Cadmium solubility in suspension during long-term generation of CdS aerosols. In: Merian, E. & Haerdi, W., eds, *Metal Compounds in Environment and Life*, 4, Northwood/Wilmington, DE, Science and Technology Letters/Science Reviews, pp. 237–241

Greene, G.U. (1974) Cadmium compounds. In: Kirk, R.E. & Othmer, D.F., eds, *Encyclopedia of Chemical Technology*, 2nd Ed., Vol. 3, New York, John Wiley & Sons, pp. 899–911

Gunn, S.A., Gould, T.C. & Anderson, W.A.D. (1961) Zinc protection against cadmium injury to rat testis. *Arch. Pathol.*, 71, 274–281

Gunn, S.A., Gould, T.C. & Anderson, W.A.D. (1963) Cadmium-induced interstitial-cell tumors in rats and mice and their prevention by zinc. *J. natl Cancer Inst.*, 31, 745–759

Gunn, S.A., Gould, T.C. & Anderson, W.A.D. (1964) Effect of zinc on cancerogenesis by cadmium. *Proc. Soc. exp. Biol. Med.*, 115, 653–657

Gunn, S.A., Gould, T.C. & Anderson, W.A.D. (1965) Comparative study of interstitial cell tumors of rat testis induced by cadmium injection and vascular ligation. *J. natl Cancer Inst.*, 35, 329–337

Gunn, S.A., Gould, T.C. & Anderson, W.A.D. (1967) Specific response of mesenchymal tissue to cancerogenesis by cadmium. *Arch. Pathol.*, 83, 493–499

Haddow, A., Dukes, C.E. & Mitchley, B.C.V. (1961) Carcinogenicity of iron preparations and metal–carbohydrate complexes. *Ann. Rep. Br. Emp. Cancer Campaign*, 39, 74–76

Haddow, A., Roe, F.J.C., Dukes, C.E. & Mitchley, B.C.V. (1964) Cadmium neoplasia: sarcomata at the site of injection of cadmium sulphate in rats and mice. *Br. J. Cancer*, **18**, 667–673

Hamilton-Koch, W., Snyder, R.D. & Lavelle, J.M. (1986) Metal-induced DNA damage and repair in human diploid fibroblasts and Chinese hamster ovary cells. *Chem.-biol. Interactions*, **59**, 17–28

Han, C., Wu, G., Yin, Y. & Shen, M. (1992) Inhibition by germanium oxide of the mutagenicity of cadmium chloride in various genotoxicity assays. *Food chem. Toxicol.*, **30**, 521–524

Hansen, K. & Stern, R.M. (1984) A survey of metal-induced mutagenicity *in vitro* and *in vivo*. *J. Am. Coll. Toxicol.*, **3**, 381–430

Harrison, P.T.C. & Heath, J.C. (1986) Apparent synergy in lung carcinogenesis: interactions between *N*-nitrosoheptamethyleneimine, particulate cadmium and crocidolite asbestos fibres in rats. *Carcinogenesis*, **7**, 1903–1908

Hartwig, A. & Beyersmann, D. (1989) Comutagenicity and inhibition of DNA repair by metal ions in mammalian cells. *Biol. Trace Elem. Res.*, **21**, 359–365

Hassler, E., Lind, B. & Piscator, M. (1983) Cadmium in blood and urine related to present and past exposure. A study of workers in an alkaline battery factory. *Br. J. ind. Med.*, **40**, 420–425

Health and Safety Executive (1992) *EH40/92. Occupational Exposure Limits 1992*, London, Her Majesty's Stationary Office, p. 11

Heath, J.C. & Daniel, M.R. (1964) The production of malignant tumours by cadmium in the rat. *Br. J. Cancer*, **18**, 124–129

Heath, J.C., Daniel, M.R., Dingle, J.T. & Webb, M. (1962) Cadmium as a carcinogen. *Nature*, **193**, 592–593

Heinrich, U. (1992) Pulmonary carcinogenicity of cadmium by inhalation in animals. In: Nordberg, G.F., Herber, R.F.M. & Alessio, L., eds, *Cadmium in the Human Environment: Toxicity and Carcinogenicity* (IARC Scientific Publications No. 118), Lyon, IARC, pp. 405–413

Heinrich, U., Peters, L., Ernst, H., Rittinghausen, S., Dasenbrock, C. & König, H. (1989) Investigation of the carcinogenic effects of various cadmium compounds after inhalation exposure in hamsters and mice. *Exp. Pathol.*, **37**, 253–258

Hellman, B. (1986) Evidence for stimulatory and inhibitory effects of cadmium on the [^{3}H]-thymidine incorporation into various organs of the mouse. *Toxicology*, **40**, 13–23

Herber, R.F.M., Stoeppler, M. & Tonks, D.B. (1990a) Cooperative interlaboratory surveys of the determination of cadmium in whole blood. *Fresenius' J. anal. Chem.*, **338**, 269–278

Herber, R.F.M., Stoeppler, M. & Tonks, D.B. (1990b) Cooperative interlaboratory surveys of cadmium analysis in urine. *Fresenius' J. anal. Chem.*, **338**, 279–286

Hoffmann, L., Putzke, H.-P., Simonn, C., Gase, P., Russbült, R., Kampehl, H.-J., Serfling, D., Erdmann, T. & Huckstorf, C. (1985a) Does cadmium play a role in the aetiology and pathogenesis of prostate carcinoma? (Ger.) *Z. ges. Hyg.*, **31**, 224–227

Hoffmann, L., Putzke, H.-P., Kampehl, H.-J., Russbült, R., Gase, P., Simonn, C., Erdmann, T. & Huckstorf, C. (1985b) Carcinogenic effects of cadmium on the prostate of the rat. *J. Cancer Res. clin. Oncol.*, **109**, 193–199

Hoffmann, L., Putzke, H.-P., Bendel, L., Erdmann, T. & Huckstorf, C. (1988) Electron microscopic results on the ventral prostate of the rat after $CdCl_2$ administration. A contribution towards etiology of the cancer of the prostate. *J. Cancer Res. clin. Oncol.*, **114**, 273–278

Holden, H. (1980a) Further mortality studies on workers exposed to cadmium fume. In: *Proceedings of the Seminar on Occupational Exposure to Cadmium, London, 20 March 1980*, London, Cadmium Association, pp. 23–24

Holden, H. (1980b) A mortality study of workers exposed to cadmium fumes. In: *Edited Proceedings of the Second International Cadmium Conference, Cannes, 6–8 February 1979*, London, Metal Bulletin Ltd, p. 211–215

Holden, H.A. (1982) Manufacture of cadmium–copper alloy. In: Wilson, D. & Volpe, R.A., eds, *Edited Proceedings of the Third International Cadmium Conference, Miami, FL, 3–5 February 1981*, London/New York, Cadmium Association/Cadmium Council, pp. 49–50

Hollander, M.L. & Carapella, S.C., Jr (1978) Cadmium and cadmium alloys. In: Mark, H.F., Othmer, D.F., Overberger, C.G., Seaborg, G.T. & Grayson, N., eds, *Kirk–Othmer Encyclopedia of Chemical Technology*, 3rd Ed., Vol. 4, New York, John Wiley & Sons, pp. 387–396

Holt, D. & Webb, M. (1987) Teratogenicity of ionic cadmium in the Wistar rat. *Arch. Toxicol.*, **59**, 443–447

Howard, W., Leonard, B., Moody, W. & Kochhar, T.S. (1991) Induction of chromosome changes by metal compounds in cultured CHO cells. *Toxicol. Lett.*, **56**, 179–186

Hubermont, G., Buchet, J.P., Roels, H. & Lauwerys, R. (1978) Placental transfer of lead, mercury and cadmium in women living in a rural area. Importance of drinking water in lead exposure. *Int. Arch. occup. environ. Health*, **41**, 117–124

IARC (1973) *IARC Monographs on the Evaluation of Carcinogenic Risk of Chemicals to Man*, Vol. 2, *Some Inorganic and Organometallic Compounds*, Lyon, pp. 74–99

IARC (1976) *IARC Monographs on the Evaluation of Carcinogenic Risk of Chemicals to Man*, Vol. 11, *Cadmium, Nickel, Some Epoxides, Miscellaneous Industrial Chemicals and General Considerations on Volatile Anaesthetics*, Lyon, pp. 39–74

IARC (1986a) *IARC Monographs on the Evaluation of the Carcinogenic Risk of Chemicals to Humans*, Vol. 38, *Tobacco Smoking*, Lyon

IARC (1986b) *IARC Monographs on the Evaluation of the Carcinogenic Risk of Chemicals to Humans*, Vol. 40, *Some Naturally Occurring and Synthetic Food Components, Furocoumarins and Ultraviolet Radiation*, Lyon, pp. 161–206

IARC (1987a) *IARC Monographs on the Evaluation of Carcinogenic Risks to Humans*, Suppl. 7, *Overall Evaluations of Carcinogenicity: An Updating of* IARC Monographs *Volumes 1 to 42*, Lyon, pp. 139–142

IARC (1987b) *IARC Monographs on the Evaluation of Carcinogenic Risks to Humans*, Suppl. 7, *Overall Evaluations of Carcinogenicity: An Updating of* IARC Monographs *Volumes 1 to 42*, Lyon, pp. 230–232

IARC (1987c) *IARC Monographs on the Evaluation of Carcinogenic Risks to Humans*, Suppl. 6, *Genetic and Related Effects: An Updating of Selected IARC Monographs from Volumes 1 to 42*, Lyon, pp. 100–106

IARC (1987d) *IARC Monographs on the Evaluation of Carcinogenic Risks to Humans*, Suppl. 6, *Genetic and Related Effects: An Updating of Selected IARC Monographs from Volumes 1 to 42*, Lyon, pp. 252–254

IARC (1989) *IARC Monographs on the Evaluation of Carcinogenic Risks to Humans*, Vol. 47, *Some Organic Solvents, Resin Monomers and Related Compounds, Pigments and Occupational Exposures in Paint Manufacture and Painting*, Lyon, pp. 329–442

IARC (1990a) *IARC Monographs on the Evaluation of Carcinogenic Risks to Humans*, Vol. 49, *Chromium, Nickel and Welding*, Lyon, pp. 257–445

IARC (1990b) *IARC Monographs on the Evaluation of Carcinogenic Risks to Humans*, Vol. 49, *Chromium, Nickel and Welding*, Lyon, pp. 447–525

IARC (1990c) *IARC Monographs on the Evaluation of Carcinogenic Risks to Humans*, Vol. 49, *Chromium, Nickel and Welding*, Lyon, pp. 49–256

IARC (1992) *IARC Monographs on the Evaluation of Carcinogenic Risks to Humans*, Vol. 54, *Occupational Exposures to Mists and Vapours from Strong Inorganic Acids; and Other Industrial Chemicals*, Lyon, pp. 189–211

Impens, R.A., Delcarte, E. & Fagot, J. (1989) Sources, pathways, and transfer of cadmium in the environment: practical possibilities of controlling its dispersion. In: Hiscock, S.A. & Volpe, R.A., eds, *Edited Proceedings of the Sixth International Cadmium Conference, Paris, 19–21 April 1989*, London/Greenwich, CT, Cadmium Association/Cadmium Council, pp.20–23

Inoue, Y. & Watanabe, T.K. (1978) Toxicity and mutagenicity of cadmium and furylfuramide in *Drosophila melanogaster*. *Jpn. J. Genet.*, **53**, 183–189

International Labour Office (1991) *Occupational Exposure Limits for Airborne Toxic Substances: Values of Selected Countries* (Occupational Safety and Health Series No. 37), 3rd Ed., Geneva, pp. 68–71

Järup, L., Rogenfelt, A., Elinder, C.-G., Nogawa, K. & Kjellström, T. (1983) Biological half-time of cadmium in the blood of workers after cessation of exposure. *Scand. J. Work Environ. Health*, **9**, 327–331

Jin, P. & Ringertz, N.R. (1990) Cadmium induces transcription of proto-oncogenes c-*jun* and c-*myc* in rat L6 myoblasts. *J. biol. Chem.*, **265**, 14061–14064

J.T. Baker (1989) *1989/90 Catalog—Laboratory Reagents and Chromatography Products*, Phillipsburg, NJ, pp. 31–32

Kanematsu, N., Hara, M. & Kada, T. (1980) *rec* Assay and mutagenicity studies on metal compounds. *Mutat. Res.*, **77**, 109–116

Kanematsu, N., Nakamine, H., Fukuta, Y., Yasuda, J.-I., Kurenuma, S. & Shibata, K.-I. (1990) Mutagenicity of cadmium, platinum and rhodium compounds in cultured mammalian cells. *J. Gifu dent. Soc.*, **17**, 575–582

Kanisawa, M. & Schroeder, H.A. (1969) Life term studies on the effect of trace elements on spontaneous tumors in mice and rats. *Cancer Res.*, **29**, 892–895

Kasuya, M., Teranishi, H., Kubota, M., Katoh, T., Aoshima, K., Saijo, Y., Iwata, K. & Kanai, M. (1986) Low molecular weight protein in blood and urine of itai-itai disease patients and their family members (Jpn). *Kankyo Hoken Rep.*, **52**, 176–180

Kasuya, M., Aoshima, K., Katoh, T., Teranishi, H., Horiguchi, H., Kitagawa, M. & Hagino, S. (1992) Natural history of itai-itai disease: a long-term observation on the clinical and laboratory findings in patients with itai-itai disease. In: Cook, M.E., Hiscock, S.A., Morrow, H. & Volpe, R.A., eds, *Edited Proceedings of the Seventh International Cadmium Conference, New Orleans, LA, 6–8 April 1992*, London/Reston, VA, Cadmium Association/Cadmium Council, pp. 180–192

Kawada, T., Koyama, H. & Suzuki, S. (1989) Cadmium, NAG activity and β_2-microglobulin in the urine of cadmium pigment workers. *Br. J. ind. Med.*, **46**, 52–55

Kawada, T., Shinmyo, R.R. & Suzuki, S. (1992) Urinary cadmium and *N*-acetyl-β-D-glucosaminidase excretion of inhabitants living in a cadmium-polluted area. *Int. Arch. occup. environ. Health*, **63**, 541–546

Kazantzis, G. (1963) Induction of sarcoma in the rat by cadmium sulphide pigment. *Nature*, **198**, 1213–1214

Kazantzis, G. (1987) Cadmium. In: Fishbein, L., Furst, A. & Mehlman, M.A., eds, *Advances in Modern Environmental Toxicology*, Vol. 11, *Genotoxic and Carcinogenic Metals: Environmental and Occupational Occurrence and Exposure*, Princeton, NJ, Princeton Scientific Publishing, pp. 127–143

Kazantzis, G. & Armstrong, B.G. (1983) A mortality study of cadmium workers from seventeen plants in England. In: Wilson, D. & Volpe, R.A., eds, *Edited Proceedings of the Fourth International Cadmium Conference, Munich, 2–4 March 1983*, London/New York, Cadmium Association/Cadmium Council, pp. 139–142

Kazantzis, G. & Blanks, R.G. (1992) A mortality study of cadmium exposed workers. In: Cook, M.E., Hiscock, S.A., Morrow, H. & Volpe, R.A., eds, *Edited Proceedings of the Seventh International Cadmium Conference, New Orleans, LA, 6-8 April 1992*, London/Reston, VA, Cadmium Association/Cadmium Council, pp. 150–157

Kazantzis, G. & Hanbury, W.J. (1966) The induction of sarcoma in the rat by cadmium sulphide and by cadmium oxide. *Br. J. Cancer*, **20**, 190–199

Kazantzis, G., Lam, T.-H. & Sullivan, K.R. (1988) Mortality of cadmium-exposed workers. A five-year update. *Scand. J. Work Environ. Health*, **14**, 220–223

Kazantzis, G., Blanks, R. & Teather, S. (1989) The mortality of cadmium exposed workers. In: Vernet, J.-P., ed., *Proceedings of the International Conference on Heavy Metals in the Environment, Geneva, September 1989*, Vol. 1, Edinburgh, CEP Consultants Ltd, pp. 304–307

Kazantzis, G., Blanks, R.G. & Sullivan, K.R. (1992) Is cadmium a human carcinogen? In: Nordberg, G.F., Herber, R.F.M. & Alessio, L., eds, *Cadmium in the Human Environment: Toxicity and Carcinogenicity* (IARC Scientific Publications No. 118), Lyon, IARC, pp. 435–446

Kershaw, W.C. & Klaassen, C.D. (1991) Cadmium-induced elevation of hepatic isometallothionein concentrations in inbred strains of mice. *Chem.-biol. Interactions*, **78**, 269–282

Keyse, S.M. & Tyrrell, R.M. (1989) Heme oxygenase is the major 32-kDa stress protein induced in human skin fibroblasts by UVA radiation, hydrogen peroxide, and sodium arsenite. *Proc. natl Acad. Sci USA*, **86**, 99–103

Kido, T., Honda, R., Tsuritani, I., Yamaya, H., Ishizaki, M., Yamada, Y. & Nogawa, K. (1988) Progress of renal dysfunction in inhabitants environmentally exposed to cadmium. *Arch. environ. Health*, **43**, 213–217

Kimura, M., Nomura, T., Tanioka, Y., Tanimoto, Y., Suda, T., Yashiki, S., Tazaki, H., Tata, R., Deguchi, N., Kotako, N. & Salgusa, J. (1988) Effects of nutritional factors in monkeys given cadmium: an overall view (Jpn). *Kankyo Hoken Rep.*, **54**, 116–122

King, E. (1955) An environmental study of casting copper–cadmium alloys. *Br. J. ind. Med.*, **12**, 198–205

Kipling, M.D. & Waterhouse, J.A.H. (1967) Cadmium and prostatic carcinoma (Letter to the Editor). *Lancet*, **i**, 730–731

Kjellström, T. & Nordberg, G.F. (1978) A kinetic model of cadmium metabolism in the human being. *Environ. Res.*, **16**, 248–269

Kjellström, T., Evrin, P.-E. & Rahnster, B. (1977) Dose–response analysis of cadmium-induced tubular proteinuria. A study of urinary β_2-microglobulin excretion among workers in a battery factory. *Environ. Res.*, **13**, 303–317

Kjellström, T., Friberg, L. & Rahnster, B. (1979) Mortality and cancer morbidity among cadmium-exposed workers. *Environ. Health Perspectives*, **28**, 199–204

Kleinman, M.T., Rhodes, J.R., Guinn, V.P. & Thompson, R.J. (1989a) General atomic absorption procedure for trace metals in airborne material collected on filters. In: Lodge, J.P., Jr, ed., *Methods of Air Sampling and Analysis*, 3rd Ed., Chelsea, MI, Lewis Publishers, pp. 608–618

Kleinman, M.T., Courtney, W.J., Guinn, V.P., Rains, T.C., Rhodes, J.R. & Thompson, R.J. (1989b) General method for preparation of tissue samples for analysis for trace metals. In: Lodge, J.P., Jr, ed., *Methods of Air Sampling and Analysis*, 3rd Ed., Chelsea, MI, Lewis Publishers, pp. 619–622

Knorre, D. (1970a) Induction of skin sarcomas in albino rats by cadmium chloride (Ger.). *Arch. Geschwulstforsch.*, **36**, 119–126

Knorre, D. (1970b) Local skin damage in albino rats during the latent period of sarcoma formation after cadmium chloride injection (Ger.). *Zbl. allgemein. Pathol.*, **113**, 192–197

Knorre, D. (1971) Induction of interstitial tumours of the testis in albino rats by cadmium chloride (Ger.). *Arch. Geschwulstforsch.*, **38**, 257–263

Kogan, I.G., Grozdova, T.Y. & Kholikova, T.A. (1978) Mutagenic action of cadmium chloride on the germ cells of *Drosophila melanogaster*. *Sov. Genet.*, **14**, 1484–1488

Koizumi, T., Li, Z.G. & Tatsumoto, H. (1992) DNA Damaging activity of cadmium in Leydig cells, a target cell population for cadmium carcinogenesis in the rat testis. *Toxicol. Lett.*, **63**, 211–220

Kojima, S., Furukawa, A., Kiyozumi, M. & Shimada, H. (1991) Comparative renal toxicity of metallothineins with different cadmium/zinc ratios in rats. *Toxicol. Lett.*, **56**, 197–205

Kollmeier, H., Seemann, J., Wittig, P., Rothe, G. & Müller, K.-M. (1990) Cadmium in human lung tissue. *Int. Arch. occup. environ. Health*, **62**, 373–377

König, H.P., Heinrich, U., Koch, H. & Peters, L. (1992) Effect of photocorrosion on cadmium sulfide suspensions applied in animal inhalation studies with CdS particles. *Arch. environ. Contam. Toxicol.*, **22**, 30–35

Konishi, N., Ward, J.M. & Waalkes, M.P. (1990) Pancreatic hepatocytes in Fischer and Wistar rats induced by repeated injections of cadmium chloride. *Toxicol. appl. Pharmacol.*, **104**, 149–156

Kowal, N.E., Johnson, D.E., Kraemer, D.F. & Pahren, H.R. (1979) Normal levels of cadmium in diet, urine, blood, and tissues of inhabitants of the United States. *J. Toxicol. environ. Health*, **5**, 995–1014

Kozachenko, V.I., Pashin, Y. V., Soboleva, L.S. & Salnikova, L.E. (1987) Study of the mutagenic effect of cadmium chloride on mammals (Russ.). *Biol. Nauk.*, **11**, 102–105

Kuhnert, P.M., Kuhnert, B.R., Bottoms, S.F. & Erhard, P. (1982) Cadmium levels in maternal blood, fetal cord blood, and placental tissues of pregnant women who smoke. *Am. J. Obstet. Gynecol.*, **142**, 1021–1029

Kuhnert, B.R., Kuhnert, P.M., Debanne, S. & Williams, T.G. (1987) The relationship between cadmium, zinc, and birth weight in pregnant women who smoke. *Am. J. Obstet. Gynecol.*, **157**, 1247–1251

Kurokawa, Y., Matsushima, M., Imazawa, T., Takamura, N., Takahashi, M. & Hayashi, Y. (1985) Promoting effect of metal compounds on rat renal tumorigenesis. *J. Am. Coll. Toxicol.*, **4**, 321–330

Kurokawa, Y., Takahashi, M., Maekawa, A. & Hayashi, Y. (1989) Promoting effect of metal compounds on liver, stomach, kidney, pancreas, and skin carcinogenesis. *J. Am. Coll. Toxicol.*, **8**, 1235–1239

Lakkad, B.C., Nigam, S.K., Karnik, A.B., Thakore, K.N. & Chatterjee, B.B. (1986) Effect of cadmium chloride on cell division and chromosomes in Chinese hamster ovary cells. *Bull. environ. Contam. Toxicol.*, **36**, 342–349

Lamm, S.H., Parkinson, M., Anderson, M. & Taylor, W. (1992) Determinants of lung cancer risk among cadmium-exposed workers. *Ann. Epidemiol.*, **2**, 195–211

Laskey, J.W. & Phelps, P.V. (1991) Effect of cadmium and other metal cations on in vitro Leydig cell testosterone production. *Toxicol. appl. Pharmacol.*, **108**, 296–306

Laskey, J.W., Rehnberg, G.L., Favor, M.J., Cahill, D.F. & Pietrzak-Flis, Z. (1980) Chronic ingestion of cadmium and/or tritium. II. Effects on growth, development, and reproductive function. *Environ. Res.*, **22**, 466–475

Laskey, J.W., Rehnberg, G.L., Laws, S.C. & Hein, J.F. (1984) Reproductive effects of low acute doses of cadmium chloride in adult male rats. *Toxicol. appl. Pharmacol.*, **73**, 250–255

Laskey, J.W., Rehnberg, G.L., Laws, S.C. & Hein, J.F. (1986) Age-related dose response of selected reproductive parameters to acute cadmium chloride exposure in the male Long-Evans rat. *J. Toxicol. environ. Health*, **19**, 393–401

Lauwerys, R.R., Buchet, J.P. & Roels, H. (1976) The relationship between cadmium exposure or body burden and the concentration of cadmium in blood and urine in man. *Int. Arch. occup. environ. Health*, **36**, 275–285

Lauwerys, R., Buchet, J.P., Roels, H., Bernard, A., Chettle, D.R., Harvey, T.C. & Al Haddad, I.K. (1980) Biological significance of cadmium concentration in blood and urine and their application in monitoring workers exposed to cadmium. In: *Edited Proceedings of the Second International Cadmium Conference, Cannes, 6–8 February 1979*, London, Metal Bulletin Ltd, pp. 164–167

Layton, W.M., Jr & Layton, M.W. (1979) Cadmium induced limb defects in mice: strain associated differences in sensitivity. *Teratology*, **19**, 229–236

Lehman, L.D. & Klaassen, C.D. (1986) Dosage-dependent disposition of cadmium administered orally to rats. *Toxicol. appl. Pharmacol.*, **84**, 159–167

Lehotzky, K., Ungváry, G., Polinák, D. & Kiss, A. (1990) Behavioral deficits due to prenatal exposure to cadmium chloride in CFY rat pups. *Neurotoxicol. Teratol.*, **12**, 169–172

Lemen, R.A., Lee, J.S., Wagoner, J.K. & Blejer, H.P. (1976) Cancer mortality among cadmium production workers. *Ann. N.Y. Acad. Sci.*, **271**, 273–279

Léonard, A. (1988) Mechanisms in metal genotoxicity: the significance of in vitro approaches. *Mutat. Res.*, **198**, 321–326

Levin, A.A. & Miller, R.K. (1980) Fetal toxicity of cadmium in the rat: maternal *vs* fetal injections. *Teratology*, **22**, 1–5

Levin, A.A. & Miller, R.K. (1981) Fetal toxicity of cadmium in the rat: decreased utero-placental blood flow. *Toxicol. appl. Pharmacol.*, **58**, 297–203

Levin, A.A., Kilpper, R.W. & Miller, R.K. (1987) Fetal toxicity of cadmium chloride: the pharmacokinetics in the pregnant Wistar rat. *Teratology*, **36**, 163–170

Levy, L.S. & Clack, J. (1975) Further studies on the effect of cadmium on the prostate gland. I. Absence of prostatic changes in rats given oral cadmium sulphate for two years. *Ann. occup. Hyg.*, **17**, 205–211

Levy, L.S., Roe, F.J.C., Malcolm, D., Kazantzis, G., Clack, J. & Platt, H.S. (1973) Absence of prostatic changes in rats exposed to cadmium. *Ann. occup. Hyg.*, **16**, 111–118

Levy, L.S., Clack, J. & Roe, F.J.C. (1975) Further studies on the effect of cadmium on the prostate gland. II. Absence of prostatic changes in mice given oral cadmium sulphate for eighteen months. *Ann. occup. Hyg.*, **17**, 213–220

Lewis, G.P., Jusko, W.J., Coughlin, L.L. & Hartz, S. (1972) Contribution of cigarette smoking to cadmium accumulation in man (Preliminary communication). *Lancet*, **i**, 291–292

Lide, D.R., ed. (1991) *CRC Handbook of Chemistry and Physics*, 72nd Ed., Boca Raton, FL, CRC Press, pp. 4-46–4-47

Lindegaard, P.M., Hansen, S.O., Christensen, J.E.J., Andersen, B.B. & Andersen, O. (1990) The distribution of cadmium within the human prostate. *Biol. Trace Elem. Res.*, **25**, 97–104

Litvinov, N.N., Voronin, V.M. & Kazatchkov, V.I. (1986) Evaluation of carcinogenicity of nitrosodimethylamine used in combination with benzene, cadmium, boron or ethanol (Russ.). *Vopr. Onkol.*, **32**, 80–84

Llewellyn, T.O. (1992) *Annual Review: Cadmium in 1991*, Washington DC, Bureau of Mines, US Department of the Interior

Loiacono, N.J., Graziano, J.H., Kline, J.K., Popovac, D., Ahmedi, X., Gashi, E., Mehmeti, A. & Rajovic, B. (1992) Placental cadmium and birthweight in women living near a lead smelter. *Arch. environ. Health*, **47**, 250–255

Lorke, D. (1978) New studies on cadmium toxicology. In: *Edited Proceedings of the First International Cadmium Conference, San Francisco, 31 January–2 February 1977*, London, Metal Bulletin Ltd, pp. 175–179

Löser, E. (1980a) A 2-year oral carcinogenicity study with cadmium on rats. *Cancer Lett.*, **9**, 191–198

Löser, E. (1980b) Chronic toxicity and multigeneration studies on rats with cadmium. In: *Edited Proceedings of the Second International Cadmium Conference, Cannes, 6–8 February 1979*, London, Metal Bulletin Ltd, pp. 131–134

Louekari, K., Valkonen, S., Pousi, S. & Virtanen, L. (1991) Estimated dietary intake of lead and cadmium and their concentration in blood. *Sci. total Environ.*, **105**, 87–99

Lucas, P.A., Jariwalla, A.G., Jones, J.H., Gough, J. & Vale, P.T. (1980) Fatal cadmium fume inhalation (Letter to the Editor). *Lancet*, **ii**, 205

Lucis, O.J., Lucis, R. & Aterman, K. (1972) Tumorigenesis by cadmium. *Oncology*, **26**, 53–67

Machemer, L. & Lorke, D. (1981) Embryotoxic effect of cadmium on rats upon oral administration. *Toxicol. appl. Pharmacol.*, **58**, 438–443

Magos, L. (1991) Epidemiological and experimental aspects of metal carcinogenesis: physicochemical properties, kinetics, and the active species. *Environ. Health Perspectives*, **95**, 157–189

Mailhes, J.B., Preston, R.J., Yuan, Z.P. & Payne, H.S. (1988) Analysis of mouse metaphase II oocytes as an assay for chemically induced aneuploidy. *Mutat. Res.*, **198**, 145–152

Maitani, T., Waalkes, M.P. & Klaassen, C.D. (1984) Distribution of cadmium after oral administration of cadmium-thionein to mice. *Toxicol. appl. Pharmacol.*, **74**, 237–243

Malcolm, D. (1983) *Batteries, secondary or rechargeable, or accumulator*. In: Parmeggiani, L., ed., *Encyclopaedia of Occupational Health and Safety*, 3rd rev. Ed., Vol. 1, Geneva, International Labour Office, pp. 249–253

Mandel, R. & Ryser, H.J.-P. (1984) Mutagenicity of cadmium in *Salmonella typhimurium* and its synergism with two nitrosamines. *Mutat. Res.*, **138**, 9–16

Marzin, D.R. & Phi, H.V. (1985) Study of the mutagenicity of metal derivatives with *Salmonella typhimurium* TA102. *Mutat. Res.*, **155**, 49–51

McGregor, D.B., Brown, A., Cattanach, P., Edwards, I., McBride, D., Riach, C. & Caspary, W.J. (1988) Responses of the L5178Y tk$^+$/tk$^-$ mouse lymphoma cell forward mutation assay: III. 72 coded chemicals. *Environ. mol. Mutag.*, **12**, 85–154

McLean, J.R., McWilliams, R.S., Kaplan, J.G. & Birnboim, H.C. (1982) Rapid detection of DNA strand breaks in human peripheral blood cells and animal organs following treatment with physical and chemical agents. *Prog. Mutat. Res.*, **3**, 137–141

McLellan, J.S., Flanagan, P.R., Chamberlain, M.J. & Valberg, L.S. (1978) Measurement of dietary cadmium absorption in humans. *J. Toxicol. environ. Health*, **4**, 131–138

Messerle, K. & Webster, W.S. (1982) The classification and development of cadmium-induced limb defects in mice. *Teratology*, **25**, 61–70

Miller, B.M. & Adler, I.-D. (1992) Aneuploidy induction in mouse spermatocytes. *Mutagenesis*, **7**, 69–76

Min, K.-S., Fujita, Y., Onosaka, S. & Tanaka, K. (1991) Role of intestinal metallothionein in absorption and distribution of orally administered cadmium. *Toxicol. appl. Pharmacol.*, **109**, 7–16

Mitra, R.S. & Bernstein, I.A. (1978) Single-strand breakage in DNA of *Escherichia coli* exposed to Cd^{2+}. *J. Bacteriol.*, **133**, 75–80

Morselt, A.F.W., Leene, W., De Groot, C., Kipp, J.B.A., Evers, M., Roelofsen, A.M. & Bosch, K.S. (1988) Differences in immunological susceptibility to cadmium toxicity between two rat strains as demonstrated with cell biological methods. Effect of cadmium on DNA synthesis of thymus lymphocytes. *Toxicology*, **48**, 127–139

Mortelmans, K., Haworth, S., Lawlor, T., Speck, W., Tainer, B. & Zeiger, E. (1986) *Salmonella* mutagenicity tests: II. Results from the testing of 270 chemicals. *Environ. Mutag.*, **8** (Suppl. 7)

Mukherjee, A., Sharma, A. & Talukder, G. (1988a) Effect of selenium on cadmium-induced chromosomal aberrations in bone marrow cells of mice. *Toxicol. Lett.*, **41**, 23–29

Mukherjee, A., Giri, A.K., Sharma, A. & Talukder, G. (1988b) Relative efficacy of short-term tests in detecting genotoxic effects of cadmium chloride in mice *in vivo*. *Mutat. Res.*, **206**, 285–295

Müller, W.-U., Streffer, C. & Joos, A.L. (1990) Toxicity of cadmium sulphate and methylmercuric chloride applied singly or in combination to early mouse embryos *in vitro*. *Toxicol. in vitro*, **4**, 57–61

Müller, T., Schuckelt, R. & Jaenicke, L. (1991) Cadmium/zinc-metallothionein induces DNA strand breaks *in vitro*. *Arch. Toxicol.*, **65**, 20–26

Muntau, H. & Baudo, R. (1992) Sources of cadmium, its distribution and turnover in the freshwater environment. In: Nordberg, G., Herber, R.F.M. & Alessio, L., eds, *Cadmium in the Human Environment: Toxicity and Carcinogenicity* (IARC Scientific Publications No. 118), Lyon, IARC, pp. 133–148

Murdoch, R.N. & Cowen, N.L. (1981) Foetotoxicity of cadmium in Quackenbush strain mice and the effects of the metal on uterine alkaline phosphatase during pseudopregnancy. *Aust. J. biol. Sci.*, **34**, 305–312

Nakagawa, H., Kawano, S., Okumura, Y., Fujita, T. & Nishi, M. (1987) Mortality study of inhabitants in a cadmium-polluted area. *Bull. environ. Contam. Toxicol.*, **38**, 553–560

Nakao, M. (1986) Studies on the effect of manganese and cadmium on carcinogenesis of prostatic cancer in rats (Jpn). *J. Kyoto Prefect. Univ. Med.*, **95**, 1681–1692

Naruse, I. & Hayashi, Y. (1989) Amelioration of the teratogenicity of cadmium by the metallothionein induced by bismuth nitrate. *Teratology*, **40**, 459–465

Nayak, B.N., Ray, M., Persaud, T.V.N. & Nigli, M. (1989) Embryotoxicity and in vivo cytogenetic changes following maternal exposure to cadmium chloride in mice. *Exp. Pathol.*, **36**, 75–80

Nishioka, H. (1975) Mutagenic activities of metal compounds in bacteria. *Mutat. Res.*, **31**, 185–189

Nogawa, K., Tsuritani, I., Yamada, Y., Kido, T., Honda, R., Ishizaki, M. & Kurihara, T. (1986) Sister chromatid exchanges in the lymphocytes of people exposed to environmental cadmium. *Toxicol. Lett.*, **32**, 283–288

Nogawa, K., Tsuritani, I., Kido, T., Honda, R., Ishizaki, M. & Yamada, Y. (1990) Serum vitamin D metabolites in cadmium-exposed persons with renal damage. *Int. Arch. occup. environ. Health*, **62**, 189–193

Nomiyama, K. & Nomiyama, H. (1984) Reversibility of cadmium-induced health effects in rabbits. *Environ. Health Perspectives*, **54**, 201–211

Nomiyama, K., Liu, S.-J. & Nomiyama, H. (1992) Critical levels of blood and urinary cadmium, urinary β_2-microglobulin and retinol-binding protein for monitoring cadmium health effects. In: Nordberg, G.F., Herber, R.F.M. & Alessio, G., eds, *Cadmium in the Human Environment: Toxicity and Carcinogenicity* (IARC Scientification Publications No. 118), Lyon, IARC, pp. 325–340

Nordberg, G.F. (1972) Cadmium metabolism and toxicity. Experimental studies on mice with special reference to the use of biological materials as indices of retention and the possible role of metallothionein in transport and detoxification of cadmium. *Environ. Physiol. Biochem.*, **2**, 7–36

Nordberg, G.F. & Nordberg, M. (1988) Biological monitoring of cadmium. In: Clarkson, T.W., Friberg L., Nordberg, G.F. & Sager, P.R., eds, *Biological Monitoring of Toxic Metals*, New York, Plenum Press, pp. 151–168

Nordberg, G.F., Piscator, M. & Lind, B. (1971) Distribution of cadmium among protein fractions of mouse liver. *Acta pharmacol. toxicol.*, **29**, 456–470

Nordberg, G.F., Goyer, R.A. & Nordberg, M. (1975) Comparative toxicity of cadmium-metallothionein and cadmium chloride on mouse kidney. *Arch. Pathol.*, **99**, 192–197

Nordberg, G.F., Herber, R.F.M. & Alessio, L., eds (1992) *Cadmium in the Human Environment: Toxicity and Carcinogenicity* (IARC Scientific Publications No. 118), Lyon, IARC

Nriagu, J.O. & Pacyna, J.M. (1988) Quantitative assessment of worldwide contamination of air, water and soils by trace metals. *Nature*, **333**, 134–139

Oberdörster, G. (1986) Update on animal carcinogenicity studies with cadmium: extrapolation to humans and future research needs. In: Wilson, D. & Volpe, R.A., eds, *Edited Proceedings of the Fifth International Cadmium Conference, San Francisco, CA, 4–6 February 1986*, London/New York, Cadmium Association/Cadmium Council, pp. 108–111

Oberdörster, G. (1989) Pulmonary toxicity and carcinogenicity of cadmium. *J. Am. Coll. Toxicol.*, **8**, 1251–1263

Oberdörster, G. & Cherian, M.G. (1992) Cadmium and the lung: current perspectives of carcinogenicity. In: Cook, M.F., Hiscock, S.A., Morrow, H. & Volpe, R.A., eds, *Edited Proceedings of the Seventh International Cadmium Conference, New Orleans, LA, 6–8 April 1992*, London/Reston VA, Cadmium Association/Cadmium Council, pp. 130–134

Oberdörster, G. & Cox, C. (1989) Kinetics of inhaled $CdCl_2$, CdO and CdS in rats and monkeys. In: Hiscock, S.A. & Volpe, R.A., eds, *Edited Proceedings of the Sixth International Cadmium Conference, Paris, 19–21 April 1989*, London/New York, Cadmium Association/Cadmium Council, pp. 147–154

Oberdörster, G. & Cox, C. (1990) Carcinogenicity of cadmium in animals: What is the significance for man? *Toxicol. environ. Chem.*, **27**, 181–195

Oberdörster, G., Cherian, M.G. & Baggs, R.B. (1993) Correlation between cadmium-induced pulmonary carcinogenicity, metallothionein expression and inflammatory processes: a species comparison. *Environ. Health Perspectives* (in press)

Oberly, T.J., Piper, C.E. & McDonald, D.S. (1982) Mutagenicity of metal salts in the L5178Y mouse lymphoma assay. *J. Toxicol. environ. Health*, **9**, 367–376

Ochi, T. (1991) Cadmium-resistant Chinese hamster V79 cells with decreased accumulation of cadmium. *Chem.-biol. Interactions*, **78**, 207–221

Ochi, T. & Ohsawa, M. (1983) Induction of 6-thioguanine-resistant mutants and single-strand scission of DNA by cadmium chloride in cultured Chinese hamster cells. *Mutat. Res.*, **111**, 69–78

Ochi, T. & Ohsawa, M. (1985) Participation of active oxygen species in the induction of chromosomal aberrations by cadmium chloride in cultured Chinese hamster cells. *Mutat. Res.*, **143**, 137–142

Ochi, T., Ishiguro, T. & Ohsawa, M. (1983) Participation of active oxygen species in the induction of DNA single-strand scissions by cadmium chloride in cultured Chinese hamster cells. *Mutat. Res.*, **122**, 169–175

Ochi, T., Mogi, M., Watanabe, M. & Ohsawa, M. (1984) Induction of chromosomal aberrations in cultured Chinese hamster cells by short-term treatment with cadmium chloride. *Mutat. Res.*, **137**, 103–109

Ochi, T., Takahashi, K. & Ohsawa, M. (1987) Indirect evidence for the induction of a prooxidant state by cadmium chloride in cultured mammalian cells and a possible mechanism for the induction. *Mutat. Res.*, **180**, 257–266

Odone, P., Bertelli, G., Dell'Orto, A., Castoldi, M.R. & Alessio, L. (1983) Biological monitoring of cadmium-exposed workers (Ital.). *Med. Lav.*, **74**, 182–190

Ohno, H., Hanaoka, F. & Yamada, M.-A. (1982) Inducibility of sister-chromatid exchanges by heavy-metal ions. *Mutat. Res.*, **104**, 141–145

Ohta, H., Seki, Y. & Imamiya, S. (1988) Metallothionein-like cadmium binding protein in rat testes administered with cadmium and selenium. *Bull. environ. Contam. Toxicol.*, **41**, 195–200

O'Riordan, M.L., Hughes, E.G. & Evans, H.J. (1978) Chromosome studies on blood lymphocytes of men occupationally exposed to cadmium. *Mutat. Res.*, **58**, 305–311

Osgood, C., Zimmering, S. & Mason, J.M. (1991) Aneuploidy in Drosophila, II. Further validation of the FIX and ZESTE genetic test systems employing female *Drosophila melanogaster*. *Mutat. Res.*, **259**, 147–163

Otsuka, F. & Ohsawa, M. (1991) Differential susceptibility of T- and B-lymphocyte proliferation to cadmium: relevance to zinc requirement in T-lymphocyte proliferation. *Chem.-biol. Interactions*, **78**, 193–205

Pääkkö, P., Kokkonen, P., Anttila, S. & Kalliomäki, P.-L. (1989) Cadmium and chromium as markers of smoking in human lung tissue. *Environ. Res.*, **49**, 197–207

Padmanabhan, R. & Hameed, M.S. (1990) Characteristics of the limb malformations induced by maternal exposure to cadmium in the mouse. *Reprod. Toxicol.*, **4**, 291–304

Pagano, D.A & Zeiger, E. (1992) Conditions for detecting the mutagenicity of divalent metals in *Salmonella typhimurium*. *Environ. mol. Mutag.*, **19**, 139–146

Parizek, J. (1960) Sterilization of the male by cadmium salts. *J. Reprod. Fertil.*, **1**, 294–309

Parízek, J. (1983) Cadmium and reproduction: a perspective after 25 years. In: Clarkson, T.W., Nordberg, G.F. & Sager, P.R., eds, *Reproductive and Developmental Toxicity of Metals*, New York, Plenum Press, pp. 301–313

Parker, P.D. (1978) Cadmium compounds. In: Mark, H.F., Othmer, D.F., Overberger, C.G., Seaborg, G.T. & Grayson, N., eds, *Kirk-Othmer Encyclopedia of Chemical Technology*, 3rd Ed., Vol. 4, New York, John Wiley & Sons, pp. 397–411

Parzyck, D.C., Shaw, S.M., Kessler, W.V., Vetter, R.J., Van Sickle, D.C. & Mayes, R.A. (1978) Fetal effects of cadmium in pregnant rats on normal and zinc deficient diets. *Bull. environ. Contam. Toxicol.*, **19**, 206–214

Peters, J.M., Thomas, D., Falk, H., Oberdörster, G. & Smith, T.J. (1986) Contribution of metals to respiratory cancer. *Environ. Health Perspectives*, **70**, 71–83

Plunkert, P.A. (1985) Cadmium. In: *Minerals Yearbook*, Vol. 1, *Metals and Minerals*, Washington DC, Bureau of Mines, US Department of the Interior, pp. 181–186

Pocock, S.J., Delves, H.T., Ashby, D., Shaper, A.G. & Clayton, B.E. (1988) Blood cadmium concentrations in the general population of British middle-aged men. *Hum. Toxicol.*, **7**, 95–103

Poirier, L.A., Kasprzak, K.S., Hoover, K.L. & Wenk, M.L. (1983) Effects of calcium and magnesium acetates on the carcinogenicity of cadmium chloride in Wistar rats. *Cancer Res.*, **43**, 4575–4581

Pomerantseva, M.D., Ramaiya, L.K. & Vilkina, G.A. (1980) Comparative efficiency of three different tests for estimation of mutagenicity of some factors in mammals (Russ.). *Genetika*, **8**, 1398–1403

Popenoe, E.A. & Schmaeler, M.A. (1979) Interaction of human DNA polymerase β with ions of copper, lead, and cadmium. *Arch. Biochem. Biophys.*, **196**, 109–120

Pott, F., Ziem, U., Reiffer, F.-J., Huth, F., Ernst, H. & Mohr, U. (1987) Carcinogenicity studies on fibres, metal compounds and some other dusts in rats. *Exp. Pathol.*, **32**, 129–152

Potts, C.L. (1965) Cadmium proteinuria. The health of battery workers exposed to cadmium oxide dust. *Ann. occup. Hyg.*, **8**, 55–61

Prigge, E. (1978) Inhalative cadmium effects in pregnant and fetal rats. *Toxicology*, **10**, 297–309

Princi, F. (1947) A study of industrial exposures to cadmium. *J. ind. Hyg. Toxicol.*, **29**, 315–320

Ramaiya, L.K. & Pomerantseva, M.D. (1977) A study of the mutagenic effect of cadmium on the germ cells of male mice. *Sov. Genet.*, **13**, 43–46

Ramel, C. & Magnusson, J. (1979) Chemical induction of nondisjunction in *Drosophila*. *Environ. Health Perspectives*, **31**, 59–66

Rasmuson, Å. (1985) Mutagenic effects of some water-soluble metal compounds in a somatic eye-color test system in *Drosophila melanogaster*. *Mutat. Res.*, **157**, 157–162

Reddy, J., Svoboda, D., Azarnoff, D. & Dawar, R. (1973) Cadmium-induced Leydig cell tumors of rat testis: morphologic and cytochemical study. *J. natl Cancer Inst.*, **51**, 891–903

Rehm, S. & Waalkes, M.P. (1988) Cadmium-induced ovarian toxicity in hamsters, mice, and rats. *Fundam. appl. Toxicol.*, **10**, 635–647

Richards, F.M., Watson, A. & Hickman, J.A. (1988) Investigation of the effects of heat shock and agents which induce a heat shock response on the induction of differentiation of HL-60 cells. *Cancer Res.*, **48**, 6715–6720

Ricksecker, R.E. (1979) Copper alloys. In: Mark, H.F., Othmer, D.F., Overberger, C.G., Seaborg, G.T. & Grayson, N., eds, *Kirk-Othmer Encyclopedia of Chemical Technology*, 3rd Ed., Vol. 7, New York, John Wiley & Sons, pp. 1–68

Rivai, I.F., Koyama, H. & Suzuki, S. (1990) Cadmium content in rice and its daily intake in various countries. *Bull. environ. Contam. Toxicol.*, **44**, 910–916

Rivedal, E. & Sanner, T. (1981) Metal salts as promoters of in vitro morphological transformation of hamster embryo cells initiated by benzo(a)pyrene. *Cancer Res.*, **41**, 2950–2953

Robison, S.H., Cantoni, O. & Costa, M. (1982) Strand breakage and decreased molecular weight of DNA induced by specific metal compounds. *Carcinogenesis*, **3**, 657–662

Roe, F.J.C., Dukes, C.E., Cameron, K.M., Pugh, R.C.B. & Mitchley, B.C.V. (1964) Cadmium neoplasia: testicular atrophy and Leydig cell hyperplasia and neoplasia in rats and mice following subcutaneous injection of cadmium salts. *Br. J. Cancer*, **18**, 674–681

Roe, F.J.C., Carter, R.L., Dukes, C.E. & Mitchley, B.C.V. (1968) Non-carcinogenicity of cadmium-free ferritin. *Br. J. Cancer*, **22**, 517-520

Roeleveld, N., Zielhuis, G.A. & Gabreëls, F. (1990) Occupational exposure and defects of the central nervous system in offspring: a review. *Br. J. ind. Med.*, **47**, 580-588

Roels, H.A., Lauwerys, R.R., Buchet, J.-P., Bernard, A., Chettle, D.R., Harvey, T.C. & Al-Haddad, I.K. (1981) In vivo measurement of liver and kidney cadmium in workers exposed to this metal: its significance with respect to cadmium in blood and urine. *Environ. Res.*, **26**, 217-240

Roels, H.A., Lauwerys, R.R., Buchet, J.-P., Bernard, A., Vos, A. & Oversteyns, M. (1989) Health significance of cadmium induced renal dysfunction: a five year follow up. *Br. J. ind. Med.*, **46**, 755-764

Röhr, G & Bauchinger, M. (1976) Chromosome analyses in cell cultures of the Chinese hamster after application of cadmium sulphate. *Mutat. Res.*, **40**, 125-130

Rosas, I., Carbajal, M.E., Gómez-Arroyo, S., Belmont, R. & Villalobos-Pietrini, R. (1984) Cytogenetic effects of cadmium accumulation on water hyacinth (*Eichhornia crassipes*). *Environ. Res.*, **33**, 386-395

Rosenberg, D.W. & Kappas, A. (1991) Induction of heme oxygenase in the small intestinal epithelium: a response to oral cadmium exposure. *Toxicology*, **67**, 199-210

Rossman, T.G. & Molina, M. (1986) The genetic toxicology of metal compounds: II. Enhancement of ultraviolet light-induced mutagenesis in *Escherichia coli* WP2. *Environ. Mutag.*, **8**, 263-271

Rossman, T.G., Molina, M. & Meyer, L.W. (1984) The genetic toxicology of metal compounds: I. Induction of λ prophage in *E. coli* WP2$_s$ (λ). *Environ. Mutag.*, **6**, 59-69

Rossman, T.G., Roy, N.K. & Lin, W.-C. (1992) Is cadmium genotoxic? In: Nordberg, G.F., Herber, R.F.M. & Alessio, L., eds, *Cadmium in the Human Environment: Toxicity and Carcinogenicity* (IARC Scientific Publications No. 118), Lyon, IARC, pp. 367-375

Saffiotti, U. & Bertolero, F. (1989) Neoplastic transformation of BALB/3T3 cells by metals and the quest for induction of a metastatic phenotype. *Biol. Trace Elem. Res.*, **21**, 475-482

Saillenfait, A.M., Payan, J.P., Brondeau, M.T., Zissu, D. & de Ceaurriz, J. (1991) Changes in urinary proximal tubule parameters in neonatal rats exposed to cadmium chloride during pregnancy. *J. appl. Toxicol.*, **11**, 23-27

Saito, H. (1987) Health of the inhabitants after removal of cadmium-polluted surface soil (Jpn.). *Kankyo Hoken Rep.*, **53**, 215-216

Saltzman, R.A., Miller, R.K. & di Sant'Agnese, P.A. (1989) Cadmium exposure on day 12 of gestation in the Wistar rat: distribution, uteroplacental blood flow, and fetal viability. *Teratology*, **39**, 19-30

Samarawickrama, G.P. & Webb, M. (1979) Acute effects of cadmium on the pregnant rat and embryo-fetal development. *Environ. Health Perspectives*, **28**, 245-249

Samarawickrama, G.P. & Webb, M. (1981) The acute toxicity and teratogenicity of cadmium in the pregnant rat. *J. appl. Toxicol.*, **1**, 264-269

Sanders, C.L. & Mahaffey, J.A. (1984) Carcinogenicity of single and multiple intratracheal instillations of cadmium oxide in the rat. *Environ. Res.*, **33**, 227-233

Sandhu, S.S., Dhesi, J.S., Gill, B.S. & Svendsgaard, D. (1991) Evaluation of 10 chemicals for aneuploidy induction in the hexaploid wheat assay. *Mutagenesis*, **6**, 369-373

Savitz, D. (1986) Changes in Spanish surname cancer rates relative to other whites, Denver area, 1969-71 to 1979-81. *Am. J. public Health*, **76**, 1210-1215

Sax, N.I. & Lewis, R.J. (1987) *Hawley's Condensed Chemical Dictionary*, 11th Ed., New York, Van Nostrand Reinhold, pp. 195-198

Saxena, D.K., Murthy, R.C. & Chandra, S.V. (1986) Embryotoxic and teratogenic effects of interaction of cadmium and lindane in rats. *Acta pharmacol. toxicol.*, **59**, 175-178

Schaller, K.H., Angerer, J. & Lehnert, G. (1991) Internal and external quality control in the toxicological analysis of blood and urine samples in the Federal Republic of Germany. *Int. Arch. occup. environ. Health*, **62**, 537-542

Schiestl, R.H., Gietz, R.D., Mehta, R.D. & Hastings, P.J. (1989) Carcinogens induce intrachromosomal recombination in yeast. *Carcinogenesis*, **10**, 1445-1455

Schmid, B.P., Hall, J.L., Goulding, E., Fabro, S. & Dixon, R. (1983) In vitro exposure of male and female mice gametes to cadmium chloride during the fertilization process, and its effects on pregnancy outcome. *Toxicol. appl. Pharmacol.*, **69**, 326-332

Schroeder, H.A., Vinton, W.H., Jr & Balassa, J.J. (1963) Effects of chromium, cadmium and lead on the growth and survival of rats. *J. Nutr.*, **80**, 48-54

Schroeder, H.A., Balassa, J.J. & Vinton, W.H., Jr (1964) Chromium, lead, cadmium, nickel and titanium in mice: effect on mortality, tumors and tissue levels. *J. Nutr.*, **83**, 239-250

Schroeder, H.A., Balassa, J.J. & Vinton, W.H., Jr (1965) Chromium, cadmium and lead in rats: effects on life span, tumors and tissue levels. *J. Nutr.*, **86**, 51-66

Schulte-Schrepping, K.-H. & Piscator, M. (1985) Cadmium and cadmium compounds. In: Gerhartz, W., Yamamoto, Y.S., Campbell, F.T., Pfefferkorn, R. & Rounsaville, J.F., eds, *Ullmann's Encyclopedia of Industrial Chemistry*, 5th Ed., Vol. A4, Deerfield Beach, FL, VCH Publishers, pp. 499-514

Scott, R. & Aughey, E. (1978) Methylcholanthrene and cadmium induced changes in rat prostate. *Br. J. Urol.*, **50**, 25-28

Sehgal, A., Osgood, C. & Zimmering, S. (1990) Aneuploidy in *Drosophila*. III: Aneuploidogens inhibit in vitro assembly of taxol-purified *Drosophila* microtubules. *Environ. mol. Mutag.*, **16**, 217-224

Shagarofsky-Tummers, A. (1992) The regulatory status of cadmium in the European Communities. In: Cook, M.E., Hiscock, S.A., Morrow, H. & Volpe, R.A., eds, *Edited Proceedings of the Seventh International Cadmium Conference, New Orleans, LA, 6-8 April 1992*, London/Reston, VA, Cadmium Association/Cadmium Council, pp. 106-109

Shaikh, Z.A., Ellis, K.J., Subramanian, K.S. & Greenberg, A. (1990) Biological monitoring for occupational cadmium exposure: the urinary metallothionein. *Toxicology*, **63**, 53-62

Shepard, T.H. (1992) *Catalog of Teratogenic Agents*, 7th Ed., Baltimore, MD, Johns Hopkins University Press, pp. 61-62

Shigematsu, I., Kitamaru, S., Takeuchi, J., Minowa, M., Nagai, M., Usui, T. & Fukushima, M. (1982) A retrospective mortality study on cadmium-exposed populations in Japan. In: Wilson, D. & Volpe, R.A., eds, *Edited Proceedings of the Third International Cadmium Conference, Miami, FL, 3-5 February 1981*, London/New York, Cadmium Association/Cadmium Council, pp. 115-118

Shimada, T., Watanabe, T. & Endo, A. (1976) Potential mutagenicity of cadmium in mammalian oocytes. *Mutat. Res.*, **40**, 389-395

Shiraishi, Y. (1975) Cytogenetic studies in 12 patients with itai-itai disease. *Humangenetik*, **27**, 31-44

Shiraishi, Y., Kurahashi, H. & Yosida, T.H. (1972) Chromosomal aberrations in cultured human leucocytes induced by cadmium sulfide. *Proc. Jpn. Acad.*, **48**, 133-137

Siemiatycki, J. (1991) *Risk Factors for Cancer in the Workplace*, Boca Raton, FL, CRC Press

Siemiatycki, J., Wacholder, S., Dewar, R., Wald, L., Bégin, D., Richardson, L., Rosenman, K. & Gérin, M. (1988) Smoking and degree of occupational exposure: are internal analyses in cohort studies likely to be confounded by smoking status? *Am. J. ind. Med.*, **13**, 59-69

Sina, J.F., Bean, C.L., Dysart, G.R., Taylor, V.I. & Bradley, M.O. (1983) Evaluation of the alkaline elution/rat hepatocyte assay as a predictor of carcinogenic/mutagenic potential. *Mutat. Res.*, **113**, 357–391

Skerfving, S., Christoffersson, J.-O., Shütz, A., Welinder, H., Spång, G., Ahlgren, L. & Mattsson, S. (1987) Biological monitoring, by in vivo XRF measurements, of occupational exposure to lead, cadmium and mercury. *Biol. Trace Elem. Res.*, **13**, 241–251

Smith, T.J., Anderson, R.J. & Reading, J.C. (1980) Chronic cadmium exposures associated with kidney function effects. *Am. J. ind. Med.*, **1**, 319–337

Smith, N.J., Topping, M.D., Stewart, J.D. & Fletcher, J.G. (1986) Occupational cadmium exposure in jig solderers. *Br. J. ind. Med.*, **43**, 663–666

Snow, E.T. (1992) Metal carcinogenesis: mechanistic implications. *Pharmacol. Ther.*, **53**, 31–65

Snyder, R.D. (1988) Role of active oxygen species in metal-induced DNA strand breakage in human diploid fibroblasts. *Mutat. Res.*, **193**, 237–246

Sorahan, T. (1987) Mortality from lung cancer among a cohort of nickel cadmium battery workers: 1946–84. *Br. J. ind. Med.*, **44**, 803–809

Sorahan, T. & Waterhouse, J.A. (1983) Mortality study of nickel–cadmium battery workers by the method of regression models in life tables. *Br. J. ind. Med.*, **40**, 293–300

Sorahan, T. & Waterhouse, J.A.H. (1985) Cancer of the prostate among nickel–cadmium battery workers (Letter to the Editor). *Lancet*, **i**, 459

Sorell, T.L. & Graziano, J.H. (1990) Effect of oral cadmium exposure during pregnancy on maternal and fetal zinc metabolism in the rat. *Toxicol. appl. Pharmacol.*, **102**, 537–545

Spectrum Chemical Mfg Corp. (1991) *Laboratory, Pharmaceutical, Cosmetic and Biotechnology Chemicals—ACS—USP/NF—FCC—1991-1992*, Gardena, CA, pp. 74–77

Stayner, L., Smith, R., Thun, M., Schnorr, T. & Lemen, R. (1992) A dose–response analysis and quantitative assessment of lung cancer risk and occupational cadmium exposure. *Ann. Epidemiol.*, **2**, 177–194

Stayner, L., Smith, R., Schnorr, T., Lemen, R. & Thun, M. (1993) Letter regarding cadmium and lung cancer. *Ann. Epidemiol.*, **3**, 114–116

Stoeppler, M. & Brandt, K. (1980) Contributions to automated trace analysis. Part V. Determination of cadmium in whole blood and urine by electrothermal atomic-absorption spectrophotometry. *Fresenius' Z. anal. Chem.*, **300**, 372–380

Stoner, G.D., Shimkin, M.B., Troxell, M.C., Thompson, T.L. & Terry, L.S. (1976) Test for carcinogenicity of metallic compounds by the pulmonary tumor response in strain A mice. *Cancer Res.*, **36**, 1744–1747

Strem Chemicals (1992) *Catalog No. 14—Metals, Inorganics and Organometallics for Research*, Newburyport, MA, pp. 22–23

Sunderman, F.W., Jr (1984) Recent advances in metal carcinogenesis. *Ann. clin. Lab. Sci.*, **14**, 93–122

Suter, K.E. (1975) Studies on the dominant-lethal and fertility effects of the heavy metal compounds methylmercuric hydroxide, mercuric chloride, and cadmium chloride in male and female mice. *Mutat. Res.*, **30**, 365–374

Sutou, S., Yamamoto, K., Sendota, H., Tomomatsu, K., Shimizu, Y. & Sugiyama, M. (1980a) Toxicity, fertility, teratogenicity, and dominant lethal tests in rats administered cadmium subchronically. I. Toxicity studies. *Ecotoxicol. environ. Saf.*, **4**, 39–50

Sutou, S., Yamamoto, K., Sendota, H. & Sugiyama, M. (1980b) Toxicity, fertility, teratogenicity, and dominant lethal tests in rats administered cadmium subchronically. II. Fertility, teratogenicity, and dominant lethal tests. *Ecotoxicol. environ. Saf.*, **4**, 51–56

Svensk Författningssamling (1979) *Förordning om ändring i kungörelsen (1973:334) om hälso- och miliöfarliga varor* [Directive for amendment to notification (1973:334) of products that are dangerous to health and the environment] (SFS 1979:771), Stockholm

Svensk Författningssamling (1980) *Förordning om ändring i förordningen (1979:771) om ändring i kungörelsen (1973:334) om hälso- och miljöfarliga varor* [Directive for amendment to notification (1979:771) about amendment to notification (1973:334) of products that are dangerous to health and the environment] (SFS 1980:84), Stockholm

Swierenga, S.H.H., Gilman, J.P.W. & McLean, J.R. (1987) Cancer risk from inorganics. *Cancer Metastasis Rev.*, **6**, 113–154

Takenaka, S., Oldiges, H., König, H., Hochrainer, D. & Oberdörster, G. (1983) Carcinogenicity of cadmium chloride aerosols in Wistar rats. *J. natl Cancer Inst.*, **70**, 367–373

Tang, X.-M., Chen, X.-Q., Zhang, J.-X. & Qin, W.-Q. (1990) Cytogenetic investigation in lymphocytes of people living in cadmium-polluted areas. *Mutat. Res.*, **241**, 243–249

Terracio, L. & Nachtigal, M. (1986) Transformation of prostatic epithelial cells and fibroblasts with cadmium chloride *in vitro*. *Arch. Toxicol.*, **58**, 141–151

Terracio, L. & Nachtigal, M. (1988) Oncogenicity of rat prostate cells transformed *in vitro* with cadmium chloride. *Arch. Toxicol.*, **61**, 450–456

Thomas, P.T., Ratajczak, H.V., Aranyi, C., Gibbons, R. & Fenters, J.D. (1985) Evaluation of host resistance and immune function in cadmium-exposed mice. *Toxicol. appl. Pharmacol.*, **80**, 446–456

Thun, M.J., Schnorr, T.M., Smith, A.B., Halperin, W.E. & Lemen, R.A. (1985) Mortality among a cohort of US cadmium production workers—an update. *J. natl Cancer Inst.*, **74**, 325–333

Thun, M.J., Schnorr, T.M. & Halperin, W.E. (1986) Retrospective mortality study of cadmium workers—an update. In: Wilson, D. & Volpe, R.A., eds., *Edited Proceedings of the Fifth International Cadmium Conference, San Francisco, CA, 4–6 February 1986*, London/New York, Cadmium Association/Cadmium Council, pp. 115–119

Thun, M.J., Elinder, C.-G. & Friberg, L. (1991) Scientific basis for an occupational standard for cadmium. *Am. J. ind. Med.*, **20**, 629–642

Tso, W.-W. & Fung, W.-P. (1981) Mutagenicity of metallic cations. *Toxicol. Lett.*, **8**, 195–200

Tsuchiya, K. (1967) Proteinuria of workers exposed to cadmium fume. The relationship to concentration in the working environment. *Arch. environ. Health*, **14**, 875–880

Tsuchiya, K., Seki, Y. & Sugita, M. (1976) Organ and tissue cadmium concentrations of cadavers from accidental deaths. *Keio J. Med.*, **25**, 83–90

Ulicny, L.J. (1992) What is the evidence for the carcinogenicity of cadmium sulphide pigments? In: Cook, M.E., Hiscock, S.A., Morrow, H. & Volpe, R.A., eds, *Edited Proceedings of the Seventh International Cadmium Conference, New Orleans, LA, 6–8 April 1992*, London/Reston, VA, Cadmium Association/Cadmium Council, pp. 139–144

Umeda, M. & Nishimura, M. (1979) Inducibility of chromosomal aberrations by metal compounds in cultured mammalian cells. *Mutat. Res.*, **67**, 221–229

UNEP (1984) *List of Environmentally Dangerous Chemical Substances and Processes of Global Significance* (Report of the Executive Director of UNEP to the 12th Session of Its Governing Council), Geneva, International Register of Potentially Toxic Chemicals

UNEP (1992) *Chemical Pollution: A Global Overview*, Geneva

UNEP (1993) *IRPTC PC Database*, Geneva

US Environmental Protection Agency (1986a) Method 6010. Inductively coupled plasma atomic emission spectroscopy. In: *Test Methods for Evaluating Solid Waste—Physical/Chemical Methods*, 3rd Ed., Vol. 1A (US EPA No. SW-846), Washington DC, Office of Solid Waste and Emergency Response, pp. 6010-1–6010-17

US Environmental Protection Agency (1986b) Method 7130. Cadmium (atomic absorption, direct aspiration). In: *Test Methods for Evaluating Solid Waste—Physical/Chemical Methods*, 3rd Ed., Vol. 1A (US EPA No. SW-846), Washington DC, Office of Solid Waste and Emergency Response, pp. 7130-1–7130-4

US Environmental Protection Agency (1986c) Method 7131. Cadmium (atomic absorption, furnace technique). In: *Test Methods for Evaluating Solid Waste—Physical/Chemical Methods*, 3rd Ed., Vol. 1A (US EPA No. SW-846), Washington DC, Office of Solid Waste and Emergency Response, pp. 7131-1–7131-5

US Environmental Protection Agency (1991) Maximum contaminant levels for inorganic chemicals. *US Code fed. Regul.*, **Title 40**, pp. 585–586

US Food and Drug Administration (1992) Standards of quality—bottled water. *US Code fed. Regul.*, **Title 21**, pp. 61–64

US National Cancer Institute (1986) *Cancer Among Blacks and Other Minorities: Statistical Profiles* (NIH Publication No. 86-2785), Bethesda, MD, US Department of Health and Human Services, pp. 9–10

US National Toxicology Program (1991) Cadmium and certain cadmium compounds. In: *Sixth Annual Report on Carcinogens. Summary 1991*, Research Triangle Park, NC, US Public Health Service, Department of Health and Human Services, pp. 114–121

US Occupational Safety and Health Administration (1992) Occupational exposure to cadmium: final rules. *Fed. Reg.*, **57**, 42102–42463

Vainio, H. & Sorsa, M. (1981) Chromosome aberrations and their relevance to metal carcinogenesis. *Environ. Health Perspectives*, **40**, 173–180

Verbost, P.M., Flik, G., Pang, P.K.T., Lock, R.A.C. & Bonga, S.E.W. (1989) Cadmium inhibition of the erythrocyte Ca^{2+} pump. A molecular interpretation. *J. biol. Chem.*, **264**, 5613–5615

Volkova, N.A. & Karplyuk, I.A. (1990) Cadmium mutagenic activity after oral administration (Russ.). *Vop. Pitan.*, **1**, 74–76

Waalkes, M.P. (1986) Effect of dietary zinc deficiency on the accumulation of cadmium and metallothionein in selected tissues of the rat. *J. Toxicol. environ. Health*, **18**, 301–313

Waalkes, M.P. & Goering, P.L. (1990) Metallothionein and other cadmium-binding proteins: recent developments. *Chem. Res. Toxicol.*, **3**, 281–288

Waalkes, M.P. & Oberdörster, G. (1990) Cadmium carcinogenesis. In: Foulkes, E.C., ed., *Biological Effects of Heavy Metals*, Vol. II, *Metal Carcinogenesis*, Boca Raton, FL, CRC Press, pp. 129–157

Waalkes, M.P. & Perantoni, A. (1988) In vitro assessment of target cell specificity in cadmium carcinogenesis: interactions of cadmium and zinc with isolated interstitial cells of the rat testes. *In vitro cell. dev. Biol.*, **24**, 558–565

Waalkes, M.P. & Rehm, S. (1992) Carcinogenicity of oral cadmium in the male Wistar (WF/NCr) rat: effect of chronic dietary zinc deficiency. *Fundam. appl. Toxicol.*, **19**, 512–520

Waalkes, M.P., Rehm, S., Riggs, C.W., Bare, R.M., Devor, D.E., Poirier, L.A., Wenk, M.L., Henneman, J.R. & Balaschak, M.S. (1988a) Cadmium carcinogenesis in the male Wistar [Crl:(WI)BR] rat: dose–response analysis of tumor induction in the prostate and testes and at the injection site. *Cancer Res.*, **48**, 4656–4663

Waalkes, M.P., Perantoni, A., Bhave, M.R. & Rehm, S. (1988b) Strain dependence in mice of resistance and susceptibility to the testicular effects of cadmium: assessment of the role of testicular cadmium-binding proteins. *Toxicol. appl. Pharmacol.*, **93**, 47–61

Waalkes, M.P., Rehm, S. & Perantoni, A. (1988c) Metal-binding proteins of the Syrian hamster ovaries: apparent deficiency of metallothionein. *Biol. Reprod.*, **39**, 953–961

Waalkes, M.P., Perantoni, A. & Palmer, A.E. (1988d) Isolation and partial characterization of the low-molecular-mass zinc/cadmium-binding protein from the testes of the patas monkey (*Erythrocebus patas*). Distinction from metallothionein. *Biochem. J.*, **256**, 131–137

Waalkes, M.P., Rehm, S., Riggs, C.W., Bare, R.M., Devor, D.E., Poirier, L.A., Wenk, M.L. & Henneman, J.R. (1989) Cadmium carcinogenesis in male Wistar [Crl:(WI)BR] rats: dose–response analysis of effects of zinc on tumor induction in the prostate, in the testes and at the injection site. *Cancer Res.*, **49**, 4282–4288

Waalkes, M.P., Rehm, S., Sass, B., Konishi, N. & Ward, J.M. (1991a) Chronic carcinogenic and toxic effects of a single subcutaneous dose of cadmium in the male Fischer rat. *Environ. Res.*, **55**, 40–50

Waalkes, M.P., Kovatch, R. & Rehm, S. (1991b) Effect of chronic dietary zinc deficiency on cadmium toxicity and carcinogenesis in the male Wistar [Hsd:(WI)BR] rat. *Toxicol. appl. Pharmacol.*, **108**, 448–456

Waalkes, M.P., Diwan, B.A., Weghorst, C.M., Bare, R.M., Ward, J.M. & Rice, J.M. (1991c) Anticarcinogenic effects of cadmium in B6C3F1 mouse liver and lung. *Toxicol. appl. Pharmacol.*, **110**, 327–335

Waalkes, M.P., Coogan, T.P. & Barter, R.A. (1992a) Toxicological principles of metal carcinogenesis with special emphasis on cadmium. *CRC Crit. Rev. Toxicol.*, **22**, 175–201

Waalkes, M.P., Rehm, S., Perantoni, A.O. & Coogan, T.P. (1992b) Cadmium exposure in rats and tumours of the prostate. In: Nordberg, G.F., Herber, R.F.M. & Alessio, L., eds, *Cadmium in the Human Environment: Toxicity and Carcinogenicity* (IARC Scientific Publications No. 118), Lyon, IARC, pp. 391–400

Wade, G.G., Mandel, R. & Ryser, H.J.-P. (1987) Marked synergism of dimethylnitrosamine carcinogenesis in rats exposed to cadmium. *Cancer Res.*, **47**, 6606–6613

Warner, C.W., Sadler, T.W., Tulis, S.A. & Smith, M.K. (1984) Zinc amelioration of cadmium-induced teratogenesis *in vitro*. *Teratology*, **30**, 47–53

Watanabe, T., Shimada, T. & Endo, A. (1977) Mutagenic effects of cadmium on the oocyte chromosomes of mice. *Jpn. J. Hyg.*, **32**, 472–481

Watanabe, T., Shimada, T. & Endo, A. (1979) Mutagenic effects of cadmium on mammalian oocyte chromosomes. *Mutat. Res.*, **67**, 349–356

Watanabe, M., Honda, S., Hayashi, M. & Matsuda, T. (1982) Mutagenic effects of combinations of chemical carcinogens and environmental pollutants in mice as shown by the micronucleus test. *Mutat. Res.*, **97**, 43–48

Watanabe, T., Koizumi, A., Fujita, H., Kumai, M. & Ikeda, M. (1985) Dietary cadmium intakes of farmers in nonpolluted areas in Japan, and the relation with blood cadmium levels. *Environ. Res.*, **37**, 33–43

Watanabe, T., Nakatsuka, H. & Ikeda, M. (1989) Cadmium and lead contents in rice available in various areas of Asia. *Sci. total Environ.*, **80**, 175–184

Watanabe, T., Nakatsuka, H., Satoh, H., Yamamoto, R. & Ikeda, M. (1992) Reduced dietary cadmium intake in past 12 years in a rural area in Japan. *Sci. total Environ.*, **119**, 43–50

Webb, M. & Samarawickrama, G.P. (1981) Placental transport and embryonic utilization of essential metabolites in the rat at the teratogenic dose of cadmium. *J. appl. Toxicol.*, **1**, 270–277

Webster, W.S. (1978) Cadmium-induced fetal growth retardation in the mouse. *Arch. environ. Health*, **33**, 36–42

Webster, W.S. & Messerle, K. (1980) Changes in the mouse neuroepithelium associated with cadmium-induced neural tube defects. *Teratology*, **21**, 79–88

Weischer, C.H. & Greve, J. (1979) Effects of cadmium-chloride-aerosols on three generations of Wistar rats (Ger.). *Zbl. Bakt. Hyg. I Abt. Orig. B*, **169**, 427–435

Whelton, B.D., Bhattacharyya, M.H., Carnes, B.A., Moretti, E.S. & Peterson, D.P. (1988) Female reproduction and pup survival and growth for mice fed a cadmium-containing purified diet through six consecutive rounds of gestation and lactation. *J. Toxicol. environ. Health*, **24**, 321–343

Whittaker, S.G., Zimmermann, F.K., Dicus, B., Piegorsch, W.W., Fogel, S. & Resnick, M.A. (1989) Detection of induced mitotic chromosome loss in *Saccharomyces cerevisiae* — an interlaboratory study. *Mutat. Res.*, **224**, 31–78

WHO (1980) *Recommended Health-based Limits in Occupational Exposure to Heavy Metals* (Technical Report Series 647), Geneva, pp. 21–35

WHO (1984) *Guidelines for Drinking-water Quality*, Vol. 1, *Recommendations*, Geneva, pp. 6, 54

WHO (1987) *Air Quality Guidelines for Europe* (WHO Regional Publications, Eur. Ser. No. 23), Copenhagen, pp. 206–207

WHO (1988) *Emission of Heavy Metal and PAH Compounds From Municipal Solid Waste Incinerators: Control Technology and Health Effects. Report on a WHO Meeting, Florence, 12–16 October 1987*, Copenhagen, pp. 31, 38–40

WHO (1989) *Evaluation of Certain Food Additives and Contaminants*, Geneva, pp. 28–31

WHO (1992a) *Cadmium—Environmental Aspects* (Environmental Health Criteria 135), Geneva

WHO (1992b) *Cadmium* (Environmental Health Criteria 134), Geneva

WHO (1992c) *Guidelines for Drinking-water Quality*, Geneva, p. 2

Wier, P.J., Miller, R.K., Maulik, D. & di Sant'Agnese, P.A. (1990) Toxicity of cadmium in the perfused human placenta. *Toxicol. appl. Pharmacol.*, **105**, 156–171

Williams, W.R., Kagamimori, S., Watanabe, M., Shinmura, T. & Hagino, N. (1983) An immunological study on patients with chronic cadmium disease. *Clin. exp. Immunol.*, **53**, 651–658

Wills, J.H., Groblewski, G.E. & Coulston, F. (1981) Chronic and multigeneration toxicities of small concentrations of cadmium in the diet of rats. *Ecotoxicol. environ. Saf.*, **5**, 452–464

Wolff, E.W. & Peel, D.A. (1985) The record of global pollution in polar snow and ice. *Nature*, **313**, 535–540

Wysowski, D.K., Landrigan, P.J., Ferguson, S.W., Fontaine, R.E., Tsongas, T.A. & Porter, B. (1978) Cadmium exposure in a community near a smelter. *Am. J. Epidemiol.*, **107**, 27–35

Yamagata, N., Iwashima, K. & Nagai, T. (1975) Gastrointestinal absorption of ingested ^{115m}Cd by a man. *Bull. Inst. public Health*, **24**, 1–6

Yu, H.S. & Chan, S.T.H. (1987) Effects of cadmium on preimplantation and early postimplantation mouse embryos *in vitro* with special reference to their trophoblastic invasiveness. *Pharmacol. Toxicol.*, **60**, 129–134

Yu, H.S., Tam, P.P.L. & Chan, S.T.H. (1985) Effects of cadmium on preimplantation mouse embryos *in vitro* with special reference to their implantation capacity and subsequent development. *Teratology*, **32**, 347–353

Zasukhina, G.D. & Sinelschikova, T.A. (1976) Mechanism of the action of certain mutagens on the DNA of human cells. *Dokl. biol. Sci.*, **230**, 409–411

Zenick, H., Hastings, L., Goldsmith, M. & Niewenhuis, R.J. (1982) Chronic cadmium exposure: relation to male reproductive toxicity and subsequent fetal outcome. *J. Toxicol. environ. Health*, **9**, 377–387

Zwennis, W.C.M. & Franssen, A.C. (1992) Assessment of occupational exposure to cadmium in The Netherlands, 1980–1989. *Am. J. ind. Med.*, **21**, 793–805

MERCURY AND MERCURY COMPOUNDS

1. Exposure Data

1.1 Chemical and physical data and analysis

1.1.1 *Synonyms, trade names and molecular formulae*

Synonyms, trade names and molecular formulae for mercury and certain mercury compounds are presented in Table 1. The list of mercury compounds is not exhaustive, nor are those compounds necessarily the most commercially important mercury-containing substances; it includes the mercury compounds for which data on carcinogenicity are considered in this volume.

Table 1. Synonyms (Chemical Abstracts Service [CAS] names are in italics), trade names and atomic or molecular formulae of mercury and mercury compounds

Chemical name	CAS Reg. No.[a]	Synonyms and trade names	Formula
Mercury metal	7439-97-6 (8030-64-6; 51887-47-9; 92355-34-5; 92786-62-4; 123720-03-6)	Colloidal mercury; hydrargyrum; liquid silver; quecksilber; quicksilver	Hg
Mercuric acetate	1600-27-7 (6129-23-3; 7619-62-7; 19701-15-6)	*Acetic acid, mercury (2+) salt*; bis(acetyloxy)mercury; diacetoxymercury; mercuri, diacetic acid; mercury acetate; mercuric diacetate; mercury diacetate	$$Hg(O-\overset{\overset{O}{\|}}{C}-CH_3)_2$$
Mercuric chloride	7487-94-7	Abavit B; bichloride of mercury; Calochlor; corrosive sublimate; corrosive mercury chloride; CRC; dichloromercury; mercuric bichloride; mercuric chloride; mercuric dichloride; mercury bichloride; *mercury chloride*; mercury(2+) chloride; mercury(II) chloride; mercury dichloride; mercury perchloride; Sublimate; Sulem	$HgCl_2$
Mercuric oxide	21908-53-2 (1344-45-2; 8028-34-0)	Mercuric oxide (HgO); mercury monoxide; mercury oxide; *mercury oxide (HgO)*; mercury(II) oxide; mercury(2+) oxide; red mercuric oxide; santar; yellow mercuric oxide	HgO

Table 1 (contd)

Chemical name	CAS Reg. No.[a]	Synonyms and trade names	Formula
Dimethylmercury	593-74-8	Methyl mercury	$(CH_3)_2Hg$
Methylmercury chloride	115-09-3	Caspan; *chloromethylmercury*; mercury methyl chloride; methylmercuric chloride; methylmercury monochloride; monomethyl mercury chloride	CH_3ClHg
Phenylmercury acetate	62-38-4 (1337-06-0; 8013-47-4; 61840-45-7; 64684-45-3)	*Acetato-O-phenylmercury*; acetatophenylmercury; acetatophenylmercury; acetic acid, phenyl mercury derivative; (acetoxymercurio)benzene; acetoxyphenylmercury; mercuriphenyl acetate; phenylmercuric acetate; phenylmercury(II) acetate	$C_6H_5-Hg-O-\underset{\underset{O}{\parallel}}{C}-CH_3$

[a]Replaced CAS Registry numbers are shown in parentheses

1.1.2 *Chemical and physical properties of the pure substances*

Selected chemical and physical properties of mercury and of the mercury compounds covered in this monograph are presented in Table 2.

Mercury (also called quicksilver because of its liquid state at room temperature) was known as early as 1000 BC. The discovery in 1938 of 1 kg of the metal in 2500-year-old sand layers on the eastern coast of Greece indicates that mercury was used in the extraction of gold at an early date. Mercury was mentioned about 200 BC in India as well as in China (Han dynasty). As early as 1556 AD, five different methods for extracting mercury from its ores were reported (Simon *et al.*, 1990).

Inorganic mercury exists in three oxidation states: 0 (metallic), +1 (mercurous) and +2 (mercuric); mercurous ions usually occur as dimers (Hg_2^{2+}). The mercurous and mercuric states form numerous inorganic and organic chemical compounds. Organomercury compounds are those in which mercury is attached covalently to at least one carbon atom (Aylett, 1973; Simon *et al.*, 1990; WHO, 1990, 1991).

In its elemental form, mercury is a dense, silvery-white, shiny metal, which is liquid at room temperature and boils at 357 °C. At 20 °C, the vapour pressure of the metal is 0.17 Pa (0.0013 mm Hg). A saturated atmosphere at 20 °C contains 14 mg/m^3 (Simon *et al.*, 1990).

Mercury compounds differ greatly in solubility: for example, in water, the solubility of metallic mercury is 60 µg/L at 25 °C, 250 µg/L at 50 °C and 1100 µg/L at 90 °C (Simon *et al.*, 1990); the solubility of mercurous chloride is 2 mg/L at 25 °C and that of mercuric chloride is 69 g/L at 20 °C (Lide, 1991). Methylmercury chloride is more soluble in water than mercurous chloride by about three orders of magnitude, owing to the very high solubility of the methylmercury cation in water. Certain species of mercury, including metallic mercury and the halide compounds of alkylmercury compounds, are soluble in non-polar solvents

Table 2. Chemical and physical properties of mercury and mercury compounds

Chemical name	Relative atomic/ molecular mass	Melting-point (°C)	Typical physical description	Density	Solubility
Mercury metal	200.59	−38.87	Silvery-white, heavy, mobile, liquid metal	13.546 (20 °C)	Soluble in nitric acid, sulfuric acid upon heavy boiling, lipids, pentane; insoluble in dilute hydrochloric, hydrobromic and hydroiodic acids, water (2 μg/L at 30 °C), ethanol, diethyl ether, cold sulfuric acid
Mercuric acetate	318.7	178–180 (decomposes)	White crystals or crystalline powder	3.27	Soluble in water (250 g/L at 10 °C), ethanol, acetic acid
Mercuric chloride	271.50	276	Colourless, rhombic, odourless, crystal or white powder	5.44 (25 °C)	Soluble in water (69 g/L at 20 °C), methanol, ethanol, amyl alcohol, acetone, formic acid, acetic acid, the lower acetate esters, diethyl ether, benzene, glycerol; slightly soluble in carbon disulfide and pyridine
Mercuric oxide	216.6	500 (decomposes)	Yellow or red, *ortho*-rombic, odourless crystalline powder	11.14	Insoluble in water (53 mg/L at 25 °C), soluble in acids; insoluble in ethanol, diethyl ether, acetone, alkali, ammoniac
Dimethylmercury	230.66	NR	Colourless liquid with a sweet odour	3.19 (20 °C)	Soluble in ethanol and diethyl ether; insoluble in water
Methylmercury chloride	251.10	167–168	White crystalline solid with a disagreeable odour	4.06	Slightly soluble in water
Phenylmercury acetate	336.75	150	White to cream-coloured, small, odourless, lustrous crystalline solid (prism, powder, leaflet)	2.4	Soluble in ethanol, benzene, glacial acetic acid, acetone, ammonium acetate, chloroform, diethyl ether; slightly soluble in water (4.37 g/L) at 25 °C)

From Aylett (1973); Lide (1991); Alfa Products (1990); Budavari (1989); Sax & Lewis (1987); Drake (1981); Singer & Nowak (1981); Worthing (1987); Strem Chemicals (1992). NR, not reported

(WHO, 1991). Mercury vapour is more soluble in plasma, whole blood and haemoglobin than in distilled-water or isotonic saline (Hursh, 1985).

Mercury forms monovalent and divalent compounds with the halogens fluorine, chlorine, bromine and iodine. It also forms monovalent and divalent compounds with sulfur. From the biochemical point of view, the most important chemical property of mercuric mercury and alkylmercury compounds may be their high affinity for sulfhydryl groups (Simon et al., 1990; WHO, 1991).

The main volatile mercury species in air is metallic mercury, but dimethylmercury may also occur. Mercury compounds such as mercuric chloride and methylmercury hydroxide are also relatively stable in fresh water, including snow, rain and standing and flowing water. $HgCl_4^{2-}$ is the dominant form of mercury in seawater (WHO, 1991).

1.1.3 Technical products and impurities

Metallic mercury—purities: triple-distilled grade, $\geq$ 99.99% (4N); ACS reagent grade, 99.995–99.9995%; electronic grade, 99.9998%; ultra-high purity grade, 99.99999–99.999999% (Alfa Products, 1990; CERAC, Inc., 1991; Aldrich Chemical Co., 1992; Strem Chemicals, 1992; Atomergic Chemetals Corp., undated; D.F. Goldsmith Chemical & Metal Corp., undated); impurities (%): Ag, 0.0001; Fe, 0.00005; Pb, 0.00001; Cu, 0.00001; Cd, 0.00001; Zn, 0.00005 (Janssen Chimica, 1990).

Mercuric acetate—purities: 97–99.9%; ACS reagent grade, $\geq$ 98% (Janssen Chimica, 1990; CERAC, Inc., 1991; Aldrich Chemical Co., 1992; Strem Chemicals, 1992).

Mercuric chloride—purities: ACS reagent grade, 99%; 99.9–99.9995%; impurities (%): Fe, 0.002; Pb, 0.002; Cu, 0.002; Ca, max. 0.002 (Janssen Chimica, 1990; CERAC, Inc., 1991; Aldrich Chemical Co., 1992; Strem Chemicals, 1992).

Mercuric oxide—purities: high-purity, 99.999%; ACS grade (yellow or red), 99% (CERAC, Inc., 1991; Aldrich Chemical Co., 1992).

Dimethylmercury— purities, 95–98% (Aldrich Chemical Co., 1992; Strem Chemicals, 1992)

Methylmercury chloride—purity: $\geq$ 95% (Alfa Products, 1990)

Phenylmercury acetate—purities: 97–97.5%; practical, US Pharmacopeia and National Formulary grades (Janssen Chimica, 1990; Aldrich Chemical Co., 1992; Strem Chemicals, 1992; D.F. Goldsmith Chemical & Metal Corp., undated). Some of the trade names associated with phenylmercuric acetate include: Agrosan D; Agrosan GN5; Algimycin; Aligimycin 200; Anticon; Antimucin WBR; Antimucin WDR; Bufen; Bufen 30; Caswell No. 656; Cekusil; Celmer; Ceresan; Ceresol; Contra Creme; Dyanacide; Femma; FMA; Fungicide R; Fungitox OR; Gallotox; Hexasan; HL-331; Hostaquick; Intercide 60; Intercide PMA 18; Kwiksan; Lerophyn; Leytosan; Liquiphene; Lorophyn; Meracen; Mercron; Mercuron; Mergal A 25; Mersolite; Mersolite 8; Mersolite D; Metasol 30; Neantina; Norforms; Nuodex PMA 18; Nylmerate; Pamisan; Panomatic; Phenmad; Phix; PMA; PMA 220; PMAC; PMAcetate; PMAL; PMAS; Programin; Purasan-SC-10; Puraturf 10; Quicksan; Quicksan 20; Riogen; Ruberon; Samtol; Sanitized SPG; Sanitol; Sanmicron; Scutl; SC-110; Seed Dressing R; Seedtox; Setrete; Shimmerex; Spor-Kl; Spruce Seal; Tag; Tag 331; Tag Fungicide; Tag HL-331; Trigosan; Troysan 30; Troysan PMA 30; Verdasan; Volpar; Zaprawa Nasienna R; Ziarnik

Impurities of mercury compounds that are the subjects of other monographs are lead (IARC, 1987a) and cadmium (this volume, p. 119).

1.1.4 *Analysis*

Selected methods for the determination of mercury in various media are presented in Table 3. Other methods have been reviewed (WHO, 1990, 1991).

Table 3. Methods for the analysis of mercury in various media

Sample matrix	Sample preparation	Assay procedure	Limit of detection	Reference
Air	Collect on Hydrar sorbent; desorb with nitric then hydrochloric acids	CVAA	0.03 µg/sample	Eller (1989)
Drugs	Digest in water-hydrochloric acid-nitric acid; heat; cool; add potassium dichromate	AAS	NR	Helrich (1990a)
Liquid waste, groundwater	Digest with sulfuric and nitric acids; add potassium permanganate and potassium persulfate solutions; heat; cool; reduce with sodium chloride-hydroxylamine sulfate; add stannous sulfate and aerate	CVAA AAS	0.2 µg/L NR	US Environmental Protection Agency (1986a) (Method 7470); Helrich (1990b)
Soil, sediment, solid and semisolid waste	Digest with distilled water and aqua-regia; heat; cool; add potassium permanganate and heat; cool; add sodium chloride-hydroxylamine sulfate; or digest as above	CVAA	0.2 µg/L	US Environmental Protection Agency (1986b) (Method 7471)
Blood, urine	Reduce inorganic and organic mercury to Hg^o with reducing agents (e.g., SnCl$_2$); estimate organic mercury as difference between total and inorganic	CVAA	0.5 µg/L	Magos & Clarkson (1972)
	Reduce total mercury with sodium borohydride; enrich with an amalgamation device (Au/Pt gauze)	CVAA	0.3 µg/L urine or blood	Angerer & Schaller (1988)
Blood, urine, hair, tissues	Automated form of the method of Magos and Clarkson (1972)	CVAA	2.5 µg/kg	Farant *et al.* (1981)

Abbreviations: CVAA, flameless cold vapour atomic absorption spectroscopy; AAS, flame or flameless atomic absorption spectroscopy; NR, not reported

The original 'dithizone' method has been replaced by atomic absorption spectrometry, neutron activation analysis, atomic fluorescence spectrometry, inductively coupled plasma emission spectrometry and spark source spectrometry. Cold vapour atomic absorption is the most popular and reliable technique. Metallic mercury and inorganic mercury compounds and organomercury compounds in biological and environmental specimens are converted by reducing agents (tin chloride, cadmium chloride–tin chloride, sodium borohydride) to metallic mercury and released as mercury vapour, which is either pumped directly through the quartz cell of the atomic absorption spectrophotometer or analysed after amalgamation on a silver–platinum gauze. The organic mercury content of the sample is given by the difference between total and inorganic compounds. For routine analysis, especially for blood and urine samples, the total mercury content is determined using sodium borohydride as the reducing agent, avoiding time-consuming decomposition of the samples (Angerer & Schaller, 1988).

The neutron activation procedure for analysis in urine is regarded as the most accurate and sensitive procedure and is usually used as the reference method (WHO, 1991).

Helrich (1990a) described several methods (atomic absorption spectrometry, gravimetry, titrimetry) for the determination of mercury and mercury compounds in various forms of drugs (solutions of organomercury compounds, ointments, calomel tablets, tablets containing purgative drugs). Helrich (1990c) described methods (flameless atomic absorption spectrometry, colorimetric dithizone) for the determination of mercury in food and fish and gas chromatographic methods for the determination of methylmercury compounds in fish and shellfish. Helrich (1990d) described methods (volatilization, precipitation, titrimetry, gravimetry) for the determination of mercury in organomercury seed disinfectants.

Pre-analytical and analytical procedures involve the risk of losing mercury from the sample, or contamination. Owing to the small amounts of mercury (in nanogram or even subnanogram ranges) in specimens, especially of biological materials, careful quality control must be undertaken. Control materials (blood and urine) are commercially available for intralaboratory quality control, and national and international intercomparison programmes are offered for external quality control. Reference materials covering the range of samples obtained for monitoring are commercially available for both environmental and biological samples (see WHO, 1991); however, the available control materials for daily use and reference materials do not cover the demand for different mercury species.

(a) *Metallic mercury*

Analytical methods for mercury in air can be divided into instant reading methods and methods with separate sampling and analysis stages. One direct ('instant') reading method is based on the 'cold vapour atomic absorption' technique, which measures the absorption of mercury vapour by ultraviolet light at a wavelength of 253.7 nm. Most of the atomic absorption spectroscopy procedures have a detection limit in the range of 2–5 $\mu g/m^3$ mercury (WHO, 1991).

Another direct reading method employed increasingly is a special gold amalgamation technique, which has been used in a number of studies to evaluate the release of metallic mercury vapour into the oral cavity from amalgam fillings (WHO, 1991). The method is based on an increase in the electrical resistance of a thin gold film after absorption of mercury vapour. The detection limit is 0.05 ng mercury (McNerney *et al.*, 1972).

In an analytical method based on separate sampling and analysis, air is sampled in two bubblers in series containing sulfuric acid and potassium permanganate. The mercury is subsequently determined by cold vapour atomic absorption. With this method, the total mercury in the air, and not just mercury vapour, can be measured. Another sampling technique involves solid absorbents. Amalgamation techniques using gold have been shown to collect mercury vapour efficiently (WHO, 1991).

Air can be sampled for the analysis of mercury by static samplers or by personal monitoring (WHO, 1991). In a comparison of results obtained using static samplers and personal samplers, the latter yielded higher time-weighted average concentrations than the former in most work places (Roels *et al.*, 1987).

(b) Mercuric chloride and mercuric acetate

A dual-stage differential atomization atomic absorption technique was developed to allow speciation of 10 mercury-containing compounds, including mercuric chloride and mercuric acetate, in aqueous solution and biological fluids (Robinson & Skelly, 1982).

(c) Methylmercury compounds

Gas chromatography is usually used for selective measurement of methylmercury compounds and other organomercury compounds, particularly in fish tissues. An alternative approach is to separate methylmercury compounds from inorganic mercury compounds by volatilization, ion exchange or distillation and to estimate them by nonselective methods (e.g. atomic absorption) (WHO, 1990).

(d) Phenylmercury acetate

Phenylmercury acetate was determined in pharmaceutical products by reverse-phase high-performance liquid chromatography of a morpholinedithiocarbamate derivative. The method is specific and sensitive and has been used to determine a number of phenylmercury salts in pharmaceutical products (Parkin, 1987).

1.2 Production and use

1.2.1 *Production*

Worldwide production data for mercury are presented in Table 4. Over the last 10 years, production figures have changed only slightly. Current production in the USA is approximately 53% of the potential capacity: Because of reduced demand, many mines and smelting plants are no longer operating or have greatly cut back production. A large proportion of Mexican production has been exported to Brazil and Argentina. China claims to have the largest mercury resources in the world; most of the Chinese production is exported to the USA. Italy, once a large producer of mercury, now imports it from Algeria and Yugoslavia. The Almadén mercury mine in Spain accounted for 90% of the total output of the European Economic Community for many years, and most of the production has been exported to Belgium, France, Luxembourg and the USA. Whereas in 1986 the former USSR exported most of its mercury, almost the entire production is now reserved for domestic use (Simon *et al.*, 1990; WHO, 1991).

(a) Metallic mercury

All mercury ores are relatively low-grade, the average mercury content being about 1%. Mercury ores lie close to the Earth's surface, so that the required mining depth is about 800 m

Table 4. Worldwide production of mercury (tonnes)

Country	1977	1978	1979	1980	1981	1982	1983	1984	1985	1986	1987	1988	1989	1990	1991
Algeria	1049	1055	506	841	877	386	828	587	795	690	773	690	586	637	431
China[a]	700	600	700	800	800	800	850	800	800	850	900	940	880	800	700
Czechoslovakia	183	196	171	159	153	151	144	152	158	168	164	168	131	126	120
Dominican Republic	18	17	21	6	3	2	4	2	1	NR	< 0.5	< 0.5	< 0.5	NR	NR
Finland	22	39	46	75	67	71	65	80	130	147	147	130	159	141	125
Germany	99	84	91	56	76	53	NR	NR	NR	NR	NR	NR	NR	NR	NR
Italy	14	3	NR	3	252	159	NR	NR	NR	NR	NR	NR	NR	NR	NR
Mexico	333	76	68	145	240	295	221	384	264	345	124	345	651	735	720
Russia[a]	2200	2000	2000	1800	1700	1700	1700	1600	1600	1500	1650	2300	2300	2100	1900
Spain	926	1020	1116	1721	1560	1540	1416	1520	1539	1471	1553	1716	1380[a]	425[a]	450
Turkey	162	173	163	154	204	246	162	182	226	262	202	97	197	60	60
USA	974	834	1018	1058	962	888	864	657	570	470	34	379	414	NR	NR
Former Yugoslavia	108	NR	NR	NR	NR	NR	52	72	88	75	67	70	51	37	30
Total[b]	6788	6097	5900	6818	6894	6291	6306	6036	6171	5978	5906	6835	6749	5061	4536

From Simon et al. (1990); Reese (1992a). NR, not reported
[a]Estimated values
[b]Totals may not add up because some values are estimates.

at most. The most important ore for mercury extraction is α-mercuric sulfide (red) (cinnabar, cinnabarite). The ore is heated with lime in retorts or furnaces to liberate the metal as vapour, which is cooled in a condensing system to form metallic mercury. Other methods include leaching of ores and concentrates with sodium sulfide and sodium hydroxide and subsequent precipitation with aluminium or by electrolysis; alternatively, mercury in ore is dissolved in a sodium hypochlorite solution, the mercury-laden solution is then passed through activated carbon to absorb the mercury, and the activated carbon is heated to produced metallic mercury. The latter methods are, however, no longer used (Drake, 1981; Simon et al., 1990).

Industrial waste containing mercury also contributes to its production. The majority of plants using chloralkali electrolysis employ liquid mercury cathodes, resulting in residues containing 10% mercury or more. In addition to this major secondary source, mercury batteries, mercury fluorescent tubes, electrical switches, thermometer breakage and obsolete rectifiers should be regarded as sources of mercury. Scrap material and industrial and municipal wastes and sludges containing mercury are treated in much the same manner as ores to recover mercury. Scrap products are first broken down to liberate metallic mercury or its compounds. Heating in retorts vaporizes the mercury which, upon cooling, condenses to high-purity metallic mercury. Industrial and municipal sludges and wastes may be treated chemically before roasting (Drake, 1981; Simon et al., 1990). Although the overall production of mercury has decreased over the last 20 years, sufficient potential uses, and therefore secondary sources, remain for the foreseeable future owing to the unique properties of the metal (Simon et al., 1990).

Most of the metallic mercury on the market is 4N material (99.99% mercury). The most common purification methods include: *Dry oxidation*—with this method, readily oxidizable constituents such as magnesium, zinc, copper, aluminium, calcium, silicon and sodium can be removed by passing air or oxygen through the liquid metal; the oxides that form have a lower density than mercury and float on its surface, where they can be removed by filtration, scooping or by removing the mercury from the bottom. *Wet oxidation*—in an aqueous medium, mercury is dissolved by adding nitric, hydrochloric or sulfuric acid (see IARC, 1992) with dichromate, permanganate or peroxide to oxidize impurities; the aqueous solution can be separated from the mercury by decanting, and traces of water can be removed with calcium oxide. *Electrolytic refining*—perchloric acid containing mercuric oxide serves as the electrolyte. *Distillation*—mercury can be evaporated under atmospheric pressure or *in vacuo*; elements with a lower vapour pressure than mercury can be separated in this way. In many cases, mercury must be distilled repeatedly to achieve the desired purity (Simon et al., 1990).

(b) *Mercuric acetate*

Mercuric acetate is produced by dissolving mercuric oxide in dilute acetic acid and concentrating the resulting solution (Simon et al., 1990).

(c) *Mercuric chloride*

Mercuric chloride is prepared by the direct oxidation of mercury with chlorine gas, the same method (chamber method) that is used to prepare mercurous chloride, except that, for mercuric chloride, an excess of chlorine gas is used to ensure complete reaction to the higher oxidation state; the reaction is carried out at temperatures > 300 °C. The escaping sublimate vapour is condensed in cooled receivers, where it settles as fine crystals. Excess chlorine is absorbed by sodium hydroxide in a tower; a very pure product results from use of this method (Singer & Nowak, 1981; Simon et al., 1990).

Mercuric chloride can also be prepared from other mercury compounds. For example, if mercuric sulfate is heated in the dry state with sodium chloride, the evolving mercuric chloride vapour can be condensed to a solid in receivers (Simon et al., 1990).

(d) *Mercuric oxide*

Mercuric oxide can be prepared *via* the anhydrous route by reaction of mercury and oxygen at 350–420 °C under oxygen pressure or by thermal decomposition of mercury nitrates at about 320 °C. Production *via* the wet route, by precipitation, is more important commercially: The oxide is precipitated from solutions of mercuric salts by addition of caustic alkali (usually mercuric chloride solutions with sodium hydroxide). Whether the yellow or the red form is obtained depends on the reaction conditions: Slow crystal growth during heating of mercury with oxygen or during thermal decomposition of mercurous nitrate leads to relatively large crystals (i.e. the red form); rapid precipitation from solution gives finer particles (i.e. the yellow form) (Simon et al., 1990).

(e) *Dimethylmercury*

The reaction of methyl iodide with mercury–sodium amalgam gives dimethylmercury (Drake, 1981).

(f) *Methylmercury chloride*

Organomercury compounds can be synthesized by reaction of Grignard reagents with mercury halides. In order to obtain pure products, the mercury salt and the Grignard reagent must contain the same anion (R is an aromatic or aliphatic group and X is a halogen):

$$RMgX + HgX_2 \rightarrow RHgX + MgX_2$$

Organic mercury compounds can also be produced by the reaction of sulfinic acids (RSO_2H) or their sodium salts with mercury halides (Simon et al., 1990).

(g) *Phenylmercury acetate*

Phenylmercury acetate is prepared by refluxing a mixture of mercuric acetate and acetic acid in a large excess of benzene (see IARC, 1987b), in what is generally referred to as a 'mercuration reaction'. The large excess of benzene is necessary because more than one hydrogen on the benzene ring can be replaced. The technical grade of phenylmercury acetate contains about 85% pure compound; the remaining 15% is di- and tri-mercurated products, which are less soluble than phenylmercury acetate and are removed by recrystallization. The product is isolated after distillation of excess benzene and acetic acid (Singer & Nowak, 1981).

1.2.2 Use

(a) Metallic mercury

The patterns of use of mercury in Germany and in the USA in different periods are presented in Tables 5 and 6. A major use of mercury is as a cathode in the electrolysis of sodium chloride solution to produce caustic soda and chlorine gas (chloralkali industry). About 50 tonnes of liquid metal are used in each of these plants. In most industrialized countries, stringent procedures have been taken to reduce losses of mercury. Mercury is used widely in the electrical industry (in lamps, arc rectifiers and mercury battery cells), in domestic and industrial control instruments (in switches, thermostats, barometers) and in other laboratory and medical instruments. Another use of liquid metallic mercury is in the extraction of gold from ore concentrates or from recycled gold articles (Kaiser & Tölg, 1984; Sax & Lewis, 1987; Budavari, 1989; Agency for Toxic Substances and Disease Registry, 1989; Simon et al., 1990; WHO, 1991).

Table 5. Use patterns for mercury in Germany (%)

Use category	1973	1976	1979	1982	1985
Chloralkali industry	37	32	28	18	23
Catalysis	13	3	8	7	2
Paints, dyes	6	4	3	1	< 1
Pesticides	9	9	11	2	5
Electrical engineering	8	13	14	21	36
Control instruments and apparatus construction	4	3	4	7	4
Chemicals and reagents	7	14	14	21	None
Medicine	7	8	8	9	13
Miscellaneous	9	14	10	14	17
Total (tonnes)	346	325	313	257	182

From Simon et al. (1990)

Table 6. Use patterns for mercury in the USA (%)

Use category	1985	1987	1990	1991	1992
Electrical	64	56	35	33	29
Chloralkali industry	14	12	33	33	34
Paint	9	10	15		
Industrial and control instruments	6	6	7	34	37
Other	7	16	10		

From Carrico (1985, 1987); Reese (1990, 1991, 1992b)

WHO (1991) estimated that, in industrialized countries, about 3% of the total consumption of mercury is in dental amalgams. Dental amalgam is a mixture of mercury with a silver-tin alloy. Most conventional amalgams consist of approximately 45–50% mercury, 25–35% silver, 2–30% copper and 15–30% tin. In industrialized countries, the alloy with mercury is now mixed in sealed capsules and applied in the prepared tooth cavity, where excess amalgam (< 5%) is removed immediately before or during condensation of the plastic mix. The amalgam begins to set within minutes of insertion and must therefore be carved to a satisfactory anatomical form within that period of time. Polishing with rotating instruments can take place after 24 h. Amalgam has been used extensively as a tooth-filling material for more than 150 years and accounts for 75–80% of all single tooth restorations. It has been estimated that each US dentist in private practice uses an average of 0.9–1.4 kg of amalgam per year (Sax & Lewis, 1987).

(b) *Mercuric acetate*

Mercuric acetate is used in the synthesis of organomercury compounds, as a catalyst in organic polymerization reactions and as a reagent in analytical chemistry (Singer & Nowak, 1981; Simon et al., 1990).

(c) *Mercuric chloride*

Mercuric chloride is an important intermediate in the production of other mercury compounds, e.g. mercurous chloride, mercuric oxide, mercuric iodide, mercuric ammonium chloride and organomercury compounds. It is also used as a catalyst in the synthesis of vinyl chloride, as a depolarizer in dry batteries and as a reagent in analytical chemistry. It has a minor importance as a wood preservative and retains some importance as a fungicide. Other uses (e.g. as a pesticide or in seed treatment) have declined considerably (Simon et al., 1990).

(d) *Mercuric oxide*

Red mercuric oxide in particular has become increasingly important commercially in the production of galvanic cells with mercuric oxide anodes in combination with zinc or cadmium cathodes. These cells are distinguished from other systems in that their voltage remains constant during discharge: they are used mainly as small, button-shaped batteries, e.g. for hearing devices, digital watches, exposure meters, pocket calculators and security installations. Additional uses of mercuric oxide are in the production of mercury[II] salts, by treatment with the corresponding acids, and as a reagent in analytical chemistry. Its importance as an additive to antifouling paint for ships and in medicine (e.g. for eye ointment) has decreased (Simon et al., 1990).

(e) *Dimethylmercury*

Dimethylmercury is an environmental contaminant that finds limited use as a laboratory reagent (Budavari, 1989; WHO, 1990).

(f) *Phenylmercury acetate*

The primary use for phenylmercury acetate has been in latex paint; it is used at low levels as a preservative and at higher levels to protect the dry film from fungal attack or mildew. It can be used for these purposes in other aqueous systems, such as inks, adhesives and caulking compounds. Phenylmercury acetate is also used as the starting material in the preparation of many other phenylmercury compounds, which are generally prepared by double-decomposition reactions with the sodium salts of the desired acid groups in aqueous solution. It is also used as a slimicide in paper mills, as a catalyst for the manufacture of certain polyurethanes, as a research chemical (Singer & Nowak, 1981; Sax & Lewis, 1987; Budavari, 1989; Campbell et al., 1992), in contraceptive gels and foams, as a preservative (including in shampoos: see IARC, 1993), as a disinfectant and as a denaturant in ethanol.

(g) *Other mercury-containing compounds*

A number of mercury-containing compounds have been used as topical antiseptics (mercuric iodide, mercuric cyanide, ammoniated mercuric chloride, merbromin [mercurochrome] and merthiolate) and as fungicides, mildewcides, insecticides and germicides (mercurous chloride, phenylmercury oleate, phenylmercury propionate, phenylmercury naphthenate, phenylmercury lactate, phenylmercury benzoate and phenylmercury borate) (Singer & Nowak, 1981; Sax & Lewis, 1987; Budavari, 1989; Simon et al., 1990). A number of alkylmercury compounds are also used as fungicides in the treatment of seed grains (ethylmercury chloride, ethylmercury *para*-toluenesulfonanilide, ethylmercury acetate, ethylmercury 2,3-dihydroxypropyl mercaptide, bis[methylmercury]sulfate, methylmercury dicyandiamide and methoxyethylmercury acetate or chloride) (Greenwood, 1985; Sax & Lewis, 1987). Mercuric fulminate is used as a detonator in explosives (Singer & Nowak, 1981).

Mercury-containing creams and soaps have long been used by dark-skinned people in some regions to obtain a lighter skin tone. The soaps contain up to 3% mercuric iodide, and the creams contain up to 10% ammoniated mercury. Both the soap and the cream are applied to the skin, allowed to dry and left overnight (WHO, 1991).

1.3 Occurrence

1.3.1 *Natural occurrence*

Metallic mercury occurs as a part of the Earth's natural geochemistry, comprising 50 μg/kg of the Earth's crust. It is 62nd in order of abundance (Aylett, 1973). It is found in the form of the sulfide, as cinnabar ore, which has an average mercury content of 0.1–4%; it is also present in the form of geodes of liquid mercury and as impregnated schist or slate. The major source of atmospheric mercury is suggested to be degassing of the Earth's crust and the oceans (Lauwerys, 1983; Berlin, 1986; WHO, 1990).

Methylmercury compounds are formed in aquatic and terrestrial environments from the methylation of metallic mercury and mercuric mercury. Methylation is likely to occur in bacteria in sediments of sea- or lakebeds. The methylmercury compounds formed are accumulated by aquatic organisms, and dimethylmercury gases are formed by degradation and released into the air. Dimethylmercury can be decomposed in the atmosphere by acidic rainwater to monomethylmercury compounds and thus re-enter the aquatic environment (Berlin, 1986). Little is known about the quantitative aspects of these cycles, and the local load of methylmercury compounds can be increased considerably by anthropogenic sources (Clarkson et al., 1988a; WHO, 1990).

1.3.2 Occupational exposures

Approximately 70 000 workers in the USA are regularly exposed to mercury (Campbell *et al.*, 1992). Table 7 lists some potential occupational exposures to the various forms of mercury. Mercury vapour is the commonest form to which workers are exposed in industries such as mining and processing of cinnabar ore and the chloralkali industry, where brine is electrolysed in mercury cells in which the cathode is a flowing sheet of liquid mercury. The manufacture and use of liquid mercury-containing instruments constitute another source of occupational exposure to mercury vapour through breakage, spillage or careless handling. Dental personnel are exposed to mercury vapours through the preparation of dental amalgams (Stokinger, 1981; Clarkson *et al.*, 1988b).

Table 7. Products, industries and jobs in which there is potential occupational exposure to mercury

Metallic mercury	Inorganic mercury compounds	Organomercury compounds
Dental medicine	Disinfectants	Bactericides
Batteries	Paints and dyes	Embalming preparations
Barometers	Explosives	Paper manufacture
Boiler makers	Fireworks manufacture	Farmers
Calibration instruments	Fur processing	Laundry and diaper services
Caustic soda production	Ink manufacture	External antiseptics
Carbon bush production	Chemical laboratory workers	Fungicides
Ceramics	Percussion caps and detonators	Insecticides manufacture
Chloralkali production	Spermicidal jellies	Seed handling
Ultrasonic amplifiers	Tannery workers	Wood preservatives
Direct current meters	Wood preservatives	Germicides
Infrared detectors	Tatooing materials	
Electrical apparatus	Taxidermists	
Electroplating	Vinyl chloride production	
Fingerprint detectors	Embalming preparations	
Silver and gold extraction	Mercury vapour lamps	
Jewellery	Antisyphilitic agents	
Fluorescent, neon, mercury arc lamps	Thermoscopy	
Manometers	Silvering of mirrors	
Paints	Photography	
Paper pulp manufacture	Perfumery and cosmetics	
Photography	Acetaldehyde production	
Pressure gauges		
Thermometers		
Semiconductor solar cells		

From Campbell *et al.* (1992)

Mixed exposure to aerosols of organic or inorganic mercury compounds also occurs: Chlorine in combination with mercury vapour, produced in chloralkali industries, forms mercuric chloride aerosols. Another source of occupational exposure is in pathology laboratories, where mercuric chloride is used with formalin as a histological fixative. Exposure to aerosols of methyl- and ethylmercury compounds has been described in connection with the manufacture and use of mercuric salts and during seed treatment (Berlin, 1986). Disinfectant manufacturers, fungicide manufacturers, seed handlers, farmers, lumberjacks, pharmaceutical industry workers and wood preservers may be exposed to organomercury compounds (Campbell et al., 1992).

Data on exposure to mercury in air and the results of biological monitoring in various industries and occupations are described below and summarized in Tables 8 and 9 (pp. 258–260). It should be noted that the concentrations of mercury detectable in the general working environment are generally lower than those to which individual workers are exposed, as detected by personal air sampling. This is due to the fact that mercury can accumulate on the clothes, hair and skin of workers, creating a situation which has been called 'microenvironmental exposure'. In a Belgian manufacturing plant, mercury concentrations in the general work environment were between 8 and 88 $\mu g/m^3$, while personal samples from the workers showed concentrations ranging from 16 to 680 $\mu g/m^3$ (see Ehrenberg et al., 1991).

Biological monitoring of people occupationally exposed to mercury vapours and inorganic mercury compounds, by measuring mercury in urine and blood mercury, reflects recent exposure. Occupational and environmental exposure to methylmercury compounds can be estimated from blood mercury levels. Mercury in hair can be used as an indicator of environmental exposure to methylmercury compounds but not for monitoring exposure to metallic mercury and inorganic mercury compounds (Elinder et al., 1988).

(a) Chloralkali plants

Exposures in chloralkali plants have been reviewed (WHO, 1976). In recent studies, covering mainly Swedish plants, average urinary mercury concentrations of 50–100 $\mu g/L$ were reported (WHO, 1991).

In a study in the USA and Canada of 567 male workers in 21 chloralkali plants, the mean atmospheric concentration of mercury was 65 $\mu g/m^3$ (SD, 85); in 12 plants, the time-weighted average concentration was 100 $\mu g/m^3$ or less, while in the remainder some employees were exposed to higher concentrations. At an ambient air concentration of 100 $\mu g/m^3$, the concentration in blood was about 60 $\mu g/L$ and that in urine about 200 $\mu g/L$. In 117 control subjects, blood mercury concentrations were lower than 50 $\mu g/L$; in 138 controls, urinary mercury concentrations were generally less than 10 $\mu g/L$ (corrected to specific gravity) (Smith et al., 1970).

The airborne concentrations of mercury in a chloralkali plant in Italy were between 60 and 300 $\mu g/m^3$; the mean urinary concentration in 55 workers exposed for 11.5 ± 8.8 years in cell preparation rooms was 158 $\mu g/L$ (range, 0–762 $\mu g/L$) and that in 17 workers exposed to mercury irregularly for 15.2 ± 10.7 years was 40.3 $\mu g/L$ (range, 0–96 $\mu g/L$) (Foà et al., 1976).

The atmospheric concentrations of mercury in a chloralkali plant in Sweden in 1975 were 64 $\mu g/m^3$ (range, 36–112 $\mu g/m^3$); the mean blood mercury concentration in 13 workers employed for 0.5–5.5 years was 238 nmol/L (47.6 $\mu g/L$), and the mean urinary concentration in the same subjects was 808 nmol/L (range, 369–1530 nmol/L) [161 $\mu g/L$; range, 74–306 $\mu g/L$]. Two years later, after improvement of the ventilation systems in the plant, the mean concentrations of mercury were 22.6 (range, 15–43) $\mu g/m^3$ in air, 92 nmol/L

(18.4 µg/L) in blood and 196 (range, 117–327) nmol/L [39.2 µg/L; range, 23–65 µg/L] in urine in a group of 16 workers who had been employed for one to seven years (Lindstedt et al., 1979).

Exposure to mercury in a chloralkali plant in Sweden was studied during ordinary maintenance work and in workers hired for a special repair task during a temporary production shutdown. A group of 14 normal maintenance workers were exposed to mean air concentrations of mercury of 65 µg/m^3 (range, 24–123 µg/m^3) and had a mean blood mercury concentration of 73 nmol/L, ranging from 45 to 150 nmol/L [14.6 µg/L; range, 9–30 µg/L], and a mean urinary concentration of 32 nmol/mmol (57.2 µg/g) creatinine (range, 16–43 nmol/mmol; 28.6–76.9 µg/g). The 16 special repair workers were exposed to a mean air concentration of 131 µg/m^3 (range, 38–437 µg/m^3) and had a mean blood mercury concentration of 148 nmol/L, ranging from 85 to 240 nmol/L [29.6 µg/L; range, 17–48 µg/L), and a mean urinary mercury concentration of 6.1 nmol/mmol (10.9 µg/g) creatinine (range, 4.7–8.7 nmol/mmol; 8.4–15.5 µg/g) (Sällsten et al., 1992).

In an epidemiological study of 1190 workers in eight Swedish chloralkali plants (described in detail on p. 271), biological monitoring data indicated a substantial reduction in exposure to mercury with time, from about 200 µg/L in urine during the 1950s to 150 µg/L in the 1960s and less than 50 µg/L in 1990 (Barregård et al., 1990). In another Swedish chloralkali plant, the average levels of mercury in air were 25–50 µg/m^3 throughout the 1980s. The mean concentrations of mercury in 26 male workers were 252 nmol/L (50.4 µg/L) in urine, 48 nmol/L (9.6 µg/L) in plasma and 78 nmol/L (15.6 µg/L) in erythrocytes, and those in 26 unexposed workers were 19 nmol/L (3.8 µg/L) in urine, 7.5 nmol/L (1.5 µg/L) in plasma and 33 nmol/L (6.6 µg/L) in erythrocytes (Barregård et al., 1991). The mean concentrations of mercury in 1985–86 in another group of 89 chloralkali workers in Sweden, who had been exposed for 1–45 years, were 55 nmol/L (11 µg/L) in blood, 45 nmol/L (9 µg/L) in serum and 14.3 nmol/mmol (25.5 µg/g) creatinine in urine. The concentrations in a control group of 75 non-occupationally exposed workers were 15 nmol/L (3 µg/L) in blood, 4 nmol/L (0.8 µg/L) in serum and 1.1 nmol/mmol (1.95 µg/g) creatinine in urine (Langworth et al., 1991).

In chloralkali plants, exposure to asbestos can occur during various maintenance operations (Barregård et al., 1990; Ellingsen et al., 1993).

(b) *Thermometer production*

In 1979, exposure to metallic mercury vapour was studied in a small thermometer factory in Israel with generally inadequate engineering and hygiene arrangements. The mean mercury concentrations in five workers exposed to 50–99 µg/m^3 were 299 nmol/L (59.8 µg/L) in urine and 105 nmol/L (21 µg/L) in blood; those in three workers exposed to 100–149 µg/m^3 were 449 nmol/L (89.8 µg/L) in urine and 122 nmol/L (24.4 µg/L) in blood; and those in seven workers exposed to 150–200 µg/m^3 were 628 nmol/L (125.6 µg/L) in urine and 143 nmol/L (28.6 µg/L) in blood (Richter et al., 1982).

Concentrations of mercury were measured in four thermometer plants in Japan: The air concentrations ranged from 25 to 226 µg/m3; those of inorganic mercury compounds in blood ranged from 80 to 1150 nmol/L (16–230 µg/L); those of metallic mercury in blood ranged from not detected to 1.10 nmol/L (not detected–0.22 µg/L); those of inorganic mercury compounds in urine ranged from 96 to 1560 nmol/L (19.2–312 µg/L); and those of metallic mercury in urine ranged from 0.05 to 1.22 nmol/L (0.01–0.24 µg/L) (Yoshida, 1985).

In a thermometer factory in the USA, 17 personal samples showed mean air concentrations of mercury of 75.6 µg/m^3 (range, 25.6-270.6); 11 area samples showed a mean of 56.7 µg/m^3 (range, 23.7–118.5). The mean urinary mercury concentration in 79 workers employed for 65 ± 48.9 months was 73.2 ± 69.7 µg/g creatinine (range, 1.3–344.5) (Ehrenberg et al., 1991).

In a thermometer factory in Sweden, where filling with mercury was done inside a ventilated hood but with spillage of mercury during temperature conditioning and testing, the mean concentration of mercury in the air was 39 µg/m^3 (range, 15–58). In seven workers, the median blood mercury concentration was 57 nmol/L (11.4 µg/L), and in six workers, the median urinary concentration was 21 nmol/mmol (37.5 µg/g) creatinine (Sällsten et al., 1992).

(c) Hospitals

In Belgium, a group of 40 chemical and biological laboratory technicians employed for < 1–15 years were exposed to an average airborne mercury concentration of 28 µg/m^3 (range, 2–124). The mean mercury concentration in urine was 10.72 ± 1.49 µg/g creatinine, and that in whole blood was 10.0 ± 0.9 µg/L. The mean mercury concentrations in a group of 23 unexposed technicians were 2.30 ± 1.49 µg/g creatinine in urine and 6.5 ± 1.1 µg/L in blood (Lauwerys & Buchet, 1973).

In a study in Scotland, use of mercuric chloride as a histological fixative was associated with high atmospheric concentrations of mercury vapour (up to 100 µg/m^3) and of all mercury compounds (200 µg/m^3). Twenty-one technicians exposed to this environment had a median urinary mercury output of 265 nmol (53 µg)/24 h. The median urinary output among a control group of 21 subjects was 72 nmol (14.4 µg)/24 h (Stewart et al., 1977).

Hospital employees who repair sphygmomanometers or work in areas in which such machines are repaired are potentially exposed to mercury. In 13 hospitals in the USA, in which most employees had worked for less than 10 years, the airborne concentrations of mercury in repair rooms ranged from 1 to 514 µg/m^3, and 86 employees tested had a mean urinary mercury concentration of 12.4 µg/L (range, 1–200) (Goldberg et al., 1990).

(d) Dental personnel

Special interest has focused on occupational exposure to mercury in dentistry. Several studies conducted during 1960–80 reported average concentrations of mercury vapour in dental clinics ranging between 20 and 30 µg/m^3 air; in certain clinics concentrations of 150–170 µg/m^3 were measured (WHO, 1991). In some of these studies, urinary mercury concentrations of dental personnel were also reported.

An average urinary mercury concentration of 40 µg/L was found among 50 dentists in the USA, with some values exceeding 100 µg/L (Joselow et al., 1968). In a nationwide US study, the average mercury concentration in the urine of 4272 dentists sampled between 1975 and 1983 was 14.2 µg/L (range, 0–556 µg/L). In 4.9% of the samples, the concentrations were ≥ 50 µg/L, and in 1.3% they were > 100 µg/L. The wide range of values was probably due to variations in occupational exposure to amalgams with time, in addition to variations in sampling techniques and other methodological problems (Naleway et al., 1985). At the annual sessions of the American Dental Association, on-site screening for exposure to mercury showed mean urinary concentrations of 5.8 µg/L in 1042 dentists in 1985 and 7.6 µg/L in 772 dentists in 1986; 10% contained concentrations above 20 µg/L (Naleway et al., 1991).

Blood samples from a group of 130 dentists in Denmark in 1986 contained a median mercury concentration of 4.0 µg/L (range, 1.2–19.2); 2.0 µg/L (1.1–4.6) were found in controls. Practice characteristics, as stated on questionnaires, were not significantly related to blood mercury concentration, but 49 dentists who ate one or more fish meals per week had a median concentration 47% higher than that of dentists who seldom consumed fish (Möller-Madsen et al., 1988).

In 82 dental clinics in northern Sweden, the median concentration of mercury vapour in air was 1.5 µg/m^3 in public surgeries and 3.6 µg/m^3 in private ones. The urinary mercury concentrations in 505 occupationally exposed subjects ranged from 1.4 to 2.9 nmol/mmol (2.5–5.13 µg/g) creatinine, which are of the same order of magnitude as those of the Swedish population as a whole. The load derived from the amalgam fillings of the exposed subjects was estimated to be of the same order of magnitude as that from the working environment (Nilsson et al., 1990). In the offices of six dentists in Sweden, the mean concentration of mercury in air was 4.5 µg/m^3 (range, 1.7–24); the mean concentrations in 12 subjects were 17 nmol/L (range, 6–29) (3.4 µg/L; range, 1.2–5.8 µg/L) in blood and 2.6 nmol/mmol (4.6 µg/g) creatinine (range, 1.1–5.4 nmol/mmol; 2.00–9.65 µg/g) (Sällsten et al., 1992). In 224 dental personnel in Sweden, the levels of mercury in urine (1.8 nmol/mmol [3.19 µg/g] creatinine) were not significantly higher than those of 81 referents (1.1 nmol/mmol [1.95 µg/g] creatinine), and no difference was seen for the plasma or blood levels. When adjustment was made, however, for amalgam fillings in the mouths of the personnel, significant differences in urinary, plasma and blood mercury concentrations were seen (Akesson et al., 1991).

Urinary excretion of inorganic mercury compounds was determined in 50 individuals attached to Madras Dental College, India. The lowest concentration observed was 3 µg/L and the highest, 136.6 µg/L. Of those subjects who handled mercury, 70% had urinary concentrations > 20 µg/L (Karthikeyan et al., 1986).

(e) *Others*

The airborne concentrations of mercury in Idrija, Slovenia, in 1950 were reported to be 0.05–5.9 mg/m^3 in a mine and 0.17–1.1 mg/m^3 in a smelter (Vouk et al., 1950). Similar values were reported during a survey conducted in 1963: 0.1–2.0 mg/m^3 in both the mine and the smelter. The average concentration of mercury in blood from 57 asymptomatic miners in Idrija was 77 µg/L (range, 0–450); the corresponding value in 16 workers with symptoms of intoxication was 110 µg/L (range, 0–510). The concentrations in urine were 276 µg/L (range, 0–1275) in the asymptomatic miners and 255 µg/L (range, 2.0–601) in those with symptoms (Ladd et al., 1966).

Concentrations > 2.0 mg/m^3 were detected in 1964 in a mine and smelter on Palawan Island, the Philippines (Ladd et al., 1966).

The average concentrations of mercury in the air in various departments in the Italian hat manufacturing industry in 1942-52 were 0.09-2.21 mg/m^3. The concentrations were > 0.2 mg/m^3 in 13 of the 17 departments studied, and concentrations as high as 4 mg/m^3 were measured in specific locations (Baldi et al., 1953).

In a mercury distillation plant in Italy, airborne mercury concentrations ranged from 0.005 to 0.278 mg/m^3; the mean urinary concentration in 19 workers was 108.26 ± 55.61 µg/L and the mean blood concentration, 77 ± 28 µg/L. In 13 subjects in a control group, the urinary mercury concentration was < 10 µg/L, while in 11 other subjects, the mean value was 15.27 µg/L (range, 11-21) (Angotzi et al., 1980).

In a recycling distillation plant in Germany, the concentration of mercury in air in February 1984 ranged from 115 to 379 µg/m^3; in 12 workers in the plant, mercury was found at 28-153 µg/L in blood and 128-609 µg/g creatinine in urine. In previous years, the levels of both biological indicators (determined since 1978) were decidedly higher: 44-255 µg/L in blood and 143-1508 µg/g creatinine in urine. The authors cited the 'normal' values for mercury as 0.2-7.2 µg/L (mean, 0.6) in blood and 0.2-5.0 µg/g creatinine (mean, 0.8) in urine (Schaller et al., 1991).

Individual external exposure in a dry alkaline battery plant in Belgium was to 40 µg/m^3 mercury, ranging from 10 to 106 µg/m^3. Urinary mercury concentrations were usually < 50 µg/g creatinine in some parts of the plant and between 50 and 100 µg/g creatinine in others (Roels et al., 1987).

In a plant for the manufacture of fluorescent lamps in Italy, the mercury concentrations in air in maintenance areas in 1984-85 were between 2 and 5 µg/m^3; 27 workers employed for 10.96 ± 1.14 years in those areas had mean urinary concentrations of 5.15 ± 2.2 µg/L (range, 2-11). In the same plant, the concentrations in the air of production areas varied between 6 and 44 µg/m^3, and 22 workers employed for 10.34 ± 1.43 years in those areas showed mean urinary concentrations of 4.94 ± 1.62 µg/L (range, 1.9-8) (Assennato et al., 1989).

In a study of reproductive function among women employed at a mercury vapour lamp factory (described in detail on pp. 296-297), De Rosis et al. (1985) reported that time-weighted average concentrations exceeded 50 µg/m^3 in 1972-76; after modification of the ventilation system, the concentrations dropped to < 10 µg/m^3.

1.3.3 Air

The most important sources of mercury in the atmosphere are degassing of the Earth's crust, emissions from volcanoes and evaporation of mercury vapours from natural bodies of water. Recent estimates indicate that these natural emissions amount to 2700-6000 tonnes per year; however, it is difficult to determine the relative contributions of natural and anthropogenous sources to the general emission of mercury in the biosphere, since some may have been deposited in water from the atmosphere and produced by human activities (WHO, 1990). Traditional municipal solid-waste incinerators may have a significant impact on the ambient air concentration as well as on the deposition rates of mercury. Rates of emission of mercury from traditional incinerators in Europe, Canada and the USA range from 100 to 2200 µg/m3 and those from advanced incinerators, 30-200 µg/m^3. Such emissions could result in deposition rates of 0.2-4.0 and 0.02-1.0 µg/m^2 per day, respectively (WHO, 1988).

Table 8. Occupational exposure to mercury in various industries and occupations

Industry and activity (country) [year, when available]	No. of workers	Air (µg/m³) Mean±SD	Air (µg/m³) Range	Urine (µg/L, except where noted) Mean±SD	Urine (µg/L, except where noted) Range	Blood (µg/L) Mean±SD	Blood (µg/L) Range	Reference
Chloralkali plants (USA and Canada; 21 plants) Cell room	567	65±85	<10–270 (TWA) <1–2640					Smith et al. (1970)
Chloralkali plant (Italy) Cell rooms Miscellaneous	72 55 17		60–300	157.79±120.94 40.29±26.16	0–762 0–96			Foà et al. (1976)
Chloralkali plant [1975] (Sweden) [1977]	13 16	64±21.8 22.6±7	36–112 15–43	161.6±62.8 39.2±14.4	74–306 23–65	47.6±23.8 18.4±6.8		Lindstedt et al. (1979)
Chloralkali plant (Sweden)	26	NR	25–50	50.4	5–186	NR		Barregård et al. (1991)
Chloralkali plant (Sweden) [1985–86]	89	NR	NR	25.5[a]	0.5–84[a]	11		Langworth et al. (1991)
Chloralkali plant (Sweden) Normal maintenance Special maintenance	NR NR	65 (14 samples) 131 (16 samples)	24–123 38–437	57[a] (8 samples) 10.9[a] (5 samples)	29–77[a] 8.4–15[a]			Sällsten et al. (1992)
Thermometer factory (Israel) [1979]	5 3 7	NR	50–99 100–149 150–200	59.8 89.8 125.6		14.6 (8 samples) 29.6 (7 samples) 21 24.4 28.6	9–30 17–48	Richter et al. (1982)
Thermometer factories (Japan; 4 factories)	27	NR	25–226	NR	19–312	NR	16–230	Yoshida (1985)
Thermometer factory (USA)	84	75.6 (17 samples)	25.6–271	73.2±69.7[a] (79 samples)	1.3–344.5[a]			Ehrenberg et al. (1991)
Thermometer factory (Sweden)	NR	39 (13 samples)	15–58	37.5[a] (6 samples)	1.96–91[a]	11.4 (7 samples)	6–20	Sällsten et al. (1992)
Pathology laboratory (Belgium)	40	28	2–124	10.72±1.49[a]	NR	10.0±0.9		Lauwerys & Buchet (1973)

Table 8 (contd)

Industry and activity (country) [year, when available]	No. of workers	Air (μg/m³) Mean±SD	Air (μg/m³) Range	Urine (μg/L, except where noted) Mean±SD	Urine (μg/L, except where noted) Range	Blood (μg/L) Mean±SD	Blood (μg/L) Range	Reference
Pathology laboratory (United Kingdom)	21	200		26.5		NR		Stewart et al. (1977)
Sphygmomanometer repair (USA; 13 facilities)	93	86	1–514	12.4±22.2 (86 samples)	1–200	NR		Goldberg et al. (1990)
Dental staff (USA) [1975–83]	4272	NR	NR	14.2±25.4	0–556	NR		Naleway et al. (1985)
Dental staff (India)	50	NR	NR	NR	3–136.6	NR		Karthikeyan et al. (1986)
Dental staff (Sweden; 82 clinics) [1983]	505	NR	1.5–3.6	NG	2.5–5.13	NG		Nilsson et al. (1990)
Dental staff (USA) [1985] [1986]	1042 772	NR NR	NR NR	5.8±8.5 7.6±11.8	max, 84 max, 115	NR		Naleway et al. (1991)
Dental staff (Denmark) [1986]	130	NR	NR	NR	NR	4.0	1.2–19.2	Möller-Madsen et al. (1988)
Dental staff (Sweden; 6 offices)	NR	4.5 (36 samples)	1.7–24	4.6	1.96–9.65	3.4	1.2–5.8	Sällsten et al. (1992)
Mercury distillation (Italy) [1976–78] Distillation Maintenance	 19 19	 NR NR	5–279	 108.26±55.61 84.11±45.54	 NR NR	 77±28 53±16		Angotzi et al. (1980)
Recycling plant (Germany) [1984]	12	NR	115–379	128–609[a]		28–153		Schaller et al. (1991)
Dry alkaline battery plant (Belgium) [1984]	10	40 (46 samples)	10–106	< 100[a] (10 samples)				Roels et al. (1987)
Fluorescent lamps (Italy) [1984–85] Maintenance Production	 27 22	 NR NR	 2–5 6–44	 5.15±2.2 4.94±1.62	 2–11 1.9–8	 NR NR		Assennato et al. (1989)

NR, not reported
[a] μg creatinine

Table 9. Concentration of mercury in the air of work places in Finland during 1977–88 and in blood in 1987

Industrial code or work	Air concentrations (µg/m³)			Concentration in blood (µg/L)			
	No. of measurements	Mean	Range	No. of workplaces	No. of measurements	Mean	Range
Seed dressing and packing	11	4	1–13	10	27	3.6	1–9
Pesticide manufacture	8	58	29–105	1	24	10.4	3–46
Mercury production	NR	32	13–157	NR	NR	NR	NR
Welding	24	88	2–150	NR	NR	NR	NR
Manufacture of light bulbs, fluorescent tubes and batteries	133	30	1–250	5	17	5.8	2–8
Laboratory work	26	15	1–120	NR	NR	NR	NR
Dentistry	136	10	1–100	21	42	4.4	1–9
Chlorine industry	NR	NR	NR	3	518	13.6	1–69

From Anttila et al. (1992). NR, not reported

Mercury concentrations in the atmosphere range from a few nanograms per cubic metre over remote, uncontaminated areas to about 20 ng/m^3 in urbanized areas. Concentrations have been estimated to be 2 ng/m^3 in the northern hemisphere and about 1 ng/m^3 in the southern hemisphere. Concentrations of mercury up to 18 ng/m^3 have been reported in the atmosphere close to active volcanoes (Berlin, 1986; Clarkson et al., 1988a).

Mercury vapour is believed to be the predominant form in the atmosphere. There is evidence that some of the mercury in ambient air is in the form of alkylmercury, and the presence of methylmercury compounds has been reported. The particulate fraction of mercury in air (as a percentage of total mercury) is usually 4% or less (WHO, 1990).

Another source of mercury in the atmosphere is the release of metallic mercury vapour during the cremation of cadavers, when all the mercury from amalgam fillings vaporizes as the temperature reaches above 800 °C. It is difficult to estimate the global release of mercury from cremation because of the uncertainties about dental status at the time of death and about the frequency of cremation (WHO, 1991).

1.3.4 *Water*

Mercury is removed from the atmosphere mainly by precipitation. The chemical species of mercury in water is mainly ionic mercury[II]. Concentrations of mercury in surface water are very low, and accurate analysis is still a problem. Total mercury concentrations range from 0.5 to 3 ng/L in open oceans, from 2 to 15 ng/L in coastal seawater and from 1 to 3 ng/L on average in freshwater rivers and lakes (WHO, 1990). The bottom sediment of lakes and oceans may contain 20–250 µg/kg mercury (Berlin, 1986). Concentrations in drinking-water are generally less than 25 ng/L (WHO, 1990).

Concentrations of mercury in inland waters of gold-mining areas in Rondônia, Brazil, were between < 0.1 and 8.6 µg/L (Pfeiffer et al., 1989). A study of water from the Madeira River and its tributaries, in the centre of the gold rush area in Brazil, showed an average mercury level of 24.6 ng/L (Nriagu et al., 1992).

1.3.5 *Soil and plants*

The commonest form of mercury in soil is the bivalent ion. Concentrations measured in soils are generally less than 1 ppm (mg/kg). Methylation of mercury has been demonstrated in soil and is influenced by humidity, temperature and the mercury concentration of the soil (Sequi, 1980; Simon et al., 1990).

The accumulation of mercury in plants increases with increasing soil concentration. Soil type has a considerable influence on this process: a high content of organic matter decreases the uptake. Generally, the highest concentrations of mercury are found at the roots, but translocation to other organs (e.g. leaves) occurs. In contrast to higher plants, mosses take up mercury from the atmosphere (WHO, 1989a).

Mercury concentrations in bottom sediments of Brazilian polluted rivers ranged between 50 and 19 800 µg/kg (Pfeiffer et al., 1989).

1.3.6 *Food*

Environmental contamination with mercury leads to a critical concentration effect in animals that occupy higher positions in the food chain (large fish and fish-eating sea fowl)

(Simon et al., 1990). The factors that determine the methylmercury concentration in fish are the mercury content of the water and bottom sediments, the pH and redox potential of the water and the species, age and size of fish (Berlin, 1986).

The concentrations of mercury in most foods are generally below the reported limit of detection, which is usually 20 µg/kg fresh weight. A large proportion of the mercury in food—at least in animal products—is likely to be in the form of methylmercury compounds. Most of the mercury in fish is as methylmercury compounds, which are formed in the bottom sediment of the ocean and in freshwater systems and are enriched to a high degree in the aquatic food chain, with the highest levels occurring in the predatory fish: The concentrations of total mercury in edible tissues of shark and swordfish are > 1200 µg/kg, whereas anchovies and smelt have average values of < 85 µg/kg (Berlin, 1986; WHO, 1990).

In a survey sponsored by the Ministry of Food, Agriculture and Forestry of Germany, the average mercury contamination of 759 specimens of fish from German fishing grounds was < 100 µg/kg (Jacobs, 1977). The mercury concentrations in edible parts of fish from polluted rivers in Brazil were between 70 and 2700 µg/kg wet wt (Pfeiffer et al., 1989).

The average daily intake of mercury can be estimated by assuming that intake from non-fish food sources is negligible in comparison with that from fish. FAO estimated an average worldwide fish intake of 16 g per person per day but an average daily intake of 300 g in populations that are largely dependent on fish; therefore, the average daily intake of total mercury will result in 3 µg, of which 80% is methylmercury compounds and 20% inorganic mercury. The average intake of methylmercury compounds can thus be calculated as 2.4 µg per day, with 2.16 µg retained (90% absorption), and the average daily intake of inorganic mercury is 0.6 µg per day, with 60 ng retained (10% absorption) (Clarkson et al., 1988a; Table 10). Daily intake from the consumption of fish from polluted water, however, can rise to toxic levels, as occurred in Minamata and Niigata in Japan around 1953–66: Concentrations of 1–20 mg/kg in fish resulted in daily intake, in people with frequent fish consumption (200–500 g per day), of 5 mg per day (Berlin, 1986).

Table 10. Estimated average daily intake and retention of various forms of mercury in populations not occupationally exposed to mercury

Source	Estimated daily intake and retention (ng mercury/day)					
	Mercury vapour		Inorganic mercury compounds		Methylmercury compounds	
	Intake	Absorbed	Intake	Absorbed	Intake	Absorbed
Atmosphere	40	32				
Water			50	5		
Food			600	60	2400	2160
Total intake	40		650		2400	2160
Absorbed		32		65		

From Clarkson et al. (1988a)

Toxic levels have also been reached following consumption of bread prepared from wheat treated with methylmercury dicyandiamide fungicide, as occurred in Iraq in the winter of 1971–72 (Bakir et al., 1973; Greenwood, 1985).

1.3.7 Dental amalgam

Dental amalgams are a potential source of exposure to mercury vapour not only for dental staff but also for the general population. Hardening of the amalgam continues over many months, so that stress on the amalgam surface, produced by chewing or grinding of the teeth, causes breakdown of a surface barrier and release of mercury vapour into the mouth. This results in the deposition of mercury in body tissues like kidney and brain and increased urinary excretion. The release of mercury from amalgams makes a significant contribution to human exposure to inorganic mercury, including mercury vapour (Clarkson et al., 1988b; WHO, 1991; US Department of Health and Human Services, 1993).

Different concentrations of mercury are released from unstimulated amalgams (3.3–7.4 ng/min) and stimulated amalgams (16.3–163.2 ng/min) (Clarkson et al., 1988b). Average daily intake of metallic mercury vapour can thus range from 3.8 to 21 µg/day, with corresponding retentions of 3–17 µg/day (WHO, 1990, 1991).

In 147 individuals in an urban Norwegian population, correlations were found between the concentrations of mercury in urine (mean, 17.5 nmol/L [3.5 µg/L]) and in exhaled air (mean, 0.8 µg/m^3) and between both urinary and air concentrations and the number of amalgam restorations, the number of amalgam-restored surfaces and the number of amalgam-restored occlusal surfaces. The results suggested that individuals with more than 36 restored surfaces absorb 10–12 µg of mercury per day (Jokstad et al., 1992).

1.3.8 Mercury-containing creams and soaps

The mean concentration of mercury in the urine of 60 African women who used skin-lightening creams, containing 5–10% ammoniated mercury, was 109 µg/L (range, 0–220). Those in the urine of six women who had used skin-lightening creams containing 1–3% ammoniated mercury for two years ranged from 28 to 600 µg/L (WHO, 1991).

Mercury was found in the blood (91.1 µg/L) and urine (784 µg/g creatinine) of a woman who had been using soap containing 1% mercuric iodide for about 15 years. Mercury was also present in the blood (19 µg/L) and urine (274 µg/g creatinine) of her three-month-old child, who was not directly exposed to mercury (Lauwerys et al., 1987).

1.3.9 Mercury-containing paint

Air samples from 19 homes recently painted with an interior latex paint with a median mercury concentration of 754 mg/L contained a median of 2 µg/m^3 mercury, while concentrations in 10 uncoated houses were below the detection limit of 0.1 µg/m^3. The median concentration in urine was higher for 65 exposed inhabitants (8.4 µg/g creatinine) than for 28 unexposed people (1.9 µg/g creatinine) (Agocs et al., 1990; WHO, 1991).

1.3.10 Human tissues and secretions

In order to establish reference values for mercury concentrations in whole blood, blood cells and plasma, 98 publications in the international scientific literature presenting biological data on individuals not occupationally exposed to mercury were reviewed critically and graded for quality (Brune et al., 1991). The mean levels of mercury in non-fish eaters were 2.0 µg/L (10th-90th percentiles, 0-4.3) in whole blood, 3.8 (2.8-4.8) in blood cells and 1.3 (0.3-2.3) µg/L in plasma. Although the authors recognized the importance of retrieving information on the number of amalgam restorations, few data were available.

In 380 Italian subjects non-occupationally exposed to mercury, the mean urinary concentration of mercury was 3.5 µg/L (range, 0.1-6.9) (Minoia et al., 1990). Average urinary mercury concentrations in 50 male and 54 female residents of the Monte Amiata mercury mine area in Italy were greater than those in 104 controls from other regions of the country: men, 2.3 µg/g creatinine (95% CI, 1.7-3.0); women, 3.9 µg/g creatinine (95% CI, 2.2-5.6); men and women combined, 3.1 µg/g creatinine (95% CI, 2.2-4.1) (Cicchella et al., 1968).

Mercury levels in the hair of unexposed populations are generally between 0.5 and 4 mg/kg. Hair mercury is indicative of blood mercury concentration at the point of growth, so that sequential analysis of hair segments provides information on past exposure to mercury and particularly to organomercury compounds (Bakir et al., 1973; Kazantzis et al., 1976).

In Sweden, increased concentrations of mercury were found in samples from former dental staff (seven dentists and one dental assistant) of the pituitary gland (average, 9.8 µmol [1.96 mg]/kg wet weight; range, 0.7-28 [0.14-5.6]), occipital cortices (average, 0.33 µmol [0.07 mg]/kg wet weight; range, 0.07-1.43 [0.014-0.3]), renal cortices (average, 8.6 µmol [1.7 mg]/kg wet weight; range, 4.7-11.3 [0.9-2.3]), and thyroid gland (range, 0.32-140 µmol [0.06-28 mg]/kg wet weight). Mercury was found together with selenium at a rough stoichiometric ratio of 1:1. In the general population, the average concentrations were 0.12 (0.03-5.83) µmol/kg wet weight in pituitary gland, 0.053 (0.012-0.114) in occipital cortices, 1.4 (0.11-4.04) in renal cortices and 0.019 (0.004-0.047) in abdominal muscles (Nylander & Weiner, 1991).

1.4 Regulations and guidelines

Occupational exposure limits and guidelines established in different parts of the world are given in Table 11. The recommended health-based occupational exposure limit is 0.05 mg/m^3 (WHO, 1980; Simon et al., 1990). The recommended health-based limit for long-term occupational exposure to mercury vapours is 50 µg/g creatinine in urine (WHO, 1980).

The American Conference of Governmental Industrial Hygienists (1992) gave notice of their intent to establish biological exposure indices for mercury in blood and urine. The values proposed are 35 µg/g creatinine for total inorganic mercury in urine in preshift samples and 15 µg/L for total inorganic mercury in blood at the end of a working week. The German biological tolerance values for metallic mercury and inorganic mercury compounds are 50 µg/L in blood and 200 µg/L in urine; that for organomercury compounds is 100 µg/L in blood (Deutsche Forschungsgemeinschaft, 1992). The Finnish guideline values for biological measurements are 10 µg/L in blood and 25 µg/L in urine (Anttila et al., 1992).

The WHO recommended guideline for all forms of mercury in drinking-water is 1 µg/L (WHO, 1992). The maximum contaminant level of mercury in drinking-water and the permissible level in bottled water in the USA is 2 µg/L (US Environmental Protection Agency, 1991; US Food and Drug Administration, 1992).

Table 11. Occupational exposure limits and guidelines for mercury and mercury compounds

Country or region	Year	Concentration (mg/m^3)	Substances affected	Interpretation[a]
Australia	1990	0.01	Alkyl mercury compounds (as Hg)	TWA, S
		0.03	Alkyl mercury compounds (as Hg)	STEL, S
		0.05	Mercury and mercury vapour	TWA, S
		0.1	Aryl mercury compounds, inorganic mercury compounds (as Hg)	TWA, S
Austria	1982	0.1	Mercury and mercury vapour	TWA
		0.01	Organic mercury compounds (as Hg)	TWA, S
Belgium	1990	0.01	Alkyl mercury compounds (as Hg)	TWA, S
		0.03	Alkyl mercury compounds (as Hg)	STEL, S
		0.05	Mercury and mercury vapour, mercury compounds except alkyls (as Hg)	TWA, S
		0.1	Aryl mercury compounds, inorganic mercury compounds (as Hg)	TWA, S
Brazil	1978	0.04	Inorganic mercury compounds (as Hg)	TWA
Bulgaria	1984	0.01	Mercury and mercury vapour, inorganic mercury compounds (as Hg)	TWA
Chile	1983	0.008	Alkyl mercury compounds (as Hg)	TWA, S
		0.04	Mercury and mercury vapour	TWA
China	1979	0.01	Mercury and mercury vapour	TWA
		0.005	Organic mercury compounds (as Hg)	TWA, S
Former Czechoslovakia	1991	0.05	Mercury and mercury vapour, mercury compounds except mono- and dialkyls (as Hg)	TWA
		0.15	Mercury and mercury vapour, mercury compounds except mono- and dialkyls (as Hg)	Ceiling
Denmark	1990	0.01	Alkyl mercury compounds (as Hg)	TWA, S
		0.05	Mercury and mercury vapour, mercury compounds except alkyls (as hg)	TWA
Egypt	1967	0.1	Mercury and mercury vapour	TWA
Finland	1992	0.01	Alkyl mercury compounds (as Hg)	TWA, S
		0.05	Mercury and mercury vapour, inorganic mercury compounds (as Hg)	TWA
France	1990	0.01	Alkyl mercury compounds (as Hg)	TWA, S
		0.05	Mercury and mercury vapour	TWA, S
		0.1	Aryl mercury compounds, inorganic mercury compounds (as Hg)	TWA, S
Germany	1992	0.1	Mercury and mercury vapour	TWA, S
		0.01	Organic mercury compounds except methylmercury (as Hg) (total dust)	TWA, S, sensitizer
		0.01	Methylmercury (total dust)	TWA, PR1, S, sensitizer

Table 11 (contd)

Country or region	Year	Concentration (mg/m^3)	Substances affected	Interpretation[a]
Hungary	1990	0.02	Mercury and mercury vapour, inorganic mercury compounds (as Hg)	TWA, sensitizer
		0.04	Mercury and mercury vapour, inorganic mercury compounds (as Hg)	STEL
		0.01	Inorganic mercury compounds (as Hg)	STEL
		0.01	Organic mercury compounds except mono- and dialkyl compounds (as Hg)	TWA, STEL
India	1983	0.01	Alkyl mercury compounds (as Hg)	TWA, S
		0.03	Alkyl mercury compounds (as Hg)	STEL, S
		0.05	Mercury and mercury vapour	TWA
		0.15	Mercury and mercury vapour	STEL
Indonesia	1978	0.01	Organic mercury compounds (as Hg)	TWA, S
		0.1	Alkyl mercury compounds (as Hg)	TWA, S
Italy	1978	0.01	Organic mercury compounds (as Hg)	TWA, S
		0.05	Inorganic mercury compounds (as Hg)	TWA, S
Japan	1991	0.05	Mercury and mercury vapour, mercury compounds except alkyl compounds (as Hg)	TWA
Mexico	1991	0.05	Mercury compounds except alkyl compounds (Hg)	TWA
		0.01	Alkyl mercury compounds (as Hg)	TWA
		0.03	Alkyl mercury compounds (as Hg)	15-min, 4 ×/day, 1-h interval
Netherlands	1986	0.05	Inorganic mercury compounds (as Hg)	TWA
		0.01	Alkyl mercury compounds (as Hg)	TWA, S
Poland	1990	0.01	Mercury and mercury vapour, organic mercury compounds (as Hg)	TWA
		0.05	Inorganic mercury compounds (as Hg)	TWA
Republic of Korea	1983	0.05	Mercury and mercury vapours	TWA
		0.03	Alkyl mercury compounds (as Hg)	TWA
Romania	1975	0.05	Mercury and mercury vapour	TWA, S
		0.15	Mercury and mercury vapour	STEL, S
		0.01	Organic mercury compounds (as Hg)	STEL, S
Sweden	1992	0.01	Alkyl mercury compounds (as Hg)	TWA, S
		0.05	Mercury and mercury vapour, mercury compounds except alkyl compounds (as Hg)	TWA, S
Switzerland	1990	0.05	Mercury and mercury vapour	TWA, S
		0.01	Organic mercury compounds (as Hg)	TWA, S, sensitizer
		0.1	Inorganic mercury compounds (as Hg)	TWA, PR1, S, sensitizer
Taiwan	1981	0.01	Organic mercury compounds (as Hg)	TWA, S
		0.05	Inorganic mercury compounds (as Hg)	TWA, S

Table 11 (contd)

Country or region	Year	Concentration (mg/m³)	Substances affected	Interpretation[a]
United Kingdom	1992	0.01	Alkyl mercury compounds (as Hg)	TWA, S
		0.03	Alkyl mercury compounds (as Hg)	STEL, S
		0.05	Mercury and mercury vapour, mercury compounds except alkyls (as Hg)	TWA
		0.15	Mercury and mercury vapour, mercury compounds except alkyls (as Hg)	STEL (10 min)
USA				
OSHA	1992	0.01	Alkyl mercury compounds (as Hg), organic mercury compounds (as Hg)	TWA, PEL, S
		0.03	Alkyl mercury compounds (as Hg), organic mercury compounds (as Hg)	STEL, PEL, S
		0.05	Mercury and mercury vapour	TWA, PEL, S
		0.1	Aryl mercury compounds, inorganic mercury compounds (as Hg)	Ceiling, PEL, S
NIOSH	1990	0.01	Alkyl mercury compounds (as Hg), organic mercury compounds (as Hg)	TWA, REL, S
		0.03	Alkyl mercury compounds (as Hg), organic mercury compounds (as Hg)	STEL, REL, S
		0.05	Mercury and mercury vapour	TWA, REL, S
ACGIH	1992	0.01	Alkyl mercury compounds (as Hg)	TWA, TLV, S
		0.03	Alkyl mercury compounds (as Hg)	STEL, TLV, S
		0.05	Methylmercury, all forms except alkyl vapours	TWA, TLV, S
		0.1	Aryl mercury compounds, inorganic mercury compounds (as Hg)	TWA, TLV, S
Former USSR	1990	0.005	Mercury and mercury vapour	TWA
		0.05	Inorganic mercury compounds (as Hg)	TWA
		0.2	Inorganic mercury compounds (as Hg)	STEL
Venezuela	1978	0.01	Alkyl mercury compounds (as Hg)	TWA, S
		0.03	Alkyl mercury compounds (as Hg)	Ceiling, S
		0.05	Inorganic mercury compounds (as Hg)	TWA
		0.15	Inorganic mercury compounds (as Hg)	Ceiling
Former Yugoslavia	1971	0.1	Mercury and mercury vapour	TWA
		0.01	Alkyl mercury compounds (as Hg)	TWA, S

From Arbeidsinspectie (1986); Cook (1987); US Occupational Safety and Health Administration (OSHA) (1992); US National Institute for Occupational Safety and Health (1990); International Labour Office (1991); American Conference of Governmental Industrial Hygienists (ACGIH) (1992); Arbejdstilsynet (1992); Deutsche Forschungsgemeinschaft (1992); Health & Safety Executive (1992); UNEP (1993)

[a]The concentrations given may or may not have regulatory or legal status in the various countries; for interpretation of the values, the original references or other authoritative sources should be consulted. PR1, a risk of damage to the developing embryo or fetus has been demonstrated unequivocally, even when exposure limits have been adhered to; S, absorption through the skin may be a significant source of exposure; TWA, time-weighted average; STEL, short-term exposure limit; PEL, permissible exposure limit; REL, recommended exposure limit; TLV, threshold limit value.

The Joint FAO/WHO Expert Committee on Food Additives set a provisional tolerable weekly intake of 300 µg total mercury per person, of which no more than 200 µg (3.33 µg/kg bw for a 60-kg individual) should be present as methylmercury compounds (WHO, 1989b). In Japan, a provisional tolerable weekly intake of 250 µg mercury per week, with no more than 170 µg as methylmercury, was calculated from the WHO values on the basis of 50 kg body weight. This weekly intake is considered to be one-tenth of the minimum toxic dose of adults and is therefore expected to give protection against fetal damage (WHO, 1990).

Stationary sources in the USA where mercury ore is processed to recover mercury, where mercury chloralkali cells are used to produce chlorine gas and alkali metal hydroxide and where wastewater treatment plant sludge is incinerated or dried are subject to the US national emission standard for mercury. Thus, atmospheric emissions from mercury ore processing facilities and mercury-cell chloralkali plants cannot exceed 2300 g of mercury per 24-h period. Atmospheric emissions from sludge incineration plants, sludge drying plants, or a combination of these, where wastewater treatment plant sludges are processed cannot exceed 3200 g of mercury per 24-h period (US Environmental Protection Agency, 1992).

In the countries of the European Communities, no detectable quantity of mercury is allowed in colouring matter authorized for use in food intended for human consumption (Commission of the European Communities, 1981). The threshold value for mercury in tuna fish in Denmark is 0.5 mg/kg (Rasmussen, 1984). In Sweden, it was recommended that the consumption of fish caught in areas of high contamination (but below 1.0 mg/kg) be restricted to one meal per week (Swedish Expert Group, 1970).

Use of mercury compounds as cosmetic ingredients in the USA is limited to eye-area cosmetics, at concentrations not exceeding 65 ppm (0.0065%) of mercury calculated as the metal (about 100 ppm or 0.01% phenylmercury acetate or nitrate) (US Department of Health and Human Services, 1992). In the European Communities, mercury and its compounds must not be used in cosmetic products, except that thiomerosal (mercurothiolate) and phenylmercury salts (including borate) can be used for eye make-up or eye make-up remover, with a maximum concentration of 0.007% mercury (Commission of the European Communities, 1990, 1991).

2. Studies of Cancer in Humans

Many populations have low-grade or infrequent exposure to metallic mercury or mercury compounds. The Working Group restricted their review to studies specific to metallic mercury or mercury compounds and to groups who are known to have considerable exposure.

2.1 Inorganic mercury compounds

2.1.1 *Descriptive studies*

In a study in Poland, mercury was determined in the hair of leukaemia patients and in healthy relatives and unrelated healthy subjects (Janicki *et al.*, 1987). The mean content of total mercury was 1.24 ± 1.93 mg/kg hair from 23 cases of acute leukaemia and 0.49

± 0.41 mg/kg hair from 79 healthy control subjects. In 47 cases of acute leukaemia (chronic granulocytic as well as chronic lymphocytic), the mercury content was 0.92 ± 1.44 mg/kg hair. For 19 leukaemia cases of all groups and their 52 relatives, the corresponding figures were 0.69 ± 0.75 mg/kg and 0.43 ± 0.24 mg/kg, respectively. These differences between cases and control subjects were significant. [The Working Group noted that comparisons of means are inappropriate, as the distributions were highly skewed, and that the distribution of mercury may have been affected by the disease.]

In Washington State, USA, occupational mortality was studied for the period 1950-71 on the basis of death certificates (Milham, 1976). For male dentists, the proportionate mortality ratio (PMR) for all malignant neoplasms was 1.05 (127 cases [95% confidence interval (CI), 0.88-1.25]). When sites with more than five cases were considered, the PMR was 1.53 for pancreatic cancer based on 12 cases [95% CI, 0.79-2.69), 1.32 for prostatic cancer based on 20 cases [95% CI, 0.80-2.03] and 1.45 for neoplasms of the lymphatic and haematopoietic tissues based on 17 cases [95% CI, 0.84-2.33).

Occupational mortality was studied in British Columbia, Canada, by the proportionate mortality method and based on 320 423 deaths for which valid records were available among men over 20 years of age (Gallagher *et al.*, 1985). The occupational codes were those used in conjunction with the censuses of 1951 and 1961. Among dentists, there were four cases of kidney cancer (PMR, 1.94; 95% CI, 0.52-4.96) and five tumours of the brain and central nervous system (PMR, 2.36; 95% CI, 0.76-5.52). There were even fewer cases at other sites, or no more than slightly elevated PMRs.

2.1.2 *Cohort studies* (see Table 12, p. 272)

(a) *Nuclear weapons industry workers*

A cohort of 2133 white men from Oak Ridge, TN, USA, who were exposed to metallic mercury and an unexposed cohort of 3260 workers from the same plant were studied with regard to mortality in comparison with national rates for white men (Cragle *et al.*, 1984). Exposure to mercury occurred in the context of lithium production in a nuclear weapons plant, which earlier had also produced a fissionable isotope of uranium; anyone in whom mercury had ever been found in the urine, regardless of the concentration, was considered to have been exposed. A mercury monitoring programme was started in mid-1953 and became effective in late 1954. The cohorts were followed-up from 1 January 1953 until 1 January 1979, when vital status was assessable for at least 95.5% of the cohort and death certificates were available for 98% or more. Total mortality was lower than expected for both groups, and there was no excess of any non-cancer death possibly related to mercury exposure (target organs were thought to be liver, lung, brain and other central nervous system, and kidney). The cancer mortality rate was lower than expected for the exposed cohort (standardized mortality ratio [SMR], 0.94 [95% CI, 0.75-1.16]; based on 85 cases) but not for the unexposed (SMR, 1.10 [0.94-1.28]; based on 175 cases). An excess of lung cancer was seen in both cohorts (SMR, 1.34 [0.97-1.81], based on 42 cases among exposed; and 1.34 [1.05-1.69], based on 71 cases among unexposed). For cancers of the brain and central nervous system, the corresponding figures were 1.22 ([0.33-3.12]; based on 4 cases) for the exposed cohort and 2.30 ([1.22-3.94]; based on 13 cases) for the unexposed; for kidney cancer, the SMRs were reported to be 1.65 ([0.45-4.23]; based on 4 cases) for the exposed cohort and 0.72 ([0.15–2.10]; based on 3 cases) for the unexposed. In subgroups with mercury levels in urine exceeding 0.3 mg/L at least once or with more than one year of exposure, there was also no clear increase in cancer mortality rates. No definite explanation could be given for the excess of lung cancer observed in both cohorts, but life-style factors or some factor other than mercury present in the plant were mentioned.

(b) Dentists

Cohorts of 3454 male and 1125 female dentists and 4662 dental nurses identified from the Swedish census in 1960 were followed for cancer development in the period 1961–79 by linkage with cancer register data (Ahlbom *et al.*, 1986). The overall standardized incidence ratio (SIR) was 2.1 (95% CI, 1.3–3.4) for glioblastoma (astrocytoma III–IV) in comparison with national incidence rates, based on 18 cases. The SIRs for the various cohorts were 2.0 for male dentists, 2.5 for female dentists and 2.2 for dental nurses. In the combined cohorts, there were also four gliomas (astrocytoma I–II) (SIR, 1.8; 95% CI, 0.5–4.7) and six meningiomas (SIR, 1.3; 95% CI, 0.5–2.8). There was no excess of all tumours in these cohorts. For comparison, physicians and female nurses were also studied; no indication was found of an excess of glioblastomas. Exposures to amalgam, chloroform and X-radiation were mentioned as possible occupational factors.

In another analysis of this population, occupational risks for intracranial gliomas in Sweden were studied by linking cancer incidence data from the national cancer registry during 1961–79 with census data on occupation from 1960 (McLaughlin *et al.*, 1987). The expected number of cases for each occupational category was calculated on the basis of the general population in the study period, and regional adjustment was applied. There were 3394 gliomas in men and 1035 in women who had been employed in 1960. An excess risk was found for male dentists, with an SIR of 2.1 ($p < 0.05$) based on 12 cases; for female dental assistants, nine cases (SIR, 2.1; $p = 0.09$) were reported. For comparison, it may be noted also that among male physicians there were 14 cases (SIR, 1.4; nonsignificant) and among female physicians, four cases (SIR, 3.7; $p < 0.05$). Male chemists, physicists, veterinary surgeons, agricultural research scientists and pharmacists also had SIRs greater than 2.0. [The Working Group noted that no distinction was made between the various subtypes of glioma.]

Mortality risks by occupation have been studied among veterans who served in the US Armed Forces between 1917 and 1940 (Hrubec *et al.*, 1992). Occupation and smoking status were assessed through questionnaires in 1954 and 1957. Follow-up to 1980 was done using insurance and pension systems (96% complete for First World War veterans). The smoking-adjusted relative risk (RR) for each occupation was estimated by using all other occupations as the standard, and Poisson regression modelling was applied. In a subcohort of 2498 dentists with a total of 1740 deaths, there were 299 cancer deaths (RR, 0.9; 90% CI, 0.80–0.97). The risk for pancreatic cancer was 1.4 (90% CI, 0.98–1.86; 27 deaths). No excess of brain or kidney tumours was detected (RR, 0.9; 90% CI, 0.45–1.74; 6 cases; and RR, 0.8; 90% CI, 0.39–1.50; 6 cases, respectively). For a group of 267 medical and dental technicians, there was an elevated risk for all cancers among 40 nonsmokers (RR, 2.5; 90% CI, 1.36–4.73; 7 deaths). For nonsmokers and smokers in this group, the risk for all cancers was only slightly elevated (RR, 1.2; 90% CI, 0.87–1.54; 34 deaths), but there was an excess of colon cancer (RR, 1.9; 90% CI, 1.01–3.53; 7 deaths).

(c) Chloralkali workers

Mortality and cancer incidence were reported for a group of 1190 male Swedish chloralkali workers in whom mercury had been measured in the blood or urine for at least one year between 1946 and 1984 (Barregård *et al.*, 1990). Their mortality and cancer incidence were compared with those of the general male population for the periods 1958–84 and 1958–82, respectively, and the follow-up was complete. The mean level of mercury excreted in the urine had been about 200 µg/L in the 1950s, 150 µg/L in the 1960s and less than 50 µg/L in the 1980s. On the basis of crude estimates, 26% of the cohort was estimated to have had an accumulated urinary mercury dose of 1000 years·µg/L or more, 457 subjects also had some (mostly low-grade) asbestos exposure; exposure to static magnetic fields was reported to have occurred. Mortality from all causes was not significantly increased, the observed to expected mortality being 1.1 (95% CI, 0.9–1.3) based on 147 deaths with 10 or more years of latency. There were 51 incident cases of cancer observed *versus* 42 expected with a latency of 10 years or more, i.e. a rate ratio of 1.2 (95% CI, 0.9–1.6). Lung cancer was the only type of tumour in clear excess, with 10 observed and 4.9 expected with a latency of 10 years or more (rate ratio, 2.0; 95% CI, 1.0–3.8). There were slight excesses of some other cancers with a latency of 10 years or more, namely three brain tumours *versus* 1.1 expected (RR, 2.7; 95% CI, 0.5–7.7), three kidney cancers *versus* 1.9 expected (1.6; 0.3–4.7), five urinary bladder cancers *versus* 2.9 expected (1.7; 0.6–4.1) and 10 prostatic cancers *versus* 8.6 expected (1.2; 0.6–2.1). The excess of lung cancer was thought to be due to exposure to asbestos; one case of mesothelioma was observed. Smoking was considered to explain 10% of the excess of lung cancer, although information on smoking habits was available for only a 7% random sample of the cohort. The authors noted that chloralkali workers have five to 10 times the mercury exposure of dental personnel.

In a cohort study of 674 male Norwegian chloralkali workers exposed to inorganic mercury for more than one year prior to 1980, who had a mean cumulative urinary concentration of 740 µg/L, there were 204 deaths *versus* 210.7 expected (SMR, 0.97; 95% CI, 0.84–1.11) and 89 incident cases of cancer *versus* 85.0 expected (SIR, 1.05; 95% CI, 0.84–1.29) (Ellingsen *et al.*, 1993). During the follow-up period (1953–89 for incidence and 1953–88 for mortality), there were 19 incident cases of lung cancer, with 11.5 expected (SIR, 1.66; 95% CI, 1.00–2.59) on the basis of national rates. There was no correlation with cumulative mercury dose, employment or latency; a somewhat increased frequency of smoking and exposure to asbestos (one mesothelioma was found) were considered to explain the excess of lung cancer. Three kidney cancers and two brain tumours were observed *versus* 3.2 and 2.45 expected, respectively. These two sites were considered by the authors to be of primary interest with regard to exposure to mercury.

(d) Mercury miners

In a cohort study of the relationship between silicosis and mortality from lung cancer in US metal miners, the difference in risk for silicotic miners compared with nonsilicotic white metal miners was greater for mercury miners than for other miners (Amandus & Costello,

Table 12. Cohort studies of populations exposed to inorganic mercury compounds

Study population Period of follow-up	End-point		Site	No. of cases	SMR	95% CI	Reference
Nuclear weapons industry workers							
2133 Mercury exposed, 3260 unexposed male workers, USA, 1953–79	Mortality	Exposed	Lung	42	1.34	[1.0–1.8]	Cragle et al. (1984)
			Kidney	4	1.65	[0.4–4.2]	
			Brain	4	1.22	[0.3–3.1]	
		Unexposed	Lung	71	1.34	[1.0–1.7]	
			Kidney	3	0.72	[0.1–2.1]	
			Brain	13	2.30	[1.2–3.9]	
Dentists							
9201 Dentists and dental nurses, Sweden, 1961–79	Incidence		Glioblastoma	18	2.1	1.3–3.4	Ahlbom et al. (1986)
			Glioma	4	1.8	0.5–4.7	
			Meningioma	6	1.3	0.5–2.8	
2498 Dentists, US veterans, 1954–80	Mortality		Pancreas	27	1.4	0.96–1.86	Hrubec et al. (1992)
			Brain	6	0.9	0.45–1.74	
			Kidney	6	0.8	0.39–1.50	
267 Medical and dental assistants, US veterans, 1954–80	Mortality		Colon	7	1.9	1.01–3.53	Hrubec et al. (1992)
			Brain	1	1.5	NR	
			Kidney	2	2.8	NR	
Chloralkali workers							
1190 Males, Sweden, 1946–82	Incidence		Lung	13	[1.8]	[0.9–3.0]	Barregård et al. (1990)
			Kidney	4	[1.3]	[0.4–3.4]	
			Brain	4	[1.8]	[0.5–4.7]	
674 Males, Norway, 1953–89	Incidence		Lung	19	1.66	1.00–2.59	Ellingsen et al. (1993)
			Kidney	3	0.95	0.2–2.8	
			Brain	2	0.8	0.1–3.0	
Mercury miners							
274 Males, USA, 1959/61–75	Mortality	11 Silicotics	Lung	3	14.0	2.89–41.0	Amandus & Costello (1991)
		263 Nonsilicotics	Lung	8	2.66	1.15–5.24	

NR, not reported

1991). The follow-up was from date of examination in 1959–61 to 31 December 1975. For the 11 silicotic mercury miners, the SMR was 14.0 (95% CI, 2.89–41.0) based on three lung cancer deaths, whereas the SMR for the 263 nonsilicotic mercury miners was 2.66 (95% CI, 1.15–5.24) based on eight cases. For other miners (copper, lead–zinc, iron and others), the corresponding figures were 1.39 [95% CI, 0.70–2.49] based on 11 silicotic lung cancer deaths and [1.14; 95% CI, 0.93–1.37] based on 110 deaths from nonsilicotic lung cancer. The reference for calculating the SMRs was death rates in white US males. No explanation was offered for the differences seen between mercury and other miners. [The Working Group noted that the small numbers of silicotic mercury miners may make the estimate unstable.]

2.1.3 *Case–control studies* (see Table 13, p. 274)

In a case–control study of incident cases of lung cancer admitted during 1981–83, 340 male and 36 female cases and 817 male and 75 female hospital controls, all residents of metropolitan Florence, Italy, were drawn from the regional general hospital for the analyses (Buiatti *et al.*, 1985). Occupational histories were collected from each subject directly; six female cases but no control had ever worked as felt-hat makers ($p = 0.01$). Heavy exposure to mercury but also to arsenic and other chemicals was reported to have occurred in the Italian hat-making industry.

In a study described in detail in the monograph on beryllium (pp. 73–74; Carpenter *et al.*, 1988), based on 29 cases identified from information on death certificates as ever exposed to mercury, the odds ratio for cancer of the central nervous system was 1.77 [95% CI, 0.5–5.8] when compared with unexposed cases. The matched analysis by highest rank ever held *versus* rank 0 yielded odds ratios of 2.01, 1.33 and 1.19 for ranks 1, 2 and 3, respectively (all odds ratios had a p value of 0.26 or greater). When risk estimates were calculated with a 10-year latency, the odds ratios were 1.58, 0.77 and 1.57 for ranks 1, 2 and 3, respectively, with a p value of 0.47 or greater. A further analysis based on time spent in ranks 2 and 3, assuming a 10-year latency, yielded odds ratios of 0.00, 0.96, 0.00 and 1.86 for workers with > 1 year and < 3 years, 3–10 years, 11–20 years and 21 years or more in ranks 2 and 3 compared with ranks 0 and 1. The authors concluded that their study does not support the hypothesis that occupational exposures to any of the 26 chemicals studied increase appreciably the risk for cancers of the central nervous system.

The effects of a great number of exposures were considered in a case–control study from Montréal, Canada, involving all major cancer forms and population controls as well as two hospital control series, i.e. cancer cases and other cases (Siemiatycki, 1991). In total, 4576 incident cancer cases were recruited through local informants at the hospitals. Completed questionnaires and interviews on occupational exposures (293 agents were considered) were obtained for 3730 of these (response rate, 81.5%). A total of 740 population controls were drawn from electoral lists or obtained by random-digit dialling. Of these, exposure was successfully assessed for 533 (72.0%). The prevalence of exposure to metallic mercury was 0.6% and that to any mercury compound (including metallic mercury), 2%. For prostatic cancer, 14 of 449 cases were exposed to mercury compounds, resulting in an odds ratio of 1.7 (90% CI, 1.0–3.0); five cases had been exposed to metallic mercury, giving an odds ratio of 6.2 (90% CI, 1.2–33.2). For lung cancer, four of the 857 cases had been exposed to metallic mercury (odds ratio, 4.0; 90% CI, 1.2–13.0). For bladder cancer, 14 of the 484 cases had been

Table 13. Case–control studies of populations exposed to inorganic mercury compounds

Study population	End-point	Exposure	Sex	No. of exposed cases	Odds ratio	95% CI	Reference
Lung cancer							
Hospital-based, Italy	Incidence	Hat makers	F	6		$p = 0.01$	Buiatti et al. (1985)
Population-based, Canada	Incidence	Mercury, metallic	M	4	4.0	1.2–13.0[a]	Siemiatycki (1991)
Prostatic cancer							
Population-based, Canada	Incidence	Mercury, metallic	M	5	6.2	1.2–33.2[a]	Siemiatycki (1991)
		Mercury and mercury compounds[b]	M	14	1.7	1.0–3.0	
Bladder cancer							
Population-based, Canada	Incidence	Mercury and mercury compounds[b]	M	14	1.5	0.9–2.6[a]	Siemiatycki (1991)
Brain tumours							
Population-based, USA	Mortality	Nuclear facilities	Central nervous system	29	1.77	[0.5–5.8]	Carpenter et al. (1988)
Population-based, Australia	Incidence	Amalgam fillings	Glioma		0.47	0.25–0.91	Ryan et al. (1992)
			Meningioma		1.04	0.43–2.47	

[a]90% CI
[b]Including organomercury compounds

exposed to mercury compounds (odds ratio, 1.5; 90% CI, 0.9–2.6). Significant results were not obtained for cancers at other sites. [The Working Group noted that although several potential confounding factors were considered not all possible occupational confounders were addressed.]

A case–control study from Adelaide, Australia, considered incident brain tumours and exposure to amalgam fillings and diagnostic dental X-rays (Ryan et al., 1992). Cases aged 25–74 were notified by neurosurgeons in Adelaide, and there was a further check for cases in cancer and brain tumour registries. Controls were selected from the Australian electoral roll, covering 95% of the adult population. In total, 190 cases of brain tumours were identified, together with 662 controls; of these, 110 glioma cases, 60 meningioma cases and 417 controls were included in the analyses. There was a decreased odds ratio (0.47; 95% CI, 0.25–0.91) for glioma in association with self-reported amalgam fillings (at least one filling) and with diagnostic X-rays (at least one X-ray) (odds ratio, 0.42; 95% CI, 0.24–0.76); the corresponding results for meningioma were 1.04 (95% CI, 0.43–2.47) in relation to fillings, whereas the risk associated with diagnostic X-rays was slightly increased (odds ratio, 1.37; 0.68–2.73). No dose–response pattern was seen for either glioma or meningioma with regard to amalgam fillings. The authors considered a biological protective mechanism unlikely.

2.2 Organomercury compounds

2.2.1 Descriptive studies

Direct SMRs for biliary tract cancer in the Japanese prefectures in 1975 were correlated with an environmental pollution index related to use of agricultural chemical products for the years 1962–66 (Yamamoto et al., 1986). In both men and women, only weak, non-significant correlations were found for exposure to mercuric compounds (such as phenylmercury acetate, used as a fungicide in Japan until 1971) converted to the dose of inorganic mercury, whereas positive and significant correlations were obtained, especially for DDT and some phenoxy herbicides.

The mortality pattern was studied in the population of a small area of the city of Minamata, Kumamoto Prefecture, Japan, which consisted mainly of fishermen and their families (Tamashiro et al., 1986) and where 70% of the 1612 confirmed cases (including 527 deaths) of Minamata disease (see pp. 291–292) in the Prefecture through 1983 were known to have occurred. SMRs were computed for different causes of death in 1970–81 by using age-specific rates for the entire city for 1972–78. The total population of the study area in 1975 was 3887 versus 36 782 in the city. Some migration took place during the study period, and, in particular, young adults moved out of the area and former residents returned. The SMR for all causes of death was 1.05 (95% CI, 0.95–1.15, based on 412 deaths) and that for all cancers was 1.18 (95% CI, 0.96–1.46, based on 84 deaths). For the various cancers reported, the corresponding figures were: oesophagus, 2.05 (95% CI, 0.67–4.78; 5 cases); stomach, 0.77 (95% CI, 0.42–1.29; 14 cases); liver, 2.07 (95% CI, 1.16–3.42; 15 cases); pancreas, 0.99 (95% CI, 0.20–2.88; 3 cases); trachea–bronchus–lung, 1.52 (95% CI, 0.79–2.65; 12 cases); breast, 2.64 (95% CI, 0.54–7.71; 3 cases); uterus, 0.89 (95% CI, 0.24–2.28; 4 cases); leukaemia, 1.82 (95% CI, 0.50–4.66; 4 cases); and other cancers, 0.98 (95% CI, 0.63–1.46; 24 cases). An elevated SMR was also seen for chronic liver disease and cirrhosis

(2.16; 95% CI, 1.41–3.17; based on 26 cases). There was some evidence that alcohol consumption in the area was above the Japanese average. [The Working Group noted that the increased risk for liver cancer seems consistent with the increased occurrence of chronic liver disease and cirrhosis and with a higher than average alcohol consumption; the latter might also have affected the risk for oesophageal cancer.]

The effects on life expectancy of elevated exposure to methylmercury compounds were studied in five coastal towns of southern Japan in comparison with a surrounding control area (Tamashiro *et al.*, 1987). The average hair concentrations of mercury were reported to be three to six times higher in the exposed area than in the control area. The study period was from 1969 through to 1982. The crude RR for death from malignant neoplasms was [1.05].

2.2.2 *Cohort study*

It was reported in letter to the Editor that 1657 people with a licence for seed disinfection using organomercury compounds and other agents, issued between 1965 and 1976, were followed through the Swedish Cancer Registry from the date of licencing until death or December 1982 (Wiklund *et al.*, 1988). The mean follow-up time was 14.7 years, resulting in 24 429 person-years of observation. Five tumours of the nervous system were observed *versus* 4.98 expected (SIR, 1.0; 95% CI, 0.33–2.34); rates of tumours at other sites were not reported. The authors noted that the use of alkylmercury compounds was banned in Sweden in the mid-1960s, and limitations were placed on mercury disinfection.

2.2.3 *Case–control studies* (see Table 14, p. 277)

Three similarly designed studies on soft-tissue sarcomas in different parts of Sweden, mainly focusing on exposure to phenoxyacetic acid herbicides and chlorophenols, also provide data on exposure to organomercury seed dressings and other pesticides (Eriksson *et al.*, 1981; Hardell & Eriksson, 1988; Eriksson *et al.*, 1990). The first study encompassed 110 cases and 219 population controls in the five southernmost counties. The second study involved 55 cases and 220 living and 110 dead controls and a third group of 190 other cancer controls in the three northernmost counties. In the third study, there were 237 cases and 237 controls from the seven central counties, matched on vital status. Information on exposure was obtained from questionnaires to the subjects or their next-of-kin, supplemented with telephone interviews. Exposure to mercury seed dressings was reported for 8.2% of cases and 4.6% of controls in the first study; for 1.9% of cases and 3.5% of living and 2.8% of dead controls in the second study; and for 4.6% of cases and 5.2% of controls in the third study. The resulting odds ratio in the first study [not given] was said to have a 90% CI that included unity. [A calculation results in a crude odds ratio of 1.9 (95% CI, 0.65–5.3) for the first study and, for the second study, 0.52 (95% CI, 0.01–4.3) with regard to living controls and 0.66 (95% CI, 0.08–5.74) using dead controls.] The odds ratio in the third study was given as 0.89 (95% CI, 0.40–1.96).

In a study from northern Sweden on malignant lymphomas, which mainly considered exposure to organic solvents, chlorophenols and phenoxyacetic acid herbicides, exposure frequencies to organomercury seed dressings were also reported (Hardell *et al.*, 1981). The study included 169 cases (60 Hodgkin's lymphomas, 109 non-Hodgkin lymphomas) and 338

(335 used in the calculation) population controls. Information on exposure was obtained through questionnaires. For the cases and controls, 5.3 and 3.0%, respectively, exposure to mercury seed dressings co-varied with exposure to phenoxyacetic acid herbicides, whereas asbestos and glass fibre exposure co-varied with chlorophenol exposure. Exposure to phenoxyacetic acid herbicides as well as to chlorophenols appeared to be strong risk factors for lymphomas, but after exclusion of subjects with exposure to phenoxy herbicides, 128 cases and 311 controls remained, with exposure frequencies to mercury seed dressings of 4.7 and 2.9%, respectively; for DDT, the corresponding figures were 5.5 and 3.5%. [For the restricted material, a calculation results in a crude odds ratio of 1.78 (95% CI, 0.62–5.11) for mercury seed dressings and 1.6 (95% CI, 0.51–4.6) for DDT.]

Table 14. Population-based case–control studies of populations of men exposed to organomercury seed dressings in Sweden

No. of exposed cases	Odds ratio	95% CI	Reference
Soft-tissue sarcomas			
[9]	[1.9]	[0.65–5.3]	Eriksson *et al.* (1981)
[1]	[0.52][a]	[0.01–4.3]	Hardell & Eriksson (1988)
	[0.66][b]	[0.08–5.7]	
[10]	0.89	0.40–1.96	Eriksson *et al.* (1990)
Lymphomas			
[6]	1.78	[0.62–5.1]	Hardell *et al.* (1981)

[a] Living controls
[b] Dead controls

3. Studies of Cancer in Experimental Animals

3.1 Metallic mercury

Intraperitoneal administration

Rat: A group of 39 male and female BDIII and BDIV rats, three months old, received two intraperitoneal injections of 0.05 ml **metallic mercury** [purity unspecified] over 14 days (total dose, 0.1 ml); mean survival was 580 days in treated rats and 780 days in controls. Only gross lesions were investigated histopathologically. At 22 months, when 12/39 animals were still alive, one female rat had a spindle-cell sarcoma in the abdominal cavity. Two females and two males of the 11 remaining rats developed similar tumours (Druckrey *et al.*, 1957). [The Working Group noted the incomplete reporting of the study and the possibility that the lesions seen were the result of a solid-state effect.]

3.2 Mercuric chloride

3.2.1 Oral administration

(a) Mouse

A group of 54 male and 54 female Swiss mice (Charles River CD strain), 20 days old, were given drinking-water containing **mercuric chloride** (5 ppm [mg/L] mercury) [purity unspecified] for life. A control group of 54 male and 54 female mice was given the drinking-water alone. Of the controls, 50% of the males were still alive at 602 days and 10% at 789 days, and 50% of females were still alive at 539 days and 10% at 691 days. Of the treated mice, 50% of males were still alive at 540 days and 10% at 697 days, and 50% of females at 575 days and 10% at 736 days. The numbers of mice autopsied were 38 control males and 47 control females and 48 male and 41 female treated mice. The authors reported that 11/41 treated female mice and 3/47 control females developed lymphoma or leukaemia [$p = 0.09$, Fisher exact test] (Schroeder & Mitchener, 1975). [The Working Group noted the incomplete reporting of the study and that only some of the animals were autopsied.]

Groups of 60 male and 60 female B6C3F1 mice, six weeks old, received 0, 5 or 10 mg/kg bw **mercuric chloride** (purity > 99%) in deionized water by gavage (10 ml/kg bw) on five days a week for 103–104 weeks. Ten animals from each group were killed at 15 months for evaluation. Survival at the end of the two-year study was 36/50, 36/50 and 31/50 in the control, low-dose and high-dose male groups and 41/50, 35/50 and 31/50 in the corresponding female groups. Body weights of both female and male treated mice were similar to those of controls throughout. Of the high-dose male mice, 2/49 developed renal tubular adenomas and 1/49 a renal tubular adenocarcinoma. No such tumour was seen in either the control or low-dose groups. No increase in the incidence of tumours was seen in the treated female mice (US National Toxicology Program, 1993).

(b) Rat

Groups of 60 male and 60 female Fischer 344/N rats, six weeks old, received 0, 2.5 or 5 mg/kg bw **mercuric chloride** (purity, > 99%) in deionized water by gavage (5 ml/kg bw) on five days a week for 103–104 weeks. Ten animals from each group were killed at 15 months for evaluation. Body weights of low- and high-dose males and high-dose females were lower than those of controls. Survival at two years was 26/50 male controls, 10/50 low-dose and 5/50 high-dose rats and 35/50, 28/49 and 30/50 in the females. The decrease in survival in male rats was due, in part, to an increased incidence of treatment-related renal disease. High-dose males had a greater incidence of renal tubular hyperplasia than control males (12/50 versus 3/50; $p = 0.005$), but the incidence of renal tubular adenomas was similar (control, 4/50; high-dose, 5/50). In female rats, renal tubular hyperplasia occurred in 5/50 high-dose rats and 2/50 controls; two high-dose female rats had renal tubular adenomas, but none was seen in controls. Treated male rats had a dose-related increase in the incidence of forestomach hyperplasia compared to controls (control, 3/49; low-dose, 16/50; high-dose, 35/50), as did high-dose female rats (control, 5/50; low-dose, 5/49; high-dose, 20/50). In addition, there was a dose-related increase in the incidence of squamous-cell papilloma of the forestomach in treated males (control, 0/50; low-dose, 3/50; high-dose, 12/50); such tumours also occurred in 2/50 high-dose female rats. High-dose males also had an increased incidence of thyroid follicular-cell carcinoma (control, 1/50; low-dose, 2/50; high-dose, 6/50), but not of hyperplasia (control, 2/50; low-dose, 4/50; high dose, 2/50) or adenoma (control, 1/50; low-dose, 4/50; high-dose, 0/50) (US National Toxicology Program, 1993). [The Working Group noted the low survival rate of male animals.]

3.2.2 *Administration with known carcinogens*

As the purpose of the investigations described below was to study interactions with known carcinogens, the studies were limited to specific target sites, were often of short duration and were not intended to address the carcinogenicity of mercury *per se*.

(a) *Mouse*

Twenty female Sencar mice [age unspecified] received single topical applications of 0.2 ml of 10 nmol [2.6 µg] 7,12-dimethylbenz[*a*]anthracene (DMBA) followed by twice weekly topical applications of 200 µg **mercuric chloride** in 0.2 ml of a 90% acetone solution for 26 weeks. A positive control group of 20 mice, initiated with DMBA, received promotion with 12-*O*-tetradecanoylphorbol 13-acetate [dose and dosing regime unspecified]. All mice in the positive control group developed skin papillomas, and two developed carcinomas. No skin tumour occurred in the mercuric chloride-treated mice (Kurokawa *et al.*, 1989). [The Working Group noted the incomplete reporting of the study.]

(b) *Rat*

A group of 15 male Fischer 344 rats, seven weeks old, was administered *N*-nitroso-*N*-hydroxydiethylamine (NHDEA) at 500 ppm [mg/L] in the drinking-water for two weeks followed by drinking-water containing 40 ppm [mg/L] **mercuric chloride** (99.5% pure) for 25 weeks. A further group of 15 rats received only mercuric chloride at 40 ppm for 25 weeks; a control group of 15 rats received drinking-water for the 27-week experimental period; and a further group of 15 rats was given NHDEA for two weeks followed by 25 weeks of drinking-water alone. There was no significant difference in the number of renal-cell tumours in rats receiving NHDEA and mercuric chloride (5/15) and those receiving NHDEA alone (2/15), but there was a significant ($p < 0.01$, Student's t test) increase in the mean number of dysplastic foci/cm^2 in the NHDEA- plus mercuric chloride-treated group (1.09) over that in the group treated with NHDEA alone (0.23). No renal-cell tumour or dysplastic focus was reported in the group receiving mercuric chloride alone (Kurokawa *et al.*, 1985).

Groups of 20 male Fischer 344 rats [age unspecified] were given drinking-water containing 50 ppm [mg/L] *N*-nitrosodiethylamine (NDEA) for four weeks to initiate liver carcinogenesis, followed by 30 weeks of treatment with drinking-water containing 40 ppm [mg/L] **mercuric chloride** [purity unspecified], water alone or 1000 ppm [1 g/L] phenobarbital (positive control). All animals were killed at week 34. Mercuric chloride treatment did not increase the number of hepatocellular carcinomas, adenomas or hyperplastic nodules over that in rats treated with NDEA alone (Kurokawa *et al.*, 1989). [The Working Group noted the incomplete reporting of the study.]

Groups of 20 male Wistar rats [age unspecified] were given *N*-methyl-*N*'-nitro-*N*-nitrosoguanidine in the drinking-water at 100 ppm [mg/L], together with a diet supplemeted with 10% sodium chloride for eight weeks to initiate gastroduodenal carcinogenesis, followed by 32 weeks of treatment with drinking-water containing 40 ppm [mg/L] **mercuric chloride** and basal diet without the 10% sodium chloride; controls were given the nitrosamine and basal diet containing sodium chloride for eight weeks then basal diet and standard drinking-water. The incidences of carcinoma and hyperplasia of the fundic and pyloric regions of the glandular stomach and of carcinoma of the duodenum were not increased by treatment with mercuric chloride over those caused by the nitrosamine alone (Kurokawa *et al.*, 1989). [The Working Group noted the incomplete reporting of the study.]

(c) *Hamster*

A group of 20 female Syrian golden hamsters [age unspecified] received three weekly injections [site unspecified] of *N*-nitrosobis(2-oxopropyl)amine (NBOPA) at a dose of 10 mg/kg bw to initiate pancreatic carcinogenesis, followed by treatment with drinking-water containing 40 ppm [mg/L] **mercuric chloride** for a further period [presumed to be 30 weeks]. A further group of 32 hamsters received NBOPA followed by drinking-water alone for 30 weeks. At the end of the study [duration unspecified], there was no difference in the multiplicity of either pancreatic adenocarcinomas or dysplastic lesions between the two groups (Kurokawa *et al.*, 1989). [The Working Group noted the incomplete reporting of the study.]

3.3 Methylmercury chloride

3.3.1 *Oral administration*

(a) *Mouse*

Groups of 60 male and 60 female ICR mice, five weeks of age, were fed a diet containing 0, 15 or 30 ppm [mg/kg] **methylmercury chloride** (99.3% purity) for 78 weeks. All animals were examined macroscopically, but histopathological examination was carried out only on kidneys of animals that died after week 53 and on lungs of mice with renal masses. The first renal tumour was detected in a male treated with 15 ppm and necropsied at week 58. Most mice given 30 ppm had severe neurotoxic effects and died or became moribund by week 26; similar, but less marked toxic effects occurred in the group treated with 15 ppm. At 78 weeks, survival among male mice was 24/60 given 0 ppm, 8/60 given 15 ppm and 0/60 given 30 ppm; survival among female mice was 33/60 given 0 ppm, 18/60 given 15 ppm and 0/60 given 30 ppm. The numbers of male mice that died after 53 weeks with renal tumours were: 1/37 (an adenoma) in the group given 0 ppm, 13/16 (total numbers of tumours: 11 adenocarcinomas [$p < 0.001$] and five adenomas [$p < 0.01$]) in the group given 15 ppm and none in the one surviving animal treated with 30 ppm. No renal tumour was reported in the female mice (Mitsumori *et al.*, 1981). [The Working Group noted the poor survival in the groups exposed to high doses of methylmercury chloride and the limited number of tissues subjected to histopathological evaluation.]

Groups of 60 male and 60 female ICR mice, five weeks of age, were administered diets containing 0, 0.4, 2 or 10 ppm (mg/kg) **methylmercury chloride** (99.3% pure) for 104 weeks. Six males and six females from each group were killed at 26-week intervals and subjected to histological examination, as were all other animals. No neurotoxic effect was observed in the treated animals, and, although all male mice given 10 ppm were dead by week 98, there was no difference in survival rates between the control and treated groups. The first renal tumour occurred in a male treated with 10 ppm at 58 weeks. Epithelial degeneration of the renal proximal tubules was seen in both males (40/59) and females (19/60) given 10 ppm, and similar but milder degeneration was seen in males given 2 ppm (12/58). The incidence of renal tumours in male mice was 1/58 (an adenoma) at 0 ppm, 0/59 at 0.4 ppm, 0/58 at 2.0 ppm and 13/59 (10 adenocarcinomas and three adenomas) at 10 ppm. [The effective numbers of animals at risk for renal tumours could not be determined.] No such tumour was seen in treated female mice (Hirano et al., 1986).

Groups of 60 male and 60 female specific-pathogen-free (SPF) B6C3F1 mice, five weeks of age, were fed diets containing 0, 0.4, 2.0 or 10 ppm [mg/kg] **methylmercury chloride** (99.3% pure) for 104 weeks. All animals were subjected to histopathological examination. In the group treated with 10 ppm, neurotoxicity was recorded in male mice at week 59 and in females at week 80; at termination, neurological signs were seen in 33/60 males and 3/60 females. Survival was similar to that of controls (48%) in all groups except males treated with 10 ppm, which had 17% survival. The incidence of chronic nephropathy was increased in male mice treated with 2 ppm (27/60) or 10 ppm (59/60) and in females given 10 ppm (56/60). The first renal tumour was seen in a male given 10 ppm and killed at week 70. Renal epithelial tumours occurred in 0/60 control males, 0/60 given 0.4 ppm, 1/60 (an adenoma) given 2 ppm and 16/60 (13 adenocarcinomas and five adenomas) given 10 ppm; among female mice, a single adenoma (1/60) was found in those given 10 ppm (Mitsumori et al., 1990). [The Working Group noted the lower survival of high-dose males after 60 weeks.]

(b) Rat

Groups of 25 male and 25 female weanling SPF Wistar rats were administered diets containing 0, 0.1, 0.5 or 2.5 ppm [mg/kg] **methylmercury chloride** (100% pure) for two years. Apart from a slight reduction in growth of females treated with 2.5 ppm, there was no effect of treatment on growth. No clinical or neurological sign of methylmercury chloride toxicity was reported during the study; mortality at 104 weeks was: 6/25 female and 7/25 male controls, 10/25 females and 8/25 males at 0.1 ppm, 9/25 females and 13/25 males at 0.5 ppm and 11/25 females and 13/25 males at 2.5 ppm. Histopathological examination was carried out on the control and 2.5 ppm-treated animals and on all animals that died. The authors reported no difference in tumour incidence or latency among the groups [no further detail reported] (Verschuuren et al., 1976a,b). [The Working Group noted the limited nature of the study.]

Groups of 56 male and 56 female SPF Sprague-Dawley rats, five weeks of age, were administered diets containing 0, 0.4, 2 or 10 ppm [mg/kg] **methylmercury chloride** (99.3% purity) for 130 weeks. Ten animals of either sex were killed at 13 and 26 weeks and 10 at 52 and 78 weeks. Neurological signs of methylmercury chloride toxicity were apparent in the 10 ppm-treated group from week 22 in males and from week 46 in females. All animals were subjected to necropsy and histopathological examination. Survival in the groups given 10 ppm was lower than in controls or in the other two treated groups; the cause of death was related to nephrotoxicity. The incidence of tumours did not differ significantly among the treated and control groups. A single renal adenoma was found in a high-dose female (Mitsumori et al., 1983, 1984).

3.3.2 Administration with known carcinogens

As the purpose of the investigations described below was to study interactions with known carcinogens, the studies were limited to specific target sites, were often of short duration and were not intended to address the carcinogenicity of mercury *per se*.

Mouse: Groups of 16–20 female Swiss-cross mice, 21–24 days old, were given 0, 0.2, 0.5, or 2.0 μg/ml (mg/L) **methylmercury chloride** [purity unspecified] in deionized drinking-water for 15 weeks and then killed. After the first three weeks of the exposure, mice received intraperitoneal injections of 1.5 mg/g [g/kg bw] urethane in normal saline [volume unspecified] or saline alone. The lung tumour incidence in the mice injected with saline was reported to be less than one tumour per mouse in all test groups [no further detail reported]. The number of pulmonary adenomas induced by urethane alone (21.5 ± 3.0) was exceeded only in the group that received the high dose of methylmercury chloride (33.1 ± 3.8) (Blakley, 1984).

Groups of 20 female W rats were maintained either on basal diet or on basal diet containing 10 ppm [mg/kg] **methylmercury chloride** [purity unspecified] dissolved in corn oil, from weaning until they delivered pups. They were also given either 0.159, 0.318 or 0.636% ethylurea in the diet from day 14 of the breeding period to parturition or 50 or 100 mg/kg bw by gavage on days 17, 18 and 19 of gestation; at the same time, they received 0.5, 1.0 or 2.0 g/L sodium nitrite in drinking-water or 25 or 50 mg/kg bw by gavage. Control groups received either the basal diet alone or the methylmercury chloride diet alone. All dams were returned to the basal diet at parturition, and progeny (generally about 25: 13 males and 12 females) were maintained on the basal diet for their lifespan. Survival was poor in some treatment groups. The incidence of neurogenic tumours was nearly 100% in some ethylurea/sodium nitrite-treated groups; there were 0/25 neurogenic tumours in the methylmercury chloride control group. Methylmercury chloride did not increase the incidence of neurogenic tumours in the groups receiving ethylurea/sodium nitrite, but schwannomas of the central nervous system tended to appear earlier than in the group given ethylurea/sodium nitrite alone (Nixon et al., 1979). [The Working Group noted the reduced sensitivity of the study, due to the very high incidence of neurogenic tumours in ethylurea/sodium nitrite-treated groups, and the poor survival.]

3.3.3 Hormonal influences

Mouse: Groups of 50 intact male and 50 intact female SPF ICR mice, seven weeks of age, were fed basal diet or basal diet containing 10 ppm [mg/kg] **methylmercury chloride** (purity, 99.3%) for 80 weeks. Groups of 50 orchiectomized male and 50 ovarectomized female mice, operated at five weeks of age, were fed basal diet containing 10 ppm methylmercury chloride only or also received weekly subcutaneous injections of 0.2 mg/mouse testosterone propionate in a 0.2% suspension (w/v) of sesame oil for 80 weeks. All groups receiving methylmercury chloride had nephrotoxic changes and caecal ulceration. No renal tumour was seen in intact males receiving basal diet alone, but one renal adenoma was seen in an intact female mouse; renal adenocarcinomas (14/50) and an adenoma (1/50) were seen in intact male mice given the basal diet with methylmercury chloride but not in intact female mice. In addition, 6/50 intact male mice given methylmercury chloride in the diet had tubular-cell hyperplasia, a lesion that the authors considered to be preneoplastic. No renal tumour was seen in orchiectomized or ovarectomized mice receiving methylmercury chloride only, but two adenocarcinomas occurred in males and three in females that received methylmercury chloride together with testosterone propionate (Hirano et al., 1988).

4. Other Relevant Data

4.1 Absorption, distribution, metabolism and excretion

The absorption, distribution, metabolism and excretion of inorganic mercury (Nordberg & Skerfving, 1972; WHO, 1976; Berlin, 1986; Clarkson et al., 1988a; WHO, 1991; Clarkson, 1992), methylmercury compounds (Nordberg & Skerfving, 1972; WHO, 1976; Berlin, 1986; Magos, 1987; Clarkson et al., 1988a; WHO, 1990) and phenylmercury acetate (Nordberg & Skerfving, 1972; WHO, 1976; Berlin, 1986; Clarkson et al., 1988a) have been reviewed.

4.1.1 *Humans*

(a) Metallic mercury and inorganic mercury compounds

In five human volunteers who inhaled radioactive metallic mercury-197 or mercury-203 vapour for 14–24 min, an average of 74% was absorbed in the respiratory tract (Hursh et al., 1976). The half-time for whole-body elimination averaged 58 days; however, elimination rates varied for different parts of the body: lung, 1.7 days; head, 21 days; kidney region, 64 days; chest, 43 days.

Absorbed metallic mercury is dissolved in the blood. Addition of metallic mercury-203 vapour to blood *in vitro* resulted in oxidation to mercuric mercury, but rather slowly (Hursh et al., 1988). The authors concluded that metallic mercury may pass the blood–brain barrier. A man who accidentally ingested 135 g of liquid metallic mercury had raised mercury concentrations in blood, but to an extent indicating only minimal absorption (Suzuki & Tanaka, 1971). The average ratio of mercury in erythrocytes:plasma was about 2 during the first few days after a 14–24-min exposure of five volunteers by inhalation of metallic mercury-197 and mercury-203 vapour (Cherian et al., 1978).

Studies in five volunteers who exposed their forearms to metallic mercury-203 vapour for 27–43 min indicated absorption of mercury through the skin of 0.01–0.04 ng/cm^2 per min per ng Hg/cm^3 air (Hursh et al., 1989).

In five human volunteers who inhaled metallic mercury-197 vapour for 11–21 min, the kidney region accumulated the highest levels of mercury (Hursh et al., 1980). In autopsy samples from seven dentists and one dental assistant, particularly high levels of mercury were found in the renal cortex (average, 8.6 μmol [1.7 mg]/kg wet weight) and pituitary glands (average, 9.8 μmol [2 g]/kg wet weight). In 24 controls, the values were 1.4 μmol [280 μg]/kg wet weight in renal cortex and 0.12 μmol [24 μg]/kg wet weight in pituitary (Nylander & Weiner, 1991). High levels have also been recorded in the thyroid glands of deceased mercury miners (average, 35 mg/kg fresh weight) (Kosta et al., 1975).

Equimolar ratios of mercury:selenium were found in pituitary and thyroid glands, kidney and brain in subjects with occupational exposure to metallic mercury vapour (Kosta et al., 1975; Nylander & Weiner, 1991). Renal biopsy samples from two patients with inorganic mercury poisoning had inclusion bodies which contained mercury and selenium (Aoi et al., 1985).

The blood mercury concentration of nine men who had been exposed to high levels (> 100 μg/m^3) of metallic mercury vapour for three days decreased with a half-time of three days for a fast phase and 18 days for a slow phase; the half-times in the urine were 28 and 141 days, respectively (Barregård et al., 1992).

Analysis of brain samples from a deceased subject who had been exposed to metallic mercury vapour for 18 months 16 years before death showed high levels of mercury, indicating that the brain has a compartment with very slow turnover of mercury. Most of the deposited mercury was in colloidal form (Hargreaves et al., 1988).

The concentration of mercury in the blood of the infants of two women who had been exposed accidentally to metallic mercury vapour during pregnancy was similar to that in maternal blood at the time of delivery, indicating transplacental passage (WHO, 1991).

An average urinary mercury concentration of about 50 μg/g creatinine was seen in 10 workers exposed to 40 μg/m^3 of air in a dry alkaline battery factory; the concentration in blood was about 18 μg/L (Roels et al., 1987).

In 10 volunteers who received single oral doses of either ^{203}Hg-mercuric nitrate as such or added to calf-liver protein, 75–92% of the dose was excreted in the faeces during the first four to five days. The average whole-body half-time for mercury (slow component) was 42 days. No difference was seen between the two forms of administration. The ratio of mercury in red blood cells to that in plasma was 0.4 over at least the first 50 days of the experiment. At that time, approximately equal amounts of mercury were excreted in faeces and urine (Rahola et al., 1973).

In a study of two men who had accidentally inhaled aerosols of neutron-activated ^{203}Hg-mercuric oxide, the lung clearance pattern displayed two phases, with biological half-times of two and 24 days, respectively, in one man; in the second, lung clearance appears to have been more rapid. The authors stated that absorption may have occurred from the lung, gastrointestinal tract or both. The major site of systemic deposition was the kidney, the content of which decreased with half-times of 60 and 37 days, respectively, in the two subjects. After 40 days, excretion was mainly urinary (Newton & Fry, 1978).

In five human volunteers who inhaled metallic mercury-197 vapour for 11–21 min, mercury was excreted by exhalation of metallic mercury and excretion of mercury in faeces and urine (Hursh et al., 1980).

(b) Methylmercury compounds

After a single oral dose of ^{203}Hg-methylmercury nitrate was given to three volunteers, methylmercury was almost completely absorbed. A maximum of 10% of the dose was deposited in the head region, presumably in the brain. Whole-body radiolabel decline followed a first-order process, with half-times of 70–74 days. The decline in radiolabel in the head was less rapid than in the rest of the body. In two of the subjects, faecal excretion accounted for about 87 and 90% of the total elimination during the 49 days that followed administration (Åberg et al., 1969). Gastrointestinal absorption was similarly high, whether methylmercury was given as the nitrate or bound to protein (Åberg et al., 1969; Miettinen, 1973).

In six volunteers who ate a single meal of fish containing methylmercury, the ratio of the concentration of mercury in erythrocytes and plasma was 21. Incorporation of methylmercury into hair was proportional to the concentration in blood at the time of formation of the hair strand; the ratio hair:blood was 292. The average half-times in blood were 7.6 h and 52 days (Kershaw et al., 1980).

In a study of 162 subjects who had been exposed to methylmercury through consumption of contaminated fish in Sweden in 1967-72, intake was associated with concentrations of mercury in blood and hair. After cessation of eating the contaminated fish, the concentration of mercury in the blood cells of four subjects decreased with a half-time of 58-87 days; in one subject, the half-time was 164 days (Skerfving, 1974). The ratio of mercury in blood cells and in plasma was 2-12 (Skerfving, 1988).

Individuals with long-term intake of around 200 µg methylmercury per day were estimated to have blood mercury concentrations of about 200 µg/L and hair concentrations of about 50 µg/g (WHO, 1990).

After consumption of bread contaminated with methylmercury for two months in Iraq, the molar fraction of total mercury as inorganic mercury in several people was 7% in whole blood, 22% in plasma, 39% in breast milk, 73% in urine and 16-40% in liver (WHO, 1990).

The average ratio of methylmercury in cord blood and in maternal blood was 1.66 (Suzuki et al., 1984). The infants of 10 fishermen's wives who were exposed to methylmercury through consumption of fish in Sweden had about 47% higher mercury levels in erythrocytes and similar levels in plasma in comparison with their mothers. The concentration of total mercury in breast milk from 15 women was similar to that in plasma; only about 20% of the total mercury in the milk was methylmercury (Skerfving, 1988).

(c) *Phenylmercury compounds*

In 509 infants in Buenos Aires, Argentina, who were exposed to phenylmercury fungicide through contaminated diapers, the average urinary excretion of total mercury was about 20 times higher than in 166 matched controls; over 90% of the mercury was inorganic (Gotelli et al., 1985).

4.1.2 *Experimental systems*

(a) *Metallic mercury and inorganic mercury compounds*

Kostial et al. (1983) observed that the retention of orally administered ^{203}Hg-mercuric chloride in the carcass, gut and whole body was higher in newborn rats (60-70%) than in weaned rats (14-15%).

Absorption of an aqueous solution of ^{203}Hg-mercuric chloride applied under occlusion onto about 3 cm^2 of the shaved skin of guinea-pigs was dependent on the mercury concentration. A maximal rate of about 0.02% per min was recorded during 5 h after application of 16 mg/ml (as mercury) (Friberg et al., 1961).

In rats, rabbits and monkeys exposed for 4 h to 1 mg/m^3 of metallic mercury vapour or injected intravenously with an equivalent dose of mercuric nitrate, the main accumulation was in the kidney, but 10 times more mercury entered the brain after exposure to mercury vapour than after injection of mercuric nitrate (Berlin et al., 1969).

In rats exposed to metallic mercury vapour, mercury deposits were found by a histochemical technique in the nerve cells in the cerebellum and hypothalamus (Møller-Madsen, 1992). In frog nerve–muscle preparations treated with mercuric chloride (3 µM [600 µg]), mercuric ions penetrated the nerve-cell membrane through sodium and calcium channels (Miyamoto, 1983).

Khayat and Dencker (1982) found four-fold higher fetal mercury concentrations in mice after exposure to metallic mercury vapour by inhalation than after intravenous injection of mercuric chloride. The passage of metallic mercury through the blood–brain barrier is usually ascribed to its lipophilicity.

In studies of cell suspensions of erythrocytes from humans, ducks and mice exposed *in vitro* to mercury vapour, uptake was proportional to catalase activity, which shows that this enzyme is involved in oxidation of mercury vapour in the erythrocyte (Halbach & Clarkson, 1978). Catalase-mediated oxidation of the vapour has also been demonstrated in other tissues, e.g. liver (Magos et al., 1978).

Intravenous injection of rats with mercuric chloride at 0.7 mg/kg bw induced metallothionein in kidney tissue, which resulted in the binding of mercury (Nishiyama et al., 1987).

After administration of 12 or 25 daily doses of mercury at 1 mg/kg bw as ^{203}Hg-mercuric chloride, the mitochondria in the proximal convoluted tubules were found to be enlarged and there were many very fine, dense, small particles. After fragmentation of the renal tissue and centrifugation at high speed, the radiolabel was found in two fractions, corresponding to mitochondria and microsomes (Bergstrand et al., 1959).

Mice given parenteral doses of mercuric chloride exhaled metallic mercury vapour; exhalation was proportional to the body burden of mercury (Dunn et al., 1978). Following intravenous treatment of rats with mercuric chloride, mercury was excreted into bile as a low-molecular-weight complex which had gel filtration properties similar to those of a mercury–glutathione complex (Ballatori & Clarkson, 1984).

In guinea-pigs exposed for a short time to metallic mercury vapour after parturition, the mercury concentration in milk was slightly lower than that in plasma. Neonates had increased concentrations of mercury in tissues and particularly in the kidney (Yoshida et al., 1992). In rats given mercuric acetate orally, a linear relationship was observed between mercury concentrations in plasma and in milk (Sundberg et al., 1991).

Selenium affects the tissue distribution and excretion of mercuric mercury. For example, three weeks' administration of sodium selenite or seleno-L-methionine (7.5, 37.5 or 75 µmol/L in drinking water) to BOM:NMRI mice increased the whole-body retention of a single oral dose (5 or 25 µmol [1 or 5 mg]/kg bw of ^{203}Hg-mercuric chloride. The effect on organ distribution varied with the dose of mercury and the type and dose of selenium compound (Nielsen & Andersen, 1991).

Human oral bacteria caused some methylation of mercuric chloride *in vitro* (Heintze et al., 1983).

(b) Methylmercury compounds

Exposure of rats to ^{203}Hg-methylmercury chloride vapour at 10–28 mg/m^3 for 6–24 h was followed by efficient uptake of methylmercury through the lungs (0.6–7 nmol/g fresh tissue) [no data on absorbed fraction given]. Rats given a single oral dose of 0.75–2.3 mg/kg bw had several times higher mercury concentrations in organs (18.6–107.6 nmol/g fresh tissue). In liver and kidney, 42–50% of the mercury was in the soluble fraction, 32–43% in the crude nuclear fraction, 6–9% in the mitochondria and 9–11% in the microsomal fraction. In brain, 29% was in the soluble and 27% in the nuclear fraction, 31% was in mitochondria and 10% in microsomes (Fang, 1980).

Absorption of an aqueous solution of ^{203}Hg-methylmercury dicyandiamide applied under occlusion onto about 3 cm^2 of the shaved skin of guinea-pigs was dependent on concentration. A maximal disappearance of 5.9% was recorded during 5 h after application of 16 mg/ml (as mercury) (Friberg *et al.*, 1961).

Significant species differences have been observed in the distribution of methylmercury compounds in the body: The ratio between mercury concentrations in erythrocytes and plasma is about 20 in monkeys (17 in squirrel, 25 in rhesus), 25 in guinea-pigs, 7 in mice and more than 100 in rats (for review, see Magos, 1987). After prolonged administration of methylmercury compounds, the brain:blood ratios are 3–6 in squirrel monkeys (for review, see Berlin, 1986), 3.3 in pigs, 1.2 in guinea-pigs, 1.2 in mice and 0.06 in rats (for review, see Magos, 1987).

Following intraperitoneal injection of 1 mg/kg bw methylmercury chloride into four strains of mice, a significant difference in mercury concentrations was observed among strains, particularly in the blood. The rate of elimination from organs also differed: the biological half-time in blood (days) was 5.03 in BALB/c, 5.52 in C3H, 7.79 in C57Bl and 3.81 in CD-1 mice; that in kidneys was 8.73, 7.73, 7.47 and 4.54, respectively (Doi & Kobayashi, 1982). Eight days after intraperitoneal administration of ^{203}Hg-methylmercury chloride (0.4 mg/kg bw as Hg) to two strains of mice, males had significantly higher mercury concentrations in kidney than had females (C129F$_1$ strain: 5.33 and 3.34%; 129 strain: 7.47 and 3.57% of the dose in males and females, respectively). There was no sex difference in whole-body mercury retention (Doherty *et al.*, 1978).

The percentage of inorganic mercury in total mercury in tissues of squirrel monkeys that received single or repeated weekly doses of methylmercury nitrate by stomach tube at about 0.8 mg/kg bw Hg, was about 20% in liver, about 50% in kidney, 30–85% in bile and < 5% in brain, showing that methylmercury is demethylated (Berlin *et al.*, 1975). Similarly, inorganic mercury was demonstrated in the kidney and to a lesser extent in the liver of rats given daily doses of methylmercury dicyandiamide (Magos & Butler, 1972).

The relative concentration of inorganic mercury in mice increased gradually after a single intravenous injection of 25 µg methylmercury chloride and was about 30% after 22 days; the author concluded that mice obtain a lower fraction of inorganic mercury in the kidney than rats (Norseth, 1971). Cats fed either methylmercury-contaminated fish or methylmercury hydroxide added to fish accumulated inorganic mercury in the liver and kidney; 62% was recovered as methylmercury in kidney and 80% in liver. The metabolism of the methylmercury in the contaminated fish and of the added hydroxide was similar (Albanus *et al.*, 1972). Similar results were found in cats fed methylmercury-contaminated fish or methylmercury chloride (Charbonneau *et al.*, 1976), and no difference in metabolism was seen in rats given four different salts of methylmercury orally or subcutaneously (Ulfvarson, 1962).

Methylmercury added as the chloride *in vitro* to erythrocytes from humans, rabbits and mice was complexed to a low-molecular-weight compound—probably glutathione. In rats, such binding was minimal (Naganuma *et al.*, 1980). Following the addition of methylmercury chloride to erythrocytes from mice, rats and humans in another study, mercury was found to be bound to haemoglobin—probably cysteinyl residues (Doi & Tagawa, 1983). In rats, L-cysteine enhanced the uptake of mercury by the brain after administration of methylmercury chloride by intracarotid injection. There were indications of a transport system carrying methylmercury over the brain capillary endothelial cell membrane (Aschner & Clarkson, 1988).

In rats injected intravenously with methylmercury chloride, methylmercury was present in the bile as a low-molecular-weight compound complex, which was identified as methylmercury glutathione on the basis of thin-layer chromatography, gel filtration and ionic exchange (Refsvik & Norseth, 1975).

After intravenous injection into rats, methylmercury was excreted into the bile, predominantly as methylmercury cysteine, which is largely reabsorbed from the intestine. There is thus enterohepatic circulation of methylmercury (Norseth & Clarkson, 1971). In rat gut, however, a fraction of methylmercury is converted to inorganic mercury, which is then excreted mainly in the faeces (Rowland *et al.*, 1980).

Hamsters administered a single oral dose of 10 mg/kg bw methylmercury chloride excreted about 50% of the mercury (only about 10% of which was inorganic mercury) in the urine within one week. In rabbits given 0.4 mg/kg bw intravenously, < 2% was excreted in the urine (Petersson *et al.*, 1989).

After addition of 250 ng methylmercury chloride to three hydroxyl radical producing systems, copper ascorbate, xanthine oxidase hypoxanthine–ferric monosodium ethylenediaminetetraacetate and hydrogen peroxide–ultraviolet B light, analysis of inorganic mercury revealed significant dealkylation, which appeared to be unrelated to either superoxide or hydrogen peroxide production alone (Suda *et al.*, 1991). In rat liver microsomes treated with 500 ng methylmercury chloride, both inorganic mercury and hydroxy radical contents increased after addition of NADPH and were further increased by KCN (Suda & Hirayama, 1992).

Selenium affects the tissue distribution and excretion of methylmercury. For example, selenite increased the brain levels of mercury in rats treated with methylmercury (Magos & Webb, 1977).

(c) *Phenylmercury and methoxyethylmercury compounds*

Faecal excretion of 0.120 mg/kg bw Hg as phenylmercury acetate in rats was 65% during 48 h after a single oral dose and 30% after intravenous administration of the same dose, indicating that more than half of the phenylmercury salt was absorbed (Prickett *et al.*, 1950).

In rats given an intraperitoneal injection of phenylmercury acetate, the compound was metabolized rapidly to mercuric mercury (Magos *et al.*, 1982).

Daniel et al. (1971) administered a single subcutaneous dose of methoxy-^{14}C-ethylmercury chloride to rats. Within three days, about half of the radiolabel appeared in exhaled air, with 44% in ethylene and 5% in carbon dioxide (44% after pyrolysis of air). Mercury was accumulated in kidney: A few hours after dosing, inorganic mercury constituted about one-half of the total mercury in that organ; after one day, all of the mercury was inorganic. About 25% of the radiolabel was excreted in urine over 4 days and about 10% after 8 days.

4.2 Toxic effects

The toxic effects of inorganic mercury (WHO, 1976; Kark, 1979; Berlin, 1986; Clarkson et al., 1988a; Dayan et al., 1990; WHO, 1991; Clarkson, 1992), methylmercury compounds (WHO, 1976; Berlin, 1986; Clarkson et al., 1988a; Dayan et al., 1990; WHO, 1990) and phenylmercuric acetate (Skerfving & Vostal, 1972; WHO, 1976; Berlin, 1986; Clarkson et al., 1988a) have been reviewed.

4.2.1 Humans

(a) Inorganic mercury

Workers accidentally exposed for 4–8 h to metallic mercury at levels estimated to have ranged from 1 to 44 mg/m^3 developed chest pain, dyspnoeic cough, haemoptysis, impairment of pulmonary function and interstitial pneumonitis (McFarland & Reigel, 1978). Acute massive exposure to metallic mercury vapour can result in psychotic reactions with delirium (for review, see Kark, 1979).

Troen et al. (1951) reported 18 cases of human poisoning by ingestion of single doses of mercuric chloride. In nine fatal cases, the lowest estimated dose was 2 g. Gastrointestinal and renal lesions were observed at autopsy.

Roels et al. (1985) examined 131 male and 54 female workers exposed to metallic mercury vapour in several factories in Belgium and 114 and 48 unexposed control male and female workers. In responses to a questionnaire, several symptoms of central nervous system disorder (memory disturbances, depressive feelings, fatigue and irritability) were more prevalent among exposed subjects than controls. A significantly increased prevalence of hand tremor was recorded in the group of exposed men, as compared to male controls (15 versus 5%). The average concentrations of mercury in urine were 52 µg/g creatinine in exposed men and 37 µg/g creatinine in women; the corresponding levels in controls were 0.9 and 1.7 µg/g creatinine.

In a study of 89 chloralkali workers with a median urinary mercury concentration of 25 µg/g creatinine (range up to 83) and a control group of 75 workers from other industries (median concentration, 2 µg/g creatinine), an association was observed between urinary mercury concentration, self-reported symptoms—tiredness, confusion and degree of neuroticism (Langworth et al., 1992a)—and urinary excretion of N-acetyl-β-glucosaminidase, a lysosomal enzyme originating from tubular epithelial cells. No significant effect on serum titres of autoantibodies (including antiglomerular basement membrane and antilaminin) was observed (Langworth et al., 1992b). Elevated excretion of N-acetyl-β-glucosaminidase was also reported by Barregård et al. (1988) in chloralkali workers.

Of 44 African women with nephrotic syndrome, 70% used or had used mercury-containing skin-lightening creams; the corresponding fraction among other general medical female in-patients was 11% (Barr et al., 1972). In eight other cases of nephrotic syndrome, IgG and C3 complement deposits were observed in glomeruli (Lindqvist et al., 1974). Proteinuria and the nephrotic syndrome have also been described in workers exposed to mercury compounds (Kazantzis et al., 1962).

Lauwerys et al. (1983) studied 62 workers in a chloralkali plant and a zinc–mercury amalgam factory with a mean urinary mercury concentration of 56 µg/g creatinine. Eight exposed workers, but none of 60 control workers who were not occupationally exposed to heavy metals but were matched to the exposed group with respect to age and socioeconomic status, had serum antibodies towards laminin, a non-collagen glycoprotein found *inter alia* in the glomerular basal membrane. No alterations were seen in a large battery of renal function tests.

In studies of dentists and chloralkali workers exposed to metallic mercury vapour (mean urinary mercury concentration, 1.3 nmol/mmol [2.3 µg/g] creatinine in dentists and 26 nmol/mmol [46 µg/g] creatinine in chloralkali workers), no significant effect on endocrine function (pituitary, thyroid and adrenal glands, testis) was observed as compared to controls (0.4–0.6 nmol/mmol [0.7–1.06 mg/g] creatinine) without occupational exposure (Erfurth et al., 1990). Similar results were reported by Langworth et al. (1990) in dental personnel.

In a study reported in detail on p. 271, Barregård et al. (1990) studied mortality among 1190 chloralkali workers who had been monitored biologically for exposure to metallic mercury vapour for at least one year in 1946–84. For workers with > 10 years of latency, mortality from all causes was not significantly increased (SMR, 1.1; 95% CI, 0.9–1.3), but mortality from circulatory disease was slightly increased (SMR, 1.3; 95% CI, 1.0–1.5). No such elevation was reported in another study of workers exposed to metallic mercury (Cragle et al., 1984; see p. 269).

Contact dermatitis with sensitization against metallic mercury has been reported. For example, Ancona et al. (1982) reported such a case in a dentist who had a positive epicutaneous patch test. Finne et al. (1982) performed patch tests on 29 patients with amalgam fillings and oral lichen planus. Positive reactions to mercury were found in 62% as compared with 3% of controls (2300 eczema cases). After the amalgam fillings had been removed from four patients, an improvement in the oral changes was recorded.

In the 1940s, 'pink disease' (acrodynia), presenting as irritation, insomnia, sweating, photophobia and general rash in children, was reported to be associated with exposure mainly to calomel (mercurous chloride) in, e.g. teething powder and ointments (Warkany, 1966). Cases have also been associated with exposure to other chemical forms of mercury, e.g. metallic mercury vapour from broken fluorescent tubes (Tunnessen et al., 1987). The mechanism by which the condition occurs has not been elucidated. Three of six children with mucocutaneous lymph node syndrome (Kawasaki disease), including increased serum IgE and eosinophilia, had urinary concentrations of mercury (16–25 µg/24 h) higher than established normal levels (< 10 µg/24 h). The syndrome may represent a hypersensitivity reaction to environmental pollution with mercury (Orlowski & Mercer, 1980).

(b) Methylmercury compounds

The first case of 'methylmercury poisoning' was described in a worker exposed to methylmercury phosphate and nitrate for a period of four months (Hunter & Russell, 1954). Since then, numerous descriptions have been published, mainly in connection with outbreaks of poisoning in subjects consuming contaminated fish in Japan (Minamata disease) (Igata, 1991) or seeds treated with methylmercury dicyandiamide, e.g. in Iraq (Bakir et al., 1973). Its main features are that: (i) the target organ is the central nervous system; (ii) there is a latent period between exposure and onset of clinical disease; (iii) the symptoms and signs include paraesthesia in the hands, feet and lips, concentric constriction of visual fields and ataxia; and (iv) morphological changes occur in the visual and precentral cortical areas as well as in the cerebellum. There is also evidence of peripheral neuropathy (Rustam et al., 1975).

In the cohort study in two administrative subunits in the vicinity of Minamata City, Japan (Tamashiro et al., 1986; see pp. 275–276), significantly elevated SMRs were observed for cerebral haemorrhage (1.67, 95% CI; 1.24–2.24), liver disease (2.00; 1.33–2.89), senility (2.34; 1.67–3.26) and violent death (accident, poisoning, suicide) (1.48; 1.12–1.97).

(c) Phenylmercury, ethylmercury and methoxyethylmercury compounds

A study of 509 infants exposed to phenylmercury acetate from contaminated diapers showed a clear dose–response relationship between the concentration of organomercury compounds in urine and urinary excretion of γ-glutamyl transpeptidase, an enzyme in the brush borders of renal tubular cells. Children with the highest mercury excretion also had increased 24-h urine volumes. Some of the children also had 'pink disease' (Gotelli et al., 1985).

A few cases of systemic poisoning by ethylmercury and methoxyethyl compounds have been reported (for review, see Skerfving & Vostal, 1972). Most patients showed symptoms and signs of disorders in the gastrointestinal tract and kidneys (albumin, red cells and casts in urine).

4.2.2 Experimental systems

(a) Metallic mercury and inorganic mercury compounds

Application of 2 ml of a solution containing 0.24 mol [65 g] mercuric chloride resulted in the death of 3/20 guinea-pigs after two days (Wahlberg, 1965).

Ashe et al. (1953) reported damage to brain, liver, kidney, heart and lungs of rabbits exposed to mercury vapour at a concentration of 29 mg/m^3 air. Damage was seen after exposure as short as 1 h. Microscopic changes were observed in mitochondria of the renal proximal tubule after 12 or 25 daily doses of 1 mg/kg bw Hg as mercuric chloride to rats (Bergstrand et al., 1959).

In a susceptible strain of rats (Brown–Norway), subcutaneous injections of mercuric chloride caused a systemic autoimmune nephritis characterized by the production of various antibodies to self and non-self antigens and an increase in total serum IgE concentrations. A biphasic autoimmune glomerulonephritis occurred: initially, anti-glomerular basement membrane antibodies were produced, resulting in linear IgG deposition along the glomerular capillary walls. Later, granular IgG deposits appeared which are responsible for an immune-complex type glomerulonephritis (Druet et al., 1978). Mercuric chloride appears to induce a T cell-dependent polyclonal activation of B cells in Brown–Norway rats (Pelletier et al., 1986); most animals develop proteinuria, which in some animals progresses to a nephrotic syndrome that is sometimes lethal (Druet et al., 1978), while in other animals the condition is transient. There is a striking strain difference. By crossing susceptible rats with unsusceptible Lewis rats, susceptibility was shown to depend on three or four genes, one of which is located within the major histocompatibility complex (Druet et al., 1982). Certain strains of mice may develop similar glomerular conditions after injection with mercuric chloride (Hultman & Eneström, 1987).

In Lewis rats injected subcutaneously with mercuric chloride (1 mg/kg bw three times a week for up to 4 weeks), no autoimmune disorder was observed. Instead, animals showed proliferation of suppressor/cytotoxic T cells in the spleen and lymph nodes. As a consequence, they developed a non-antigen-specific immunosuppression and responded to neither classical mitogens nor alloantigens (Pelletier et al., 1987a). Mercuric chloride could also inhibit the development of an organ-specific autoimmune disorder, Heymann's nephritis (Pelletier et al., 1987b).

Micromolar concentrations of mercury have been shown to increase the release of acetylcholine in frog neuromuscular preparations (Manalis & Cooper, 1975) and that of dopamine in adult mouse brain homogenates (Bondy et al., 1979).

Significant decreases in the activities of several enzymes of the glutathione (GSH) metabolic pathway in kidney—GSH disulfide reductase, GSH-peroxidase, γ-glutamyl-cysteine synthetase and γ-glutamyl transpeptidase—were seen 24 h after subcutaneous administration of 10 μmol[2.5 ml]/kg bw mercuric chloride to Sprague–Dawley rats; in the liver, only the activity of GSH disulfide reductase was decreased. After administration of 30 μmol [7.5 mg]/kg bw, the decreases in specific enzyme activities were accompanied by large losses of cellular protein and decreased GSH concentrations in both kidney and liver. The effects could be blocked by sodium selenite (Chung et al., 1982). The mercuric ion binds to reduced sulfhydryl groups in proteins and inhibits a wide range of enzymes (for review, see Kark, 1979).

In Holtzman rats given a lethal intravenous dose of 3 mg/kg bw Hg as mercuric chloride and sacrificed after 4 h, there was extensive renal haemorrhage. Kidney mitochondria contained mercury at 4–5 nmol[0.8–1 μg]/mg protein and showed uncoupling of oxidative phosphorylation.

In mitochondrial preparations of kidney cortex from Sprague–Dawley rats, mercury at concentrations of 2 nmol/mg protein and above affected mitochondrial respiration: clear stimulation of state 4, mild stimulation of state 3 and inhibition of the 2,4-dinitrophenol-induced uncoupled respiration rate. These effects were both preventable and reversible by addition of albumin or dithioerythritol to the in-vitro system (Weinberg et al., 1982a), but not in mitochondria isolated 3 h after subcutaneous administration of mercuric chloride at 5 mg/kg bw, when the concentration of mercury in mitochondrial protein was 0.72 ± 0.10 nmol/mg (Weinberg et al., 1982b).

Addition of mercuric chloride at concentrations of 1–6 μm [0.2–1.2 mg] mercury to preparations of mitochondria from rat kidney cortex and heart in the presence of antimycin

A decreased the production of superoxide but increased hydrogen peroxide production. The authors concluded that mercuric ion caused dismutation of the superoxide, leading to increased hydrogen peroxide formation, which could lead to oxidative tissue damage. Addition of mercurous ions did not affect superoxide production (Miller *et al.*, 1991). [The Working Group noted that the mercury concentrations employed were high.]

Mercuric ions from mercuric chloride, added at 1 mM (270 mg), reacted *in vitro* with isolated DNA (Eichhorn & Clark, 1963). [The Working Group noted the very high concentration used.] No study has shown covalent binding to DNA, e.g. by isolating such an adduct from DNA after complete hydrolysis to nucleosides.

Inhibition of protein synthesis was observed in cell-free systems prepared from mouse glioma after addition of mercuric chloride at a concentration of 2×10^{-5} M [5 mg] (Nakada *et al.*, 1980). [The Working Group noted the high concentration used.] Mercuric chloride at a concentration of 10 μM [2.3 mg] reduced lipid synthesis in isolated mouse sciatic nerve (Clöez *et al.*, 1987).

Sodium selenite dramatically decreased the acute nephrotoxicity of mercuric chloride in rats, when given simultaneously or even 1 h after mercury (Pařízek & Oštádalová, 1967).

(b) Methylmercury compounds

There are clear species differences in symptoms and signs of poisoning by methylmercury compounds. Blindness has been reported in man, rats, monkeys and pigs, but not in cats (for reviews, see WHO, 1976, 1990). Man, monkeys and cats develop ataxia; but in rats dosed orally with methylmercury chloride reduced conduction velocities and histopathological changes occurred in peripheral nerves, while the central nervous system was not affected (Fehling *et al.*, 1975).

Renal damage is a typical finding in rats. Male Wistar rats fed mercury at 0.250 mg/kg bw per day as methylmercury chloride for up to 26 months developed severe renal tubular damage. The estimated mercury level in kidney was 30.2 mg/kg in males and 60 mg/kg in females (Munro *et al.*, 1980). Nuclear swelling and vacuolar degeneration of the cytoplasm were seen in SPF ICR mice fed a diet containing 10 ppm methylmercury chloride for 26 weeks (Hirano *et al.*, 1986). Treatment of monkeys with daily oral doses of 80–125 μg/kg bw methylmercury hydroxide for 3–12 months did not appear to affect the general well-being of the animals, but ultrastructural changes occurred in the kidneys, with intracytoplasmic vacuoles and electron-dense inclusion bodies in the proximal tubuli (Chen *et al.*, 1983).

In mice fed mercury at 3.9 mg/kg diet as methylmercury chloride for 12 weeks, thymus weight and cell number were decreased, the lymphoproliferative response to T and B mitogens was increased in thymus and spleen, and natural killer cell activity was decreased in the spleen and blood (Ilbäck, 1991). Mice fed methylmercury chloride at doses of 1–10 mg/kg diet for 84 days had significantly higher mortality rates when inoculated with encephalomyelitis virus (nononcogenic) than did animals not given methylmercury (Koller, 1975).

Impairment of adrenal and testicular function occurred in rats given 23 intraperitoneal injections of 0.26 mg methylmercury chloride over six weeks (Burton & Meikle, 1980); thyroid function was impaired in mice given two intraperitoneal doses of 5 mg/kg bw (Kawada *et al.*, 1980).

Female Charles River CD rats were given 3–10 mg/L methylmercury hydroxide in drinking-water four weeks prior to mating and through day 19 of pregnancy. With concentrations of 3–5 mg/L, there was decreased synthesis of mitochondrial structural proteins in the livers of the fetuses and inhibition of several mitochondrial enzymes (Fowler & Woods, 1977a). In male rats of the same strain treated similarly for six weeks, electron microscopy revealed swelling of the renal proximal tubule cell mitochondria at a dose of 5 mg/L. The respiratory control ratios were decreased (mitochondrial respiratory dysfunction), and effects were seen on enzyme activities, including decreased monoamine oxidase and cytochrome oxidase and increased δ-aminolaevulinic acid synthetase. The rats had increased urinary excretion of porphyrins but no deterioration in standard renal function tests (Fowler & Woods, 1977b).

Mouse glioma cell cultures treated with methylmercury chloride (5×10^{-6} M for 4 h) showed inhibition of cell mitosis, by blockage of the polymerization of tubulin to microtubuli, with accumulation of cells during mitosis. Electron microscopy showed an absence of microtubuli as mitotic spindle fibres and disorganization of chromosomes (Miura *et al.*, 1978).

Sodium selenite, and possibly also the chemically unknown form of selenium found in marine foods, delayed the onset of the toxic effects of methylmercury chloride in rats and reduced the severity of its effects (Chang & Suber, 1982).

Methylmercury hydroxide added to fish homogenate and methylmercury-contaminated fish were equally neurotoxic to cats (Albanus *et al.*, 1972). Similar results (ataxia, loss of balance or motor incoordination, loss of nerve cells) were found in cats fed either methylmercury chloride or methylmercury-contaminated fish (Charbonneau *et al.*, 1976).

(c) *Phenylmercury, ethylmercury and methoxyethylmercury*

Renal damage was observed in mice, rats and rabbits given phenylmercury nitrate and chloride intraperitoneally or intravenously (Weed & Ecker, 1933). Ethylmercury poisoning has been described in rats, rabbits, cats, sheep, swine and calves. The symptoms are similar to those of methylmercury poisoning (Skerfving & Vostal, 1972). In rats administered the fungicide methoxyethyl mercury chloride (2 mg/kg bw for 50 days or 0.2 mg/kg bw for 80 days) intraperitoneally, impaired weight gain, renal damage and signs of nervous system damage (e.g. tremor, ataxia) were seen (Lehotzy & Bordas, 1968).

4.3 Reproductive and prenatal effects

4.3.1 *Humans*

The effects of inorganic and organomercury compounds on human reproduction and development have been reviewed (Khera, 1979; Inskip & Piotrowski, 1985; Schardein, 1985; Burbacher *et al.*, 1990; Roeleveld *et al.*, 1990; Shepard, 1992).

(a) *Metallic mercury and inorganic mercury compounds*

(i) *Exposure of women*

Adverse pregnancy outcomes have been reported following exposure to mercuric chloride tablets (Afonso & de Alvarez, 1960), to mercuric iodide-containing soap (Lauwerys *et al.*, 1987) and in a dental surgery unit where the concentration of mercury exceeded the threshold limit value of 0.05 mg/m^3 (Gelbier & Ingram, 1989). After exposure of a woman prior to week 17 of pregnancy to metallic mercury in a contaminated carpet (24-h urinary concentration of mercury, 230 µg/L), no adverse effect was seen on birth weight, growth or on acquisition of developmental milestones in the child at the age of two (Thorp *et al.*, 1992).

Heidam (1984) conducted a historical prospective study of pregnancy outcomes in women in 12 selected occupations in the Danish county of Funen. Controls were employed in occupations with less exposure to chemicals. Dental assistants returned 94% of the 772 mailed questionnaires on pregnancy history. The incidence of spontaneous abortions in dental assistants in private clinics was 11.2% in 259 pregnancies, yielding a crude odds ratio of 1.1 (95% CI, 0.7–1.8). After control for confounding variables, including age at gravidity, pregnancy order and maternal age at pregnancy, the odds ratio was 1.0 (0.6–1.6). Dichotomization of dental assistants according to whether they reported exposure to inorganic mercury compounds also showed no increase in the spontaneous abortion rate in the exposed subgroup.

Brodsky *et al.* (1985) conducted a postal survey of 30 272 female dental assistants in California (USA) regarding the use of anaesthetic agents and mercury amalgams and health and pregnancy histories for the years 1968–78. The response rate was 70%. Exposure was categorized on the basis of the number of amalgam restorations prepared per week into no, low (0–40) or high (> 40). Outcomes were adjusted for maternal age and cigarette smoking. No relationship was observed between exposure and spontaneous abortion or congenital abnormalities.

Sikorski *et al.* (1987) evaluated reproductive function and outcome in 81 women (45 dentists, 36 dental assistants) exposed occupationally to metallic mercury and in 34 unexposed women [occupational details not given] recruited at random in the Lublin region of Poland. Exposure was ascertained by determination of mercury in samples of scalp and pubic hair; the mercury content in hair was related to duration of employment and to the number of amalgams used per week. A total of 57 exposed women had 117 pregnancies, 24% of which ended in spontaneous abortion, stillbirth or congenital malformations (including five cases of spina bifida). Thirty unexposed women had 63 pregnancies, 11% of which ended in an adverse outcome. Reproductive failure was associated with the mercury content of the hair. The frequency of menstrual disorders was also high in exposed women and was related to the number of years employed and to the mercury content of scalp hair. [The Working Group noted that temporal matching of exposure and pregnancy was not carried out, that no mention of potential confounders was made and that hair mercury levels poorly reflect exposure to metallic mercury.]

Ericson and Källén (1989) evaluated 8157 infants born to dentists, dental assistants and dental technicians in Sweden between 1976 and 1986. Outcomes were standardized for maternal age and parity, year of birth and sex of the infant. There was no suggestion of an increased rate of stillbirths or congenital malformations. The risk ratio for low birth weight (< 2500 g) was 0.9 (95% CI, 0.7–1.2) for dentists, 1.2 (1.0–1.3) for dental assistants and 0.8 (0.5–1.4) for dental technicians. Data on spontaneous abortions were available only for 1980–81, and the rates for dentists, dental assistants and dental technicians corresponded to expected figures. The authors also reported no increase in the rates of spontaneous abortion or neural tube defects among women working in dentistry, as ascertained in a small prospective study in Malmö in 1964–65. [The Working Group noted that no marker of exposure to mercury was used.]

De Rosis et al. (1985) studied the possible effects on reproductive function and outcome in women of exposure to mercury vapour in two mercury vapour lamp factories in Italy. Workers were exposed to mercury in only one plant, where time-weighted averages exceeded 0.05 mg/m^3 in 1972–76; they were subsequently reduced to < 0.01 mg/m^3. Workers in a second plant were used as the reference group. Participation was 79% (153 women) in the exposed plant and 88% (293) in the reference plant. Past health events were ascertained by interview. The prevalence and incidence of menstrual cycle disorders were higher in the exposed group, with an age-standardized ratio of abnormal cycles of 1.4. Exposed married women also had a higher prevalence of primary subfecundity. No difference in the rates of spontaneous abortion was found, but the malformation rate, particularly of dislocations of the hip, was higher in the exposed group (6/106 births) than in the unexposed group (0/218 births); however, the authors noted that the prevalence of the condition differed between northern and southern Italy.

(ii) *Exposure of men*

A questionnaire on fertility was distributed to the total male work force of three factories in which workers were exposed to mercury vapour and of two control plants with comparable work characteristics in Belgium (Lauwerys et al., 1985). Blood and urine mercury concentrations were used as indices of exposure. The mercury-exposed group consisted of 17 workers in a zinc–mercury amalgam factory, 35 workers in a chloralkali plant and 51 workers in plants for the manufacture of electrical equipment. The 50th and 95th percentiles of mercury in the urine were 36.9 and 147.1 µg/g creatinine. No difference was noted between the observed and expected numbers of children in the mercury-exposed group.

Alcser et al. (1989) conducted a retrospective study of reproductive function in 247 white male workers who had been employed for at least four months between 1953 and 1966 at a US Department of Energy plant where large quantities of metallic mercury were used in 1953–1963. Intermittent periods of potentially high exposure occurred, especially between 1955 and 1956, and a quarterly programme of urine analysis charted worker exposure from 1953 onwards. A control group was selected from unexposed workers at the same plant. Most measures of reproductive health (fertility rates, incidence of major malformations and childhood illnesses) did not differ between the two groups. The wives of the exposed men had a higher rate of miscarriages; however, this effect was also present prior to exposure to mercury.

Cordier et al. (1991) studied the rate of spontaneous abortions in wives of workers exposed to mercury vapour at a chloralkali plant in France and compared it with that of the wives of controls from the same plant. Reproductive history was ascertained by questionnaire in 1984, and exposure history was provided by a plant physician. Urinary mercury levels were measured in most potentially exposed workers at least once a year from 1968. The response to the questionnaire was about 75%, resulting in the inclusion of 118 exposed and 283 unexposed workers. Results were adjusted for maternal age, gravidity, tobacco use and alcohol consumption. The risk for spontaneous abortion increased significantly with increasing urinary mercury concentration in the three months preceding pregnancy. For example, for urinary mercury concentrations in excess of 50 µg/ml in the three-month period prior to the initiation of pregnancy, the spontaneous abortion rate was 18.4/100 pregnancies, as compared with 8.6/100 in the wives of unexposed men [RR, 2.1; 95% CI, 1.1–4.1]. No relationship between exposure to mercury and birth weight or the frequency of malformations was found.

(b) Methylmercury compounds

In a review of the literature, Inskip and Piotrowski (1985) found no evidence that miscarriage, stillbirth, major deficits in birthweight, chromosomal damage or hormonal imbalances in infants were associated with exposure to methylmercury compounds; microcephaly appeared to be the only congenital malformation associated with exposure. Most effects were expressed as clinical symptoms, such as delay in disappearance of primitive reflexes, mental disturbances, retardation of physical development, retardation in emergence of behaviour patterns, disturbances in chewing and swallowing, motility disturbances, impairment of voluntary movements and coordination (ataxia) and constriction of the visual field. Manifestations of toxicity were not always evident at birth but sometimes developed later in childhood.

In a review of autopsy reports on children exposed *in utero* to methylmercury compounds, Burbacher *et al.* (1990) concluded that high concentrations in the brain (12–20 ppm [mg/kg]) decreased brain size, damaged the cortex, basal ganglia and cerebellum and resulted in ventricular dilatation, ectopic cells, gliosis, disorganized layers, misorientated cells and loss of cells. At those tissue concentrations, the neurobehavioural effects included blindness, deafness, cerebral palsy, spasticity, mental deficiency and seizures. At concentrations of 3–11 ppm (mg/kg), mental deficiency, abnormal reflexes and muscle tone and retarded motor development occurred [no data were presented on neuropathological effects]. At low levels (< 3 ppm), delayed psychomotor development was reported.

Foldspang and Hansen (1990) studied reproductive outcomes in Godthaab (365 infants; 45.9% of total births in the period) and Thule (11 infants; 100% of total births), Greenland, between January 1983 and December 1986. Women were invited to participate in the study when they entered maternity clinics at the beginning of labour; nonparticipation was attributed to the difficulty of collecting data in the Arctic. Socioeconomic data, cigarette consumption, consumption of traditional Greenlandic foods (eating whale and seal meat was widespread) and other data were obtained by interview or from hospital records. Maternal and umbilical blood samples were collected at delivery and assayed for total mercury. The average blood mercury concentration of the infants was 21 µg/ml (range, 2–136 µg/L), while maternal levels averaged 14.9 µg/ml (range, 2–128 µg/L). Birth weights were inversely proportional to maternal and offspring blood mercury concentrations. [The Working Group noted that maternal height was not taken into account although birthplace was.]

Grandjean and Weihe (1993) studied birthweight in relation to fish consumption in residents of the Faroe Islands. A total of 1024 births that occurred between March 1986 and December 1987 were included. The average birthweights of the infants of nonsmoking mothers were 3400 g in 13 infants whose mothers consumed no fish and 3600 g ($n = 83$), 3850 ($n = 220$), 3800 ($n = 183$) and 3750 g ($n = 114$) in women who consumed 1, 2, 3 and > 4 fish dinners per week, respectively. The average total mercury concentrations in cord blood were 20, 118, 105, 133 and 138 nmol/L [4, 23.6, 21, 26.6 and 27.6 µg/L] in the same groups. Thus, elevated cord blood mercury concentrations were associated with increased birth-weight, but the authors attributed this correlation to the content of (n-3)-polyunsaturated fatty acids in fish.

4.3.2 Experimental systems

(a) Metallic mercury and inorganic mercury compounds

The reproductive and developmental effects of metallic mercury and its salts in laboratory animals have been reviewed (Khera, 1979; Barlow & Sullivan, 1982; Léonard et al., 1983; Schardein, 1985; Shepard, 1992). In a review, Barlow and Sullivan (1982) concluded that exposure to metallic mercury (e.g. inhalation of 0.3 ppm [2.5 mg/m^3] by rats for 6 h per day for three weeks prior to pregnancy and again on gestation days 7–20) and to inorganic mercury (e.g. intravenous injections of 2–4 mg/kg bw mercury into hamsters on gestation day 8) can cause fetal growth retardation and prenatal and postnatal mortality.

Altered oocyte maturation was reported after exposure of hamsters to mercuric chloride on day 1 of the oestrous cycle. The effective dose levels were as low as 1 mg/kg bw per day (Lamperti & Printz, 1973; Watanabe et al., 1982).

When mercuric chloride (at 5–80 µM [1.2–18.8 mg]) was added to freshly prepared human semen samples in vitro, a dose- and time-dependent decrease in sperm motility was observed. In addition, morphological changes and silver-enhanced mercury deposits in the sperm were noted (Ernst & Lauritsen, 1991).

Exposure of mice to mercuric chloride as 1.5 or 2.0 mg/kg bw Hg by intravenous injection on day 0 resulted in a high incidence of abnormal blastocysts when cells were examined on day 3.5 of gestation (Kajiwara & Inouye, 1986). The minimal effective doses of mercuric acetate that reduced embryonic viability and increased the incidence of malformations and growth retardation in hamsters treated on day 1 of gestation were 35, 25 and 8 mg/kg by oral administration, 8 mg/kg by subcutaneous injection, 4 mg/kg by intravenous injection and 2 mg/kg by intraperitoneal injection (Gale, 1974). Subcutaneous injection of 15 mg/kg bw mercuric acetate to six strains of hamsters on gestation day 8 caused increased resorptions and abnormal and growth retarded fetuses, the incidence of which varied slightly from strain to strain (Gale, 1981).

Exposure of mice to doses of 7.5–25 mg/kg mercuric chloride by subcutaneous injection on day 16 of gestation resulted in a 40% reduction in fetal accumulation of vitamin B$_{12}$ and α-aminobutyric acid within 4 h; no overt fetal toxicity was observed with doses up to 15 mg/kg, although some fetal deaths occurred with 20 mg/kg and maternal lethality was seen at 25 mg/kg (Danielsson et al., 1984). Reduced levels of fetal zinc, copper and iron were reported 4–24 h after exposure of pregnant rats to 0.79 mg/kg mercury by intravenous injection on gestation day 12 (Holt & Webb, 1986a). Intravenous injections of 0.5–0.6 mg/kg mercuric chloride on gestation day 7 were reported to cause fetal malformations. A slightly higher dose (0.79 mg/kg) caused resorptions when given on day 12 and growth retardation when given on days 8, 10, 12, 14 or 16. The authors attributed the fetal effects to alterations in maternal renal function resulting from exposure to mercury (Holt & Webb, 1986b).

Subcutaneous administration of 1 mg/kg bw mercuric chloride to Sprague–Dawley rats on the last eight days of gestation induced a transient increase in urinary excretion of β_2-microglobulin and albumin in both mothers and offspring. In male offspring, these effects reappeared at 180 days of age. A follow-up experiment in which females were dosed throughout pregnancy showed an effect on male offspring renal function at 3–4 months of age, but not at 10 months (Bernard et al., 1992).

Decreased embryonic growth was observed after exposure *in vitro* of day-10 rat embryos to 4 μM mercuric chloride for 48 h or to 20 μM for 24 h; the concentrations required to affect morphogenesis were 1 μM and 20 μM, respectively (Kitchin et al., 1984; Saillenfait et al., 1990).

(b) *Methylmercury compounds*

The literature on the effects of exposure to methylmercury compounds on prenatal development in experimental animals, including effects on the function of several organ systems in postnatal animals following exposure *in utero*, is extensive (for reviews, see Khera, 1979; Reuhl & Chang, 1979; Léonard et al., 1983; Inskip & Piotrowski, 1985; Mottet et al., 1985; Schardein, 1985; Burbacher et al., 1990; Shepard, 1992).

Subcutaneous injection of hamsters with 6.4 or 12.8 mg/kg bw mercury as methylmercury chloride on day 1 of the oestrous cycle did not affect the number of oocytes released (Watanabe et al., 1982).

Albino male rats received 0, 5 or 10 μg/kg bw per day methylmercury chloride by intraperitoneal injection for 15–90 days. Time- and dose-dependent decrease in seminiferous tubular diameter, numbers of Sertoli cells per tubular cross section, and numbers of spermatogonia, preleptotene spermatocytes, pachytene spermatocytes and step-7 spermatids were found. Zygotenes at stages XII through XIII and pachytenes at stages XII through early XIV of seminiferous tubules were most affected. The Sertoli cell was suggested as the target of toxicity (Vachhrajani et al., 1992). [The Working Group noted that the testes were immersed, fixed and embedded in paraffin.] In freshly prepared human semen samples to which methylmercury chloride was added *in vitro*, similar, but less rapid and pronounced changes than those seen with mercuric chloride (see above) were present; however, no silver-enhanced mercury deposition was seen in sperm (Ernst & Lauritsen, 1991).

No effect on the ability to inseminate females or produce viable young was noted in male mice exposed by oral intubation for five to seven days to up to 5 mg/kg mercury as methylmercury chloride in seven consecutive five-day breeding trials. When male Wistar rats were exposed by oral intubation at the same dose regimen for seven days and followed over 14 consecutive five-day breeding trials, a reduced incidence of pregnancy was seen at 5 mg/kg on days 0–15 after treatment and reduced numbers of viable implants were seen on days 5–20 after 2.5 or 5 mg/kg. With longer-term exposures (up to 125 days), reduced numbers of viable implants were seen 25–30 days after exposure to 1 mg/kg and 85–90 days after exposure to 0.5 mg/kg (Khera, 1973a).

A three-generation study showed a lower viability index in F_1 and F_2 generations of rats following dietary exposure to 2.5 but not to 0.5 ppm (mg/kg) methylmercury chloride.

Growth retardation was observed in F_{2a} females at 0.1, 0.5 and 2.5 ppm and in F_{2a} males at 2.5 ppm; and increased relative kidney weights were observed in P males and females, F_{1a} males and F_{2a} females and males at 2.5 ppm, in F_{2a} males and females at 0.5 ppm and in F_{2a} females and F_{1a} males at 0.1 ppm (Verschuuren et al., 1976c).

The development of mouse blastocysts *in vitro* was affected by exposure to methylmercury chloride at 1 μM (Matsumoto & Spindle, 1982) and 0.3 μM (Müller et al., 1990). Intravenous injections of 2 mg/kg bw mercury or more as methylmercury chloride to mice on day 0 of gestation (Kajiwara & Inouye, 1986) or intraperitoneal injection of 5 mg/kg bw to rats during the pre-implantation period (Giavini et al., 1985) affected embryonic development and/or viability.

Prenatal effects on offspring were reported following exposure of mice *in vivo* to methylmercuric chloride during pregnancy at doses as low as 5 mg/kg (fetal weight, Fuyuta et al., 1978; embryonic death, Curle et al., 1983, 1987); malformations commonly seen at this dose or at slightly higher doses included cleft palate and hydronephrosis. The effective dose levels in the rat fetus appear to be similar to those that cause effects in mice (Fuyuta et al., 1979); however, the manifestations vary somewhat (e.g. cleft palate is observed less frequently at 7.5 mg/kg). Reductions in embryonic growth and viability were seen in rat embryos taken on gestation day 10 and exposed *in vitro* to 30 μM methylmercury chloride for 48 h; effects on morphogenesis were reported at the lowest dose tested (3 μM) (Kitchin et al., 1984). Histological damage to the developing brain was observed following exposure *in utero* to methylmercury chloride of hamsters (10 mg/kg on gestation day 10; 2 mg/kg on gestation days 10–15; Reuhl et al., 1981), guinea-pigs (7.5 mg/kg on day 21, 28, 35, 42 or 49; Inouye & Kajiwara, 1988) and cats (0.25 mg/kg on gestation days 10–58; Khera, 1973b). Monkeys (*Macacca fascicularis*) exposed to 50 or 90 μg/kg bw methylmercury hydroxide by oral intubation for 124 days before mating appeared to have lower conception rates and smaller offspring, but small sample sizes precluded statistical significance (Burbacher et al., 1984).

Exposure of mice *in utero* to doses as low as 8 mg/kg of methylmercury compounds on single days of gestation resulted in neonatal mortality and growth impairment (Gates et al., 1986, using the chloride), hydrocephaly (Choi et al., 1988, chloride), changes in activity in the open field (Spyker et al., 1972, dicyandiamide [$CH_3HgNHC(NH)NHCN$]; Su & Okita, 1976, hydroxide) and altered swimming behaviour (Spyker et al., 1972, dicyandiamide). Snell et al. (1977, chloride) reported lower concentrations of liver glycogen in fetal (two-day prenatal) rats but higher concentrations in six-day-old rats exposed to 4 or 8 mg/kg on gestation day 9. Robbins et al. (1978, chloride) found decreased levels of cytochrome P450 and certain xenobiotic metabolizing enzymes in 26–36-week-old male but not female offspring exposed by oral intubation to 5 mg/kg on gestation day 0 or to 2.75 mg/kg on gestation day 7. Chang and Sprecher (1976a,b) reported morphological evidence of renal tubular damage (degenerative changes in epithelial cells of the proximal tubule, hyperplastic changes in distal convoluted tubules and thickening of the tubular epithelial linings) in neonatal rats after injection of dams with 1 or 4 mg/kg methylmercury chloride on day 8 of gestation. Smith et al. (1983) exposed rats to 4 mg/kg methylmercury chloride on days 8, 10 and 12 of gestation and observed reduced uptake of an organic anion (*para*-aminohippurate) by renal slices on postnatal day 42, but not on days 1 or 7, and reduced ability to eliminate sodium and water in volume-loaded rats when measured on postnatal day 42. Slotkin et al. (1986) reported slightly reduced growth rates after weaning, alteration of renal function, an increased level of liver ornithine decarboxylase and altered renal ornithine decarboxylase response to isoproterenol and vasopressin in rats injected subcutaneously with 0.5 or 1.0 mg/kg methylmercury hydroxide on days 8–21 of gestation.

Bornhausen et al. (1980) reported impaired operant behaviour performance in the offspring of rats exposed to daily doses as low as 0.01 mg/kg methylmercury chloride on days 6–9 of gestation. A large, multilaboratory evaluation of behavioural effects in rat offspring exposed to 2 or 6 mg/kg methylmercury chloride on days 6–9 of gestation found increased auditory startle response at the high dose in young offspring and dose-related effects on figure-8 maze exploratory activity and in the pharmacological response to d-amphetamine challenge in older animals (Buelke-Sam et al., 1985). In rats exposed to mercury at 3.9 mg/kg diet as methylmercury chloride via their dams during gestation and lactation and via the diet up to the age of 50 days, no histological change occurred in the brain, but increased noradrenaline levels were observed in the cerebellum (Lindström et al., 1991). Rice (1992) found deficits in fixed interval performance, but not in discrimination reversal or activity patterns, in offspring of *Macaca fascicularis* exposed to steady-state levels during gestation and subsequently of 0, 10, 25 or 50 µg/kg per day mercury as methylmercury chloride. One infant in the high-dose group showed overt signs of methylmercury toxicity.

4.4 Genetic and related effects

4.4.1 *Humans* (see also Table 15, pp. 304–305 and Appendices 1 and 2)

(a) *Dietary exposures*

Skerfving et al. (1970) examined nine Swedish subjects who ate methylmercury-contaminated fish (containing 1–7 ppm [mg/kg] mercury) at least three times a week for more than five years and four controls who ate uncontaminated fish (containing ≤ 0.05 ppm [mg/kg] mercury) less than once a week. There was no significant difference in the frequency of chromosomal aberrations between exposed subjects and controls nor any correlation between aneuploidy or polyploidy rates and concentrations of mercury in red blood cells, which were in the range of 5–17 ng/g in controls and 21–370 ng/g in exposed subjects. Mercury concentrations were, however, significantly correlated with the frequency of structural rearrangements. The study was expanded to include a total of 23 exposed subjects (including the nine subjects already reported in 1970) and 16 controls (Skerfving et al., 1974). Small differences were observed in the frequency of chromosomal aberrations in the exposed groups, and a significant correlation was seen between chromatid-type aberrations, 'unstable' chromosome-type aberrations or aneuploidy and mercury concentrations in red blood cells, which were in the range of 3–17 ng/g in controls and 12–1100 ng/g in exposed subjects. There was no correlation between the frequency of chromosomal aberrations and variations in mercury concentrations in repeated samplings.

Wulf et al. (1986) investigated the frequency of sister chromatid exchange in the lymphocytes of 147 Eskimos living in Greenland or Denmark, who were divided into three groups according to their intake of seal meat: subjects who ate seal meat at least six times a week and had an average concentration of mercury in the blood of 62.5 µg/L (range, 41.9–

65.4); subjects who ate seal meat two to five times per week and had mercury concentrations of 23.2–51.0 µg/L; subjects who ate seal meat once a week or less and had an average mercury concentration in the blood of 22.2 µg/L (range, 5.4–26.4). The mean frequency of sister chromatid exchange was 1.7-fold higher in the group that ate seal meat at least six times a week than in those who ate it less than once a week and 10.7-fold higher in the intermediary group. An increase of 10 µg/L in blood mercury corresponded to an increase of 0.2–0.3 sister chromatid exchanges per cell. [The Working Group noted that the reported results are difficult to interpret because only a series of statistical analyses is provided in the article, with limited original cytogenetic data.]

No increase in the frequency of sister chromatid exchange or numerical chromosomal alterations was detected in 16 subjects who ate fish caught from a methylmercury-contaminated area in Colombia as compared to 14 controls who ate fish from an uncontaminated area. The blood mercury ranges were 2.2–25.8 µg/L in unexposed and 10.2–97.3 µg/L in the exposed people. The frequency of structural chromosomal aberrations was increased only when achromatic lesions (chromatid and chromosome gaps) were included (Monsalve & Chiappe, 1987).

(b) Occupational exposures

Verschaeve *et al.* (1976) examined seven control subjects (blood mercury concentration, 2.5–8.4 µg/L) and 28 mercury-exposed subjects (blood mercury concentration, < 0.1–13 µg/L; urinary mercury concentration, < 0.1–114.12 µg/L) in Belgium, 10 of whom were under medical supervision for mercury intoxication, and 18 subjects working with mercury at Brussels University. An increased frequency of aneuploidy was seen in those subjects exposed to metallic mercury (14), amalgams (3), phenylmercury (8) and ethylmercury (3), while the incidence of structural chromosomal aberrations was increased only in the last (small) group. An increased rate of hyperploidy was also reported by Verschaeve *et al.* (1978) in 16 workers exposed to phenylmercury acetate (blood mercury concentration, 0–5.6 µg/L), compared to 12 unexposed controls (0–3.5 µg/L). In an abstract, Verschaeve and Susanne (1979) reported an increased rate of aneuploidy, with no increase in the frequency of structural chromosomal aberrations in 10 subjects exposed to mercury-containing amalgams in a dental practice and compared with 10 controls, but they could not rule out other factors such as X-rays. Verschaeve *et al.* (1979) failed to detect any chromosomal effect in 28 workers exposed to metallic mercury (urinary mercury concentration, 7–175 µg/L) in a chloralkali plant, as compared with 20 unexposed controls (eight from the same plant [< 5–15 µg/L] and 12 from the general population). In the discussion of the report, the authors questioned the positive findings in their previous three studies, stating that they might have been due to lack of information on exposures to agents other than mercury in the subjects. Negative results were also reported in a more recent Belgian study (Mabille *et al.*, 1984) involving cytogenetic analyses of 25 unexposed subjects (urinary mercury, < 5 µg/g creatinine, and blood mercury, < 6 µg/L) and of 22 workers exposed to metallic mercury in a chloralkali plant and in a plant in which mercury is amalgamated with zinc (urinary mercury, 8.2–286 µg/g creatinine, and blood mercury, 7.5–105.2 µg/L).

Popescu *et al.* (1979) examined peripheral blood lymphocytes from 22 workers in two departments of a chemical plant in Romania, four of whom were exposed to vapours of metallic mercury and 18 to a mixture of mercuric chloride, methylmercury chloride and ethylmercury chloride. During the year before the study, atmospheric mercury concentrations ranged from 0.15 to 0.44 mg/m3. Urinary analysis demonstrated high concentrations of mercury (100–896 µg/L). When compared with 10 unexposed controls, neither exposed group had an increased rate of aneuploidy or of total structural chromosomal aberrations; however, both had a significant increase in the frequency of acentric fragments.

In an abstract, Mottironi et al. (1986) reported an increased rate of sister chromatid exchange in somatic cells [presumably lymphocytes] from 29 workers exposed to metallic mercury and inorganic mercury in two plants [presumably in the USA] (blood mercury, 6.7–103.9 µg/L) over that in 26 unexposed controls (blood mercury, 1.5–6.1 µg/L). The increase was significant in 'exposed workers with high mercury levels' in the blood [no detail given] and was enhanced by cigarette smoking. An increased rate of sister chromatid exchange, related to time since exposure, was detected in Argentina in the lymphocytes of 38 children, aged one month to five years, who had been intoxicated by the use of phenylmercury acetate to disinfect diapers. Nineteen unexposed children served as controls. The increased rate of sister chromatid exchange disappeared nine months after exposure ceased (Mudry de Pargament et al., 1987).

Barregård et al. (1991) compared the incidence of lymphocytic micronuclei in 26 chloralkali workers (air mercury concentration, 25–50 µg/m^3) and 26 unexposed controls in Sweden. No difference was found between the two groups, and no correlation was found with current mercury concentrations in erythrocytes, plasma or urine (exposed, 4.8–64.6 µg/L, 2.8–40 µg/L and 5–186 µg/L; controls, 2.4–20.2 µg/L, 0.8–2.6 µg/L and 0.2–9.6 µg/L, respectively). A significant association was found between the number of micronuclei in phytohaemagglutinin-stimulated blood and previous exposure to mercury (measured either by a cumulative exposure index, i.e. integrated yearly mean blood mercury over employment time, or number of occasions when blood mercury peaks were > 150 nmol/L [30 µg/L]), suggesting an accumulation of cytogenetic effects in T lymphocytes. No such association was seen in pokeweed mitogen-stimulated blood. Anwar and Gabal (1991) examined 29 workers in an explosives factory in Egypt (mean urinary mercury concentration, 123 µg/L) who were exposed to mercury fulminate [$Hg(CNO)_2$] (which results from the reaction between mercuric nitrate, ethanol and nitric acid) and 29 controls (mean urinary mercury concentration, 39 µg/L). The frequencies of both micronuclei and chromosomal aberrations (gaps, breaks and fragments) were increased in the exposed group. The authors reported, however, that the increases were not correlated with urinary concentration of mercury or duration of exposure, putting in question the role of mercury in the observed clastogenic effect. In addition, there was no increased incidence of either aneuploidy or polyploidy.

4.4.2 *Experimental systems*

The genetic and related effects of mercury compounds have been reviewed (Ramel, 1972; Léonard et al., 1983; Kazantzis & Lilly, 1986).

(a) *Inorganic mercury compounds* (see also Table 16, pp. 307–309 and Appendices 1 and 2)

Almost all of the studies reported were carried out with mercuric chloride.

Table 15. Genetic and related effects of mercury in humans

Test system	Result without exogenous metabolic system	Dose[a] (LED/HID)	Reference
Food contaminated with organomercury compounds[b]			
SLH, Sister chromatid exchange, human lymphocytes in vivo	(+)[c]	0.042	Wulf et al. (1986)
SLH, Sister chromatid exchange, human lymphocytes in vivo	–	0.040	Monsalve & Chiappe (1987)
CLH, Chromosomal aberrations, human lymphocytes in vivo	(+)	0.126	Skerfving et al. (1970)
CLH, Chromosomal aberrations, human lymphocytes in vivo	(+)	0.12	Skerfving et al. (1974)
CLH, Chromosomal aberrations, human lymphocytes in vivo	–[d]	0.040	Monsalve & Chiappe (1987)
AVH, Aneuploidy, human lymphocytes in vivo	–	0.126	Skerfving et al. (1970)
AVH, Aneuploidy, human lymphocytes in vivo	(+)	0.12	Skerfving et al. (1974)
Occupational and environmental exposures to mercury			
Metallic mercury			
SLH, Sister chromatid exchange, human lymphocytes in vivo[e]	+	0.027	Mottironi et al. (1986) abstract
MVH, Micronucleus induction, phytohaemaglutinin-stimulated human (T) lymphocytes in vivo	(+)	0.025	Barregård et al. (1991)
MVH, Micronucleus induction, pokeweed mitogen-stimulated human (T/B) lymphocytes in vivo	–	0.025	Barregård et al. (1991)
CLH, Chromosomal aberrations, human lymphocytes in vivo	–	NR	Verschaeve et al. (1976)
CLH, Chromosomal aberrations, human lymphocytes in vivo	+	NR	Popescu et al. (1979)
CLH, Chromosomal aberrations, human lymphocytes in vivo	–	NR	Verschaeve et al. (1979)
CLH, Chromosomal aberrations, human lymphocytes in vivo	–	0.031	Mabille et al. (1984)
AVH, Aneuploidy, human lymphocytes in vivo	?	NR	Verschaeve et al. (1976)
AVH, Aneuploidy, human lymphocytes in vivo	–	NR	Popescu et al. (1979)
AVH, Aneuploidy, human lymphocytes in vivo	–	NR	Verschaeve et al. (1979)
Amalgams			
CLH, Chromosomal aberrations, human lymphocytes in vivo	–	NR	Verschaeve et al. (1976)
CLH, Chromosomal aberrations, human lymphocytes in vivo	–	NR	Verschaeve & Susanne (1979) abstract
AVH, Aneuploidy, human lymphocytes in vivo	?	NR	Verschaeve et al. (1976)
AVH, Aneuploidy, human lymphocytes in vivo	?	NR	Verschaeve & Susanne (1979) abstract

Table 15 (contd)

Test system	Result without exogenous metabolic system	Dose[a] (LED/HID)	Reference
Ethylmercury compounds [unspecified]			
CLH, Chromosomal aberrations, human lymphocytes *in vivo*	?	NR	Verschaeve *et al.* (1976)
AVH, Aneuploidy, human lymphocytes *in vivo*	?	NR	Verschaeve *et al.* (1976)
Mercury fulminate [Hg(CNO)$_2$]			
MVH, Micronuclei, human lymphocytes *in vivo*	?	NR	Anwar & Gabal (1991)
CLH, Chromosomal aberrations, human lymphocytes *in vivo*	?	NR	Anwar & Gabal (1991)
AVH, Aneuploidy, human lymphocytes *in vivo*	–	NR	Anwar & Gabal (1991)
Methylmercury chloride/ethylmercury chloride/mercuric chloride mixture			
CLH, Chromosomal aberrations, human lymphocytes *in vivo*	+	NR	Popescu *et al.* (1979)
AVH, Aneuploidy, human lymphocytes *in vivo*	–	NR	Popescu *et al.* (1979)
Phenylmercury compounds [unspecified]			
CLH, Chromosomal aberrations, human lymphocytes *in vivo*	–	0.008	Verschaeve *et al.* (1976)
AVH, Aneuploidy, human lymphocytes *in vivo*	(+)	0.008	Verschaeve *et al.* (1976)
Phenylmercury acetate			
CLH, Chromosomal aberrations, human lymphocytes *in vivo*	–	0.002	Verschaeve *et al.* (1978)
AVH, Aneuploidy, human lymphocytes *in vivo*	?	0.002	Verschaeve *et al.* (1978)
SCE, Sister chromatid exchange, human lymphocytes *in vivo*	+	NR	Mudry de Pargament *et al.* (1987)

+, positive; (+), weakly positive; +?, positively questioned by the authors themselves; –, negative; ?, inconclusive
[a]Mean concentration of Hg in blood; µg/ml. NR, not reported
[b]Organic mercury of alimentary source (seal or fish meat)
[c]Also contaminated with lead, cadmium and selenium
[d]Excluding gaps; positive if gaps are included
[e]Exposure to metallic mercury mixed with organic mercury

In bacteria, assays for differential toxicity suggest that mercuric chloride induces DNA damage very weakly in *Bacillus subtilis* and not in *Escherichia coli*. No studies of bacterial mutation were available to the Working Group.

Mercuric chloride weakly induced mitotic recombination and induced mitochondrial mutations in *Saccharomyces cerevisiae*. It induced various types of mutations in the plant, *Anacharis canadensis*.

Mercuric chloride did not increase the frequency of micronuclei in cultured fish cells, even when tested at doses 10 times higher than those that were effective for some organomercury compounds.

In cultured mammalian cells, mercuric chloride inhibited DNA repair induced by X-rays but not that induced by ultraviolet radiation. Gene mutations at the *tk* locus were induced in a single study with mouse lymphoma L5178Y cells, but only in the presence of an exogenous metabolic system from rat liver. Sister chromatid exchange was induced in cultured Chinese hamster ovary cells and in human lymphocytes. Spindle disturbance and chromosomal aberrations were induced by mercuric chloride in most studies with cultured mammalian cells, including human lymphocytes, and by mercuric acetate in mouse oocytes *in vitro*.

Mercuric chloride enhanced cell transformation produced by simian adenovirus SA7 in Syrian hamster embryo primary cell cultures. Mercuric acetate did not induce anchorage-dependent growth of human fibroblasts.

In larvae of the newt, *Pleurodeles waltl*, mercuric chloride induced chromosomal aberrations and micronuclei in erythrocytes. Studies of mammals exposed to mercuric chloride *in vivo* have given negative or conflicting results. Neither chromosomal aberrations nor aneuploidy were observed in Syrian hamster bone marrow or oocytes following a single subcutaneous dose of 12.8 mg/kg mercuric chloride. In mice, the frequency of chromosomal aberrations in bone-marrow cells was increased in one study after a single oral dose of 3 mg/kg but not in another study by intraperitoneal injection of a dose of 6 mg/kg. In a second study in mice, chromosomal aberrations were not induced in spermatogonia. Weak dominant lethal effects have been described in rats and mice. Mercuric acetate did not induce chromosomal aberrations in mouse oocytes after subcutaneous or intravenous dosing.

(b) *Organomercury compounds* (see also Table 17, pp. 312–320 and Appendices 1 and 2)

Very weak differential toxicity was induced in *B. subtilis* by methylmercury chloride, but negative results were obtained with phenylmercury chloride and bis(ethylmercury)hydrogen phosphate. Mutations were not induced in *Salmonella typhimurium* by methylmercury chloride or methylmercury acetate.

Methylmercury chloride did not induce gene conversion or mitotic recombination in *S. cerevisiae*, but conflicting results were obtained for induction of mutations, mitochondrial mutations and aneuploidy.

Phenylmercury nitrate induced mutations in seedlings of *Zea mays*, and phenylmercury hydroxide induced mutations in seedlings of a number of different plants. Chromosomal aberrations and/or spindle disturbances were induced in *Allium cepa* roots by all of eight compounds tested.

Table 16. Genetic and related effects of inorganic mercury compounds in experimental systems

Test system	Result without exogenous metabolic system	Result with exogenous metabolic system	Dose[a] (LED/HID)	Reference
Mercuric chloride (74% Hg)				
PRB, Lambda-prophage induction, *E. coli*	–	0		Rossman *et al.* (1991)
BSD, *Bacillus subtilis* rec strains, differential toxicity	(+)	0	0.036	Kanematsu *et al.* (1980)
ERD, *Escherichia coli* rec strains, differential toxicity	–	0	10 000	Brandi *et al.* (1990)
SCH, *Saccharomyces cerevisiae* D7, mitotic crossing-over	(+)	0	0.5	Fukunaga *et al.* (1981)
SCR, *Saccharomyces cerevisiae* N123, petite mutation	(+)	0	60	Fukunaga *et al.* (1981)
PLM, *Anacharis canadensis*, mutation	+	0	20	MacFarlane & Messing (1953)
***, Micronuclei, fish (*Lepomis macrochirus*)[b] cells *in vitro*	–	0	740	Babich *et al.* (1990)
***, Inhibition of X-ray-induced DNA repair, Chinese hamster ovary cells *in vitro*	+	0	0.8	Christie *et al.* (1986)
***, Inhibition of UV-induced DNA repair, Chinese hamster ovary cells *in vitro*	–	0	0.2	Christie *et al.* (1986)
DIA, DNA strand breaks, Chinese hamster ovary cells *in vitro*	+	0	10	Cantoni *et al.* (1982)
DIA, DNA strand breaks, Chinese hamster ovary cells *in vitro*	+	0	5.0	Robison *et al.* (1982)
DIA, DNA strand breaks, Chinese hamster ovary cells *in vitro*	+	0	2.0	Cantoni & Costa (1983)
DIA, DNA strand breaks, Chinese hamster ovary cells *in vitro*	+	0	5.0	Cantoni *et al.* (1984a)
DIA, DNA strand breaks, Chinese hamster ovary cells *in vitro*	+	0	5.0	Cantoni *et al.* (1984b)
DIA, DNA strand breaks, Chinese hamster ovary cells *in vitro*	+	0	1.0	Robison *et al.* (1984)
DIA, DNA strand breaks, mouse embryo fibroblasts *in vitro*	+	0	10	Zasukhina *et al.* (1983)
DIA, DNA strand breaks, rat embryo fibroblasts *in vitro*	+	0	0.02	Zasukhina *et al.* (1983)
RIA, DNA repair, Syrian hamster cells *in vitro*	(+)	0	0.02	Robison *et al.* (1984)
GST, Gene mutation, mouse lymphoma L5178Y cells, *tk* locus, *in vitro*	–	(+)	2.0	Oberly *et al.* (1982)
SIC, Sister chromatid exchange, Chinese hamster ovary cells *in vitro*	(+)	0	4.44	Howard *et al.* (1991)
CIC, Chromosomal aberrations, Chinese hamster ovary cells *in vitro*	+	0	2.0	Howard *et al.* (1991)
			0.2	

Table 16 (contd)

Test system	Result		Dose[a] (LED/HID)	Reference
	Without exogenous metabolic system	With exogenous metabolic system		
Mercuric chloride (contd)				
***, Spindle disturbances, Indian muntjac fibroblasts *in vitro*	+	0	0.1	Verschaeve et al. (1984)
***, Spindle disturbances, human lymphocytes *in vitro*	+	0	0.2	Verschaeve et al. (1984)
T7S, Cell transformation, SA7/Syrian hamster embryo cells *in vitro*	+	0	10	Casto et al. (1979)
SHL, Sister chromatid exchange, human lymphocytes *in vitro*	+	0	0.08	Morimoto et al. (1982)
CHL, Chromosomal aberrations, human lymphocytes *in vitro*	+	0	4.0	Verschaeve et al. (1985)
CHT, Chromosomal aberrations, human HeLa cells *in vitro*	−	0	7.4	Umeda et al. (1969)
***, Chromosomal condensation, human lymphocytes *in vitro*	+	0	2.0	Andersen et al. (1983)
***, Micronuclei in red blood cells, newt larvae *in vivo*	+		0.012	Zoll et al. (1988)
CBA, Chromosomal aberrations, mouse bone-marrow cells *in vivo*	−		4.44, ip × 1	Poma et al. (1981)
CBA, Chromosomal aberrations, Syrian hamster bone-marrow cells *in vivo*	(+)		4.74, sc × 1	Watanabe et al. (1982)
CBA, Chromosomal aberrations, mouse bone-marrow cells *in vivo*	+		2.22, po × 1	Ghosh et al. (1991)
CGG, Chromosomal aberrations, mouse spermatogonia *in vivo*	−		4.44, ip × 1	Poma et al. (1981)
COE, Chromosomal aberrations, Syrian hamster oocytes *in vivo*	−		9.47, sc × 1	Watanabe et al. (1982)
***, Chromosomal aberrations, newt larvae and embryos *in vivo*	+		0.06, water × 4 days	Zoll et al. (1988)
AVA, Aneuploidy, Syrian hamster bone-marrow cells *in vivo*	−		9.47, sc × 1	Watanabe et al. (1982)
AVA, Aneuploidy, Syrian hamster oocytes *in vivo*	−		9.47, sc × 1	Watanabe et al. (1982)
DLM, Dominant lethal mutation, mice	(+)		1.48, ip × 1	Suter (1975)
DLR, Dominant lethal mutation, rats	(+)		0.0003, po/day × 12 months	Zasukhina et al. (1983)
Mercurous chloride				
BSD, *Bacillus subtilis rec* strains, differential toxicity	+	0	10 000	Kanematsu et al. (1980)

Table 16 (contd)

Test system	Result		Dose[a] (LED/HID)	Reference
	Without exogenous metabolic system	With exogenous metabolic system		
Mercuric acetate (63% Hg)				
CIA, Chromosomal aberrations, mouse oocytes *in vitro*	+	0	35	Jagiello & Lin (1973)
TIH, Anchorage-independent growth, human foreskin fibroblasts *in vitro*	−	0	2.0	Biedermann & Landolph (1987)
COE, Chromosomal aberrations, mouse oocytes *in vivo*	−		2, iv × 1	Jagiello & Lin (1973)
COE, Chromosomal aberrations, mouse oocytes *in vivo*	−		10, sc × 1	Jagiello & Lin (1973)

+, considered to be positive; (+), considered to be weakly positive in an inadequate study; −, considered to be negative; ?, considered to be inconclusive (variable responses in several experiments within an adequate study); 0, not tested

[a]LED, lowest effective dose; HID, highest ineffective dose. In-vitro tests, μg/ml; in-vivo tests, mg/kg bw. Doses given as concentration of element, not concentration of compound; ip, intraperitoneally; sc, subcutaneously; iv, intravenously; po, orally by gavage

[b]Bluegill sunfish

***Not displayed on profile

Methylmercury hydroxide induced sex-linked recessive lethal mutations, but not chromosomal aberrations or meiotic crossing-over, in *Drosophila melanogaster*. It induced chromosomal aberrations in *Stethophyma grossum*. Methylmercury chloride, methylmercury hydroxide, phenylmercury hydroxide and phenylmercury acetate consistently induce aneuploidy in *D. melanogaster*. Methylmercury chloride did not induce aneuploidy in silkworms.

Studies of gene mutations in cultured mammalian cells have yielded varying responses. In one study, both methylmercury chloride and methoxyethylmercury chloride induced ouabain-resistance and *hprt* locus mutations in Chinese hamster V79 cells, whereas in another study with the same cells methylmercury hydroxide did not induce mutations at the *hprt* locus.

The induction of spindle disturbances and chromosomal aberrations has been studied extensively in cultured mammalian cells, including human lymphocytes. Significant responses were obtained consistently with methylmercury chloride in a number of studies of both end-points. In addition, chromosomal aberrations and/or spindle disturbances have been induced by methylmercury hydroxide, methoxyethylmercury chloride, dimethyl mercury, ethylmercury chloride and phenylmercury chloride in independent studies using Chinese hamster V79 cells, human HeLa cells and lymphocytes *in vitro*. The frequency of micronuclei, which may be an expression of either spindle disturbances or chromosomal breakage, was increased in cultured cells from *Lepomis macrochinus* (bluegill sunfish) after treatment with methylmercury chloride, ethylmercury chloride or phenylmercury chloride.

Methylmercury chloride induced chromosomal aberrations in larvae and embryos of the newt, *Pleurodeles waltl*, and micronuclei in peripheral erythrocytes of the larvae. Treatment of pregnant rats with methylmercury chloride induced chromosomal aberrations in the livers of the fetuses, but it did not induce chromosomal aberrations in the bone marrow of Syrian hamsters and rats or in oocytes of Syrian hamsters. Intraperitoneal injection of methylmercury acetate did not induce micronuclei in mouse bone-marrow cells. Spindle disturbances were induced by methylmercury chloride in fetal lung and liver cells after treatment of mice *in vivo* in two studies and in killifish (*Fundulus heteroclitus*) embryo cells. Aneuploidy was seen in bone-marrow cells and oocytes of Syrian hamsters in one study but not in another. Methylmercury chloride appears therefore to be more active as a clastogen in fetal than in adult tissues of mice and more active as a spindle poison in Syrian hamster bone marrow than in Syrian hamster oocytes.

Dominant lethal mutation has been demonstrated in male rats and female mice, but not in male mice, treated with methylmercury chloride. Methylmercury hydroxide induced either weak or no dominant lethal effect in male mice. Methylmercury acetate did not induce sperm-head abnormalities in mice.

Few studies have been conducted on nonionized organomercury compounds; those that have been performed reflect the properties described above. Thus, dimethylmercury induced DNA fragmentation in the slime mould *Physarum polycephalum* and chromosomal aberrations and aneuploidy in cultured human lymphocytes; it induced chromosomal aberrations in mouse oocytes *in vitro* but not *in vivo*.

Several fungicides containing organomercury compounds have been tested for genotoxic activity in various plant systems. Spindle disturbances were induced by Panogen 5, 8 and 15, while chromosomal aberrations were induced by Agrimax M, Granosan, Ceresan M, Betoxin and New Improved Ceresan. [The Working Group noted that the different results may not reflect different properties, as various authors were involved.] In *D. melanogaster*, sex-linked recessive lethal mutation was induced by Ceresan and Ceresan M, but not by Agallol 3, and neither Ceresan nor Agallol 3 induced dominant lethal effects.

The azo dye, mercury orange, was not mutagenic to strains of *S. typhimurium*.

Considerations with regard to genotoxic mechanisms

Mercury has not only a direct effect on chromosomes, resulting in clastogenic effects in eukaryotes, but also causes disturbance of the spindle mechanism, owing to its high affinity for the sulfhydryl groups contained in spindle fibre proteins. Organomercury compounds inhibit the spindle mechanism even more strongly than colchicine, but, in contrast to colchicine, produce a gradual transition to c-mitosis at sub-lethal doses, which may result in aneuploidy and/or polyploidy.

In general, inorganic mercury compounds are less effective than ionizable organomercury compounds in inducing genetic effects *in vitro*. Similarities in the effects of different mercury compounds may suggest similar modes of action, while differences may be due to variations in solubility and bioavailability and in the rate of formation of a common toxic entity.

The possible contribution of reactive oxygen species to the genotoxicity of inorganic mercury compounds has also been addressed. ^{203}Hg-Mercuric chloride is taken up by Chinese hamster ovary cells and was reported to bind to the DNA in these cells in a temperature-dependent manner; however, DNA strand breaks were induced at 37 °C, but not at 4 °C, even though there was uptake and DNA binding of mercury at the lower temperature. It therefore appears that DNA strand breaks induced by Hg^{2+} require cellular metabolic processes. Mercuric chloride induced single-strand breaks in DNA of Chinese hamster ovary cells, and the effect was related linearly to leakage of superoxide into the medium. DNA damage induced by mercuric chloride can be increased by the addition of diethyldithiocarbamate, which inhibits superoxide dismutase, as well as by diethyl maleate, which depletes glutathione. Single strand breakage was inhibited by superoxide dismutase, catalase, glycerol and ascorbate (Cantoni *et al.*, 1984b).

5. Summary of Data Reported and Evaluation

5.1 Exposure data

Mercury occurs at low concentrations in the Earth's crust, mainly in sulfide ores (cinnabar), from which it has been extracted for a variety of uses for many centuries. Common applications of metallic mercury are as a cathode in the electrolytic production of chlorine, in dental amalgams, in the extraction of gold from ore concentrates, in electrical equipment and in devices for measuring temperature and pressure. Mercury compounds have been used as fungicides in paints and on seeds and grains, as antiseptics, in electrical applications, and as catalysts and intermediates.

Table 17. Genetic and related effects of organomercury compounds in experimental systems

Test system	Result		Dose[a] (LED/HID)	Reference
	Without exogenous metabolic system	With exogenous metabolic system		
Methylmercury chloride (80% Hg)				
BSD, *Bacillus subtilis* rec strains, differential toxicity	+	0	1000	Kanematsu *et al.* (1980)
SA0, *Salmonella typhimurium* TA100, reverse mutation (spot test)	–	0	NR	Kanematsu *et al.* (1980)
SA5, *Salmonella typhimurium* TA1535, reverse mutation (spot test)	–	0	NR	Kanematsu *et al.* (1980)
SA7, *Salmonella typhimurium* TA1537, reverse mutation (spot test)	–	0	NR	Kanematsu *et al.* (1980)
SA8, *Salmonella typhimurium* TA1538, reverse mutation (spot test)	–	0	NR	Kanematsu *et al.* (1980)
SA9, *Salmonella typhimurium* TA98, reverse mutation (spot test)	–	0	NR	Kanematsu *et al.* (1980)
EC2, *Escherichia coli* WP2, reverse mutation (spot test)	–	0	NR	Kanematsu *et al.* (1980)
ECR, *Escherichia coli* WP2 B/r, reverse mutation (spot test)	–	0	NR	Kanematsu *et al.* (1980)
SCG, *Saccharomyces cerevisiae*, gene conversion	–	0	NR	Nakai & Machida (1973) abstract
SCH, *Saccharomyces cerevisiae*, mitotic recombination	–	0	NR	Nakai & Machida (1973) abstract
SCH, *Saccharomyces cerevisiae* D7, mitotic recombination	–	0	10.0	Phipps & Miller (1982)
SCF, *Saccharomyces cerevisiae*, forward mutation	+	0	NR	Phipps & Miller (1983)
SCR, *Saccharomyces cerevisiae*, reverse mutation	–	0	NR	Nakai & Machida (1973) abstract
SCR, *Saccharomyces cerevisiae*, petite mutation	+	0	NR	Nakai & Machida (1973) abstract
SCR, *Saccharomyces cerevisiae*, petite mutation	–	0	10.0	Phipps & Miller (1983)
SCN, *Saccharomyces cerevisiae*, aneuploidy	?	0	NR	Nakai & Machida (1973) abstract
PLI, Water hyacinth (*Eichhornia crassipes*), micronuclei	+	0	0.1 (acute exposure)	Panda *et al.* (1988)
***, *Allium cepa*, spindle disturbances	+	0	1.0	Fiskesjö (1969)
***, Silkworm, aneuploidy	–		NR	Tazima (1974) abstract
DMN, *Drosophila melanogaster* aneuploidy (FIX system)	+		5.0	Osgood *et al.* (1991)
DMN, *Drosophila melanogaster* aneuploidy (ZESTE system)	–		100	Osgood *et al.* (1991)

Table 17 (contd)

Test system	Result		Dose[a] (LED/HID)	Reference
	Without exogenous metabolic system	With exogenous metabolic system		
Methylmercury chloride (contd)				
G9O, Gene mutation, Chinese hamster lung V79 cells, ouabain resistance, in vitro	+	0	0.32	Fiskesjö (1979)
G9H, Gene mutation, Chinese hamster lung V79 cells, 8-azaguanine resistance, in vitro	+	0	0.16	Fiskesjö (1979)
***, Micronucleus test, fish (*Lepomis macrochirus*) cells in vitro	+	0	0.08	Babich et al. (1990)
CIC, Chromosomal aberrations, Chinese hamster brain cells in vitro	+	0	NR	Kato (1976) abst.
***, Spindle disturbances, Indian muntjac fibroblasts in vitro	+	0	1.0	Verschaeve et al. (1984)
SHL, Sister chromatid exchange, human lymphocytes in vitro	+	0	0.016	Morimoto et al. (1982)
***, Spindle disturbances, human lymphocytes in vitro	+	0	0.4	Fiskesjö (1970)
CHL, Chromosomal aberrations, human lymphocytes in vitro	+	0	0.04	Kato (1976) abstract; Kato et al. (1976) abstract
***, Spindle disturbances, human lymphocytes in vitro	+	0	0.08	Tournamille et al. (1982)
CHL, Chromosomal aberrations, human lymphocytes in vitro	+	0	1.0	Verschaeve et al. (1985)
CHL, Chromosomal aberrations, human lymphocytes in vitro	+	0	0.12	Betti et al. (1992)
AIH, Aneuploidy, human lymphocytes in vitro	+	0	0.12	Betti et al. (1992)
SVA, Sister chromatid exchange, mouse fetal lung and liver cells in vivo	+		8.0, po × 1	Curle et al. (1987)
***, Micronuclei, newt (*Pleurodeles waltl*) larvae red blood cells, in vivo	+		0.012, in water × 12 days	Zoll et al. (1988)
***, Nuclear abnormalities, cat bone-marrow cells in vivo	+		0.008, po × 39 months	Miller et al. (1979)
***, Spindle disturbances, mouse fetal lung and liver cells in vivo	+		4.0, po × 1	Curle et al. (1983)
AVA, Aneuploidy, Syrian hamster bone-marrow cells in vivo	+		4.74, sc × 1	Watanabe et al. (1982)
***, Spindle disturbances, mouse fetal lung and liver cells in vivo	+		4.0, po × 1	Curle et al. (1987)
***, Spindle disturbances, killifish (*Fundulus heteroclitus*) embryos in vivo	+		0.04, in water	Perry et al. (1988)
CBA, Chromosomal aberrations, Syrian hamster bone-marrow cells in vivo	(+)		9.47, sc × 1	Watanabe et al. (1982)

Table 17 (contd)

Test system	Result Without exogenous metabolic system	Result With exogenous metabolic system	Dose[a] (LED/HID)	Reference
Methylmercury chloride (contd)				
CBA, Chromosomal aberrations, rat bone-marrow cells *in vivo*	+		4.64, ip × 1	Li & Lin (1991)
AVA, Aneuploidy, Syrian hamster oocytes *in vivo*	−		9.47, sc × 1	Watanabe *et al.* (1982)
AVA, Aneuploidy, Syrian hamster bone-marrow cells *in vivo*	+		4.47, sc × 1	Watanabe *et al.* (1982)
COE, Chromosomal aberrations, Syrian hamster oocytes *in vivo*	−		9.47, sc × 1	Watanabe *et al.* (1982)
COE, Chromosomal aberrations, Syrian hamster oocytes *in vivo*	−		8.0, ip × 1	Mailhes (1983)
***, Chromosomal aberrations, newt (*Pleurodeles walt*) larvae or embryos *in vivo*	+		0.04, in water × 4 days	Zoll *et al.* (1988)
COE, Chromosomal aberrations, rat embryo liver cells *in vivo*	+		1.52, ip × 1	Li & Lin (1991)
DLM, Dominant lethal mutation, male mice *in vivo*	−		5, po × 7 days	Khera (1973a)
DLM, Dominant lethal mutation, female mice *in vivo*	+		2.0, ip × 1	Verschaeve & Léonard (1984)
DLR, Dominant lethal mutation, male rats *in vivo*	+		2.5, po × 7 days	Khera (1973a)
DLR, Dominant lethal mutation, male rats *in vivo*	+		0.5, po × 90 days	Khera (1973a)
AVA, Aneuploidy, Syrian hamster oocytes *in vivo*	+		8.0, ip × 1	Mailhes (1983)
Methylmercury hydroxide [CH$_3$HgOH] (86% Hg)				
ACC, *Allium cepa*, chromosomal aberrations	+	0	0.05	Ramel (1969)
***, *Allium cepa*, spindle disturbances	+	0	0.05	Ramel (1969)
***, *Vicia faba*, spindle disturbances	+	0	0.02	Ramel (1972)
DMG, *Drosophila melanogaster*, meiotic crossing-over	−		4.3	Ramel (1972)
DMX, *Drosophila melanogaster*, sex-linked recessive lethal mutations	(+)		4.3	Ramel (1972)
DMX, *Drosophila melanogaster*, sex-linked recessive lethal mutations	+		8.6, diet	Magnusson & Ramel (1986)
***, *Drosophila melanogaster*, effect on radiation-induced chromosomal aberrations	−		4.3	Ramel (1972)
***, *Stethophyma grossum*, chromosomal aberrations	+		8 ng/animal	Klášterská & Ramel (1978)

Table 17 (contd)

Test system	Result		Dose[a] (LED/HID)	Reference
	Without exogenous metabolic system	With exogenous metabolic system		
Methylmercury hydroxide (contd)				
DMN, *Drosophila melanogaster*, aneuploidy	+		0.25, diet	Ramel & Magnusson (1969)
DMN, *Drosophila melanogaster*, aneuploidy	+		0.25, diet	Ramel & Magnusson (1979)
DMN, *Drosophila melanogaster*, aneuploidy	+		0.43, diet	Magnusson & Ramel (1986)
***, Spindle disturbances, Chinese hamster lung V79 cells *in vitro*	+	0	0.42	Önfelt (1983)
G9H, Gene mutation, Chinese hamster lung V79 cells, *hprt* locus, *in vitro*	−	0	0.16	Önfelt & Jenssen (1982)
DLM, Dominant lethal mutation, (SEC×C57Bl)F$_1$ male mice *in vivo*	(+)		7.4, ip × 1	Suter (1975)
DLM, Dominant lethal mutation, (101×C3H)F$_1$ male mice *in vivo*	−		7.4, ip × 1	Suter (1975)
Methylmercury acetate [CH$_3$HgCO$_2$CH$_3$] (73% Hg)				
SA0, *Salmonella typhimurium* TA100, reverse mutation	−	−	183	Bruce & Heddle (1979)
SA5, *Salmonella typhimurium* TA1535, reverse mutation	−	−	183	Bruce & Heddle (1979)
SA7, *Salmonella typhimurium* TA1537, reverse mutation	−	−	183	Bruce & Heddle (1979)
SA9, *Salmonella typhimurium* TA98, reverse mutation	−	−	183	Bruce & Heddle (1979)
MVM, Micronuclei, B6C3F1 mouse bone-marrow cells *in vivo*	−		11.0, ip × 5	Bruce & Heddle (1979)
SPM, Sperm-head abnormalities, B6C3F1 mice *in vivo*	−		11.0, ip × 5	Bruce & Heddle (1979)
Methylmercury dicyandiamide [CH$_3$HgNHC(NH)NHCN] (67% Hg)				
***, *Allium cepa*, spindle disturbances	+		0.5	Ramel (1969)
DLM, Dominant lethal mutation, mice *in vivo*	−	0	2.0	Ramel (1972)
Ethylmercury chloride [CH$_3$CH$_2$HgCl]				
***, *Allium cepa*, spindle disturbances	+	0	0.4	Fiskesjö (1969)
***, Micronuclei, fish (*Lepomis macrochirus*) cells *in vitro*	+	0	0.08	Babich *et al.* (1990)
***, Spindle disturbances, human HeLa cells *in vitro*	+	0	1	Umeda *et al.* (1969)

Table 17 (contd)

Test system	Result		Dose[a] (LED/HID)	Reference
	Without exogenous metabolic system	With exogenous metabolic system		
Bis(ethylmercury)hydrogen phosphate [(CH$_3$CH$_2$Hg)$_2$HPO$_4$]				
BSD, *Bacillus subtilis* rec strains, differential toxicity	–	0	14.4	Shirasu *et al.* (1976)
Butylmercury bromide [(CH$_3$(CH$_2$)$_3$HgBr]				
***, *Allium cepa*, spindle disturbances	+	0	0.2	Fiskesjö (1969)
Methoxyethylmercury chloride [(CH$_3$O)CH$_2$CH$_2$HgCl)]				
***, *Allium cepa*, spindle disturbance	+	0	0.63	Ramel (1969)
***, *Allium cepa*, spindle disturbances	+	0	2.0	Fiskesjö (1969)
DMN, *Drosophila melanogaster*, aneuploidy	–		20, diet	Ramel & Magnusson (1969)
DMN, *Drosophila melanogaster*, aneuploidy	–		2.5, larval diet	Ramel & Magnusson (1979)
G9O, Gene mutation, Chinese hamster lung V79 cells, ouabain resistance, *in vitro*	+	0	0.07	Fiskesjö (1979)
G9A, Gene mutation, Chinese hamster lung V79 cells, 8-azaguanine resistance, *in vitro*	+	0	0.07	Fiskesjö (1979)
***, Spindle disturbances, human lymphocytes *in vitro*	+	0	2.0	Fiskesjö (1970)
Phenylmercury chloride [◯–HgCl]				
BSD, *Bacillus subtilis* rec strains, differential toxicity	–	0	12.8	Shirasu *et al.* (1976)
***, Micronucleus test, fish (*Lepomis macrochirus*) cells *in vitro*	+	0	0.03	Babich *et al.* (1990)
***, Spindle disturbances, human HeLa cells *in vitro*	+	0	1.0	Umeda *et al.* (1969)
Phenylmercury hydroxide [◯–HgOH]				
PLM, *Anacharis canadensis*, mutation	+	0	6.8	MacFarlane & Messing (1953)

Table 17 (contd)

Test system	Result		Dose[a] (LED/HID)	Reference
	Without exogenous metabolic system	With exogenous metabolic system		
Phenylmercury hydroxide (contd)				
PLM, *Coleus blumei*, mutation	+	0	0.5	MacFarlane & Messing (1953)
PLM, *Raphanus sativus*, mutation	+	0	68	MacFarlane & Messing (1953)
PLM, *Ruppia maritima*, mutation	+	0	6.8	MacFarlane & Messing (1953)
PLM, *Zea mays*, mutation	+	0	6.8	MacFarlane & Messing (1953)
ACC, *Allium cepa*, chromosomal aberrations	+	0	6.8	MacFarlane (1956)
ACC, *Allium cepa*, chromosomal aberrations	+	0	0.24	Ramel (1969)
***, *Allium cepa*, spindle disturbances	+	0	0.16	Ramel (1969)
Phenylmercury nitrate [⌬–HgNO$_3$]				
PLM, *Zea mays*, mutation	+	0	2.4	MacFarlane & Messing (1953)
ACC, *Allium cepa*, chromosomal aberrations	+	0	5.9	MacFarlane (1956)
Phenylmercury acetate [⌬–HgCO$_2$CH$_3$]				
BSD, *Bacillus subtilis* rec strains, differential toxicity	–	0	12	Shirasu et al. (1976)
BSD, *Bacillus subtilis* rec strains, differential toxicity	+	0	200	Kanematsu et al. (1980)
DMN, *Drosophila melanogaster*, aneuploidy	(+)[b]		0.32	Ramel & Magnusson (1969)
Dimethylmercury [CH$_3$HgCH$_3$]				
***, *Physarum polycephalum* (slime mould), DNA fragments	+	0	500	Yatscoff & Cummins (1975)

Table 17 (contd)

Test system	Result		Dose[a] (LED/HID)	Reference
	Without exogenous metabolic system	With exogenous metabolic system		
Dimethylmercury (contd)				
CIM, Chromosomal aberrations, mouse oocytes *in vitro*	+	0	10	Jagiello & Lin (1973)
CHL, Chromosomal aberrations, human lymphocytes *in vitro*	+	0	8.7	Betti *et al.* (1992)
AIH, Aneuploidy, lymphocytes *in vitro*	+	0	0.34	Betti *et al.* (1992)
COE, Chromosomal aberrations, mouse oocytes *in vivo*	–		140, iv × 1	Jagiello & Lin (1973)
Mercury-containing fungicides (denomination and composition as reported by authors)				
Panogen 5 (containing methylmercury dicyandiamide; Hg, 5 g/L)				
***, *Allium cepa*, spindle disturbances	+	0	0.05	Ramel (1969)
Panogen 8 (containing methylmercury dicyandiamide; Hg, 6.4 g/L)				
***, *Allium cepa*, spindle disturbances	+	0	0.16	Ramel (1969)
Panogen 15 (containing 2.3% methylmercury dicyandiamide; 1.54% Hg)				
***, *Vicia faba*, spindle disturbances	+	0	0.015	Ahmed & Grant (1972)
***, *Tradescantia* species, spindle disturbances	+	0	0.015	Ahmed & Grant (1972)
Ceresan (containing phenylmercury acetate; 1% Hg)				
DMX, *Drosophila melanogaster*, sex-linked recessive lethal mutations	+		200, diet, adult	Gayathri & Krishnamurthy (1985)
DML, *Drosophila melanogaster*, dominant lethal mutations	–		200, diet, adult	Gayathri & Krishnamurthy (1985)
Agrimax M (containing phenylmercury dinaphthylmethanedisulfonate; % Hg not known)				
***, *Avena sativa*, polyploidy	+	0	NR	Bruhin (1955)
***, *Crepis capillaris*, polyploidy	+	0	NR	Bruhin (1955)

Table 17 (contd)

Test system	Result		Dose[a] (LED/HID)	Reference
	Without exogenous metabolic system	With exogenous metabolic system		
Granosan (2% ethylmercury chloride [EMC] + 98% talc; 1.5% Hg)				
•••, *Crepis capillaris*, nuclear abnormalities	–	0	15	Bruhin (1955)
•••, *Linum usitatissimum*, nuclear abnormalities	–	0	75	Kostoff (1940)
•••, *Pisum sativum*, nuclear abnormalities	+	0	75	Kostoff (1940)
•••, *Secale cereale*, nuclear abnormalities	+	0	15	Kostoff (1939, 1940)
•••, *Triticum aegilopodes*, nuclear abnormalities	+	0	15	Kostoff (1939, 1940)
•••, *Triticum durum*, nuclear abnormalities	+	0	15	Kostoff (1939, 1940)
•••, *Triticum persicum*, nuclear abnormalities	+	0	15	Kostoff (1939, 1940)
•••, *Triticum polonicum*, nuclear abnormalities	+	0	15	Kostoff (1939, 1940)
•••, *Triticum vulgare*, nuclear abnormalities	+	0	15	Kostoff (1939, 1940)
Ceresan M[c] (containing ethylmercury *para*-toluenesulfonanilide)				
DMX, *Drosophila melanogaster*, sex-linked recessive lethal mutations	+		14.3, diet	Mathew & Al-Doori (1976)
Agallol 3 (containing methoxyethylmercury chloride; 3% Hg)				
DMX, *Drosophila melanogaster*, sex-linked recessive lethal mutations	–		600, diet, adult	Gayathri & Krishnamurthy (1985)
DML, *Drosophila melanogaster*, dominant lethal mutations	–		600, diet, adult	Gayathri & Krishnamurthy (1985)
Betoxin (containing 90% ethylmercury halogenide; % Hg not known)				
ACC, *Allium cepa*, chromosomal aberrations	+	0	NR	Fiskesjö (1969)
•••, *Allium cepa*, spindle disturbances	+	0	NR	Fiskesjö (1'969)
New improved Ceresan (containing ethylmercury phosphate)				
PLC, *Zea mays*, chromosomal aberrations	+	0	NR	Sass (1937)

Table 17 (contd)

Test system	Result		Dose[a] (LED/HID)	Reference
	Without exogenous metabolic system	With exogenous metabolic system		
Azo dye				
Mercury orange (41% Hg) [N=N–⌬–HgCl, OH]				
SA0, *Salmonella typhimurium* TA100, reverse mutation	–	–	103	Brown *et al.* (1978)
SA5, *Salmonella typhimurium* TA1535, reverse mutation	–	–	103	Brown *et al.* (1978)
SA7, *Salmonella typhimurium* TA1537, reverse mutation	–	–	103	Brown *et al.* (1978)
SA8, *Salmonella typhimurium* TA1538, reverse mutation	–	–	103	Brown *et al.* (1978)
SA9, *Salmonella typhimurium* TA98, reverse mutation	–	–	103	Brown *et al.* (1978)

+, considered to be positive; (+), considered to be weakly positive in an inadequate study; –, considered to be negative; ?, considered to be inconclusive (variable responses in several experiments within an adequate study); 0, not tested

[a]LED, lowest effective dose; HID, highest ineffective dose. In-vitro tests, μg/ml; in-vivo tests, mg/kg bw. Doses given as concentration of element, not concentration of compound; NR, not reported; po, orally, by gavage; sc, subcutaneously; ip, intraperitoneally; iv, intravenously

[b]Statistically significant, but may be due to control values lower than those in other experiments

[c]Claimed to be responsible for two outbreaks of poisoning in 1956 and 1960 in Iraq

***Not displayed on profile

Workers are exposed to mercury by inhalation, principally to metallic mercury but also to inorganic and organic mercury compounds. Occupations in which the highest exposures occur include mercury mining, work in chloralkali and alkaline battery plants and production of devices for measuring temperature and pressure. Lower exposures have been measured for people employed in hospital laboratories and dental clinics. Exposures have been measured by both ambient air monitoring and biological monitoring.

Nonoccupational sources of exposure to mercury include food (methylmercury compounds, mainly in aquatic organisms) and dental amalgam fillings (metallic mercury). These exposure levels are usually lower than those typically detected in occupational settings.

5.2 Human carcinogenicity data

Metallic mercury and inorganic mercury compounds

A cohort study in a nuclear weapons factory in the USA on exposure to metallic mercury showed no difference in risk for lung cancer in exposed and unexposed subcohorts from the same factory. In a nested case–control study at two nuclear facilities in the USA, the risk for cancers of the central nervous system was not associated with estimated levels of exposure to mercury.

A cohort study of chloralkali workers in Sweden identified a two-fold, significant excess risk for lung cancer and some nonsignificant excess risks for cancers of the brain and kidney. Lung cancers also occurred in an almost two-fold excess in Norwegian chloralkali workers, whereas the numbers of cases of cancer of the brain and kidney were close to those expected. In both studies, asbestos and smoking were judged to be the main determinants of the excess risk for lung cancer.

In a study of male and female dentists and female dental nurses in Sweden, a two-fold risk for brain tumours was found in each of the three cohorts. No such risk appeared among dentists or medical and dental technicians in a US study of military veterans; these groups had excess risks for pancreatic and colon cancer, respectively. In an Australian case–control study of brain tumours and amalgam fillings, there was a decreased risk for gliomas and no effect was seen with regard to meningiomas.

The risk for lung cancer was found to be higher among individuals with silicosis who had been working in US mercury mines than in subjects with silicosis who had worked elsewhere. This finding was based on small numbers, however, and the confidence limits overlapped.

A case–control study in Italy indicated an excess risk for lung cancer among women in the felt-hat industry who had heavy exposure to mercury but also to arsenic.

In a population-based case–control study from Canada, risk for prostatic cancer was associated with exposure to mercury compounds in general and the risk for lung cancer with exposure to metallic mercury.

Organomercury compounds

Studies in Minamata, Japan, on causes of death in populations with high exposure to mercury included areas with a high prevalence of methylmercury poisoning. The only clear indication of an increased cancer risk was in the most informative of these studies, in which excess mortality from cancer of the liver and cancer of the oesophagus was found in the area with the highest exposure, together with an increased risk for chronic liver disease and cirrhosis. Consumption of alcoholic beverages was known to be higher than average in the area.

A cohort study of individuals in Sweden with a licence for seed disinfection with mercury compounds and other agents found no excess of brain cancer. Of the three Swedish case-control studies on exposure to mercury seed dressings and soft-tissue sarcomas, only one showed an odds ratio above unity; in all three studies, the confidence intervals included unity. For malignant lymphomas, there was a slightly but nonsignificantly elevated odds ratio for exposure to mercury seed dressings, but other exposures had higher odds ratios and, consequently, potential confounding.

5.3 Animal carcinogenicity data

Mercuric chloride was tested for carcinogenicity in two studies in mice, by oral gavage and by administration in the drinking-water; only the study by gavage was adequate for an evaluation of carcinogenicity. Mercuric chloride was also tested in one study in rats by oral gavage. In mice, a few renal adenomas and adenocarcinomas occurred in males only. In rats, a few renal adenomas occurred in females; there was a dose-related increase in the incidence of squamous-cell papilloma of the forestomach in males, and a few papillomas were seen in females. Dose-related hyperplasia of the forestomach was seen in both males and females.

Methylmercury chloride was tested for carcinogenicity in three studies in mice and two studies in rats by oral administration in the diet. In all three studies in mice, the incidence of renal adenomas and adenocarcinomas was increased in males. In the two studies in rats, no increase in tumour incidence was reported. In another study in mice given methylmercury chloride, a significant number of renal tumours was found in intact male mice and a few renal tumours were found in gonadectomized male and female mice that also received testosterone propionate; no renal tumour was found in male or female gonadectomized mice that did not receive testosterone propionate.

5.4 Other relevant data

After inhalation, about 70–80% of metallic mercury vapour is retained and absorbed. Little metallic mercury is taken up in the gastrointestinal tract, and less than 10% is absorbed. Metallic mercury passes into the brain and fetus. In the body, metallic mercury is oxidized to mercuric mercury, which binds to reduced sulfhydryl groups. The kidney is the main depository following exposure to both metallic and mercuric mercury. Mercuric mercury is eliminated mainly in urine and faeces; it is also excreted in milk. In humans, inorganic mercury compounds have two half-times: one lasts for days or weeks and the other much longer. Mercury concentrations in urine, blood and plasma are useful for biological monitoring.

Methylmercury compounds present in seafood are almost completely absorbed from the gastrointestinal tract and are distributed to most tissues. The methylmercury compounds bind to reduced sulfhydryl groups; a fraction is converted to mercuric mercury, the extent of conversion differing among species. Methylmercury compounds are excreted mainly in the bile; in the intestine, some mercury is biotransformed into inorganic mercury compounds and excreted in the faeces. Methylmercury compounds pass into the fetus and are excreted in milk. In humans, methylmercury compounds have a single biological half-time of approximately two months. Concentrations in blood and hair are useful for monitoring exposure to methylmercury compounds.

Following intense exposure to metallic mercury vapour, lung damage occurs; gastrointestinal and renal tubular necrosis occur after ingestion of mercuric mercury. Long-term exposure to metallic mercury causes encephalopathy and renal damage; chronic exposure to mercuric mercury causes renal tubular damage. Immunologically based glomerulonephritis can occur. In rats, mercuric chloride may cause immunosuppression. Effects on the immune system vary considerably among rodent strains. Inorganic mercury is a cause of allergic contact dermatitis. The nervous system is the main target organ for methylmercury compounds, but interspecies differences exist; in some species, there are also effects on the kidney. Some selenium compounds affect the kinetics of inorganic and methylmercury compounds and have a protective effect against their toxicity.

In several studies of female dental assistants, no increased risk for spontaneous abortion or birth defects was seen. Parenteral administration of mercury salts to pregnant rodents induces fetal growth retardation, malformations and death; altered placental transport of nutrients may be involved. Methylmercury compounds induce adverse effects on human development—most notably microcephaly and deficits in neurological development. Similar effects have been shown in many laboratory species. The conceptus appears to be more sensitive than the maternal organism. The dose levels of methylmercury compounds that affect reproduction and development are generally lower than those of inorganic mercury and affect a wider range of end-points.

The findings of 14 studies of cytogenetic effects, such as sister chromatid exchange, micronucleus formation, structural chromosomal aberrations, aneuploidy and polyploidy, in peripheral lymphocytes of individuals exposed to metallic mercury and various mercury compounds are controversial and uncertain. Thus, four studies involving subjects exposed to methylmercury compounds from contaminated seal or fish meat were either inconclusive or indicated slight chromosomal effects. Nine studies in individuals exposed from occupational sources to metallic mercury, amalgams, alkyl- and arylmercury compounds or mercury fulminate gave either negative or borderline results, or the exact role of mercury in any positive result was uncertain. A slight yet significant increase in the frequency of sister chromatid exchange was observed in only one subset of children intoxicated with phenylmercury acetate used for disinfecting diapers.

Several organomercury compounds and fungicides containing organomercury compounds were assayed in a variety of short-term tests. Tests for unscheduled DNA synthesis, sister chromatid exchange, chromosomal aberrations and dominant lethal mutations in mammals *in vivo* gave conflicting results. Tests for clastogenicity in fish and amphibians gave more convincingly positive results. All studies of induction of c-mitosis (spindle disturbances), sister chromatid exchange, structural chromosomal aberrations and aneuploidy in cultured human lymphocytes gave positive results. The results of the majority of studies of the induction of forward mutations, c-mitosis and polyploidy in cultured mammalian (non-human) cells were positive, and those of one study on micronucleus induction in cultured fish cells were also positive. In *Drosophila melanogaster* and other insects, the majority of mercury compounds induced sex-linked recessive lethal mutation and nondisjunction (aneuploidy) but did not induce dominant lethal mutation. The assessment of nuclear or mitochondrial DNA mutations, mitotic recombination and gene conversion in the yeast *Saccharomyces cerevisiae* led to conflicting results. Most of the few studies available in bacteria (investigating differential killing in rec^- *Bacillus subtilis* or reversion in his^- *Salmonella typhimurium* or trp^- *Escherichia coli*) gave negative results.

There were fewer studies of inorganic mercury compounds (mostly mercuric chloride), and a minority compared inorganic and organic compounds. No experimental study was available on metallic mercury. As in studies with organomercury compounds, studies in rodents treated *in vivo* with mercuric chloride gave weakly positive results for dominant lethal mutation. Studies on the induction of chromosomal aberrations in rodents yielded conflicting results. One study on chromosomal effects in amphibians gave positive results for mercuric chloride and methylmercury chloride at similar doses. Chromosomal alterations were reported in cultured human lymphocytes. The dose of mercuric chloride required to induce sister chromatid exchange in cultured human lymphocytes was 5–25 times higher than those needed of methylmercury chloride. Mercuric acetate did not induce anchorage-independent growth in human cells. Five to ten times higher doses of mercuric chloride than methylmercury chloride were required to induce polyploidy. DNA damage has been induced repeatedly in mammalian cells by mercuric chloride. Although the information comes from single studies, this compound also induced sister chromatid exchange, chromosomal aberrations, aneuploidy (spindle disturbances) and enhancement of virus-induced morphological transformation. Unlike organomercury compounds, mercuric chloride failed to enhance the frequency of micronuclei in cultured fish cells. Mercuric chloride failed to enhance lethality in a DNA repair-deficient strain of *E. coli*.

5.5 Evaluation[1]

There is *inadequate evidence* in humans for the carcinogenicity of mercury and mercury compounds.

There is *inadequate evidence* in experimental animals for the carcinogenicity of metallic mercury.

There is *limited evidence* in experimental animals for the carcinogenicity of mercuric chloride.

There is *sufficient evidence* in experimental animals for the carcinogenicity of methylmercury chloride.

In making the overall evaluation, the Working Group took into account evidence that methylmercury compounds are similar with regard to absorption, distribution, metabolism, excretion, genotoxicity and other forms of toxicity.

---

[1]For definition of the italicized terms, see Preamble, pp. 26-30.

Overall evaluation

Methylmercury compounds *are possibly carcinogenic to humans (Group 2B)*.

Metallic mercury and inorganic mercury compounds *are not classifiable as to their carcinogenicity to humans (Group 3)*.

6. References

Åberg, B., Ekman, L., Falk, R., Greitz, U., Persson, G. & Snihs, J.-O. (1969) Metabolism of methylmercury (^{203}Hg) compounds in man. Excretion and distribution. *Arch. environ. Health*, **19**, 478–484

Afonso, J.F. & de Alvarez, R.R. (1960) Effects of mercury on human gestation. *Am. J. Obstet. Gynecol.*, **80**, 145–154

Agency for Toxic Substances and Disease Registry (1989) *Toxicological Profile for Mercury* (US NTIS PB90-181256), Atlanta, GA, US Public Health Service

Agocs, M.M., Etzel, R.A., Parrish, R.G., Paschal, D.C., Campagna, P.R., Cohen, D.S., Kilbourne, E.M. & Hesse, J.L. (1990) Mercury exposure from interior latex paint. *New Engl. J. Med.*, **323**, 1096–1101

Ahlbom, A., Norell, S., Rodvall, Y. & Nylander, M. (1986) Dentists, dental nurses, and brain tumours. *Br. med. J.*, **292**, 662

Ahmed, M. & Grant, W.F. (1972) Cytological effects of the mercurial fungicide Panogen 15 on *Tradescantia* and *Vicia faba* root tips. *Mutat. Res.*, **14**, 391–396

Akesson, I., Schutz, A., Attewell, R., Skerfving, S. & Glantz, P.-O. (1991) Status of mercury and selenium in dental personnel: impact of amalgam work and own fillings. *Arch. environ. Health*, **46**, 102–109

Albanus, L., Frankenberg, L., Grant, C., von Haartman, U., Jernelöv, A., Nordberg, G., Rydälv, M., Schütz, A. & Skerfving, S. (1972) Toxicity for cats of methylmercury in contaminated fish from Swedish lakes and of methylmercury hydroxide added to fish. *Environ. Res.*, **5**, 425–442

Alcser, K.H., Brix, K.A., Fine, L.J., Kallenbach, L.R. & Wolfe, R.A. (1989) Occupational mercury exposure and male reproductive health. *Am. J. ind. Med.*, **15**, 517–529

Aldrich Chemical Co. (1992) *Aldrich Catalog/Handbook of Fine Chemicals 1992–1993*, Milwaukee, WI, pp. 507, 793–794, 1001

Alfa Products (1990) *Alfa Catalog—Research Chemicals and Accessories*, Ward Hill, MA, pp. 250, 258, 294, 530

Amandus, H. & Costello, J. (1991) Silicosis and lung cancer in US metal miners. *Arch. environ. Health*, **46**, 82–89

American Conference of Governmental Industrial Hygienists (1992) *1992–1993 Threshold Limit Values for Chemical Substances and Physical Agents and Biological Exposure Indices*, Cincinnati, OH, p. 25

Ancona, A., Ramos, M., Suarez, R. & Macotela, E. (1982) Mercury sensitivity in a dentist (Short communication). *Contact Derm.*, **8**, 218

Andersen, O., Rønne, M. & Nordberg, G.F. (1983) Effects of inorganic metal salts on chromosome length in human lymphocytes. *Hereditas*, **98**, 65–70

Angerer, J. & Schaller, K.H., eds (1988) *Analyses of Hazardous Substances in Biological Materials*, Vol. 2, *Methods for Biological Monitoring*, Weinheim, VCH Verlagsgesellschaft, pp. 195–207

Angotzi, G., Cassitto, M.G., Camerino, D., Cioni, R., Desideri, E., Franzinelli, A., Gori, R., Loi, F. & Sartorelli, E. (1980) Relationship between mercury exposure and health in workers of a mercury distillation plant in the Province of Siena (Ital.). *Med. Lav.*, **6**, 463–480

Anttila, A., Jaakkola, J., Tossavainen, A. & Vainio, H. (1992) *Occupational Exposure to Chemicals in Finland* (Altisteet Työssä 34), Helsinki, Institute of Occupational Health & Finnish Work Environmental Fund

Anwar, W.A. & Gabal, M.S. (1991) Cytogenetic study in workers occupationally exposed to mercury fulminate. *Mutagenesis*, **6**, 189–192

Aoi, T., Higuchi, T., Kidokoro, R., Fukumura, R., Yagi, A., Ohguchi, S., Sasa, A., Hayashi, H., Sakamoto, N. & Hanaichi, T. (1985) An association of mercury with selenium in inorganic mercury intoxication. *Hum. Toxicol.*, **4**, 637–642

Arbeidsinspectie [Labour Inspection] (1986) *De Nationale MAC-Lijst 1986* [National MAC List 1986], Voorburg, p. 15

Arbejdstilsynet [Labour Inspection] (1992) *Graensevaerdier for Stoffer og Materialer* [Limit Values for Compounds and Materials] (No. 3.1.0.2), Copenhagen, p. 22

Aschner, M. & Clarkson, T.W. (1988) Uptake of methylmercury in the rat brain: effects of amino acids. *Brain Res.*, **462**, 31–39

Ashe, W.F., Largent, E.J., Dutra, F.R., Hubbard, D.M. & Blackstone, M. (1953) Behavior of mercury in the animal organism following inhalation. *Arch. ind. Hyg. occup. Med.*, **7**, 19–43

Assennato, G., Porro, A., Longo, G., Longo, F. & Ambrosi, L. (1989) Effects of low mercury concentrations on the nervous system among workers employed in the manufacture of fluorescent lamps (Ital.). *Med. Lav.*, **80**, 307–315

Atomergic Chemetals Corp. (undated) *High Purity Metals Brochure*, Farmingdale, NY

Aylett, B.J. (1973) Mercury. In: Bailar, J.C., Jr, Eméleus, H.J., Nyholm, R. & Trotman-Dickenson, A.F., eds, *Comprehensive Inorganic Chemistry*, Vol. 3, Oxford, Pergamon Press, pp. 275–328

Babich, H., Goldstein, S.H. & Borenfreund, E. (1990) In vitro cyto- and genotoxicity of organo-mercurials to cells in culture. *Toxicol. Lett.*, **50**, 143–149

Bakir, F., Damluji, S.F., Amin-Zaki, L., Murtadha, M., Khalidi, A., Al-Rawi, N.Y., Tikriti, S., Dhahir, H.I., Clarkson, T.W., Smith, J.C. & Doherty, R.A. (1973) Methylmercury poisoning in Iraq. An interuniversity report. *Science*, **181**, 230–241

Baldi, G., Vigliani, E.C. & Zurlo, N. (1953) Chronic mercurialism in felt hat industries (Ital.). *Med. Lav.*, **44**, 161–198

Ballatori, N. & Clarkson, T.W. (1984) Inorganic mercury secretion into bile as a low molecular weight complex. *Biochem. Pharmacol.*, **33**, 1087–1092

Barlow, S.M. & Sullivan, F.M. (1982) *Reproductive Hazards of Industrial Chemicals. An Evaluation of Animal and Human Data*, London, Academic Press, pp. 386–406

Barr, R.D., Rees, P.H., Cordy, P.E., Kungu, A., Woodger, B.A. & Cameron, H.M. (1972) Nephrotic syndrome in adult Africans in Nairobi. *Br. med. J.*, **ii**, 131–134

Barregård, L., Hultberg, B., Schütz, A. & Sällsten, G. (1988) Enzymuria in workers exposed to inorganic mercury. *Int. Arch. occup. environ. Health*, **61**, 65–69

Barregård, L., Sällsten, G. & Järvholm, B. (1990) Mortality and cancer incidence in chloralkali workers exposed to inorganic mercury. *Br. J. ind. Med.*, **47**, 99–104

Barregård, L., Högstedt, B., Schütz, A., Karlsson, A., Sällsten, G. & Thiringer, G. (1991) Effects of occupational exposure to mercury vapor on lymphocyte micronuclei. *Scand. J. Work Environ. Health*, **17**, 263–268

Barregård, L., Sällsten, G., Schütz, A., Attewell, R., Skerfving, S. & Järvholm, B. (1992) Kinetics of mercury in blood and urine after brief occupational exposure. *Arch. environ. Health*, **47**, 176–184

Bergstrand, A., Friberg, L., Mendel, L. & Odeblad, E. (1959) The localization of subcutaneously administered radioactive mercury in the rat kidney (Abstract No. 8). *J. ultrastruct. Res.*, **3**, 238

Berlin, M. (1986) Mercury. In: Friberg, L., Nordberg, G.F. & Vouk, V.B., eds, *Handbook on Toxicology of Metals*, Vol. II, *Specific Metals*, 2nd ed., Amsterdam, Elsevier, pp. 387–445

Berlin, M., Fazackerley, J. & Nordberg, G.F. (1969) The uptake of mercury in the brains of mammals exposed to mercury vapor and to mercuric salts. *Arch. environ. Health*, **18**, 719–729

Berlin, M., Carlson, J. & Norseth, T. (1975) Dose-dependence of methylmercury metabolism. A study of distribution: biotransformation and excretion in the squirrel monkey. *Arch. environ. Health*, **30**, 307–313

Bernard, A.M., Collette, C. & Lauwerys, R. (1992) Renal effects of in utero exposure to mercuric chloride in rats. *Arch. Toxicol.*, **66**, 508–513

Betti, C., Davini, T. & Barale, R. (1992) Genotoxic activity of methyl mercury chloride and dimethyl mercury in human lymphocytes. *Mutat. Res.*, **281**, 255–260

Biedermann, K.A. & Landolph, J.R. (1987) Induction of anchorage independence in human diploid foreskin fibroblasts by carcinogenic metal salts. *Cancer Res.*, **47**, 3815–3823

Blakley, B.R. (1984) Enhancement of urethan-induced adenoma formation in Swiss mice exposed to methylmercury. *Can. J. comp. Med.*, **48**, 299–302

Bondy, S.C., Anderson, C.L., Harrington, M.E. & Prasad, K.N. (1979) The effects of organic and inorganic lead and mercury on neurotransmitter high-affinity transport and release mechanisms. *Environ. Res.*, **19**, 102–111

Bornhausen, M., Müsch, H.R. & Greim, H. (1980) Operant behavior performance changes in rats after prenatal methylmercury exposure. *Toxicol. appl. Pharmacol.*, **56**, 305–310

Brandi, G., Schiavano, G.F., Albano, A., Cattabeni, F. & Cantoni, O. (1990) Growth delay and filamentation of *Escherichia coli* wild-type and *rec A* cells in response to hexavalent chromium and other metal compounds. *Mutat. Res.*, **245**, 201–204

Brodsky, J.B., Cohen, E.N., Whitcher, C., Brown, B.W., Jr & Wu, M.L. (1985) Occupational exposure to mercury in dentistry and pregnancy outcome. *J. Am. dent. Assoc.*, **111**, 779–780

Brown, J.P., Roehm, G.W. & Brown, R.J. (1978) Mutagenicity testing of certified food colors and related azo, xanthene and triphenylmethane dyes with the *Salmonella*/microsome system. *Mutat. Res.*, **56**, 249–271

Bruce, W.R. & Heddle, J.A. (1979) The mutagenic activity of 61 agents as determined by the micronucleus, *Salmonella*, and sperm abnormality assays. *Can. J. genet. Cytol.*, **21**, 319–334

Bruhin, A. (1955) Polyploidizing action of a seed corrosive (Ger.). *Phytopathol. Z.*, **23**, 381–394

Brune, D., Nordberg, G.F., Vesterberg, O., Gerhardsson, L. & Wester, P.O. (1991) A review of normal concentrations of mercury in human blood. *Sci. total Environ.*, **100**, 235–282

Budavari, S., ed. (1989) *The Merck Index*, 11th ed., Rahway, NJ, Merck & Co., pp. 512, 923–927

Buelke-Sam, J., Kimmel, C.A., Adams, J., Nelson, C.J., Vorhees, C.V., Wright, D.C., St Omer, V., Korol, B.A., Butcher, R.E., Geyer, M.A., Holson, J.F., Kutscher, C.L. & Wayner, M.J. (1985) Collaborative behavioral teratology studies: results. *Neurobehav. Toxicol. Teratol.*, **7**, 591–624

Buiatti, E., Kriebel, D., Geddes, M., Santucci, M. & Pucci, N. (1985) A case control study of lung cancer in Florence, Italy. I. Occupational risk factors. *J. Epidemiol. Community Health*, **39**, 244–250

Burbacher, T.M., Monnett, C., Grant, K.S. & Mottet, N.K. (1984) Methylmercury exposure and reproductive dysfunction in the nonhuman primate. *Toxicol. appl. Pharmacol.*, **75**, 18–24

Burbacher, T.M., Rodier, P.M. & Weiss, B. (1990) Methylmercury developmental neurotoxicity: a comparison of effects in humans and animals. *Neurotoxicol. Teratol.*, **12**, 191–202

Burton, G.V. & Meikle, A.W. (1980) Acute and chronic methyl mercury poisoning impairs rat adrenal and testicular function. *J. Toxicol. environ. Health*, **6**, 597–606

Campbell, D., Gonzales, M. & Sullivan, J.B., Jr (1992) Mercury. In: Sullivan, J.B., Jr & Krieger, G.R., eds, *Hazardous Materials Toxicology. Clinical Principles of Environmental Health*, Baltimore, Williams & Wilkins, pp. 824–833

Cantoni, O. & Costa, M. (1983) Correlations of DNA strand breaks and their repair with cell survival following acute exposure to mercury(II) and X-rays. *Mol. Pharmacol.*, **24**, 84–89

Cantoni, O., Evans, R.M. & Costa, M. (1982) Similarity in the acute cytotoxic response of mammalian cells to mercury(II) and X-rays: DNA damage and glutathione depletion. *Biochem. biophys. Res. Commun.*, **108**, 614–619

Cantoni, O., Christie, N.T., Robison, S.H. & Costa, M. (1984a) Characterization of DNA lesions produced by $HgCl_2$ in cell culture systems. *Chem.-biol. Interactions*, **49**, 209–224

Cantoni, O., Christie, N.T., Swann, A., Drath, D.B. & Costa, M. (1984b) Mechanisms of $HgCl_2$ cytotoxicity in cultured mammalian cells. *Mol. Pharmacol.*, **26**, 360–368

Carpenter, A.V., Flanders, W.D., Frome, E.L., Tankersley, W.G. & Fry, S.A. (1988) Chemical exposures and central nervous system cancers: a case–control study among workers at two nuclear facilities. *Am. J. ind. Med.*, **13**, 351–362

Carrico, L.C. (1985) Mercury. In: *Mineral Commodity Summaries 1985*, Washington DC, Bureau of Mines, US Department of the Interior, pp. 98–99

Carrico, L.C. (1987) Mercury. In: *Mineral Commodity Summaries 1987*, Washington DC, Bureau of Mines, US Department of the Interior, pp. 100–101

Casto, B.C., Meyers, J. & DiPaolo, J.A. (1979) Enhancement of viral transformation for evaluation of the carcinogenic or mutagenic potential of inorganic metal salts. *Cancer Res.*, **39**, 193–198

CERAC, Inc. (1991) *Advanced Specialty Inorganics*, Milwaukee, WI, p. 149

Chang, L.W. & Sprecher, J.A. (1976a) Hyperplastic changes in the rat distal tubular epithelial cells following in utero exposure to methylmercury. *Environ. Res.*, **12**, 218–223

Chang, L.W. & Sprecher, J.A. (1976b) Degenerative changes in the neonatal kidney following in-utero exposure to methylmercury. *Environ. Res.*, **11**, 392–406

Chang, L.W. & Suber, R. (1982) Protective effect of selenium on methylmercury toxicity: a possible mechanism. *Bull. environ. Contam. Toxicol.*, **29**, 285–289

Charbonneau, S.M., Munro, I.C., Nera, E.A., Armstrong, F.A.J., Willes, R.F., Bryce, F. & Nelson, R.F. (1976) Chronic toxicity of methylmercury in the adult cat. Interim report. *Toxicology*, **5**, 337–349

Chen, W.-J., Body, R.L. & Mottet, N.K. (1983) Biochemical and morphological studies of monkeys chronically exposed to methylmercury. *J. Toxicol. environ. Health*, **12**, 407–416

Cherian, M.G., Hursh, J.B., Clarkson, T.W. & Allen, J. (1978) Radioactive mercury distribution in biological fluids and excretion in human subjects after inhalation of mercury vapor. *Arch. environ. Health*, **33**, 109–114

Choi, B.H., Kim, R.C. & Peckham, N.H. (1988) Hydrocephalus following prenatal methylmercury poisoning. *Acta neuropathol.*, **75**, 325–330

Christie, N.T., Cantoni, O., Sugiyama, M., Cattabeni, F. & Costa, M. (1986) Differences in the effects of Hg(II) on DNA repair induced in Chinese hamster ovary cells by ultraviolet or X-rays. *Mol. Pharmacol.*, **29**, 173–178

Chung, A.-S., Maines, M.D. & Reynolds, W.A. (1982) Inhibition of the enzymes of glutathione metabolism by mercuric chloride in the rat kidney: reversal by selenium. *Biochem. Pharmacol.*, **31**, 3093–3100

Cicchella, G., Focardi, L. & Rossaro, R. (1968) Urinary excretion of mercury in healthy people living in mercury mine regions and elsewhere (Ital.). *Lav. Um.*, **20**, 3–9

Clarkson, T. (1992) The uptake and disposition of inhaled mercury vapor. In: *Potential Biological Consequences of Mercury Released from Dental Amalgam*, Stockholm, Swedish Medical Research Council, pp. 59–75

Clarkson, T.W., Hursh, J.B., Sager, P.R. & Syversen, T.L.M. (1988a) Mercury. In: Clarkson, T.W., Friberg, L., Nordberg, G.F. & Sager, P.R., eds, *Biological Monitoring of Toxic Metals*, New York, Plenum Press, pp. 199–246

Clarkson, T.W., Friberg, L., Hursh, J.B. & Nylander, M. (1988b) The prediction of intake of mercury vapor from amalgams. In: Clarkson, T.W., Friberg, L., Nordberg, G.F. & Sager, P.R., eds, *Biological Monitoring of Toxic Metals*, New York, Plenum Press, pp. 247–264

Cloëz, I., Dumont, O., Piciotti, M. & Bourre, J.M. (1987) Alterations of lipid synthesis in the normal and dysmyelinating trembler mouse sciatic nerve by heavy metals (Hg, Pb, Mn, Cu, Ni). *Toxicology*, **46**, 65–71

Commission of the European Communities (1981) Council Directive on the approximation of the rules of the Member States concerning the colouring matters authorised for use in foodstuffs intended for human consumption. *Off. J. Eur. Comm.*, **L43**, 11

Commission of the European Communities (1990) Proposal for a Council Directive on the approximation of the laws of the Member States relating to cosmetic products. *Off. J. Eur. Comm.*, **C322**, 29–77

Commission of the European Communities (1991) Thirteenth Commission Directive of 12 March 1991 (91/814/EEC) on the approximation of the laws of the Member States relating to cosmetic products. *Off. J. Eur. Commun.*, **L91**, 59–62

Cook, W.A. (1987) *Occupational Exposure Limits—Worldwide*, Akron, OH, American Industrial Hygiene Association, pp. 123, 145, 197

Cordier, S., Deplan, F., Mandereau, L. & Hemon, D. (1991) Prenatal exposure to mercury and spontaneous abortions. *Br. J. ind. Med.*, **48**, 375–381

Cragle, D.L., Hollis, D.R., Qualters, J.R., Tankersley, W.G. & Fry, S.A. (1984) A mortality study of men exposed to elemental mercury. *J. occup. Med.*, **26**, 817–821

Curle, D.C., Ray, M. & Persaud, T.V.N. (1983) Methylmercury toxicity: in vivo evaluation of teratogenesis and cytogenetic changes. *Anat. Anz. Jena*, **153**, 69–82

Curle, D.C., Ray, M. & Persaud, T.V.N. (1987) In vivo evaluation of teratogenesis and cytogenetic changes following methylmercuric chloride treatment. *Anat. Rec.*, **219**, 286–295

Daniel, J.W., Gage, J.C. & Lefevre, P.A. (1971) The metabolism of methoxyethylmercury salts. *Biochem. J.*, **121**, 411–415

Danielsson, B.R.G., Dencker, L., Khayat, A. & Orsén, L. (1984) Fetotoxicity of inorganic mercury in the mouse: distribution and effects of nutrient uptake by placenta and fetus. *Biol. Res. Pregn.*, **5**, 102–109

Dayan, A.D., Hertel, R.F., Heseltine, E., Kazantzis, G., Smith, E.M. & Van der Venne, M.-T., eds (1990) *Immunotoxicity of Metals and Immunotoxicology*, New York, Plenum Press

De Rosis, F., Anastasio, S.P., Selvaggi, L., Beltrame, A. & Moriani, G. (1985) Female reproductive health in two lamp factories: effects of exposure to inorganic mercury vapour and stress factors. *Br. J. ind. Med.*, **42**, 488–494

Deutsche Forschungsgemeinschaft (1992) *MAK and BAT Values 1992. Maximum Concentrations at the Workplace and Biological Tolerance Values for Working Materials* (Report No. 28), Weinheim, VCH Verlagsgesellschaft, pp. 47, 50, 103

D.F. Goldsmith Chemical & Metal Corp. (undated) *High Purity Elements; Fine Inorganic Chemicals; Precious Metals; Mercury*, Evanston, IL, p. 18

Doherty, R.A., Gates, A.H., Sewell, C.E. & Freer, C. (1978) Methylmercury sexual dimorphism in the mouse. *Experientia*, **34**, 871

Doi, R. & Kobayashi, T. (1982) Organ distribution and biological half-time of methylmercury in four strains of mice. *Japan J. exp. Med.*, **52**, 307–314

Doi, R. & Tagawa, M. (1983) A study on the biochemical and biological behavior of methylmercury. *Toxicol. appl. Pharmacol.*, **69**, 407–416

Drake, H.J. (1981) Mercury. In: Mark, H.F., Othmer, D.F., Overberger, C.G., Seaborg, G.T. & Grayson, N., eds, *Kirk–Othmer Encyclopedia of Chemical Technology*, 3rd Ed., Vol. 15, New York, John Wiley & Sons, pp. 143–156

Druckrey, H., Hamperl, H. & Schmähl, D. (1957) Carcinogenic action of metallic mercury after intraperitoneal administration in rats (Ger.). *Z. Krebsforsch.*, **61**, 511–519

Druet, P., Druet, E., Potdevin, F. & Sapin, C. (1978) Immune type glomerulonephritis induced by $HgCl_2$ in the Brown–Norway rat. *Ann. Immunol.*, **129C**, 777–792

Druet, E., Sapin, C., Fournie, G., Mandet, C., Günther, E. & Druet, P. (1982) Genetic control of susceptibility to mercury-induced immune nephritis in various strains of rat. *Clin. Immunol. Immunopathol.*, **25**, 203–212

Dunn, J.D., Clarkson, T.W. & Magos, L. (1978) Ethanol-increased exhalation of mercury in mice. *Br. J. ind. Med.*, **35**, 241–244

Ehrenberg, R.L., Vogt, R.L., Smith, A.B., Brondum, J., Brightwell, W.S., Hudson, P.J., McManus, K.P., Hannon, W.H. & Phipps, F.C. (1991) Effects of elemental mercury exposure at a thermometer plant. *Am. J. ind. Med.*, **19**, 495–507

Eichhorn, G.L. & Clark, P. (1963) The reaction of mercury (II) with nucleosides. *Am. J. chem. Soc.*, **85**, 4020–4024

Elinder, C.-G., Gerhardsson, L. & Oberdoerster, G. (1988) Biological monitoring of metals. In: Clarkson, T.W., Friberg, L., Nordberg, G.F. & Sager, P., eds, *Biological Monitoring of Toxic Metals*, New York, Plenum Press, pp. 1–71

Eller, P.M., ed. (1989) *NIOSH Manual of Analytical Methods*, 3rd Ed., Suppl. 3, (DHHS (NIOSH) Publ. No. 84-100), Washington DC, US Government Printing Office, pp. 6009-1–6009-4

Ellingsen, D.G, Andersen, A., Nordhagen, H.P., Efskind, J. & Kjuus, H. (1993) Incidence of cancer and mortality among workers exposed to mercury vapour in the Norwegian chloralkali industry. *Br. J. ind. Med.*, **50** (in press)

Erfurth, E.M., Schütz, A., Nilsson, A., Barregård, L. & Skerfving, S. (1990) Normal pituitary hormone response to thyrotrophin and gonadotrophin releasing hormones in subjects exposed to elemental mercury vapour. *Br. J. ind. Med.*, **47**, 639–644

Ericson, A. & Källén, B. (1989) Pregnancy outcome in women working as dentists, dental assistants or dental technicians. *Int. Arch. occup. environ. Health*, **61**, 329–333

Eriksson, M., Hardell, L., Berg, N.O., Möller, T. & Axelson, O. (1981) Soft-tissue sarcomas and exposure to chemical substances: a case–referent study. *Br. J. ind. Med.*, **38**, 27–33

Eriksson, M., Hardell, L. & Adami, H.-O. (1990) Exposure to dioxins as a risk factor for soft tissue sarcoma: a population-based case–control study. *J. natl Cancer Inst.*, **82**, 486–490

Ernst, E. & Lauritsen, J.G. (1991) Effect of organic and inorganic mercury on human sperm motility. *Pharmacol. Toxicol.*, **69**, 440–444

Fang, S.C. (1980) Comparative study of uptake and tissue distribution of methylmercury in female rats by inhalation and oral routes of administration. *Bull. environ. Contam. Toxicol.*, **24**, 65–72

Farant, J.-P., Brissette, D., Moncion, L., Bigras, L. & Chartrand, A. (1981) Improved cold-vapor atomic absorption technique for the microdetermination of total and inorganic mercury in biological samples. *J. anal. Toxicol.*, **5**, 47–51

Fehling, C., Abdulla, M., Brun, A., Dictor, M., Schütz, A. & Skerfving, S. (1975) Methylmercury poisoning in the rat: a combined neurological, chemical, and histopathological study. *Toxicol. appl. Pharmacol.*, **33**, 27–37

Finne, K., Göransson, K. & Winckler, L. (1982) Oral lichen planus and contact allergy to mercury. *Int. J. oral Surg.*, **11**, 236–239

Fiskesjö, G. (1969) Some results from *Allium* tests with organic mercury halogenides. *Hereditas*, **62**, 314–322

Fiskesjö, G. (1970) The effect of two organic mercury compounds on human leukocytes *in vitro*. *Hereditas*, **64**, 142–146

Fiskesjö, G. (1979) Two organic mercury compounds tested for mutagenicity in mammalian cells by use of the cell line V 79-4. *Hereditas*, **90**, 103–109

Foà, V., Caimi, L., Amante, L., Antonini, C., Gattinoni, A., Tettamanti, G., Lombardo, A. & Giuliani, A. (1976) Patterns of some lysosomal enzymes in the plasma and of proteins in urine of workers exposed to inorganic mercury. *Int. Arch. occup. environ. Health*, **37**, 115–124

Foldspang, A. & Hansen, J.C. (1990) Dietary intake of methylmercury as a correlate of gestational length and birth weight among newborns in Greenland. *Am. J. Epidemiol.*, **132**, 310–317

Fowler, B.A. & Woods, J.S. (1977a) The transplacental toxicity of methyl mercury to fetal rat liver mitochondria. Morphometric and biochemical studies. *Lab. Invest.*, **36**, 122–130

Fowler, B.A. & Woods, J.S. (1977b) Ultrastructural and biochemical changes in renal mitochondria during chronic oral methyl mercury exposure. The relationship to renal function. *Exp. mol. Pathol.*, **27**, 403–412

Friberg, L., Skog, E. & Wahlberg, J.E. (1961) Resorption of mercuric chloride and methyl mercury dicyandiamide in guinea-pigs through normal skin and through skin pre-treated with acetone, alkylaryl-sulphonate and soap. *Acta dermatovener.*, **41**, 40–52

Fukunaga, M., Kurachi, Y., Ogawa, M., Mizuguchi, Y., Kodama, Y. & Chihara, S. (1981) The genetic effects of environmental pollutants on eukaryotic cells. Mutagenicity on nuclear and mitochondrial genes of yeast by metals (Jpn.). *J. Univ. occup. environ. Health. Jpn*, **3**, 245–254

Fuyuta, M., Fujimoto, T. & Hirata, S. (1978) Embryotoxic effects of methylmercuric chloride administered to mice and rats during organogenesis. *Teratology*, **18**, 353–366

Fuyuta, M., Fujimoto, T. & Kiyofuji, E. (1979) Teratogenic effects of a single oral administration of methylmercuric chloride in mice. *Acta anat.*, **104**, 356–362

Gale, T. (1974) Embryopathic effects of different routes of administration of mercuric acetate in the hamster. *Environ. Res.*, **8**, 207–213

Gale, T.F. (1981) The embryotoxic response produced by inorganic mercury in different strains of hamsters. *Environ. Res.*, **24**, 152–161

Gallagher, R.P., Threlfall, W.J., Band, P.R. & Spinelli, J.J. (1985) *Occupational Mortality in British Columbia 1950–1984*, Vancouver, BC, Cancer Control Agency of British Columbia and Workers' Compensation Board of British Columbia

Gates, A.H., Doherty, R.A. & Cox, C. (1986) Reproduction and growth following prenatal methylmercuric chloride exposure in mice. *Fundam. appl. Toxicol.*, **7**, 486–493

Gayathri, M.V. & Krishnamurthy, N.B. (1985) Investigations on the mutagenicity of two organomercurial pesticides, Ceresan and Agallol 3, in *Drosophila melanogaster*. *Environ. Res.*, **36**, 218–229

Gelbier, S. & Ingram, J. (1989) Possible foetotoxic effects of mercury vapour: a case report. *Public Health*, **103**, 35–40

Ghosh, A.K., Sen, S., Sharma, A. & Talukder, G. (1991) Effect of chlorophyllin on mercuric chloride-induced clastogenicity in mice. *Food chem. Toxicol.*, **29**, 777–779

Giavini, E., Vismara, C. & Broccia, M.L. (1985) Effects of methylmercuric chloride administered to pregnant rats during the preimplantation period. *Ecotoxicol. environ. Saf.*, **9**, 189–195

Goldberg, M., Klitzman, S., Payne, J.L., Nadig, R.J., McGrane, J.-A. & Goodman, A.K. (1990) Mercury exposure from the repair of blood pressure machines in medical facilities. *Appl. occup. environ. Hyg.*, **5**, 604–610

Gotelli, C., Astolfi, E., Cox, C., Cernichiari, E. & Clarkson, T.W. (1985) Early biochemical effects of an organic mercury fungicide on infants: 'dose makes the poison'. *Science*, **227**, 638–640

Grandjean, P. & Weihe, P. (1993) Neurobehavioral effects of intrauterine mercury exposure: potential sources of bias. *Environ. Res.*, **61**, 176–183

Greenwood, M.R. (1985) Methylmercury poisoning in Iraq. An epidemiological study of the 1971–1972 outbreak. *J. appl. Toxicol.*, **5**, 148–159

Halbach, S. & Clarkson, T.W. (1978) Enzymatic oxidation of mercury vapor by erythrocytes. *Biochim. biophys. Acta*, **523**, 522–531

Hardell, L. & Eriksson, M. (1988) The association between soft tissue sarcomas and exposure to phenoxyacetic acids. A new case-referent study. *Cancer*, **62**, 652–656

Hardell, L., Eriksson, M., Lenner, P. & Lundgren, E. (1981) Malignant lymphoma and exposure to chemicals, especially organic solvents, chlorophenols and phenoxy acids: a case–control study. *Br. J. Cancer*, **43**, 169–176

Hargreaves, R.J., Evans, J.G., Janota, I., Magos, L. & Cavanagh, J.B. (1988) Persistent mercury in nerve cells 16 years after metallic mercury poisoning. *Neuropathol. appl. Neurobiol.*, **14**, 443–452

Health & Safety Executive (1992) *EH40/92 Occupational Exposure Limits 1992*, London, Her Majesty's Stationary Office, p. 21

Heidam, L.Z. (1984) Spontaneous abortions among dental assistants, factory workers, painters, and gardening workers: a follow up study. *J. Epidemiol. Community Health*, **38**, 149–155

Heintze, U., Edwardsson, S., Dérand, T. & Birkhed, D. (1983) Methylation of mercury from dental amalgam and mercuric chloride by oral streptococci *in vitro*. *Scand. J. dent. Res.*, **91**, 150–152

Helrich, K., ed. (1990a) *Official Methods of Analysis of the Association of Official Analytical Chemists*, 15th Ed., Vol. 1, Arlington, VA, Association of Official Analytical Chemists, pp. 508–511

Helrich, K., ed. (1990b) *Official Methods of Analysis of the Association of Official Analytical Chemists*, 15th Ed., Vol. 1, Arlington, VA, Association of Official Analytical Chemists, pp. 326–327

Helrich, K., ed. (1990c) *Official Methods of Analysis of the Association of Official Analytical Chemists*, 15th Ed., Vol. 1, Arlington, VA, Association of Official Analytical Chemists, pp. 262–269

Helrich, K., ed. (1990d) *Official Methods of Analysis of the Association of Official Analytical Chemists*, 15th Ed., Vol. 1, Arlington, VA, Association of Official Analytical Chemists, pp. 162–163

Hirano, M., Mitsumori, K., Maita, K. & Shirasu, Y. (1986) Further carcinogenicity study on methylmercury chloride in ICR mice. *Jpn. J. vet. Sci.*, **48**, 127–135

Hirano, M., Ueda, H., Mitsumori, K., Maita, K. & Shirasu, Y. (1988) Hormonal influence on carcinogenicity of methylmercury in mice. *Jpn. J. vet. Sci.*, **50**, 886–893

Holt, D. & Webb, M. (1986a) Comparison of some biochemical effects of teratogenic doses of mercuric mercury and cadmium in the pregnant rat. *Arch. Toxicol.*, **58**, 249–254

Holt, D. & Webb, M. (1986b) The toxicity and teratogenicity of mercuric mercury in the pregnant rat. *Arch. Toxicol.*, **58**, 243–248

Howard, W., Léonard, B., Moody, W. & Kochhar, T.S. (1991) Induction of chromosome changes by metal compounds in cultured CHO cells. *Toxicol. Lett.*, **56**, 179–186

Hrubec, Z., Blair, A.E., Rogot, E. & Vaught, J. (1992) *Mortality Risks by Occupation among US Veterans of Known Smoking Status 1954–1980*, Vol. 1 (NIH Publication No. 92-3407), Washington DC, National Cancer Institute

Hultman, P. & Eneström, S. (1987) The induction of immune complex deposits in mice by peroral and parenteral administration of mercuric chloride: strain dependent susceptibility. *Clin. exp. Immunol.*, **67**, 283–292

Hunter, D. & Russell, D.S. (1954) Focal cerebral and cerebellar atrophy in a human subject due to organic mercury compounds. *J. Neurol. Neurosurg. Psychiatr.*, **17**, 235–241

Hursh, J.B. (1985) Partition coefficients of mercury (^{203}Hg) vapor between air and biological fluids. *J. appl. Toxicol.*, **5**, 327–332

Hursh, J.B., Clarkson, T.W., Cherian, M.G., Vostal, J.J. & Mallie, R.V. (1976) Clearance of mercury (Hg-197, Hg-203) vapor inhaled by human subjects. *Arch. environ. Health*, **31**, 302–309

Hursh, J.B., Greenwood, M.R., Clarkson, T.W., Allen, J. & Demuth, S. (1980) The effect of ethanol on the fate of mercury vapor inhaled by man. *J. Pharmacol. exp. Ther.*, **214**, 520–527

Hursh, J.B., Sichak, S.P. & Clarkson, T.W. (1988) In vitro oxidation of mercury by the blood. *Pharmacol. Toxicol.*, **63**, 266–273

Hursh J.B., Clarkson, T.W., Miles, E.F. & Goldsmith, L.A. (1989) Percutaneous absorption of mercury vapor by man. *Arch. environ. Health*, **44**, 120–127

IARC (1987a) *IARC Monographs on the Evaluation of Carcinogenic Risks to Humans*, Suppl. 7, *Overall Evaluations of Carcinogenicity: An Updating of IARC Monographs Volumes 1 to 42*, Lyon, pp. 230–232

IARC (1987b) *IARC Monographs on the Evaluation of Carcinogenic Risks to Humans*, Suppl. 7, *Overall Evaluations of Carcinogenicity: An Updating of IARC Monographs Volumes 1 to 42*, Lyon, pp. 120–122

IARC (1992) *IARC Monographs on the Evaluation of Carcinogenic Risks to Humans*, Volume 54, *Occupational Exposures to Mists and Vapours from Strong Inorganic Acids; and Other Industrial Chemicals*, Lyon

IARC (1993) *IARC Monographs on the Evaluation of Carcinogenic Risks to Humans*, Vol. 57, *Occupational Exposures of Hairdressers and Barbers and Personal Use of Hair Colourants; Some Hair Dyes, Cosmetic Colourants, Industrial Dyestuffs and Aromatic Amines*, Lyon, p. 55

Igata, A. (1991) Epidemiological and clinical features of Minamata disease. In: Susuki, T., ed, *Advances in Mercury Toxicology*, New York, Plenum Press, pp. 439–457

Ilbäck, N.-G. (1991) Effects of methyl mercury exposure on spleen and blood natural killer (NK) cell activity in the mouse. *Toxicology*, **67**, 117–124

Inouye, M. & Kajiwara, Y. (1988) Developmental disturbances of the fetal brain in guinea-pigs caused by methylmercury. *Arch. Toxicol.*, **62**, 15–21

Inskip, M.J. & Piotrowski, J.K. (1985) Review of the health effects of methylmercury. *J. appl. Toxicol.*, **5**, 113–133

International Labour Office (1991) *Occupational Exposure Limits for Airborne Toxic Substances: Values of Selected Countries* (Occupational Safety and Health Series No. 37), 3rd Ed., Geneva, pp. 252–255, 270–271

Jacobs, G. (1977) Total and organically bound mercury content in fish from German fishing grounds (Ger.). *Z. Lebensmittel. Untersuch.-Forsch.*, **164**, 71–76

Jagiello, G. & Lin, J.S. (1973) An assessment of the effects of mercury on the meiosis of mouse ova. *Mutat. Res.*, **17**, 93–99

Janicki, K., Dobrowolski, J. & Krásnicki, K. (1987) Correlation between contamination of the rural environment with mercury and occurrence of leukaemia in men and cattle. *Chemosphere*, **16**, 253–257

Janssen Chimica (1990) *1991 Catalog Handbook of Fine Chemicals*, Beerse, pp. 754–755, 954

Jokstad, A., Thomassen, Y., Bye, E., Clench-Aas, J. & Aaseth, J. (1992) Dental amalgam and mercury. *Pharmacol. Toxicol.*, **70**, 308–313

Joselow, M.M., Goldwater, L.J., Alvarez, A. & Herndon, J. (1968) Absorption and excretion of mercury in man. XV. Occupational exposure among dentists. *Arch. environ. Health*, **17**, 39–43

Kaiser, G. & Tölg, G. (1984) Mercury. In: Hutzingter, O., ed., *The Handbook of Environmental Chemistry*, Vol. 3, Part A, *Anthropogenic Compounds*, New York, Springer-Verlag, pp. 1–58

Kajiwara, Y. & Inouye, M. (1986) Effects of methylmercury and mercuric chloride on preimplantation mouse embryos *in vivo*. *Teratology*, **33**, 231–237

Kanematsu, N., Hara, M. & Kada, T. (1980) *rec* Assay and mutagenicity studies on metal compounds. *Mutat. Res.*, **77**, 109–116

Kark, P. (1979) Clinical and neurochemical aspects of inorganic mercury intoxication. In: Vinken, P.J. & Bruyn, G.W., eds, *Handbook of Clinical Neurology*, Vol. 36, Amsterdam, Elsevier, pp. 147–197

Karthikeyan, K.S., Parameswaran, A. & Rajan, B.P. (1986) Mercury toxicity in dental personnel. *J. Indian Dent. Assoc.*, **58**, 215–220

Kato, R. (1976) Chromosome breakage associated with organic mercury in Chinese hamster cells *in vitro* (Abstract No. 10). *Mutat. Res.*, **58**, 340–341

Kato, R., Nakamura, A. & Sawai, T. (1976) Chromosome breakage associated with organic mercury in human leukocytes *in vitro* and *in vivo* (Abstract). *Jpn. J. Hum. Genet.*, **20**, 256–257

Kawada, J., Nishida, M., Yoshimura, Y. & Mitani, K. (1980) Effects of organic and inorganic mercurials on thyroidal functions. *J. Pharm. Dyn.*, **3**, 149–159

Kazantzis, G. & Lilly, L.J. (1986) Mutagenic and carcinogenic effects of metals. In: Friberg, L., Nordberg, G.F. & Vouk, W.B., eds, *Handbook on the Toxicology of Metals*, Vol. 1, 2nd Ed, Amsterdam, Elsevier, pp. 319–390

Kazantzis, G., Schiller, K.F.R., Asscher, A.W. & Drew, R.G. (1962) Albuminuria and the nephrotic syndrome following exposure to mercury and its compounds. *Q. J. Med. New Ser.*, **31**, 403–418

Kazantzis, G., Al-Mufti, A.W., Al-Jawad, A., Al-Shahwani, Y., Majid, M.A., Mahmoud, R.M., Soufi, M., Tawfiq, K., Ibrahim, M.A. & Dabagh, H. (1976) Epidemiology of organomercury poisoning in Iraq. II. Relationship of mercury levels in blood and hair to exposure and to clinical findings. *Bull. WHO*, **53** (Suppl.), 37–48

Kershaw, T.G., Clarkson, T.W. & Dhahir, P.H. (1980) The relationship between blood levels and dose of methylmercury in man. *Arch. environ. Health*, **35**, 28–36

Khayat, A. & Dencker, L. (1982) Fetal uptake and distribution of metallic mercury vapor in the mouse: influence of ethanol and aminotriazole. *Biol. Res. Pregn.*, **3**, 38–46

Khera, K.S. (1973a) Reproductive capability of male rats and mice treated with methyl mercury. *Toxicol. appl. Pharmacol.*, **24**, 167–177

Khera, K.S. (1973b) Teratogenic effects of methylmercury in the cat: note on the use of this species as a model for teratogenicity studies. *Teratology*, **8**, 293–303

Khera, K.S. (1979) Teratogenic and genetic effects of mercury toxicity. In: Nriagu, J.O., ed., *The Biogeochemistry of Mercury in the Environment*, Amsterdam, Elsevier, pp. 503–518

Kitchin, K.T., Ebron, M.T. & Svendsgaard, D. (1984) In vitro study of embryotoxic and dysmorphogenic effects of mercuric chloride and methylmercury chloride in the rat. *Food Chem. Toxicol.*, **22**, 31–37

Klášterská, I. & Ramel, C. (1978) The effect of methyl mercury hydroxide on meiotic chromosomes of the grasshopper *Stethophyma grossum*. *Hereditas*, **88**, 255–262

Koller, L.D. (1975) Methylmercury: effect on oncogenic and nononcogenic viruses in mice. *Am. J. vet. Dis.*, **36**, 1501–1504

Kosta, L., Byrne, A.R. & Zelenko, V. (1975) Correlation between selenium and mercury in man following exposure to inorganic mercury. *Nature*, **254**, 238–239

Kostial, K., Šimonović, I., Rabar, I., Blanuša, M. & Landeka, M. (1983) Age and intestinal retention of mercury and cadmium in rats. *Environ. Res.*, **31**, 111–115

Kostoff, D. (1939) Effect of the fungicide 'Granosan' on atypical growth and chromosome doubling in plants (Short communication). *Nature*, **144**, 334

Kostoff, D. (1940) Atypical growth, abnormal mitosis and polyploidy induced by ethylmercurychloride. *J. Phytopathol.*, **2**, 91–96

Kurokawa, Y., Matsushima, M., Imazawa, T., Takamura, N., Takahashi, M. & Hayashi, Y. (1985) Promoting effect of metal compounds on rat renal tumorigenesis. *J. Am. Coll. Toxicol.*, **4**, 321–330

Kurokawa, Y., Takahashi, M., Maekawa, A. & Hayashi, Y. (1989) Promoting effect of metal compounds on liver, stomach, kidney, pancreas and skin carcinogenesis. *J. Am. Coll. Toxicol.*, **8**, 1235–1239

Ladd, A.C., Zuskin, E., Valic, F., Almonte, J.B. & Gonzales, T.V. (1966) Absorption and excretion of mercury in miners. *J. occup. Med.*, **8**, 127–131

Lamperti, A.A. & Printz, R.H. (1973) Effects of mercuric chloride on the reproductive cycle of the female hamster. *Biol. Reprod.*, **8**, 378–387

Langworth, S., Röjdmark, S. & Åkesson, A. (1990) Normal pituitary response to thyrotrophin releasing hormone in dental personnel exposed to mercury. *Swed. Dent. J.*, **14**, 101–103

Langworth, S., Elinder, C.-G., Göthe, C.J. & Vesterberg, O. (1991) Biological monitoring of environmental and occupational exposure to mercury. *Int. Arch. occup. environ. Health*, **63**, 161–167

Langworth, S., Almkvist, O., Söderman, E. & Wilkström, B.-O. (1992a) Effects of occupational exposure to mercury vapour on the central nervous system. *Br. J. ind. Med.*, **49**, 545–555

Langworth, S., Elinder, C.-G., Sundquist, K.G. & Vesterberg, O. (1992b) Renal and immunological effects of occupational exposure to inorganic mercury. *Br. J. ind. Med.*, **49**, 394–401

Lauwerys, R.R. (1983) Mercury. In: Parmeggiani, L., ed., *Encyclopedia of Occupational Health and Safety*, 3rd rev. Ed., Vol. 2, Geneva, International Labour Office, pp. 1332–1335

Lauwerys, R.R. & Buchet, J.P. (1973) Occupational exposure to mercury vapors and biological action. *Arch. environ. Health*, **27**, 65–68

Lauwerys, R., Bernard, A., Roels, H., Buchet, J.P., Gennart, J.P., Mahieu, P. & Foidart, J.M. (1983) Anti-laminin antibodies in workers exposed to mercury vapour. *Toxicol. Lett.*, **17**, 113–116

Lauwerys, R., Roels, H., Genet, P., Toussaint, G., Bouckaert, A. & De Cooman, S. (1985) Fertility of male workers exposed to mercury vapor or to manganese dust: a questionnaire study. *Am. J. ind. Med.*, **7**, 171–176

Lauwerys, R., Bonnier, C., Evrard, P., Gennart, J.P. & Bernard, A. (1987) Prenatal and early postnatal intoxication by inorganic mercury resulting from the maternal use of mercury containing soap. *Hum. Toxicol.*, **6**, 253–256

Lehotzky, K. & Bordas, S. (1968) Study on the subacute neurotoxic effect of methoxy-ethyl mercury chloride (MEMC) in rats. *Med. Lav.*, **59**, 241–249

Léonard, A., Jacquet, P. & Lauwerys, R.R. (1983) Mutagenicity and teratogenicity of mercury compounds. *Mutat. Res.*, **114**, 1–18

Li, Y.-H. & Lin, X.-W. (1991) The transplacental effect of methylmercury on the chromosome of embryo liver cells in rat (Chin.). *Chin. J. prev. Med.*, **25**, 220–221

Lide, D.R., ed. (1991) *CRC Handbook of Chemistry and Physics*, 72nd Ed., Boca Raton, FL, CRC Press, pp. 4-74–4-75

Lindqvist, K.J., Makene, W.J., Shaba, J.K. & Nantulya, V. (1974) Immunofluorescence and electron microscopic studies of kidney biopsies from patients with nephrotic syndrome, possibly induced by skin lightening creams containing mercury. *East Afr. med. J.*, **51**, 168–169

Lindstedt, G., Gottberg, I., Holmgren, B., Jonsson, T. & Karlsson, G. (1979) Individual mercury exposure of chloralkali workers and its relation to blood and urinary mercury levels. *Scand. J. Work Environ. Health*, **5**, 59–69

Lindström, H., Luthman, J., Oskarsson, A., Sundberg, J. & Olson, L. (1991) Effects of long-term treatment with methyl mercury on the developing rat brain. *Environ. Res.*, **56**, 158–169

Mabille, V., Roels, H., Jacquet, P., Léonard, A. & Lauwerys, R.R. (1984) Cytogenetic examination of leukocytes of workers exposed to mercury vapour. *Int. Arch. occup. environ. Health*, **53**, 257–260

MacFarlane, E.W.E. (1956) Cytological conditions in root tip meristem after gross antagonism of phenylmercuric poisoning. *Exp. Cell Res.*, **5**, 375–385

MacFarlane, E.W.E. & Messing, A.M. (1953) Shoot chimeras after exposure to mercurial compounds. *Bot. Gaz.*, **115**, 66–76

Magnusson, J. & Ramel, C. (1986) Genetic variation in the susceptibility to mercury and other metal compounds in *Drosophila melanogaster*. *Teratog. Carcinog. Mutag.*, **6**, 289–305

Magos, L. (1987) The absorption, distribution and excretion of methyl mercury. In: Eccles, C.U. & Annau, Z., eds, *The Toxicity of Methylmercury*, Baltimore, MD, Johns Hopkins University Press, pp. 24–44

Magos, L. & Butler, W.H. (1972) Cumulative effects of methylmercury dicyandiamide given orally to rats. *Food Cosmet. Toxicol.*, **10**, 513–517

Magos, L. & Clarkson, T.W. (1972) Atomic absorption determination of total, inorganic and organic mercury in blood. *J. Assoc. off. anal. Chem.*, **55**, 966–971

Magos, L. & Webb, M. (1977) The effects of selenium on the brain uptake of methylmercury. *Arch. Toxicol.*, **38**, 201–207

Magos, L., Halbach, S. & Clarkson, T.W. (1978) Role of catalase in the oxidation of mercury vapor. *Biochem. Pharmacol.*, **27**, 1373–1377

Magos, L., Sparrow, S. & Snowden, R. (1982) The comparative renotoxicology of phenylmercury and mercuric chloride. *Arch. Toxicol.*, **50**, 133–139

Mailhes, J.B. (1983) Methylmercury effects on Syrian hamster metaphase II oocyte chromosomes. *Environ. Mutag.*, **5**, 679–686

Manalis, R.S. & Cooper, G.P. (1975) Evoked transmitter release increased by inorganic mercury at frog neuromuscular junction. *Nature*, **257**, 690–691

Mathew, C. & Al-Doori, Z. (1976) The mutagenic effect of the mercury fungicide Ceresan M in *Drosophila melanogaster*. *Mutat. Res.*, **40**, 31–36

Matsumoto, N. & Spindle, A. (1982) Sensitivity of early mouse embryos to methylmercury toxicity. *Toxicol. appl. Pharmacol.*, **64**, 108–117

McFarland, R.B. & Reigel, H. (1978) Chronic mercury poisoning from a single brief exposure. *J. occup. Med.*, **20**, 532–534

McLaughlin, J.K., Malker, H.S.R., Blot, W.J., Malker, B.K., Stone, B.J., Weiner, J.A., Ericsson, J.L.E. & Fraumeni, J.F., Jr (1987) Occupational risks for intracranial gliomas in Sweden. *J. natl Cancer Inst.*, **78**, 253–257

McNerney, J.J., Buseck, P.R. & Hanson, R.C. (1972) Mercury detection by means of thin gold films. *Science*, **178**, 611–612

Miettinen, J.K. (1973) Absorption and elimination of dietary mercury (Hg^{++}) and methyl mercury in man. In: Miller, M.W. & Clarkson, T.W., eds, *Mercury, Mercurials and Mercaptans*, Springfield, IL, C.C. Thomas, pp. 233–243

Milham, S., Jr (1976) *Occupational Mortality in Washington State 1950–1971*, Vols I and II, Washington DC, US Department of Health, Education, and Welfare

Miller, C.T., Zawidzka, Z., Nagy, E. & Charbonneau, S.M. (1979) Indicators of genetic toxicity in leucocytes and granulocytic precursors after chronic methylmercury ingestion by cats. *Bull. environ. Contam. Toxicol.*, **21**, 296–303

Miller, D.M., Lund, B.-O. & Woods, J.S. (1991) Reactivity of Hg(II) with superoxide: evidence for the catalytic dismutation of superoxide by Hg(II). *J. Biochem. Toxicol.*, **6**, 293–298

Minoia, C., Sabbioni, E., Apostoli, P., Pietra, R., Pozzoli, L., Gallorini, M., Nicolaou, G., Alessio, L. & Capodaglio, E. (1990) Trace elements reference values in tissues from inhabitants of the European Community. I. A study of 46 elements in urine, blood and serum of Italian subjects. *Sci. total Environ.*, **95**, 89–105

Mitsumori, K., Maita, K., Saito, T., Tsuda, S. & Shirasu, Y. (1981) Carcinogenicity of methylmercury chloride in ICR mice: preliminary note on renal carcinogenesis. *Cancer Lett.*, **12**, 305–310

Mitsumori, K., Takahashi, K., Matano, O., Goto, S. & Shirasu, Y. (1983) Chronic toxicity of methylmercury chloride in rats: clinical study and chemical analysis. *Jpn. J. vet. Sci.*, **45**, 747–757

Mitsumori, K., Maita, K. & Shirasu, Y. (1984) Chronic toxicity of methylmercury chloride in rats: pathological study. *Jpn. J. vet. Sci.*, **46**, 549–557

Mitsumori, K., Hirano, M., Ueda, H., Maita, K. & Shirasu, Y. (1990) Chronic toxicity and carcinogenicity of methylmercury chloride in B6C3F$_1$ mice. *Fundam. appl. Toxicol.*, **14**, 179–190

Miyamoto, M.D. (1983) Hg^{2+} causes neurotoxicity at an intracellular site following entry through Na and Ca channels. *Brain Res.*, **267**, 375–379

Møller-Madsen, B. (1992) Localization of mercury in CNS of the rat. V. Inhalation exposure to metallic mercury. *Arch. Toxicol.*, **66**, 79–89

Møller-Madsen, B., Hansen, J.C. & Kragstrup, J. (1988) Mercury concentrations in blood from Danish dentists. *Scand. J. dent. Res.*, **96**, 56–59

Monsalve, M.V. & Chiappe, C. (1987) Genetic effects of methylmercury in human chromosomes: I. A cytogenetic study of people exposed through eating contaminated fish. *Environ. mol. Mutag.*, **10**, 367–376

Morimoto, K., Iijima, S. & Koizumi, A. (1982) Selenite prevents the induction of sister-chromatid exchanges by methyl mercury and mercuric chloride in human whole-blood cultures. *Mutat. Res.*, **102**, 183–192

Mottet, N.K., Shaw, C.-M. & Burbacher, T.M. (1985) Health risks from increases in methylmercury exposure. *Environ. Health Perspectives*, **63**, 133–140

Mottironi, V.D., Harrison, B., Pollara, B., Gooding, R. & Banks, S. (1986) Possible synergistic effect of mercury and smoking on sister-chromatid exchange (SCE) rates in humans (Abstract No. 1669). *Fed. Proc.*, **45**, 441

Mudry de Pargament, M.D., Larripa, I., Labal de Vinuesa, M., Barlotti, M., De Biase, P. & Brieux de Salum, S. (1987) Sister chromatid exchange and accidental exposure to phenylmercury acetate (Fr.). *Bol. Estud. méd. biol. Méx.*, **35**, 207–211

Müller, W.-U., Streffer, C. & Joos, A.L. (1990) Toxicity of cadmium sulphate and methylmercuric chloride applied singly or in combination to early mouse embryos *in vitro*. *Toxicol. in vitro*, **4**, 57–61

Munro, I.C., Nera, E.A., Charbonneau, S.M., Junkins, B. & Zawidzka, Z. (1980) Chronic toxicity of methylmercury in the rat. *J. environ. Pathol. Toxicol.*, **3**, 437–447

Naganuma, A., Koyama, Y. & Imura, N. (1980) Behavior of methylmercury in mammalian erythrocytes. *Toxicol. appl. Pharmacol.*, **54**, 405–410

Nakada, S., Nomoto, A. & Imura, N. (1980) Effect of methylmercury and inorganic mercury on protein synthesis in mammalian cells. *Ecotoxicol. environ. Saf.*, **4**, 184–190

Nakai, S. & Machida, I. (1973) Genetic effect of organic mercury on yeast (Abstract No. 7). *Mutat. Res.*, **21**, 348

Naleway, C., Sakaguchi, R., Mitchell, E., Muller, T., Ayer, W.A. & Hefferren, J.J. (1985) Urinary mercury levels in US dentists, 1975–1983: review of health assessment program. *J. Am. Dent. Assoc.*, **111**, 37–42

Naleway, C., Chou, H.-N., Muller, T., Dabney, J., Roxe, D. & Siddiqui, F. (1991) On-site screening for urinary Hg concentrations and correlation with glomerular and renal tubular function. *J. public Health Dent.*, **51**, 12–17

Newton, D. & Fry, F.A. (1978) The retention and distribution of radioactive mercuric oxide following accidental inhalation. *Ann. occup. Hyg.*, **21**, 21–32

Nielsen, J.B. & Andersen, O. (1991) A comparison of the effects of sodium selenite and seleno-L-methionine on disposition of orally-administered mercuric chloride. *J. Trace Elem. Electrolytes Health Dis.*, **5**, 245–250

Nilsson, B., Gerhardsson, L. & Nordberg, G.F. (1990) Urine mercury levels and associated symptoms in dental personnel. *Sci. total Environ.*, **94**, 179–185

Nishiyama, S., Taguchi, T. & Onosaka, S. (1987) Induction of zinc-thionein by estradiol and protective effects on inorganic mercury-induced renal toxicity. *Biochem. Pharmacol.*, **36**, 3387–3391

Nixon, J.E., Koller, L.D. & Exon, J.H. (1979) Effect of methylmercury chloride on transplacental tumors induced by sodium nitrite and ethylurea in rats. *J. natl Cancer Inst.*, **63**, 1057–1063

Nordberg, G.F. & Skerfving, S. (1972) Metabolism. In: Friberg, L. & Vostal, J., eds, *Mercury in the Environment. An Epidemiological and Toxicological Appraisal*, Cleveland, OH, CRC Press, pp. 29–91

Norseth, T. (1971) Biotransformation of methyl mercuric salts in the mouse studied by specific determination of inorganic mercury. *Acta pharmacol. toxicol.*, **29**, 375–384

Norseth, T. & Clarkson, T.W. (1971) Intestinal transport of ^{203}Hg-labeled methyl mercury chloride. Role of biotransformation in rats. *Arch. environ. Health*, **22**, 568–577

Nriagu, J.O., Pfeiffer, W.C., Malm, O., de Souza, C.M.M. & Mierle, G. (1992) Mercury pollution in Brazil (Letter to the Editor). *Nature*, **356**, 389

Nylander, M. & Weiner, J. (1991) Mercury and selenium concentrations and their interrelations in organs from dental staff and the general population. *Br. J. ind. Med.*, **48**, 729–734

Oberly, T.J., Piper, C.E. & McDonald, D.S. (1982) Mutagenicity of metal salts in the L5178Y mouse lymphoma assay. *J. Toxicol. environ. Health*, **9**, 367–376

Önfelt, A. (1983) Spindle disturbances in mammalian cells. I. Changes in the quantity of free sulfhydryl groups in relation to survival and c-mitosis in V79 Chinese hamster cells after treatment with colcemid, diamide, carbaryl and methyl mercury. *Chem.-biol. Interactions*, **46**, 201–217

Önfelt, A. & Jenssen, D. (1982) Enhanced mutagenic response of MNU by post-treatment with methylmercury, caffeine or thymidine in V79 Chinese hamster cells. *Mutat. Res.*, **106**, 297–303

Orlowski, J.P. & Mercer, R.D. (1980) Urine mercury levels in Kawasaki disease. *Pediatrics*, **66**, 633–636

Osgood, C., Zimmering, S. & Mason, J.M. (1991) Aneuploidy in Drosophila. II. Further validation of the FIX and ZESTE genetic test systems employing female *Drosophila melanogaster*. *Mutat. Res.*, **259**, 147–163

Panda, B.B., Das, B.L., Lenka, M. & Panda, K.K. (1988) Water hyacinth (*Eichhornia crassipes*) to biomonitor genotoxicity of low levels of mercury in aquatic environment. *Mutat. Res.*, **206**, 275–279

Parizek, J. & Ostádalová, I. (1967) The protective effect of small amounts of selenite in sublimate intoxication. *Experientia*, **23**, 142–143

Parkin, J.E. (1987) Assay of phenylmercury salts in pharmaceutical products by high-performance liquid chromatography of the morpholinedithiocarbamate derivative. *J. Chromatogr.*, **407**, 389–392

Pelletier, L., Pasquier, R., Hirsch, F., Sapin, C. & Druet, P. (1986) Autoreactive T cells in mercury-induced autoimmune disease: in vitro demonstration. *J. Immunol.*, **137**, 2548–2554

Pelletier, L., Pasquier, R., Rossert, J. & Druet, P. (1987a) HgCl$_2$ induced nonspecific immunosuppression in Lewis rats. *Eur. J. Imunol.*, **17**, 49–54

Pelletier, L., Galceran, M., Pasquier, R., Ronco, P., Verroust, P., Bariety, J. & Druet, P. (1987b) Down modulation of Heymann's nephritis by mercuric chloride. *Kidney int.*, **32**, 227–232

Perry, D.M., Weis, J.S. & Weis, P. (1988) Cytogenetic effects of methylmercury in embryos of the killifish, *Fundulus heteroclitus*. *Arch. environ. Contam. Toxicol.*, **17**, 569–574

Petersson, K., Dock, L. & Vahter, M. (1989) Metabolism of methylmercury in rabbits and hamsters. *Biol. Trace Elem. Res.*, **21**, 219–226

Pfeiffer, W.C., de Lacerda, L.D., Malm, O., Souza, C.M.M., da Silveira, E.G. & Bastos, W.R. (1989) Mercury concentrations in inland waters of gold-mining areas in Rondônia, Brazil. *Sci. total Environ.*, **87/88**, 233–240

Phipps, J. & Miller, D.R. (1982) Some aspects of the genetic toxicity of methylmercury in yeasts (Fr.). *C.R. Acad. Sci. Paris Ser. III*, **295**, 683–686

Phipps, J. & Miller, D.R. (1983) Genetic toxicity of methylmercury chloride (CH$_3$HgCl) on mitochondria of *Saccharomyces cerevisiae* (Fr.). *Can. J. Microbiol.*, **29**, 1149–1153

Poma, K., Kirsch-Volders, M. & Susanne, C. (1981) Mutagenicity study on mice given mercuric chloride. *J. appl. Toxicol.*, **1**, 314–316

Popescu, H.I., Negru, L. & Lancranjan, I. (1979) Chromosomal aberrations induced by occupational exposure to mercury. *Arch. environ. Health*, **34**, 461–463

Prickett, C.S., Laug, E.P. & Kunze, F.M. (1950) Distribution of mercury in rats following oral and intravenous administration of mercuric acetate and phenylmercuric acetate. *Proc. Soc. exp. Biol. Med.*, **73**, 585–588

Rahola, T., Hattula, T., Korolainen, A. & Miettinen, J.K. (1973) Elimination of free and protein-bound ionic mercury ($^{203}Hg^{2+}$) in man. *Ann. clin. Res.*, **5**, 214–219

Ramel, C. (1969) Genetic effects of organic mercury compounds. I. Cytological investigations on *Allium* roots. *Hereditas*, **61**, 208–230

Ramel, C. (1972) Genetic effects. In: Friberg, L. & Vostal, D., eds, *Mercury in the Environment: Toxicological Effects and Epidemiological and Toxicological Appraisal*, Cleveland, OH, CRC Press, pp. 169–181

Ramel, C. & Magnusson, J. (1969) Genetic effects of organic mercury compounds. II. Chromosome segregation in *Drosophila melanogaster*. *Hereditas*, **61**, 231–254

Ramel, C. & Magnusson, J. (1979) Chemical induction of nondisjunction in *Drosophila*. *Environ. Health Perspectives*, **31**, 59–66

Rasmussen, G. (1984) *Kviksølv: Tunkonserves 1988* [Mercury in Tinned Tuna Fish 1983], Copenhagen, National Food Agency (in Danish)

Reese, R.G., Jr (1990) Mercury. In: *Mineral Commodity Summaries 1990*, Washington DC, Bureau of Mines, US Department of the Interior, pp. 108–109

Reese, R.G., Jr (1991) Mercury. In: *Mineral Commodity Summaries 1991*, Washington DC, Bureau of Mines, US Department of the Interior, pp. 102–103

Reese, R.G., Jr (1992a) *Mineral Industry Surveys: Annual Review—Mercury in 1991*, Washington DC, Bureau of Mines, US Department of the Interior

Reese, R.G., Jr (1992b) Mercury. In: *Mineral Commodity Summaries 1992*, Washington DC, Bureau of Mines, US Department of the Interior, pp. 112–113

Refsvik, T. & Norseth, T. (1975) Methyl mercuric compounds in rat bile. *Acta pharmacol. toxicol.*, **36**, 67–78

Reuhl, K.R. & Chang, L.W. (1979) Effects of methylmercury on the development of the nervous system: a review. *Neurotoxicology*, **1**, 21–55

Reuhl, K.R., Chang, L.W. & Townsend, J.W. (1981) Pathological effects of in utero methylmercury exposure on the cerebellum of the golden hamster. I. Early effects upon the neonatal cerebellar cortex. *Environ. Res.*, **26**, 281–306

Rice, D.C. (1992) Effects of pre- plus postnatal exposure to methylmercury in the monkey on fixed interval and discrimination reversal performance. *NeuroToxicology*, **13**, 443–452

Richter, E.D., Peled, N. & Luria, M. (1982) Mercury exposure and effects at a thermometer factory. *Scand. J. Work Environ. Health*, **8** (Suppl. 1), 161–166

Robbins, M.S., Hughes, J.A., Sparber, S.B. & Mannering, G.J. (1978) Delayed teratogenic effect of methylmercury on hepatic cytochrome P-450-dependent monooxygenase systems of rats. *Life Sci.*, **22**, 287–293

Robinson, J.W. & Skelly, E.M. (1982) Speciation of mercury compounds by differential atomization-atomic absorption spectroscopy. *J. environ. Health Sci.*, **A17**, 391–425

Robison, S.H., Cantoni, O. & Costa, M. (1982) Strand breakage and decreased molecular weight of DNA induced by specific metal compounds. *Carcinogenesis*, **3**, 657–662

Robison, S.H., Cantoni, O. & Costa, M. (1984) Analysis of metal-induced DNA lesions and DNA-repair replication in mammalian cells. *Mutat. Res.*, **131**, 173–181

Roeleveld, N., Zielhuis, G.A. & Gabreëls, F. (1990) Occupational exposure and defects of the central nervous system in offspring: review. *Br. J. ind. Med.*, **47**, 580–588

Roels, H., Gennart, J.-P., Lauwerys, R., Buchet, J.-P., Malchaire, J. & Bernard, A. (1985) Surveillance of workers exposed to mercury vapour: validation of a previously proposed biological threshold limit value for mercury concentration in urine. *Am. J. ind. Med.*, 7, 45–71

Roels, H., Abdeladim, S., Ceulemans, E. & Lauwerys, R. (1987) Relationships between the concentrations of mercury in air and in blood or urine in workers exposed to mercury vapour. *Ann. occup. Hyg.*, 31, 135–145

Rossman, T.G., Molina, M., Meyer, L., Boone, P., Klein, C.B., Wang, Z., Li, F., Lin, W.C. & Kinney, P.L. (1991) Performance of 133 compounds in the lambda prophage induction endpoint of the Microscreen assay and a comparison with *S. typhimurium* mutagenicity and rodent carcinogenicity assays. *Mutat. Res.*, 260, 349–367

Rowland, I.R., Davies, M.J. & Evans, J.G. (1980) Tissue content of mercury in rats given methylmercuric chloride orally: influence of intestinal flora. *Arch. environ. Health*, 35, 155–160

Rustam, H., Von Burg, R., Amin-Zaki, L. & El Hassani, S. (1975) Evidence for a neuromuscular disorder in methylmercury poisoning. Clinical and electrophysiological findings in moderate to severe cases. *Arch. environ. Health*, 30, 190–195

Ryan, P., Lee, M.W., North, B. & McMichael, A.J. (1992) Amalgam fillings, diagnostic dental x-rays and tumours of the brain and meninges. *Oral Oncol. Eur. J. Cancer*, 28B, 91–95

Saillenfait, A.M., Langonne, I., Sabate, J.P. & de Ceaurriz, J. (1990) Interaction between mercuric chloride and zinc in rat whole-embryo culture. *Toxicol. in vitro*, 4, 129–136

Sällsten, G., Barregård, L., Langworth, S. & Vesterberg, O. (1992) Exposure to mercury in industry and dentistry: a field comparison between diffusive and active samplers. *Appl. occup. environ. Hyg.*, 7, 434–440

Sass, J.E. (1937) Histological and cytological studies of ethyl mercury phosphate poisoning in corn seedlings. *Phytopathology*, 27, 95–99

Sax, N.I. & Lewis, R.J. (1987) *Hawley's Condensed Chemical Dictionary*, 11th Ed., New York, Van Nostrand Reinhold, pp. 741–742, 745–746, 904

Schaller, K.-H., Triebig, G., Schiele, R. & Valentin, H. (1991) Biological monitoring and health surveillance of workers exposed to mercury. In: Dillon, H.K. & Ho, M.H., eds, *Biological Monitoring of Exposure to Chemical Metals*, New York, John Wiley & Sons, pp. 3–9

Schardein, J.L. (1985) *Chemically Induced Birth Defects*, New York, Marcel Dekker, pp. 622–632

Schroeder, H.A. & Mitchener, M. (1975) Life-term effects of mercury, methyl mercury and nine other trace metals on mice. *J. Nutr.*, 105, 452–458

Sequi, P. (1980) The behaviour of chromium and mercury in soil (Ital.). In: Frigerio A., ed., *Rischi e Tossicita' dell'Inquinamento da Metalli: Cromo e Mercurio*, Milan, DiEsseTi Publications, pp. 27–50

Shepard, T.H. (1992) *Catalog of Teratogenic Agents*, 7th Ed., Baltimore, MD, Johns Hopkins University Press, pp. 249–251

Shirasu, Y., Moriya, M., Kato, K., Furuhashi, A. & Kada, T. (1976) Mutagenicity screening of pesticides in the microbial system. *Mutat. Res.*, 40, 19–30

Siemiatycki, J., ed. (1991) *Risk Factors for Cancer in the Workplace*, Boca Raton, FL, CRC Press

Sikorski, R., Juszkiewicz, T., Paszkowski, T. & Szprengier-Juszkiewicz, T. (1987) Women in dental surgeries: reproductive hazards in occupational exposure to metallic mercury. *Int. Arch. occup. environ. Health*, 59, 551–557

Simon, M., Jönk, P., Wühl-Couturier, G. & Daunderer, M. (1990) Mercury, mercury alloys, and mercury compounds. In: Elvers, B., Hawkins, S. & Schulz, G., eds, *Ullmann's Encyclopedia of Industrial Chemistry*, Vol. A16, *Magnetic Materials to Mutagenic Agents*, New York, VCH Publishers, pp. 269–298

Singer, W. & Nowak, M. (1981) Mercury compounds. In: Mark, H.F., Othmer, D.F., Overberger, C.G., Seaborg, G.T. & Grayson, N., eds, *Kirk–Othmer Encyclopedia of Chemical Technology*, 3rd Ed., Vol. 15, New York, John Wiley & Sons, pp. 157–171

Skerfving, S. (1974) Methylmercury exposure, mercury levels in blood and hair, and health status in Swedes consuming contaminated fish. *Toxicology*, **2**, 3–23

Skerfving, S. (1988) Mercury in women exposed to methylmercury through fish consumption, and in their newborn babies and breast milk. *Bull. environ. Contam. Toxicol.*, **41**, 475–482

Skerfving, S. & Vostal, J. (1972) Symptoms and signs of intoxication. In: Friberg, L. & Vostal, J., eds, *Mercury in the Environment*, Cleveland, OH, CRC Press, pp. 93–107

Skerfving, S., Hansson, K. & Lindsten, J. (1970) Chromosome breakage in humans exposed to methyl mercury through fish consumption. Preliminary communication. *Arch. environ. Health*, **21**, 133–139

Skerfving, S., Hansson, K., Mangs, C., Lindsten, J. & Ryman, N. (1974) Methylmercury-induced chromosome damage in man. *Environ. Res.*, **7**, 83–98

Slotkin, T.A., Kavlock, R.J., Cowdery, T., Orband, L., Bartolome, M., Gray, J.A., Rehnberg, B.F. & Bartolome, J. (1986) Functional consequences of prenatal methylmercury exposure: effects on renal and hepatic responses to trophic stimuli and on renal excretory mechanisms. *Toxicol. Lett.*, **34**, 231–345

Smith, R.G., Vorwald, A.J., Patil, L.S. & Mooney, T.F., Jr (1970) Effects of exposure to mercury in the manufacture of chlorine. *Am. ind. Hyg. Assoc. J.*, **31**, 687–700

Smith, J.H., McCormack, K.M., Braselton, W.E., Jr & Hook, J.B. (1983) The effect of prenatal methylmercury administration on postnatal renal functional development. *Environ. Res.*, **30**, 63–71

Snell, K., Ashby, S.L. & Barton, S.J. (1977) Disturbances of perinatal carbohydrate metabolism in rats exposed to methylmercury *in utero*. *Toxicology*, **8**, 277–283

Southard, J.H. & Nitisewojo, P. (1973) Loss of oxidative phosphorylation in mitochondria isolated from kidneys of mercury poisoned rats. *Biochem. biophys. Res. Commun.*, **52**, 921–927

Spyker, J.M., Sparber, S.B. & Goldberg, A.M. (1972) Subtle consequences of methylmercury exposure: behavioral deviations in offspring of treated mothers. *Science*, **177**, 621–623

Stewart, W.K., Guirgis, H.A., Sanderson, J. & Taylor, W. (1977) Urinary mercury excretion and proteinuria in pathology laboratory staff. *Br. J. ind. Med.*, **34**, 26–31

Stokinger, H.E. (1981) Mercury, Hg. In: Clayton, G.D. & Clayton, F.L., eds, *Patty's Industrial Hygiene and Toxicology*, 3rd rev. Ed., Vol. 2A, New York, John Wiley & Sons, pp. 1769–1792

Strem Chemicals (1992) *Catalog No. 14 — Metals, Inorganics and Organometallics for Research*, Newburyport, MA, pp. 70–72

Su, M.-Q. & Okita, G.T. (1976a) Behavioral effects on the progeny of mice treated with methylmercury. *Toxicol. appl. Pharmacol.*, **38**, 195–205

Suda, I. & Hirayama, K. (1992) Degradation of methyl and ethyl mercury into inorganic mercury by hydroxyl radical produced from rat liver microsomes. *Arch. Toxicol.*, **66**, 398–402

Suda, I., Totoki, S. & Takahashi, H. (1991) Degradation of methyl and ethyl mercury into inorganic mercury by oxygen free radical-producing systems: involvement of hydroxyl radical. *Arch. Toxicol.*, **65**, 129–134

Sundberg, J., Oskarsson, A. & Bergman, K. (1991) Milk transfer of inorganic mercury to suckling rats. Interaction with selenite. *Biol. Trace Elem. Res.*, **28**, 27–38

Suter, K.E. (1975) Studies on the dominant-lethal and fertility effects of the heavy metal compounds methylmercuric hydroxide, mercuric chloride, and cadmium chloride in male and female mice. *Mutat. Res.*, **30**, 365–374

Suzuki, T. & Tanaka, A. (1971) Absorption of metallic mercury from the intestine after rupture of Miller–Abbot balloon. *Jpn. J. ind. Health*, **13**, 222–223

Suzuki, T., Yonemoto, J., Satoh, H., Naganuma, A., Imura, N. & Kigawa, T. (1984) Normal organic and inorganic mercury levels in the human feto-placental system. *J. appl. Toxicol.*, **4**, 249–252

Swedish Expert Group (1970) Metallic mercury in fish. A toxicological–epidemiological risk evaluation. Report from an expert group. *Nord. Hyg. Tidskr.*, Suppl. 3

Tamashiro, H., Arakaki, M., Futatsuka, M. & Lee, E.S. (1986) Methylmercury exposure and mortality in southern Japan: a close look at causes of death. *J. Epidemiol. Community Health*, **40**, 181–185

Tamashiro, H., Fukutomi, K. & Lee, E.S. (1987) Methylmercury exposure and mortality in Japan: a life table analysis. *Arch. environ. Health*, **42**, 100–107

Tazima, Y. (1974) Attempts to induce non-disjunction by means of irradiation and chemical treatment in the silkworm (Abstract No. E-15-8). *Radiat. Res.*, **59**, 267–268

Thorp, J.M., Jr, Boyette, D.D., Watson, W.J. & Cefalo, R.C. (1992) Elemental mercury exposure in early pregnancy. *Obstet. Gynecol.*, **79**, 874–876

Tournamille, J., Caporiccio, B., Michel, R. & Sentein, P. (1982) Action of methylmercury chloride on mitosis of human lymphocytes in culture: ultrastructural study (Fr.). *C.R. Soc. Biol.*, **176**, 194–203

Troen, P., Kaufman, S.A. & Katz, K.H. (1951) Mercuric bichloride poisoning. *New Engl. J. Med.*, **244**, 459–463

Tunnessen, W.W., Jr, McMahon, K.J. & Baser, M. (1987) Acrodynia: exposure to mercury from fluorescent light bulbs. *Pediatrics*, **79**, 786–789

Ulfvarson, U. (1962) Distribution and excretion of some mercury compounds after long term exposure. *Int. Arch. Gewerbepathol. Gewerbehyg.*, **19**, 412–422

Umeda, M., Saito, K., Hirose, K. & Saito, M. (1969) Cytotoxic effect of inorganic, phenyl, and alkyl mercuric compounds on HeLa cells. *Jpn. J. exp. Med.*, **39**, 47–58

UNEP (1993) *IRPTC PC Database*, Geneva

US Department of Health and Human Services (1992) *Cosmetics Handbook*, Washington DC, p. 16

US Department of Health and Human Services (1993) *Dental Amalgam: A Scientific Review and Recommended Public Health Service Strategy for Research, Education and Regulation*, Washington DC, US Public Health Service

US Environmental Protection Agency (1986a) Method 7470. Mercury in liquid waste (manual cold-vapor technique). In: *Test Methods for Evaluating Solid Waste — Physical/Chemical Methods*, 3rd Ed. (US EPA No. SW-846), Vol. 1A, Washington DC, Office of Solid Waste and Emergency Response, pp. 7470-1–7470-8

US Environmental Protection Agency (1986b) Method 7471. Mercury in solid or semisolid waste (manual cold-vapor technique). In: *Test Methods for Evaluating Solid Waste — Physical/Chemical Methods*, 3rd Ed. (US EPA No. SW-846), Vol. 1A, Washington DC, Office of Solid Waste and Emergency Response, pp. 7471-1–74701-10

US Environmental Protection Agency (1991) Maximum contaminant levels for inorganic chemicals. *US Code fed. Regul.*, **Title 40**, pp. 585–586

US Environmental Protection Agency (1992) National emission standard for mercury. *US Code fed. Regul.*, **Title 40**, pp. 26–32

US Food and Drug Administration (1992) Standards of quality—bottled water. *US Code fed. Regul.*, **Title 21**, pp. 61-64

US National Institute for Occupational Safety and Health (1990) *NIOSH Pocket Guide to Chemical Hazards* (DHHS (NIOSH) Publication No. 90-117), Cincinnati, OH, pp. 140-141

US National Toxicology Program (1993) *Toxicology and Carcinogenesis Studies of Mercuric Chloride (CAS No. 7487-14-7) in F344 Rats and B6C3F$_1$ Mice (Gavage Studies)* (NTP TR 408; NIH Publication No. 93-3139), Research Triangle Park, NC, US Department of Health and Human Services

US Occupational Safety and Health Administration (1989) Air contaminants—permissible exposure limits. *US Code fed. Regul.*, **Title 29**, p. 601

Vachhrajani, K.D., Chowdhury, A.R. & Dutta, K.K. (1992) Testicular toxicity of methylmercury: analysis of cellular distribution pattern at different stages of the seminiferous epithelium. *Reprod. Toxicol.*, **6**, 355-361

Verschaeve, L. & Léonard, A. (1984) Dominant lethal test in female mice treated with methyl mercury chloride. *Mutat. Res.*, **136**, 131-136

Verschaeve, L. & Susanne, C. (1979) Genetic hazards of mercury exposure in dental surgery (Abstract No. 81). *Mutat. Res.*, **64**, 149

Verschaeve, L., Kirsch-Volders, M., Susanne, C., Groetenbriel, C., Haustermans, R., Lecomte, A. & Roossels, D. (1976) Genetic damage induced by occupationally low mercury exposure. *Environ. Res.*, **12**, 306-316

Verschaeve, L., Kirsch-Volders, M., Hens, L. & Susanne, C. (1978) Chromosome distribution studies in phenylmercury acetate exposed subjects and in age-related controls. *Mutat. Res.*, **57**, 335-347

Verschaeve, L., Tassignon, J.-P., Lefevre, M., De Stoop, P. & Susanne, C. (1979) Cytogenetic investigation of leukocytes of workers exposed to metallic mercury. *Environ. Mutag.*, **1**, 259-268

Verschaeve, L., Kirsch-Volders, M. & Susanne, C. (1984) Mercury-induced segregational errors of chromosomes in human lymphocytes and in Indian muntjac cells. *Toxicol. Lett.*, **21**, 247-253

Verschaeve, L., Kirsch-Volders, M., Hens, L. & Susanne, C. (1985) Comparative in vitro cytogenetic studies in mercury-exposed human lymphocytes. *Mutat. Res.* **157**, 221-226

Verschuuren, H.G., Kroes, R., Den Tonkelaar, E.M., Berkvens, J.M., Helleman, P.W., Rauws, A.G., Schuller, P.L. & Van Esch, G.J. (1976a) Toxicity of methylmercury chloride in rats. I. Short-term study. *Toxicology*, **6**, 85-96

Verschuuren, H.G., Kroes, R., Den Tonkelaar, E.M., Berkvens, J.M., Helleman, P.W., Rauws, A.G., Schuller, P.L. & Van Esch, G.J. (1976b) Toxicity of methylmercury chloride in rats. III. Long-term toxicity study. *Toxicologist*, **6**, 107-123

Verschuuren, H.G., Kroes, R., Den Tonkelaar, E.M., Berkvens, J.M., Helleman, P.W., Rauws, A.G., Schuller, P.L. & Van Esch, G.J. (1976c) Toxicity of methylmercury chloride in rats. II. Reproduction study. *Toxicology*, **6**, 97-106

Vouk, V.B., Fugaš, M. & Topolnik, Z. (1950) Environmental conditions in the mercury mine of Idria. *Br. J. Med.*, **7**, 168-176

Wahlberg, J.E. (1965) Percutaneous toxicity of metal compounds. A comparative investigation in guinea pigs. *Arch. environ. Health*, **11**, 201-204

Warkany, J. (1966) Acrodynia—postmortem of a disease. *Am. J. Dis. Child.*, **112**, 147-156

Watanabe, T., Shimada, T. & Endo, A. (1982) Effects of mercury compounds on ovulation and meiotic and mitotic chromosomes in female golden hamsters. *Teratology*, **25**, 381-384

Weed, L.A. & Ecker, E.E. (1933) Phenyl-mercuric compounds. Their action on animals and their preservative values. *J. infect. Dis.*, **52**, 354-362

Weinberg, J.M., Harding, P.G. & Humes, H.D. (1982a) Mitochondrial bioenergetics during the initiation of mercuric chloride-induced renal injury. I. Direct effects of in-vitro mercuric chloride on renal cortical mitochondrial function. *J. biol. Chem.*, 257, 60–67

Weinberg, J.M., Harding, P.G. & Humes, H.D. (1982b) Mitochondrial bioenergetics during the initiation of mercuric chloride-induced renal injury. II. Functional alterations of renal cortical mitochondria isolated after mercuric chloride treatment. *J. biol. Chem.*, 257, 68–74

WHO (1976) *Mercury* (Environmental Health Criteria 1), Geneva

WHO (1980) *Exposure to Heavy Metals* (Tech. Rep. Series 647), Geneva, p. 128

WHO (1988) *Emission of Heavy Metal and PAH Compounds from Municipal Solid Waste Incinerators: Control Technology and Health Effects*, Copenhagen, pp. 23, 40

WHO (1989a) *Mercury—Environmental Aspects* (Environmental Health Criteria 86), Geneva

WHO (1989b) *Evaluation of Certain Food Additives and Contaminants* (Tech. Rep. Series 776), Geneva, pp. 33–34

WHO (1990) *Methylmercury* (Environmental Health Criteria 101), Geneva

WHO (1991) *Inorganic Mercury* (Environmental Health Criteria 118), Geneva

WHO (1992) *Guidelines for Drinking-water Quality. Tables of Guideline Values*, Geneva, p. 2

Wiklund, K., Dich, J., Holm, L.-E. & Eklund, G. (1988) Risk of tumors of the nervous system among mercury and other seed disinfectant applicators in Swedish agriculture (Letter to the Editor). *Acta oncol.*, 27, 865

Worthing, C.R., ed. (1987) *The Pesticide Manual. A World Compendium*, 8th Ed., Thornton Heath, British Crop Protection Council, pp. 658–659

Wulf, H.C., Kromann, N., Kousgaard, N., Hansen, J.C., Niebuhr, E. & Albøge, K. (1986) Sister chromatid exchange (SCE) in Greenlandic Eskimos. Dose–response relationship between SCE and seal diet, smoking, and blood cadmium and mercury concentrations. *Sci. total Environ.*, 48, 81–94

Yamamoto, M., Endoh, K., Toyama, S., Sakai, H., Shibuya, N., Takagi, S., Magara, J. & Fujiguchi, K. (1986) Biliary tract cancers in Japan: a study from the point of view of environmental epidemiology. *Acta med. biol.*, 34, 65–76

Yatscoff, R.W. & Cummins, J.E. (1975) DNA breakage caused by dimethylmercury and its repair in a slime mould, *Physarum polycephalum*. *Nature*, 257, 422–423

Yoshida, M. (1985) Relation of mercury exposure to elemental mercury levels in the urine and blood. *Scand. J. Work Environ. Health*, 11, 33–37

Yoshida, M., Satoh, H., Kishimoto, T. & Yamamura, Y. (1992) Exposure to mercury *via* breast milk in suckling offspring of maternal guinea pigs exposed to mercury vapor after parturition. *J. Toxicol. environ. Health*, 35, 135–139

Zasukhina, G.D., Vasilyeva, I.M., Sdirkova, N.I., Krasovsky, G.N., Vasyukovich, L.Y., Kenesariev, U.I. & Butenko, P.G. (1983) Mutagenic effect of thallium and mercury salts on rodent cells with different repair activities. *Mutat. Res.*, 124, 163–173

Zoll, C., Saouter, E., Boudou, A., Ribeyre, F. & Jaylet, A. (1988) Genotoxicity and bioaccumulation of methyl mercury and mercuric chloride *in vivo* in the newt *Pleurodeles waltl*. *Mutagenesis*, 3, 337–343

EXPOSURES IN THE GLASS MANUFACTURING INDUSTRY

1. Exposure Data

1.1 Historical overview

Morey (1938) defined glass as 'an inorganic substance in a condition which is continuous with, and analogous to, the liquid state of that substance but which, as the result of having been cooled from a fused condition, has attained so high a degree of viscosity as to be, for all practical purposes, rigid.' Similarly, the American Society for Testing Materials defines glass as 'an inorganic product of fusion that has cooled to a rigid condition without crystallizing' (de Jong, 1989).

While the precise origin of glass manufacture is unknown, glasses occur abundantly in nature and may have been a source of inspiration for development of the technology. Obsidian, pumice (a natural foam glass) and tektites (glassy bodies probably of meteoric origin) are examples of naturally occurring glass. The earliest tektites worked by humans date from the Magdalenian period about 25 000 years ago (de Jong, 1989). Knowledge of smelting glass was developed in the period 3500–2000 BC. Techniques for melting the raw materials in glass manufacture played an important role in the development of glass.

Glass melting technology passed through four stages: (i) glass manufacture in open pits ca. 3000 BC, until the invention of the blowpipe in about 250 BC; (ii) use of mobile wood-fired melting-pot furnaces, until about the seventeenth century, by travelling glass manufacturers; (iii) use of local pot furnaces, fired by wood and coal (1600–1850); and (iv) use of gas-heated melting-pot and tank furnaces from 1860, followed by the electric furnace of 1910 (de Jong, 1989).

A major breakthrough in glass production was the invention of the blowpipe by the Romans, which was used to its finest expression by the Venetian glass-blowers of Murano. With regard to art glass, the method of blowing glass seems to be much the same today as it probably was more than a millenium ago. The flexibility of this technique still makes it popular in fabricating complicated special items. The blowpipe is a hollow, stainless-steel pipe; a gob of glass is collected in the pipe by dipping it into the melt, and blowing air through the pipe swells the gob, provided the viscosity of the glass is still sufficiently low. The gob may then be placed in an iron or wooden mould and blown to the shape of the mould, or it may be worked into the desired shape without the aid of a mould.

1.2 Description of the industry (from de Jong, 1989, except where indicated)

1.2.1 *Introduction*

There are five main sectors in the glass manufacturing industry: flat glass, containers and pressed ware, art glass, special glass (e.g. optical, ophthalmic, electronic) and fibre glass.

Fibre glass was considered in a previous monograph (IARC, 1988) and is not included here (see General Remarks, p. 36, for evaluations). Figure 1 illustrates the basic principles of glass manufacture. The modern production of flat glass is the most highly automated and usually involves tank melting with continuous feeding of batch ingredients and the float (Pilkington) process (Grundy, 1990) for forming. The production of containers and similar products has also become increasingly mechanized. Modern production techniques involve tank melting with continuous feeding of batch ingredients and mechanical blowing or pressing of molten glass. The production of art and special glass can involve a variety of modern and traditional techniques, including manual loading of melting pots and mouth blowing. The production processes currently used to produce glass, other than fibre glass, are discussed below.

1.2.2 Raw materials

Glass has some of the physical properties of both liquids and solids: when cooled from the hot molten state, it gradually increases in viscosity without crystallization over a wide temperature range until it assumes its characteristic hard, brittle form; cooling is controlled to prevent high strain (Boyd & Thompson, 1980).

Any mixture with those physical properties is theoretically a glass. Glass has a very large number of chemical compositions, which fall into four main types:

(i) **Soda-lime–silica glasses**: These are the most important glasses in terms of quantity produced and variety of use, including almost all flat glass, containers, low-cost mass-produced domestic glassware and electric light bulbs.

(ii) **Lead–potash–silica glasses**: These contain a varying but often high proportion of lead oxide (see IARC, 1987a). For example, in the production of heavy crystal glass, the glass batch contains about 30% lead (Andersson et al., 1990), while in semi-crystal glass production the amount of lead is less than 10%. Fabrication of optical glass and hand-blown domestic and decorative glassware depends on the high refractive index and ease of cutting and polishing leaded glass. The high electrical resistivity and radiation protection of leaded glass are important in electrical and electronic applications.

(iii) **Borosilicate glasses**: Borosilicate glasses, with low thermal expansion, are resistant to thermal shock, making them useful for domestic oven and laboratory glassware (Cameron & Hill, 1983).

(iv) **Other glasses**: There are many other glass-forming systems, with a variety of compositions.

The raw materials for glass are mainly: silica (see IARC, 1987b), in the form of sand or crushed rock quartz; soda ash, or in some cases salt cake (sodium sulfate); potassium carbonate or nitrate; crushed limestone or dolomite; red lead or litharge; boric acid or borax; and cullet, which consists of broken or crushed glass (Cameron & Hill, 1983).

The major proportion of almost all glass batches is silica sand. Waste glass, or cullet, is an almost universal addition to the batch melted in glass furnaces. The advantages of this raw material are that it facilitates the melting of other components, requires up to 25% less heat to melt than an isochemical batch of raw materials and normally reduces dust during the batching. Batches with optimal melting efficiency may contain about 30–40 wt% cullet. Recycled bottles constitute about 15% of the cullet used in the container glass industry. This

Fig. 1. Processes and materials involved in the manufacture of glass

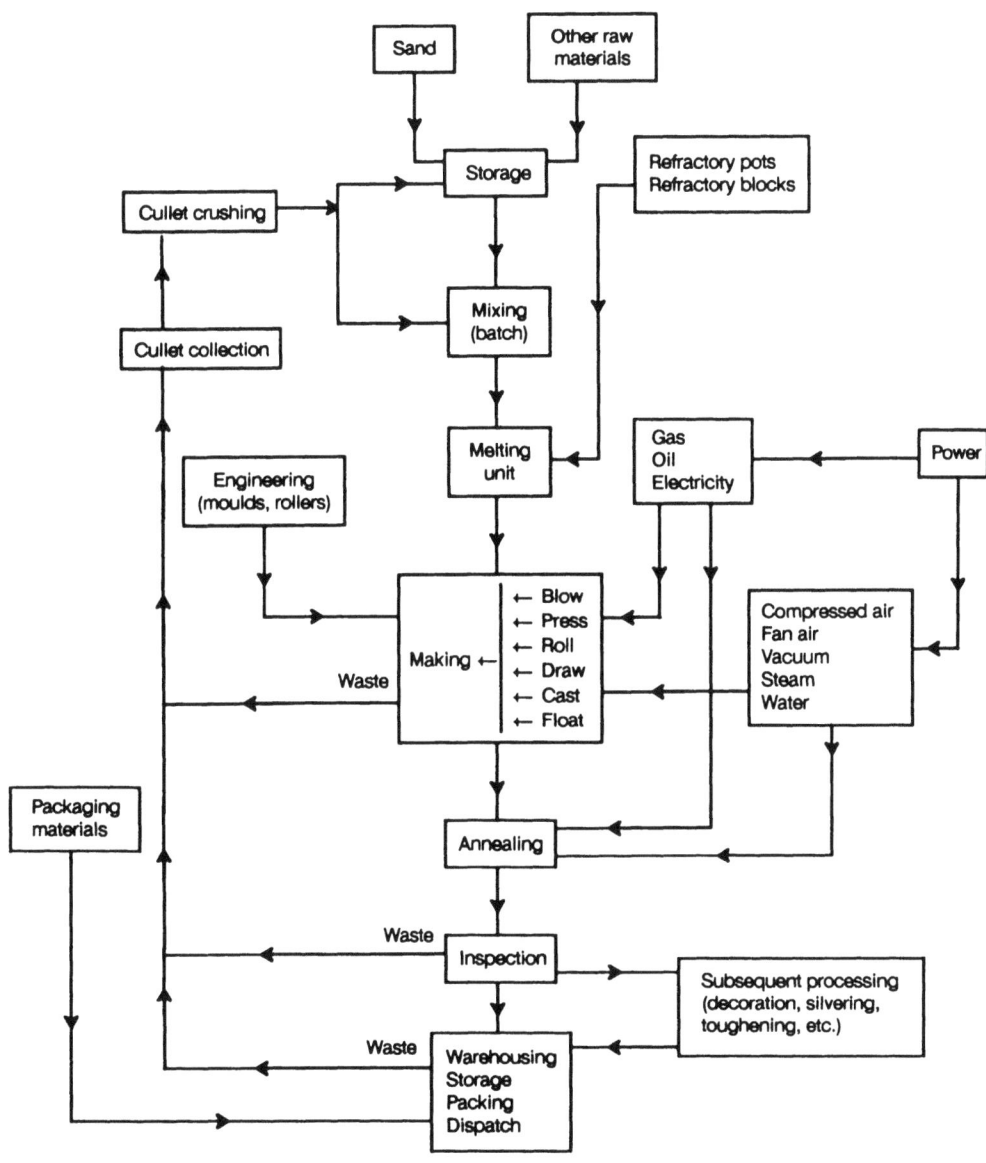

From Cameron & Hill (1983)

amount is expected to increase with the increasing introduction of recycling laws. Raw materials are selected according to purity, consistency, grain size, water content, supply, pollution potential, ease of mixing and melting and cost. The commonest ingredients in glass production are listed in Table 1; not all of the constituents are contained in every type of glass.

Table 1. Raw materials used in glass production

Raw material	Chemical composition	Glass-making oxide
Sand	SiO_2[a]	SiO_2
Soda ash	Na_2CO_3	Na_2O
Trona	$Na_2CO_3 \cdot NaHCO_3 \cdot 2H_2O$	Na_2O
Limestone	$CaCO_3$	CaO
Dolomite	$CaCO_3 \cdot MgCO_3$	CaO MgO
Feldspar	$(K,Na)_2O \cdot Al_2O_3 \cdot 6SiO_2$[a]	SiO_2 Al_2O_3 $(K,Na)_2O$
Nepheline Syenite	$NaAlSiO_4$[b]	SiO_2 Al_2O_3 $(K,Na)_2O$
Petalite	$LiAlSi_4O_{10}$	Li_2O Al_2O_3 SiO_2
Borax (5 mol)	$Na_2B_4O_7 \cdot 5H_2O$	Na_2O B_2O_3
Boric acid	H_3BO_3	B_2O_3
Colemanite	$Ca_2B_6O_{11} \cdot 5H_2O$	CaO B_2O_3
Ulexite	$NaCaB_5O_9 \cdot 8H_2O$	Na_2O CaO B_2O_3
Red lead[b]	Pb_3O_4	PbO
Litharge	PbO	PbO
Anhydrous potash	K_2CO_3	K_2O
Fluorspar	CaF_2	CaO
Zinc oxide	ZnO	ZnO
Barium carbonate	$BaCO_3$	BaO

From de Jong (1989)
[a]Refractory components
[b]Added by the Working Group

Contaminants and other chemicals are added in small amounts for special purposes. The primary contaminants of sand used in glass-making are ferric oxide (see IARC, 1987c), followed by titanium dioxide (see IARC, 1989a), zirconium dioxide and chromium oxides (see IARC, 1990a). The acceptable limits for ferric oxide in glass are 0.005–0.03 wt%, depending on the product. Oxides of transition metals, such as copper, cobalt (see IARC, 1991), nickel (see IARC, 1990b), vanadium and tungsten, are also often present and normally not desired.

Chemical or physical decoloration of such glasses is therefore important. Chemical decoloration is used to oxidize iron to its weakly coloured trivalent state by increasing the oxygen content of the melt, usually by adding oxygen-producing compounds such as potassium nitrate and sodium sulfate. Physical decoloration is often used when the melt contains a higher concentration of iron. In this case, the addition of other colouring agents compensates for the yellow-green colour of the glass. Common compensating agents are selenium (see IARC, 1975) and oxides of manganese, cobalt and nickel.

Conversely, when coloration of glass is desired, oxides of transition elements are the main colouring agents used. Common transition-metal oxides used in the glass industry include cobalt, nickel, chromium, iron, manganese, copper, vanadium and cadmium. Concentrations are typically 0.5–5 wt%. Oxidation conditions affect the colour achieved.

Other chemicals may be added for different purposes: e.g. fluorides to reduce viscosity and aid melting, zirconium dioxide to raise the softening-point and cerium oxide to stabilize glass against ultraviolet discoloration.

1.2.3 *Mixing and melting*

The three steps involved in the production of glass are melting, fining and homogenization. The cold batch is placed in the tank and melted at 1200–1650 °C. Decarbonation, desulfurization and dehydration are the first chemical processes used, followed by partial melting. Silicate formation occurs at about 500–800 °C.

Fining is the process of removing bubbles from the glass melt. This is accomplished in two ways:

(i) by the addition of chemical fining agents. Sodium sulfate or arsenic (see IARC, 1987d) and antimony trioxides (see IARC, 1989b) are generally used. Typically, about 0.3 wt% arsenic oxides or arsenates are added to the batch, although for some glass types up to 1.5 wt% arsenic trioxide may be used; and

(ii) by varying the melt temperature, either by raising the tank temperature, with an attendant decrease of melt viscosity and increase in bubble expulsion, or by lowering the temperature and increasing gas resorption.

Homogenization of the batch is generally assured by mechanical stirring.

Accuracy and precision in weighing the various batch constituents are important, as are thorough mixing of the ingredients and prevention of subsequent segregation. Batch handling systems vary widely throughout the industry, from manual to fully automatic. Wet mixing and batch agglomeration–pelletizing, briquetting and compaction are becoming popular, especially for the addition of lead and arsenic compounds.

1.2.4 *Pot processing*

The older pot process now serves mainly for the manufacture of high-quality glass, such as optical glass, and for small quantities of special glass, such as hand-blown crystal. The pots vary in size, up to those capable of holding nearly 2 tonnes of ingredients. The pots are made from a number of different types of clay combined with flint or silica flour. Pot melting of glass often involves the hazards inherent in hand shovelling and filling. The pots are tempered slowly at 900 °C by electrical heating, fired at 1200 °C and vitrified at 1400 °C in the pot furnace. Open pots containing 150–1000 kg of melt have been used, especially in Europe, to manufacture coloured and optical glasses as well as crystal glass. Closed pots surrounded by refractory brick walls are the system of choice in the USA. The largest pot furnaces could contain 8–10 pots, each with a diameter of 1 m. Special, valuable products (e.g. specially coloured glass) may be produced in tanks built from refractory brick and heated directly, producing 1–5 tonnes of glass daily. This process is particularly well suited for the manufacture of soft (i.e. low viscosity) glass, such as crystal or soda lime glass, which require special production techniques. Modern techniques for special glasses may involve the use of induction heating with the melt contained in platinum crucibles; this technique also involves manual handling of batch materials.

1.2.5 Tank processing

Large volumes of glass are produced exclusively in tanks capable of holding up to 2000 tonnes of melt. Producers of flat glass have always used the largest tanks, formerly for the vertical drawn sheet process and now for the rolled plate and float processes. The tank is divided into two sections, either by a permanent bridge wall or by floating refractory baffles. The larger section into which the fill (i.e. the batch with cullet) is introduced is called the melting end. Most of the tanks provide for enclosed continuous feeding of batch ingredients. The other section, in which the melt starts to cool towards its working viscosity, is called the working or refining end. Partitioning of the tank allows continuous production of glass. The fuel usually used is oil or natural gas.

1.2.6 Forming/making

Glass objects are formed from molten glass by blowing, pressing, drawing and casting. 'Hand-blowing' is the classic method of glass fabrication and is used in modern glass plants only for the manufacture of art objects, large objects in low demand that cannot be fabricated by machine, and complicated technical shapes. Partial automation is being introduced into hand-forming operations, where the glassblower blows gobs of the proper viscosity into moulds.

Deep items (e.g. bottles) are formed mechanically by blowing glass into moulds with compressed air. Hinged moulds, which can be opened to remove the ware, are generally used for the blowing operation. These moulds are lined with a water-absorbent coating, which develops a steam cushion between the coating and glass during blowing. A second type of mould is the hinged hot-iron mould, in which the glass comes directly into contact with the mould surface on blowing. Narrow-mouth containers are manufactured in a two-stage process.

Although blowing is used in the manufacture of deep items, pressing is used for relatively flat items, such as dinnerware, optical and sealed-beam lenses, filter glass and television tube panels. Press moulds are commonly made of cast iron, bronze steel or superalloys with galvanized surfaces. Moulds (including hand moulds) are sometimes lubricated with mineral oils (see IARC, 1987f), graphited oils or, occasionally, other organic materials, such as tallow and oleic acid. Hand pressing is now being replaced by machine pressing.

The traditional process for producing sheet glass is to draw it from the furnace by a vertical process which gives it a fire-finished surface. Owing to the combined effects of drawing and gravity, some minor distortion is inevitable. The plate glass passes through water-cooled rollers into an annealing oven. Surface damage must be removed by grinding and polishing. Patterned glasses are still made by this method.

The vertical drawn process has largely been replaced by the float process for flat glass. The Pilkington float process has made possible the manufacture of a glass that combines the advantages of both sheet and plate. Float glass has a fire-finished surface and is free from distortion. Molten glass floats from the huge melting tank (up to 2000 tonnes of glass) along the surface of a bath of molten tin, in which an inert atmosphere of nitrogen prevents oxidation. The glass conforms to the perfect surface of the molten tin. As the glass passes over the tin, the temperature is reduced until the glass is sufficiently hard to be fed on to the rollers of the annealing oven without marking its under-surface. Sulfur dioxide may be applied at this point to reduce further the risk of marking. After annealing, the glass requires no further treatment and is ready for automatic cutting and packing. The advantage of the float process, apart from the mirror quality of the glass surface, is its high production capacity.

1.2.7 *Annealing and other processing*

Annealing of a glass product is nearly always necessary after any forming operation. The glass is heated uniformly to a temperature sufficiently high to relieve any internal stress, without causing deformation of the object under its own weight. The ware is subsequently cooled slowly to prevent formation of new stresses. Glassware is normally annealed in long, continuous ovens called lehrs, which are usually heated electrically.

After production in different processes, glass may undergo secondary processes, including cutting, grinding, polishing, heat processing, chemical treatment and surface coating. Workers may be exposed to chemical agents during grinding, polishing, chemical treatment and surface coating.

The purpose of grinding is to remove the upper layer of the glass surface. An abrasive produces a small check or crack in the glass, the dimensions of which depend on the grain size of the abrasive: increasingly finer abrasives produce a relatively smooth surface. Natural abrasive grits (e.g. quartz, sandstone, corundum, garnet and diamond) are used as well as synthetic grits (e.g. silicon carbide, aluminium oxide and boric oxide). Water or a suitable cutting fluid is used in grinding.

Polishing is done either mechanically or chemically. Mechanical polishing requires finely powdered abrasives such as rouge (ferric oxide) and cerium oxide. These abrasives operate on the same principle as those in grinding. Chemical polishing includes acid polishing and flame polishing. In acid polishing, the glass may be submerged in a mixture of hydrofluoric and concentrated sulfuric acids or in other acids; hydrofluoric acid is also used for etching glass.

Vitreous enamels are applied by spraying, silk screening and the application of decals. They may be fused to the ware at high temperature. Metallic coatings are produced either by applying a liquid suspension of metal to the surface and then firing it or by evaporation of metal on the glass. These coatings are used on flat glass as a means of controlling transmission and reflection of light, as electrical semiconductors in tin oxide films, as resistors in electronic circuits, as defrosting agents and in aircraft glazing. Lacquers are applied to glass for decorative purposes.

1.3 Exposures in the workplace

1.3.1 *Introduction*

A number of potential occupational health hazards are present in the glass industry, including silica dust and certain metallic compounds. Exposure to silica has been evaluated previously (see IARC, 1987b).

The production of glass involves the use of many metals, usually as oxides; nearly every element in the periodic table has been used in modern glass technology (see section 1.2). In particular, exposure to lead has been noted in the past: In the production of heavy crystal glass (about 30% lead) and semi-crystal glass (< 10% lead), lead is an important source of occupational exposure. Other elements to which workers are exposed include antimony, arsenic, cadmium (see monograph, p. 119), manganese, selenium, nickel and chromium (Andersson *et al.*, 1990); they may be exposed to either dusts or fumes. Glass-blowing offers special opportunities for exposure to the metallic compounds in glass and alloy materials, which may migrate up the pipe into the worker's mouth. In Sweden, samples from blowpipes contained lead, manganese, nickel (Andersson *et al.*, 1990; Wingren & Englander, 1990) and arsenic (Andersson *et al.*, 1990).

For chemical polishing and matting of glass surfaces, sulfuric (see IARC, 1992) and hydrofluoric acids are used. Some processes also involve potential exposure to polycyclic aromatic hydrocarbons (see IARC, 1983) and asbestos (see IARC, 1987e). The working environment around a glass furnace is hot, and most of the heat is in the form of radiant energy. Significant heat problems also arise during maintenance and emergency repair work: temperatures in areas where men do routine maintenance is frequently in the range of 120–160 °C; under emergency repair conditions it may reach 200 °C (Cameron & Hill, 1983). In the past, asbestos was used as a thermoinsulator in hot structures, as well as in protective clothing. The workers who were exposed to the largest quantities of asbestos were probably construction and maintenance workers rather than those engaged in the actual production of glass (Lucas, 1981; Sankila *et al.*, 1990; Kronenberg *et al.*, 1991).

Very few surveys involving ambient and biological monitoring of workers exposed to chemicals have been reported from the glass industry, and almost all the quantitative data available to the Working Group were for exposure to lead and other metals. In particular, no quantitative data on past exposures were available for the mortality and cancer morbidity cohort studies carried out in Italy and Finland (Cordioli *et al.*, 1987; Sankila *et al.*, 1990).

1.3.2 *Exposure to lead*

Air measurements in glass manufacturing industries showed concentrations of < 0.001–0.11 mg/m^3 lead, with the highest levels in a heavy crystal glassworks (Andersson *et al.*, 1990; Wingren & Englander, 1990).

Because blood lead levels give better information about total lead exposure than lead concentrations in ambient air, biological monitoring was chosen for the evaluation of individual exposures in the studies described below.

Between 1970 and 1973, 49 workers in three Finnish crystal glass plants were investigated for blood lead: The median concentration was [410 µg/L] (range, 120–820 µg/L). At that time, the recommended limit for blood lead in Finland was 700 µg/L (Tola et al., 1976).

Exposure to lead and other substances was evaluated among workers grinding, polishing and glueing leaded crystal glass art objects. Five of six measurements in the breathing zone in the grinding department exceeded the US National Institute for Occupational Safety and Health (NIOSH) criterion of 50 µg/m^3. The average of all six samples was 60 µg/m^3 (range, 30–80 µg/m^3); however, no blood sample contained more than 400 µg/L. The mean blood lead concentration in the grinding department was 291 µg/L (range, 220–360 µg/L) (Gunter & Thoburn, 1985).

Lüdersdorf et al. (1987) examined blood lead concentrations in a group of 109 male workers at two glass-producing factories in Germany. The group was divided into four subgroups, according to their specific activities: melter, batch mixer, craftsman and glass washer. The medians and ranges for blood lead concentrations are given in Table 2, which shows that the highest values occurred in blood specimens from batch mixers.

Table 2. Concentrations of lead in blood in workers in two German glass factories: comparison of subgroups

Specific activity	No.	Blood lead (µg/L)	
		Median	Range
Melter	32	220	130–600
Batch mixer	45	340	200–680
Craftsman	8	275	190–410
Glass washer	24	170	70–430
Total	109	250	70–680

From Lüdersdorf et al. (1987)

Schaller et al. (1988) studied blood lead levels, determined by flame atomic absorption spectrometry, in the German crystal glass industry for the period 1978–86. A total of 6080 determinations were performed for 1625 men and 269 women. The median concentrations (and 68% ranges) varied from 470 µg/L (275–665 µg/L) for men to 255 µg/L (115–415 µg/L) for women ≤ 45 years of age and 270 µg/L (135–455 µg/L) for women > 45 years of age. Table 3 presents the blood lead concentrations in relation to period of examination; it shows a general decrease in internal exposure with time. For men, 764 (14%) of the determinations exceeded the German 'biological tolerance value' of 700 µg/L blood. [The Working Group noted that the large decrease between 1978 and 1979 may have been related, in part, to the phasing out of lead in gasoline in Germany and the resultant decrease in environmental exposures.]

Table 3. Blood lead concentrations (µg/L) in the German glass industry for the period 1978–86

Year	Median	68% range	99% range
1978	545	325/775	165/1300
1979	485	265/725	85/1085
1980	420	235/635	90/1020
1981	440	245/685	75/1065
1982	445	245/635	105/1045
1983	430	215/675	70/1100
1984	435	255/635	50/ 955
1985	440	245/635	65/1010
1986	445	205/605	25/ 880

From Schaller *et al.* (1988)

In a British lead crystal manufacturing plant, 87 people were monitored for concentrations of lead in blood and tibia *in vivo*, the latter reflecting cumulative exposure. The duration of exposure to lead was 10.0 ± 1.1 years. The mean concentration of lead was 481 ± 18 µg/L in blood (non-occupationally exposed, 131 ± 16 µg/L) and 17.5 ± 1.9 µg/g wet weight in tibia (non-occupationally exposed, 9.4 ± 2.1 µg/g wet weight) (Somervaille *et al.*, 1988).

Andersson *et al.* (1990) collected 36 personal air samples in three Swedish glassworks, one producing heavy crystal glass and two producing semi-crystal glass. The results are presented in Table 4. The glassworks producing heavy crystal had a higher air concentration of lead, especially in the foundry area, than those producing semi-crystal. Of the 28 samples from the semi-crystal glassworks, only four contained concentrations above the present Swedish threshold limit value of 50 µg/m^3, whereas in the heavy crystal glassworks 7/12 samples exceeded that limit. Lead was also detected in slag from inside the blowpipes at concentrations (geometric mean) of 6.93 µg/mg slag in the heavy crystal glassworks and 0.72 µg/mg slag in the semi-crystal glass industry (see Table 7, p. 359).

Although stained-glass workers are not involved in the manufacture of glass, they may be exposed to lead during soldering. Landrigan *et al.* (1980) measured blood lead concentrations in 12 professional stained-glass workers, in five hobbyists and in four family members of workers in the USA. The concentrations in professional workers (mean, 207 µg/L) were higher than those of hobbyists (116 µg/L) and family members (113 µg/L). The mean lead concentration in settled dust samples from a stained-glass workshop was 11 000 ppm (mg/kg).

Baxter *et al.* (1985) surveyed 47 workers in the four largest stained-glass workshops in the United Kingdom. The mean blood lead concentration was 300 µg/L (range, 100–700 µg/L); nine workers had concentrations of 400 µg/L or more. The mean concentration of lead in personal air samples of five glaziers inside the workshop was 30 µg/m^3 (range, 10–50 µg/m^3), and samples of general air all contained 10 µg/m^3. All results were well below the current standard for lead in air in the United Kingdom of 150 µg/m^3.

Table 4. Concentrations of lead (μg/m³) in the air of three Swedish glass factories, presented as geometric means (GM) with 95% confidence intervals (95% CI)

Work area	Semi-crystal glassworks			Heavy crystal glassworks		
	GM	95% CI	No. of samples	GM	95% CI	No. of samples
Foundry	6	3–11	16	61	48–79	7
Oven inlay	72	-	4	71	-	2
Other	8	2–22	8	10	-	3

From Andersson et al. (1990)

1.3.3 Exposure to other metals

Exposures in the production of hypodermic syringes from glass containing small amounts of antimony and cerium oxide were studied. Environmental concentrations of antimony, stibine (antimony hydride) and cerium were approximately 1% of the NIOSH recommended maximal concentration at the time of the study: 500 μg/m³, 0.1 ppm and 5000 μg/m³ (Burroughs & Horan, 1981).

Lüdersdorf et al. (1987) studied external and internal exposure to antimony of 109 male workers in two German glass-producing factories. Airborne, blood and urinary concentrations of antimony are presented in Table 5. The airborne concentrations in the batch area exceeded the German 'technical exposure limit' value of 300 μg/m³ (Deutsche Forschungsgemeinschaft, 1992), and the highest concentrations of antimony in blood and urine were found in workers in the batch area.

Chrostek et al. (1980) investigated 35 crystal glassworkers working in the mix and melt area and batch house who were exposed to various compounds, including arsenic trioxide, selenium and silica flour. Personal air monitoring of eight workers revealed arsenic concentrations of 2–11 μg/m³, all of which were in excess of the NIOSH recommended standard of 2 μg/m³, although only one exceeded the US Occupational Safety and Health Administration standard of 10 μg/m³. All eight personal samples indicated exposure to selenium (0.04–7.92 μg/m³) below the US Occupational Safety and Health Administration standard of 200 μg/m3 [no NIOSH standard given]. The personal samples for respirable dust indicated exposures of 0.14–0.99 mg/m³. The quartz content of bulk dust samples was 10%. The results of clinical examinations and interviews revealed no arsenic-related health complaint or symptom and no arsenic-related skin disorder. All blood samples contained concentrations of arsenic below the detection limit of 10 μg/kg; however, blood was considered to be a less reliable specimen than urine for assessing exposure to arsenic.

Roels et al. (1982) measured total airborne arsenic in a Belgian glassware factory where arsenic trioxide was used to produce uncoloured glass, determined urinary inorganic arsenic and its metabolites and evaluated hand and mouth contamination by arsenic before and after the workshift in 10 workers. The results suggested that the high urinary arsenic

Table 5. Time-weighted average airborne concentrations of antimony in total dust and antimony concentrations in blood and in urine in two German glass factories

Field of activity	Air sampling technique	No. of samples	Antimony trioxide ($\mu g/m^3$)	Antimony concentration ($\mu g/L$)[a]			
				Blood		Urine	
				Median	Range	Median	Range
Melting area							
Melter	Personal	32	< 50	0.8	0.4–1.8	0.9	0.2–2.9
Batch mixer	Stationary	45	< 5–5	1.1	0.5–2.4	5.0	1.5–15.7
Batch bunker							
Craftsman	Personal	8	< 50–840	0.7	0.5–1.0	0.9	0.4–3.7
Glass washer	Stationary	24	40–290	1.1	0.4–3.1	1.2	0.6–6.3
Total		109		1.0	0.4–3.1	1.9	0.2–15.7

From Lüdersdorf et al. (1987); detection limits: personal air monitoring, 50 $\mu g/m^3$; stationary sampling, 5 $\mu g/m^3$
[a]Antimony levels in non-occupationally exposed population: 0.3–1.7 $\mu g/L$ blood, 0.2–0.7 $\mu g/L$ urine

concentrations found (mean, around 300 μg/g creatinine; range, 10–941 μg/g) were probably more closely related to oral intake from contaminated hands than to absorption from the lungs. Urinary arsenic excretion in control workers ranged from 7.6 to 59 μg/L.

In two German cross-sectional studies (in 1976 and 1981) to evaluate internal exposure of employees in the heavy crystal industry, urinary arsenic concentrations of 3–114 μg/g creatinine were found. In 33% (1976) and 16% (1981) of the cases, urinary arsenic elimination exceeded the upper limit of normal (25 μg/g creatinine) (Schaller et al., 1982).

In a study in the United Kingdom, two cases of subacute arsenic poisoning were reported among decorative glass workers. Although air levels in most cases were below the recommended limit of 0.2 mg/m^3 (Table 6), excessive uptake seemed to have occurred in some workers (Ide & Bullough, 1988).

Farmer and Johnson (1990) reported exposure to airborne arsenic trioxide, used as a decolourizing agent, in a specialist glass manufacturing industry during the weighing of constituents for glass batches and during mixing of chemicals. Inorganic arsenic (As[V], As[III]) and its metabolites (mono- and dimethylarsonic acid) were determined in 18 first-void urine samples by direct hydride generation–atomic absorption spectrometry. The mean urinary arsenic concentration was 79.4 μg/g creatinine, in comparison with 4.4 μg/g creatinine for controls.

In Swedish heavy crystal and semi-crystal glass industries, Andersson et al. (1990) detected only a very small amount (< 6 μg/m^3) of arsenic; nickel and manganese were not detected (< 1 μg/m^3). Arsenic, nickel and manganese were detected in microgram per milligram concentrations in slag from inside blowpipes (Table 7).

Table 6. Results of personal and background sampling of arsenic in air of decorative glassworks in the United Kingdom (mg/m^3)

Site	Personal		Environment	
	Sample	8-h TWA	Sample	8-h TWA
Factory A				
Mixer 80 min	0.67	0.11	0.69	0.11
Charger 15 min	0.11	0.02	0.71	0.12
20 min	0.03	0.005		
Factory B				
Mixer 76 min	2.40	0.38	0.12	0.02
			0.26	0.04
			4.55	0.72

From Ide & Bullough (1988). TWA, time-weighted average; recommended exposure limit for arsenic: 0.2 mg/m^3

Table 7. Content of some metals (µg/mg slag) in blowpipes, presented as geometric means (GM) with 95% confidence intervals (95% CI)

Metal	Semi-crystal glassworks			Heavy crystal glassworks		
	No. of samples	GM	95% CI	No. of samples	GM	95% CI
Arsenic	79	0.26	0.22–0.31	39	0.27	0.23–0.32
Manganese	79	3.61	3.15–4.13	39	5.44	4.02–7.38
Nickel	75	0.57	0.44–0.73	39	4.99	3.42–7.28

From Andersson et al. (1990)

Raithel et al. (1991) found very high external and internal exposure to nickel in German shops in which nickel-armoured hollow-glass moulds were produced or repaired. Hollow-glass moulds used in automatic machines are plated with nickel and nickel alloys (70–98%) by flame spraying with nickel-containing powder (75–99%); the moulds also undergo abrasive buffing and polishing with grinding disks, lathes and emery paper. The airborne nickel levels in three factories in 1981 and 1984 are summarized in Table 8. The German technical exposure limit of 500 µg/m^3 for nickel and its compounds was exceeded at three of 24 measuring stations (range, 3.4–623 µg/m^3). Between 1981 and 1984, dust control and working conditions were improved. Urinary nickel excretion of workers in 24 German hollow-glass factories ranged from 0.2 to 60.2 µg/g creatinine (mean, 4.5) in pre-shift samples and were 0.5–211 µg/g creatinine (median, 6.9) in post-shift samples. The highest urinary nickel concentrations were detected in flame sprayers (median, 25.3 µg/L). Lower internal exposure was found for craftsmen, i.e. polishers and chasers (median, 7.4 µg/L).

Table 8. Measurements of nickel fine dust in three German hollow-glass mould repair shops in 1981 and 1984

1981		1984	
Description	Nickel fine dust ($\mu g/m^3$)	Description	Nickel fine dust ($\mu g/m^3$)
Mechanical work (chase) with ventilation	190	Mechanical work (grinding) with ventilation	18
	141	Grinding, polishing and thermal spraying with ventilation	410
Electrowelding with ventilation	20	Emery frame with ventilation	180
Flame spraying with ventilation	114	Flame spraying with ventilation	569
Flame spraying with ventilation	444		75
	413	Flame spraying without ventilation	85
	302	Electrowelding with ventilation	50
	243	Mechanical work with ventilation	6.8
Mechanical work with ventilation	145	Flame spraying with ventilation	10.2
	550		3.4
Mechanical work without ventilation	623		
Flame spraying with ventilation	500		
	260		
Mechanical work and flame spraying with ventilation	300		

From Raithel et al. (1991)

1.3.4 Other exposures

Exposure may occur to polycyclic aromatic hydrocarbons in fumes generated by oil-fired furnaces and in mineral oils used for lubricating moulds. Workers were exposed by inhalation to oil aerosols during casting, where contact of oil with hot moulds at ca. 300–700 °C produces mists and fumes, in two Italian plants. In a plant producing bottles and jars for foods, moulds were lubricated manually with graphited oil; in a crystal glass plant, the moulds were lubricated automatically every few seconds with graphited oil. Typical concentrations of polycyclic aromatic hydrocarbons in the oils were 0.1–5 ppm. A number of airborne compounds (benzo[a]anthracene and chrysene) were detected in close proximity to their source during aerosol emission (i.e. during mould lubrication) at concentrations in the order of 1 $\mu g/m^3$ in both plants. Such levels decreased to about 0.1 $\mu g/m^3$ in personal air samples. Exposures to oil mist were in the range 0.7–2.4 mg/m^3 (time-weighted average), thus complying with the generally accepted limit of 5 mg/m^3 (Menichini et al., 1990).

Gunter and Thoburn (1985) measured exposures to airborne petroleum distillate in a US crystal facility, where leaded crystal was cut, grinded, polished and glued together into various art objects. The environmental concentrations were well below the NIOSH evaluation criteria, as were the concentrations of 1,1,1-trichloroethane and toluene in the breathing zone.

Interleaving materials, such as Lucor® (50:50 mixture of Lucite® beads, a polymer of the acrylic monomer methyl methacrylate, and adipic acid) and wood flour or a combination of the two, are used in the flat glass industry to prevent window panes from adhering to each other during packing and unpacking. In a study of a flat glass industry in the USA, exposures to adipic acid were below the detection limit (2 µg per sample). Results of sampling for particulates (< 2 mg/m^3) showed that all samples were below the threshold limit values of the American Conference of Governmental Industrial Hygienists and the permissible exposure limits of the US Occupational Safety and Health Administration for both total (10–15 mg/m^3) and respirable (5 mg/m^3) nuisance dusts (Almaguer, 1985).

2. Studies of Cancer in Humans

2.1 Descriptive studies

In a Nordic, census-based record-linkage study (Lynge *et al.*, 1986) on the relationship between possible exposure to silica dust and lung cancer in male occupational groups, the authors found an excess among Danish glass-makers (occupational code 356), based on three cases *versus* 1.85 expected (standardized incidence ratio [SIR], 1.62; 95% confidence interval [CI], 0.33–4.74). No such excess was found in the other Nordic countries.

In a Swedish record-linkage study between the National Cancer–Environment Registry and national cancer registries for 1961–79, McLaughlin *et al.* (1987a) studied the risk for intracranial gliomas in various occupations. A significant excess SIR of 1.60 was found [95% CI, 1.03–2.36] among 'potters, kilnmen, and glass workers' (code 81), based on two-digit selection of the work titles and on 25 cases. After selection on the basis of three-digit occupational titles, the number of remaining cases in glass-makers (code 811) was reduced to six with an SIR of 1.7 (not significant). In a second, similar study, McLaughlin *et al.* (1987b) found an SIR of 5.20 [95% CI, 1.90–11.4] for meningiomas among 'glass makers' (code 811), based on six cases. [The Working Group noted that an excess of brain cancer was found in other occupational categories in the area in which glass-works were located (Wingren & Axelson, 1992).]

In a similar record-linkage study on nasopharyngeal cancer in Sweden, Malker *et al.* (1990) found a significant excess risk among glass-makers (code 811) (3 cases; SIR, 6.2 [95% CI, 1.3–18.3]).

In an ecological study (Dolin, 1992) of bladder cancer in England and Wales, the numbers of deaths from that cancer in 1969–73 and 1974–80 were obtained for 400 districts, and the percentages of workers in 220 different occupations were collected from the 1971 census tracts for the same districts. In the 'high-risk' areas identified, there were significantly higher percentages of workers in 23 occupations as compared with the average for England and Wales. Among these occupations were male glass process workers [not further specified] (relative risk [RR], 4.79; 95% CI, 2.79–7.67) and glass formers and finishers (RR, 5.47; 95% CI, 3.79–7.64).

2.2 Cohort studies (see Table 9, p. 364)

Cordioli *et al.* (1987) performed a cohort mortality study in Italy of 468 workers who had been employed for at least one year between 1953 and 1967 at a plant producing 'low-quality' glass containers. Prior to mechanization of the plant in 1967, melting pots were loaded manually, the initial blow was by mouth, and there was no division between work areas. Although the exact nature of the exposures was not known, exposures to mineral-oil fumes, arsenic and dyes containing chromium, nickel, iron, manganese, cobalt, titanium and cadmium were suspected. The cohort was followed through the end of 1985, and 28 deaths due to cancer were observed (RR, 1.27 [95% CI, 0.84–1.84]), including 13 from lung cancer (RR, 2.09 [95% CI, 1.1–3.6]) and four from cancer of the larynx (RR, 4.49 [95% CI, 1.2–11.4]). Although based upon small numbers, the risk for laryngeal cancer appeared to increase with duration of employment, while the risk for lung cancer did not. All laryngeal cancers and 12 of the lung cancers occurred at least 10 years after first employment (RR, 5.72 [95% CI, 1.54–14.6]; and RR, 2.32 [95% CI, 1.20–4.06], respectively). [The Working Group noted that information on smoking was not given.]

Neuberger and Kundi (1990) recruited two cohorts of 1626 men who had been exposed or unexposed to high concentrations of silica dust of any type in 1089 Viennese (Austria) plants and examined during 1950–60; they were followed up through 1985. By the end of follow-up, 87 and 84% had died; 179 lung cancer deaths had occurred in the exposed cohort (RR compared to local rates, 1.69 [95% CI, 1.45–1.96]) and 141 in the unexposed cohort (RR, 1.18 [0.99–1.39]). In the exposed cohort, 28 lung cancer deaths (RR, 2.37 [1.58–3.43]) occurred among subjects with the occupational title 'ceramics and glass' [not further specified]. The authors noted that the cross-sectional recruitment of the study participants is heavily influenced by selection. [The Working Group noted the high risk for lung cancer in the control group and that no data were available on smoking.]

Wingren and Englander (1990) investigated a Swedish cohort of 625 male art glass-workers employed for more than one month between 1964 and 1985. There was a slight excess of all cancers, and mortality from lung cancer was in excess: six deaths *versus* 4.2 (RR, 1.44 [95% CI, 0.52–3.11]) and 2.5 (RR, 2.36 [0.88–5.22]) expected, based on national and county referents, respectively. There was also a small excess mortality from colon cancer: four cases *versus* 1.6 (RR, 2.45 [0.67–6.40]; national rates), and there were two pharyngeal cancers *versus* 0.2 expected (RR, 9.87 [1.2–36.10]; national rates). Similar excesses were seen in comparison with county rates. The excesses of lung cancer occurred mainly in men working in the foundry producing heavy crystal glass (RR, 3.9 [0.8–11.4]) and in refinement workers (grinders, etchers, polishers and controllers) (RR, 2.8 [0.6–8.2]) exposed for more than 15 years. Cancer of the prostate also occurred in slight excess: four cases *versus* 3.0 based on national rates (RR, 1.34 [0.36–3.41]); two were in glass-blowers and workers manufacturing heavy crystal glass and two in refinement workers. The authors had information confirming that smoking was less prevalent in the study group than in the reference population. The smoking-adjusted RR for lung cancer, based on a survey of smoking among 10% of the glass-workers, was 3.5 [1.3–7.7] (based on national rates), assuming a latency of 10 years.

In a Finnish study, the incidence of cancer was studied in a cohort of 1803 men and 1946 women with at least three months of continuous employment in two plain glass manufacturing factories [processes unspecified] and followed from 1953 through 1986 (Sankila *et al.*, 1990). An excess of skin cancer (melanomas and basal-cell carcinomas excluded) was found among male oral glass-blowers (two cases; 0.25 expected; SIR, 8.00; 95% CI, 0.97–28.9), and an excess of lung cancer was found among men in the two plants combined

(62 cases; 47.7 expected; SIR, 1.30; 95% CI, 1.00–1.67). The risk for lung cancer was also increased among glass-blowers using automated methods (SIR, 1.60) but not among oral glass-blowers (SIR, 0.29). The risk for stomach cancer was increased in oral glass-blowers (3 cases; RR, 2.16; 0.44–6.26). [The Working Group noted that no information was given on smoking.]

2.3 Case–control studies (see Table 10, p. 367)

2.3.1 *Cancer of the urinary bladder*

In a Canadian population-based study of 480 male and 152 female incident cases in 1974–76 (Howe *et al.*, 1980), an odds ratio of 6.0 (95% CI, 0.7–276) was found for male 'glass processors'.

A group of 303 incident cases of carcinoma (or papilloma not specified as benign) of the lower urinary tract in white males and 296 white male referent subjects were studied in Detroit (USA) in 1977–78. Patients and controls were interviewed to obtain lifetime work histories: Six case subjects and one referent subject (odds ratio, 5.9; 95% CI, 0.7–49.8) had ever been employed in glass or glass products manufacture (Silverman *et al.*, 1983).

In a hospital-based case–control study on work-related cancer of the urinary bladder in France in 1984–87 (Cordier *et al.*, 1993), 15 of 658 cases among men occurred in 'glass formers and potters' *versus* seven among the referents (odds ratio adjusted for smoking, 1.82; 95% CI, 0.73–4.53). [The Working Group noted that specific information on exposure was not given.]

2.3.2 *Cancers of the respiratory organs*

Milne *et al.* (1983) carried out a case–control study of 925 lung cancer deaths in Alameda County, California, USA, in 1958–62, comparing their occupations with those of 6420 deaths from other cancers in the same County, as identified from death certificates. They found a significant ($p < 0.05$) positive association with employment in glass, clay and stone manufacture (11 cases; odds ratio, 1.9). [The Working Group noted the limitations of using information on occupation derived solely from death certificates.]

Buiatti *et al.* (1985) reported a study comprising 376 incident, histologically confirmed cases of lung cancer in Florence, Italy, admitted to a regional hospital between 1981 and 1983. A total of 892 referent subjects were recruited from among patients who were admitted to the same hospital and who did not have lung cancer. Detailed work histories were compiled directly for each subject. Only one case but five referents had glass-work in their work histories [crude odds ratio, 0.5; 95% CI, 0.1–3.9].

Levin *et al.* (1988) studied the lifetime work histories, smoking histories and other exposure factors among 733 male Chinese with lung cancer in Shanghai in 1984–85 and among 760 male referents selected from the general population. Information was compiled by the use of a structured questionnaire administered in the subjects' homes, in hospital or at work sites. About 35 major occupational categories were examined. A deficit (odds ratio, 0.6; 95% CI, 0.3–1.5; adjusted for each occupation) of lung cancer was found among males working in 'glass, ceramic and enamelled product manufacture'. A parallel study was

Table 9. Cohort studies of exposures in the glass manufacturing industry

Study population	Site	No. of cases	RR	95% or 90% CI	Reference
468 Italian male glass-workers, producing glass containers, 1953–67 (mortality)	Lung	13	2.09	[1.1–3.6]	Cordioli et al. (1987)
	Larynx	4	4.49	[1.2–11.4]	
	Stomach	2	0.61	[0.07–2.2]	
191 male ceramics and glass-workers, not otherwise specified, but with occupational histories of exposure to high concentrations of silica dust, Austria, 1950–60 (mortality)	Lung	28	2.37	[1.58–3.43]	Neuberger & Kundi (1990)
	Stomach	6	1.16	[0.42–2.53]	
	Intestine	7	1.50	[0.60–3.09]	
625 Swedish male art glass-workers (mortality)	Lung[a]	6	2.4[b]	[0.9–5.2]	Wingren & Englander (1990)
	Colon[a]	4	2.5	[0.7–6.4]	
	Prostate[a]	4	1.7	[0.5–4.2]	
	Pharynx[a]	2	15.9	[1.8–57.4]	
3749 male and female Finnish glass-workers, unspecified as to process or product, 1953–86 (incidence)	Skin[c]	11	1.53	0.76–2.73	Sankila et al. (1990)
	Lung	69	1.28	0.99–1.62	
	Stomach	34	0.93	0.64–1.29	
	Colon	7	0.46	0.19–0.96	
	Bladder	9	0.97	0.44–1.84	
140 male oral glass-blowers	Skin[c]	2	8.00	0.97–28.9	
	Lung	1	0.29	0.01–1.64	
	Stomach	3	2.16	0.44–6.26	

[a]RR based on local county death rates
[b]Smoking-adjusted RR for lung cancer, 3.5 [1.3–7.7], with 10-year latency requirement
[c]Melanoma and basal-cell carcinomas excluded

performed among 672 female cases and 735 referent subjects, but small numbers in each occupational group precluded detailed analyses. The largest excess (odds ratio, 5.1; CI, 1.3–23.5) was found among female glass and glass product manufacturing workers, based on 15 cases and three referents. When 20 years of employment in the industry was applied as an inclusion criterion, the excess was more than seven fold.

2.3.3 Tumours at multiple sites

A preliminary study in three parishes with glass industries in southeastern Sweden (Wingren & Axelson, 1985) revealed an excess of deaths from stomach cancer in 1951–79 among glass-blowers (odds ratio, 6.4; 95% CI, 3.0–14.0), based on eight cases. For unspecified glass-workers [known to include glass-blowers], the odds ratio for stomach cancer was 1.5 (0.68–3.2), based on nine cases. Lung cancer was also seen in unspecified glass-workers, with an odds ratio of 2.4 (1.0–5.8), based on seven exposed cases. The same authors (Wingren & Axelson, 1987) expanded the study on mortality among workers in Swedish glass-works by selective causes of deaths, i.e. for total cancer, stomach cancer, colon cancer, lung cancer and cardiovascular deaths. Cases with these causes of death were considered in males aged 45 and over in the registers of deaths and burials in 11 parishes (including the three studied previously) in 1950–82; the eight new parishes were also analysed separately. Control subjects were taken as other causes of death among males aged 45 years and over in the same parishes. Information on exposure to various metal compounds was obtained from seven existing glass-works in the area. Stomach cancer appeared in excess for glass-blowers (odds ratio, 2.6 [95% CI, 1.4–4.9]) based on 11 exposed cases, as did colon cancer (odds ratio, 3.1 [95% CI, 1.2–7.7]), based on five exposed cases, and lung cancer (odds ratio, 2.3 [95% CI, 0.8–6.3]), based on four exposed cases. For unspecified glass-workers, the odds ratio for for stomach cancer was 1.4 [95% CI, 0.8–2.4], based on 18 exposed cases, and that for colon cancer was 1.8 [95% CI, 0.9–3.7], based on nine exposed cases; for lung cancer, the odds ratio was 1.9 [95% CI, 1.0–3.7], based on 11 exposed cases. On the basis of the information on exposure obtained from the glass-works, the authors later made an attempt to identify certain exposures as determinants of the cancer risks found (Wingren & Axelson, 1993) through further case–control evaluations in the art glass industry. The risk for stomach cancer in particular was associated with exposure to arsenic, copper, nickel, manganese and to some extent lead and chromium. For colon cancer, an increasing trend in risk was seen with increasing use of antimony and lead, the two elements being strongly correlated. For lung cancer, no obvious trend with exposure to any metal could be found.

In a case–control study based on death certificates, 9663 white and 3253 black men in Illinois (USA), aged 35–74, who had cancers of the stomach, pancreas, lung, prostate, urinary bladder or brain or non-Hodgkin's lymphomas (Mallin et al., 1989) were compared with control groups chosen by sampling randomly among non-cancer deaths from the same age groups. Occupation was coded on the basis of the 1980 census. A three-fold excess risk for brain cancer was found, based on eight cases among manufacturers of glass and glass products. [The Working Group noted the limitations of using information on occupation derived solely from death certificates.]

A case–control study conducted in the Montréal (Canada) metropolitan area (Siemiatycki, 1991) included all males aged 35–70 with a histologically confirmed diagnosis of cancer at 20 selected sites made between September 1979 and June 1985. A total of 3730 cases were interviewed. Occupational exposure to 293 substances potentially present in the work environment was assessed by a group of experts on the job description in the questionnaires. Cases of cancer at each site were compared with all other cancer cases. Age, cigarette smoking and a number of other potential confounders were controlled for in the analyses. 'Glass dust' was one of the exposure categories with a prevalence of 1% in the total sample and was associated with stomach cancer (5 exposed cases; odds ratio, 1.8 [90% CI, 0.7–4.8]) and lung cancer (18 exposed cases; odds ratio, 2.2 [90% CI, 1.0–5.0]). When only substantial exposure was considered, the figures were: stomach cancer, four exposed cases; odds ratio, 2.7 [90% CI, 0.8–8.6] and lung cancer, six exposed cases; odds ratio, 1.0 [90% CI, 0.3–3.6].

2.4 Childhood cancer

In a proportionate mortality study of the distribution of the occupations of fathers of children who died from neoplasms in the United Kingdom, Sanders *et al.* (1981) found no indication of a relationship with glass and ceramics work (proportionate mortality ratio, 1.02), on the basis of 21 cancer deaths occurring in the period 1959–63. In 1970–72, the proportionate mortality ratio was 0.98, based on nine cancer deaths.

3. Other Relevant Data

3.1 Absorption, distribution, metabolism and excretion

No relevant data were available to the Working Group.

3.2 Toxic effects

Mortality from cardiovascular disease among Swedish glass-workers was studied in a case–control study, described in detail on p. 365 (Wingren & Axelson, 1987). The odds ratio for glass-workers who died of cardiovascular disease was 1.2 [95% CI, 1.0–1.4]. The crude odds ratio was highest (1.3 [95% CI, 0.9–1.8] for glass-blowers.

In a cohort study in the same area of Sweden, where glassworks are prevalent, described on p. 362 (Wingren & Englander, 1990), the SMR for all deaths was 0.98, based on 97 observed deaths, using national rates for comparison and 1.17 when county death rates were used for the comparison. The SMRs for cardiovascular deaths were 1.21 and 1.26 (39 deaths), respectively, and those for cerebrovascular disease, 1.50 and 1.68 (11 deaths). Neither was significantly different from unity. The SMR for cardiovascular disease increased to 1.8 (based on national rates) ($p < 0.01$) when adjustment for smoking was attempted.

[The Working Group noted that it is not clear how many of the cases from the case–control study were included in the cohort study.]

In a cross-sectional study in Germany (Wagner 1975) involving 131 glass-blowers aged 29–76 who had been exposed for 10–46 years, symptoms of chronic bronchitis [not specified]

Table 10. Case–control studies of exposures in the glass manufacturing industry

Study population	Exposure	Sex	No. of exposed cases	Odds ratio	95% CI	Remarks	Reference
Bladder cancer (incidence)							
Population-based, Canada	Glass-workers	M	6	6.0	0.7–276		Howe *et al.* (1980)
Population-based, USA	Glass-workers	M	6	5.9	0.7–50		Silverman *et al.* (1983)
Lung cancer							
Hospital-based, Italy (incidence)	Glass-workers	M	1	[0.5]	[0.1–3.9]	Crude odds ratio	Buiatti *et al.* (1985)
Population-based, China (incidence)	Glass, ceramics and enamelled product workers	M	12	0.6	0.3–1.5	Odds ratio adjusted for other occupation	Levin *et al.* (1988)
	Glass products workers	F	15	5.1	1.3–23.5		
Population-based, Sweden (mortality)	All glass-workers	M	21	1.7	[1.0–2.8]	Mantel–Haenszel odds ratio	Wingren & Axelson (1987)
	Glass-blowers	M	4	2.3	[0.8–6.3]		
	Unspecified	M	11	1.9	[1.0–3.7]		
Population-based, Canada (incidence)	Glass dust (any)	M	18	2.2	[1.0–5.0]	Mantel–Haenszel odds ratio	Siemiatycki (1991)
	Substantial	M	6	1.0	[0.3–3.6]		
Stomach cancer							
Population-based, Sweden	All glass-workers	M	44	1.5	[1.0–2.1]	Mantel–Haenszel odds ratio	Wingren & Axelson (1987)
	Glass-blowers	M	11	2.6	[1.4–4.9]		
	Unspecified	M	18	1.4	[0.8–2.4]		
Population-based, Canada	Glass dust (any)	M	5	1.8	[0.7–4.8]	Mantel–Haenszel odds ratio	Siemiatycki (1991)
	Substantial	M	4	2.7	[0.8–8.6]		
Colon cancer							
Population-based, Sweden	All glass-workers	M	18	1.6	[0.9–2.8]	Mantel–Haenszel odds ratio	Wingren & Axelson (1987)
	Glass-blowers	M	5	3.1	[1.2–7.7]		
	Unspecified	M	9	1.8	[0.9–3.7]		

were reported by 11. Thirty had abnormal lung function tests, and of these, 11 were considered to have emphysema; eight of the 11 smoked 10–30 cigarettes daily. No control group was studied.

Of 47 art glass-blowers (mean age, 34.5 years), 21% reported having usual cough and 31% reported wheezing in a questionnaire study in the USA (Braun & Tsiatis, 1979); 34 of the 47 studied were smokers or ex-smokers. [The Working Group noted that the basis of selection and the number of workers who refused to participate in the study were not indicated.] The frequency of different indicators of abnormal lung function (vital capacity, forced expiratory volume in one second [FEV_1], maximal mid-expiratory flow, maximal flow at 50% vital capacity) ranged from 2 to 19% in 42 art glass-blowers.

Munn *et al.* (1990) studied lung function (forced vital capacity, FEV_1, mid-expiratory flow rate, maximal voluntary ventilation, maximal expiratory and inspiratory muscle pressure) in 87 volunteers (64 were smokers) from three glass factories in the USA. The participants were divided into non-glass-blowers, part-time glass-blowers and full-time glass-blowers. All function measurements were on average no lower than 95% of the predicted value; full-time glass-blowers had significantly higher FEV_1, forced vital capacity and muscle pressure values than their colleagues. [The Working Group noted the possibility of selection bias; reasons for participating and not participating in the study were not elucidated.]

Srivastava *et al.* (1988) studied the etiological factors in chronic bronchitis in a 'representative sample' of 373 glass-bangle workers in a case–control study in India [selection criteria not indicated]. Eighty-nine of the workers were judged to have chronic bronchitis. The risk for chronic bronchitis increased with age, tobacco smoking, low socioeconomic status and duration of employment in the glass-bangle industry. The odds ratio for workers with chronic bronchitis to have worked > 25 years in the glass-bangle industry was 2.30 ($p < 0.1$) (corrected for age but not for socioeconomic status or smoking), compared with those with exposure < 16 years.

In a cross-sectional study of lung function in India, Rastogi *et al.* (1991) observed that 220 asymptomatic glass-bangle workers (123 smokers) [selection criteria not indicated; exposed workers with tuberculosis, bronchial asthma or chronic bronchitis excluded] had lower lung function variables than 88 unexposed controls (37 smokers). A number of heavy metals, such as arsenic, lead, cadmium, zinc, copper, cobalt and selenium are used as colouring agents in the manufacture of glass bangles and are mixed manually with soda ash and silica sand in varying proportions. The difference in forced expiratory flow rate over 75 and 85% of the spirogram reached statistical significance in both smokers and nonsmokers.

In an effort to identify cases of asbestos-related diseases in a glass bottle manufacturing factory in Texas, USA, employees were offered a medical examination. The average duration of employment was 17 years, ranging from 6 months to 36 years. Pleural plaques or pleural fibrosis were observed in 38/334 (224 smokers) workers, fibrosis in 22 and restrictive pulmonary function in 19. Because less than half of the eligible workforce volunteered for the study, thereby resulting in possible selection bias, the authors stated that these figures do not represent the true prevalence of these diseases (Kronenberg *et al.*, 1991). [The Working Group noted that previous employment history of the cases was not described.]

The occurrence of cataract due to heat was first described in the eighteenth century; a nineteenth-century report stated that glass-blowers frequently developed cataracts (Keatinge et al., 1955). In a review of company records and examination of seven workers (10% of the exposed workforce) with long duration of employment, Dunn (1950) found no case of cataract. In a study of 20 Swedish glass-works (Lydahl & Philipson 1984), the risk of people exposed to infrared of having lowered visual acuity was 2.5 times higher than that of controls (95% CI, 1.4–4.4); the probability of having been operated for a cataract was 12 times as high (95% CI, 2.6–54).

3.3 Reproductive and developmental effects

No relevant data were available to the Working Group.

3.4 Genetic and related effects

Šrám et al. (1985) performed a cytogenetic analysis on the peripheral blood lymphocytes of 31 workers in a glass factory in the Czech Republic and of 23 unexposed controls. The authors noted exposure to mineral oil mists containing polycyclic aromatic hydrocarbons. Although exposure did not exceed the national maximum allowable concentration for mineral oil aerosols (5 mg/m^3 air), a significant increase in the frequency of aberrant cells and chromosome breaks per cell was detected in exposed workers, with no significant difference between smokers and nonsmokers in either group. In particular, higher rates of dicentrics, reciprocal translocations and cells with pulverization were observed in exposed workers. [The Working Group noted that exposures to other compounds were not taken into account.]

4. Summary of Data Reported and Evaluation

4.1 Exposure data

There are five main sectors in the glass manufacturing industry: flat glass, container and pressed ware, art glass, special glass (e.g. optical, ophthalmic, electronic) and fibre glass (which is not considered here). The basic steps in the manufacture of glass products are melting, fining, homogenization, annealing and forming. Art and special glasses are produced by pot processes, involving manual batch handling. Art glass production has changed little with time and, for the most part, still involves blowing by mouth. During the twentieth century, the production of flat glass and container glass has evolved from traditional batch processes to highly automated processes. The modern production of flat glass is the most highly automated and usually utilizes tank melting with the continuous feeding of batch ingredients and the float (Pilkington) process for forming. The production of containers and pressed ware has also become increasingly mechanized, with mechanical blowing or pressing of the molten glass.

Exposure to lead, arsenic and antimony oxides occurs primarily in sectors of the industry where traditional, non-mechanized techniques are used, such as in the production of crystal and other art glasses. Other potential exposures in glass manufacture include silica, asbestos, other metal oxides and polycyclic aromatic hydrocarbons.

4.2 Human carcinogenicity data

Four cohort studies of workers involved in glass manufacture—at a plant in Italy producing glass containers, among ceramics and glass workers in Austria, at two glass factories in Finland and among art glass-workers in Sweden—found increased risks for lung cancer. Population-based case–control studies in Sweden and Canada also found increased risks for lung cancer in glass-workers; a population-based case–control study in China found a significantly increased risk for lung cancer in female glass-workers and a nonsignificantly decreased risk in male glass, ceramics and enamelled product workers. None of the studies was specifically informative with respect to work in the flat-glass manufacturing industry. It is unlikely that the increased risk for lung cancer can be explained by nonoccupational risk factors such as smoking, in view of the consistency and magnitude of the findings, which were obtained in studies of various designs in different countries. When smoking habits were addressed in one of the studies, the estimated relative risk for lung cancer was increased.

In general, no distinction was made in these studies between different components of the glass manufacturing industry. The only subgroup of glass-workers for whom specific findings were available was glass-blowers. Population-based case–control studies in Sweden on glass-workers and in Canada on people exposed to glass dust found small increased risks for stomach cancer, whereas in three cohort studies of glass-workers in Italy, Austria and Finland the risks for stomach cancer were not increased; in two of the cohort studies, the numbers of cases were small. Only the cohort study in Finland and the case–control study in Sweden specifically reported findings on stomach cancer in glass-blowers; both showed stronger increases in risk in glass-blowers than in glass-workers in general.

The three cohort studies in Austria, Finland and Sweden showed little evidence of an increased risk for intestinal cancer. A Swedish population-based case–control study of colon cancer found a small increase in risk in glass-workers in general but a stronger increase in glass-blowers.

Two population-based case–control studies, in Canada and the USA, showed nonsignificantly increased risks for urinary bladder cancer in glass-workers, but the numbers of cases were small. An Italian cohort study showed an increased risk for laryngeal cancer in glass-workers. In the Finnish cohort study, an increased risk was seen for basal-cell carcinomas of the skin in male workers.

The evidence that favours a causal association between exposures in the glass manufacturing industry and cancer is: a reasonably consistent association with lung cancer in all four cohort studies; a similar though less consistent association with lung cancer in three case–control studies; a larger lung cancer risk than can reasonably be explained by non-occupational confounding factors; the presence of human lung carcinogens in some components of the glass manufacturing industry; and the finding of an increased risk for stomach cancers in several cohort and case–control studies. Findings that limit the interpretation of causality include: the poorly characterized and heterogeneous exposures of workers in the glass manufacturing industry, which are likely to result in a weak or null association between exposure and cancer risk in some studies; the absence of demonstrated dose–response relationships; the fact that, in some studies, risk estimates were made for the combination of glass-workers and workers in other industries, thereby diminishing the degree to which results can be interpreted for the glass manufacturing industry itself; and the relatively few studies of workers in the glass manufacturing industry.

4.3 Other relevant data

A single study reported an increased frequency of chromosomal aberrations in peripheral blood lymphocytes of subjects working in a glass factory in the Czech Republic.

4.4 Evaluation[1]

There is *limited evidence* that occupational exposures in the manufacture of art glass, glass containers and pressed ware are carcinogenic[2].

There is *inadequate evidence* that occupational exposures in flat-glass and special glass manufacture are carcinogenic.

Overall evaluations

The manufacture of art glass, glass containers and pressed ware entails exposures *that are probably carcinogenic to humans (Group 2A)*.

Occupational exposures in flat-glass and special glass manufacture *are not classifiable as to their carcinogenicity to humans (Group 3)*.

5. References

Almaguer, D. (1985) *Health Hazard Evaluation Report. PPG Industries, Mt Zion, IL* (HETA 84-050-1595), Cincinnati, OH, National Institute for Occupational Safety and Health

Andersson, L., Wingren, G. & Axelson, O. (1990) Some hygienic observations from the glass industry. *Int. Arch. occup. environ. Health*, **62**, 249–252

Baxter, P.J., Samuel, A.M. & Holkham, M.P.E. (1985) Lead hazard in British stained glass workers (Short report). *Br. med. J.*, **291**, 383

Boyd, D.C. & Thompson, D.A. (1980) Glass. In: Mark, H.F., Othmer, D.F., Overberger, C.G., Seaborg, G.T. & Grayson, N., eds, *Kirk–Othmer Encyclopedia of Chemical Technology*, Vol. 11, New York, John Wiley & Sons, pp. 807–880

Braun, S.R. & Tsiatis, A. (1979) Pulmonary abnormalities in art glassblowers. *J. occup. Med.*, **21**, 487–489

---

[1]For definition of the italicized terms, see Preamble, pp. 26–30.
[2]This evaluation does not apply to glass fibre, which was evaluated previously (see General Remarks, p. 36). The Working Group could not identify the specific exposure, process or activity that is most likely to be responsible for the excess risk.

Buiatti, E., Kriebel, D., Geddes, M., Santucci, M. & Pucci, N. (1985) A case control study of lung cancer in Florence, Italy. I. Occupational risk factors. *J. Epidemiol. Community Health*, **39**, 244–250

Burroughs, G.E. & Horan, J. (1981) *Health Hazard Evaluation Report. Becton–Dickinson Company, Columbus, Nebraska* (HHE 80-023-804), Cincinnati OH, National Institute for Occupational Safety and Health

Cameron, J.D. & Hill, J.W. (1983) In: Parmeggiani, L., ed., *Encyclopaedia of Occupational Health and Safety*, 3rd rev. Ed., Vol. 1, Geneva, International Labour Office, pp. 966–970

Chrostek, W.J., Elesh, E. & Taylor, J.S. (1980) *Health Hazard Evaluation Report. Jeannette Glass Company, Jeannette, PA* (HE 80-19-765), Cincinnati, OH, National Institute for Occupational Safety and Health

Cordier, S., Clavel, J., Limasset, J.-C., Boccon-Gibod, L., Le Moual, N., Mandereau, L. & Hemon, D. (1993) Occupational risks of bladder cancer in France: a multicentre case–control study. *Int. J. Epidemiol.*, **22**, 403–411

Cordioli, G., Cuoghi, L., Solari, P.L., Berrino, F., Crosignani, P. & Riboli, E. (1987) Mortality from tumours in a cohort of workers in the glass industry (Ital.). *Epidemiol. Prevenz.*, **30**, 16–18

Deutsche Forschungsgemeinschaft (1992) *MAK and BAT Values 1992. Maximum Concentrations at the Workplace and Biological Tolerance Values for Working Materials*, Weinheim, VCH Verlagsgesellschaft, p. 84

Dolin, P.J. (1992) A descriptive study of occupation and bladder cancer in England and Wales. *Br. J. Cancer*, **65**, 476–478

Dunn, K.L. (1950) Cataract from infra-red rays (glass workers' cataract). A preliminary study on exposures. *Arch. occup. Hyg.*, **1**, 166–180

Farmer, J.G. & Johnson, L.R. (1990) Assessment of occupational exposure to inorganic arsenic based on urinary concentrations and speciation of arsenic. *Br. J. ind. Med.*, **47**, 342-348

Grundy, T. (1990) *The Global Miracle of Flat Glass: A Tribute to St Helens and its Glassworkers*, St Helens, Merseyside

Gunter, B.J. & Thoburn, T.W. (1985) *Health Hazard Evaluation Report. Crystal Zoo, Boulder, CO* (HETA 84-384-1580), Cincinnati, OH, National Institute for Occupational Safety and Health

Howe, G.R., Burch, J.D., Miller, A.B., Cook, G.M., Esteve, J., Morrison, B., Gordon, P., Chambers, L.W., Fodor, G. & Winsor G.M. (1980) Tobacco use, occupation, coffee, various nutrients, and bladder cancer. *J. natl Cancer Inst.*, **64**, 701–713

IARC (1975) *IARC Monographs on the Evaluation of Carcinogenic Risk of Chemicals to Man*, Vol. 9, *Some Aziridines, N-, S- and O-Mustards and Selenium*, Lyon, pp. 245–260

IARC (1983) *IARC Monographs on the Evaluation of the Carcinogenic Risk of Chemicals to Humans*, Vol. 32, *Polynuclear Aromatic Compounds, Part 1, Chemical, Environmental and Experimental Data*, Lyon

IARC (1987a) *IARC Monographs on the Evaluation of Carcinogenic Risks to Humans*, Suppl. 7, *Overall Evaluations of Carcinogenicity: An Updating of* IARC Monographs *Volumes 1 to 42*, Lyon, pp. 230-232

IARC (1987b) *IARC Monographs on the Evaluation of the Carcinogenic Risk of Chemicals to Humans*, Vol. 42, *Silica and Some Silicates*, Lyon, pp. 39–143

IARC (1987c) *IARC Monographs on the Evaluation of Carcinogenic Risks to Humans*, Suppl. 7, *Overall Evaluations of Carcinogenicity: An Updating of* IARC Monographs *Volumes 1 to 42*, Lyon, pp. 216–219

IARC (1987d) *IARC Monographs on the Evaluation of Carcinogenic Risks to Humans*, Suppl. 7, *Overall Evaluations of Carcinogenicity: An Updating of* IARC Monographs *Volumes 1 to 42*, Lyon, pp. 100–106

IARC (1987e) *IARC Monographs on the Evaluation of Carcinogenic Risks to Humans*, Suppl. 7, *Overall Evaluations of Carcinogenicity: An Updating of* IARC Monographs *Volumes 1 to 42*, Lyon, pp. 106–116

IARC (1987f) *IARC Monographs on the Evaluation of Carcinogenic Risks to Humans*, Suppl. 7, *Overall Evaluations of Carcinogenicity: An Updating of* IARC Monographs *Volumes 1 to 42*, Lyon, pp. 252–254

IARC (1988) *IARC Monographs on the Evaluation of Carcinogenic Risks to Humans*, Vol. 43, *Man-made Mineral Fibres and Radon*, Lyon, pp. 39–171

IARC (1989a) *IARC Monographs on the Evaluation of Carcinogenic Risks to Humans*, Vol. 47, *Some Organic Solvents, Resin Monomers and Related Compounds, Pigments and Occupational Exposures in Paint Manufacturing and Painting*, Lyon, pp. 307–326

IARC (1989b) *IARC Monographs on the Evaluation of Carcinogenic Risks to Humans*, Vol. 47, *Some Organic Solvents, Resin Monomers and Related Compounds, Pigments and Occupational Exposures in Paint Manufacturing and Painting*, Lyon, pp. 291–305

IARC (1990a) *IARC Monographs on the Evaluation of Carcinogenic Risks to Humans*, Vol. 49, *Chromium, Nickel and Welding*, pp. 49–256

IARC (1990b) *IARC Monographs on the Evaluation of Carcinogenic Risks to Humans*, Vol. 49, *Chromium, Nickel and Welding*, pp. 257–445

IARC (1991) *IARC Monographs on the Evaluation of Carcinogenic Risks to Humans*, Vol. 52, *Chlorinated Drinking-water; Chlorination By-products; Some Other Halogenated Compounds; Cobalt and Cobalt Compounds*, pp. 363–472

IARC (1992) *IARC Monographs on the Evaluation of Carcinogenic Risks to Humans*, Vol. 54, *Occupational Exposures to Mists and Vapours from Strong Inorganic Acids; and Other Industrial Chemicals*, Lyon, pp. 41–130

Ide, C.W. & Bullough, G.R. (1988) Arsenic and old glass. *J. Soc. occup. Med.*, **38**, 85–88

de Jong, B.H.W.S. (1989) Glass. In: *Ullmann's Encyclopedia of Industrial Chemistry*, Vol. A12, Weinheim, VCH Verlagsgesellschaft

Keatinge, G.F., Pearson, J., Simons, J.P. & White, E.E. (1955) Radiation cataract in industry. *Arch. ind. Health*, **11**, 305–314

Kronenberg, R.S., Levin, J.L., Dodson, R.F., Garcia, J.G.N. & Griffith, D.E. (1991) Asbestos-related disease in employees of a steel mill and a glass bottle manufacturing plant. *Toxicol. ind. Health*, **7**, 73–79

Landrigan, P.J., Tamblyn, P.B., Nelson, M., Kerndt, P., Kronoveter, K.J. & Zack, M.M. (1980) Lead exposure in stained glass workers. *Am. J. ind. Med.*, **1**, 177–180

Levin, L.I., Zheng, W., Blot, W.J., Goa, Y.-T. & Fraumeni, J.F., Jr (1988) Occupational and lung cancer in Shanghai: a case–control study. *Br. J. ind. Med.*, **45**, 450–458

Lucas, C. (1981) *Health Hazard Evaluation Report. Pilgrim Glass Company, Ceredo, West Virginia* (HETA 81-209-891), Cincinnati, OH, National Institute for Occupational Safety and Health

Lüdersdorf, R., Fuchs, A., Mayer, P., Skulsuksai, G. & Schäcke, G. (1987) Biological assessment of exposure to antimony and lead in the glass-producing industry. *Int. Arch. occup. environ. Health*, **59**, 469–474

Lydahl, E. & Philipson, B. (1984) Infrared radiation and cataract II. Epidemiologic investigation of glass workers. *Acta ophthalmol.*, **62**, 976–992

Lynge, E., Kurppa, K., Kristofersen, L., Malker, H. & Sauli, H. (1986) Silica dust and lung cancer: results from the Nordic occupational mortality and cancer incidence registers. *J. natl Cancer Inst.*, **77**, 883–889

Malker, H.S.R., McLaughlin, J.K., Weiner, J.A., Silverman, D.T., Blot, W.J., Ericsson, J.L.E. & Fraumeni, J.F., Jr (1990) Occupational risk factors for nasopharyngeal cancer in Sweden. *Br. J. ind. Med.*, **47**, 213–214

Mallin, K., Rubin, M. & Joo, E. (1989) Occupational cancer mortality in Illinois white and black males, 1979–1984, for seven cancer sites. *Am. J. ind. Med.*, **15**, 699–717

McLaughlin, J.K., Malker, H.S.R., Blot, W.J., Malker, B.K., Stone, B.J., Weiner, J.A., Ericsson, J.L.E. & Fraumeni, J.F., Jr (1987a) Occupational risks for intracranial gliomas in Sweden. *J. natl Cancer Inst.*, **78**, 253–257

McLaughlin, J.K., Thomas, T.L., Stone, B.J., Blot, W.J., Malker, H.S.R., Wiener, J.A., Ericsson, J.L.E. & Malker, B.K. (1987b) Occupational risks for meningiomas of the CNS in Sweden. *J. occup. Med.*, **29**, 66–68

Menichini, E., Bonanni, L. & Merli, F. (1990) Determination of polycyclic aromatic hydrocarbons in mineral oils and oil aerosols in glass manufacturing. *Toxicol. environ. Chem.*, **28**, 37–51

Milne, K.L., Sandler, D.P., Everson, R.B. & Brown, S.M. (1983) Lung cancer and occupation in Alameda county: a death certificate case–control study. *Am. J. ind. Med.*, **4**, 565–575

Morey, G.W. (1938) *The Properties of Glass* (ACS Monograph No. 77), New York, Reinhold

Munn, N.J., Thomas, S.W. & DeMesquita, S. (1990) Pulmonary function in commercial glass blowers. *Chest*, **98**, 871–874

Neuberger, M. & Kundi, M. (1990) Occupational dust exposure and cancer mortality—results of a prospective cohort study. In: Simonato, L., Fletcher, A.C., Saracci, R. & Thomas, T.L., eds, *Occupational Exposure to Silica and Cancer Risk* (IARC Scientific Publications No. 97), Lyon, IARC, pp. 65–73

Raithel, H.J., Schaller, K.H. & Valentin, H. (1991) Biological monitoring of nickel in different industrial areas in the Federal Republic of Germany. In: Dillon, H.K. & Ho, M.H., eds, *Biological Monitoring of Exposure to Chemicals: Metals*, New York, John Wiley & Sons, pp. 27–38

Rastogi, S.K., Gupta, B.N., Husain, T., Chandra, H., Mathur, N., Pangtey, B.S., Chandra, S.V. & Garg, N. (1991) A cross-sectional study of pulmonary function among workers exposed to multimetals in the glass bangle industry. *Am. J. ind. Med.*, **20**, 391–399

Roels, H., Buchet, J.-P., Truc, J., Croquet, F. & Lauwerys, R. (1982) The possible role of direct ingestion on the overall absorption of cadmium or arsenic in workers exposed to CdO and As_2O_3 dust. *Am. J. ind. Med.*, **3**, 53–65

Sanders, B.M., White, G.C. & Draper, G.J. (1981) Occupations of fathers of children dying from neoplasms. *J. Epidemiol. Community Health*, **35**, 245–250

Sankila, R., Karjalainen, S., Pukkala, E., Oksanen, H., Hakulinen, T., Teppo, L. & Hakama, M. (1990) Cancer risk among glass factory workers: an excess of lung cancer? *Br. J. ind. Med.*, **47**, 815–818

Schaller, K.H., Schiele, R. & Valentin, H. (1982) Questions on the action of arsenic in mixing, melting and charging in the lead crystal industry (Ger.). In: *Arbeitsmedizinische Untersuchungen zur Einwirkung von Fremdstoffen und Schadstoffen in der keramischen und Glas-Industrie* [Medical Study at Work of the Action of Impurities and Hazardous Substances in the Ceramics and Glass Industry], Heft 31, Würzburg, Berufsgenossenschaft der keramischen und Glas-Industrie [Professional Association of the Ceramics and Glass Industry], pp. 25–28

Schaller, K.H., Schiele, R., Weltle, D. & Valentin, H. (1988) Lead burden in the ceramics and glass industry. Evaluation of the results of the study from 1978 to 1986 (Ger.). In: *Berufskrankheiten in der keramischen und Glas-Industrie* [Occupational Diseases in the Ceramics and Glass Industry], Heft 35, Würzburg, Berufsgenossenschaft der keramischen und Glas-Industrie [Professional Association of the Ceramics and Glass Industry], pp. 7–43

Siemiatycki, J., ed. (1991) *Risk Factors for Cancer in the Workplace*, Boca Raton, FL, CRC Press

Silverman, D.T., Hoover, R.N., Albert, S. & Graff, K.M. (1983) Occupation and cancer of the lower urinary tract in Detroit. *J. natl Cancer Inst.*, **70**, 237–245

Somervaille, L.J., Chettle, D.R., Scott, M.C., Tennant, D.R., McKiernan, M.J., Skilbeck, A. & Trethowan, W.N. (1988) In vivo tibia lead measurements as an index of cumulative exposure in occupationally exposed subjects. *Br. J. ind. Med.*, **45**, 174–181

Šrám, R.J., Holá, N., Kotěšovec, F. & Novákova, A. (1985) Cytogenetic analysis of peripheral blood lymphocytes in glass workers occupationally exposed to mineral oils. *Mutat. Res.*, **144**, 277–280

Srivastava, A.K., Mathur, N., Rastogi, S.K. & Gupta, B.N. (1988) Case control study of chronic bronchitis in glass bangle workers. *J. Soc. occup. Med.*, **38**, 134–136

Tola, S., Hernberg, S. & Vesanto, R. (1976) Occupational lead exposure in Finland. VI. Final report. *Scand. J. Work Environ. Health*, **2**, 115–127

Wagner, F. (1975) Lung emphysema in glass blowers (Ger.). *Arbeitsmed.-Inf.*, **2**, 28–32

Wingren, G. & Axelson, O. (1985) Mortality pattern in a glass producing area in SE Sweden. *Br. J. ind. Med.*, **42**, 411–414

Wingren, G. & Axelson, O. (1987) Mortality in the Swedish glassworks industry. *Scand. J. Work Environ. Health*, **13**, 412–416

Wingren, G. & Axelson, O. (1992) Cluster of brain cancers spuriously suggesting occupational risk among glassworkers. *Scand. J. Work Environ. Health*, **18**, 85–89

Wingren, G. & Axelson, O. (1993) Epidemiological studies of occupational cancer as related to complex mixtures of trace elements in the art glass industry. *Scand. J. Work Environ. Health* (in press)

Wingren, G. & Englander, V. (1990) Mortality and cancer morbidity in a cohort of Swedish glassworkers. *Int. Arch. occup. environ. Health*, **62**, 253–257

SUMMARY OF FINAL EVALUATIONS

Agent	Degree of evidence of carcinogenicity		Overall evaluation of carcinogenicity to humans
	Human	Animal	
Beryllium and beryllium compounds	S	S	1[a]
Cadmium and cadmium compounds	S		1[a]
Cadmium compounds		S	
Cadmium metal		L	
Mercury and mercury compounds			
Methylmercury compounds	I		2B[a]
Methylmercury chloride		S	
Metallic mercury and inorganic mercury compounds	I		3
Metallic mercury		I	
Mercuric chloride		L	
Occupational exposures in the glass manufacturing industry			
Art glass, glass containers and pressed ware, manufacture of	L		2A
Flat-glass and special glass, manufacture of	I		3

S, sufficient evidence; L, limited evidence; I, inadequate evidence; for definitions, see preamble, pp. 26–30
[a]Other relevant data were taken into consideration in making the overall evaluation.

APPENDIX 1

SUMMARY TABLES OF
GENETIC AND RELATED EFFECTS

APPENDIX 1

Summary table of genetic and related effects of beryllium compounds

Compound	Nonmammalian systems														Mammalian systems																				
	Prokaryotes		Lower eukaryotes			Plants				Insects					In vitro														In vivo							
															Animal cells							Human cells							Animals							Humans
	D	G	D	R	G	A	D	G	C	R	G	C	G	A	D	G	S	M	C	A	T	D	G	S	M	C	A	T	D	G	S	M	C	DL	A	D	S	M	C	A
Beryllium chloride	–	–																																						
Beryllium nitrate	+¹	–																																						
Beryllium oxides	–¹	–¹													+¹		–¹				+¹																			
Beryllium sulfate	+	–			–¹										–¹	+¹	–¹	+¹	?		+				+¹	?						–¹								

A, aneuploidy; C, chromosomal aberrations; D, DNA damage; DL, dominant lethal mutation; G, gene mutation; I, inhibition of intercellular communication; M, micronuclei; R, mitotic recombination and gene conversion; S, sister chromatid exchange; T, cell transformation

In completing the tables, the following symbols indicate the consensus of the Working Group with regard to the results for each end-point:

+ considered to be positive for the specific end-point and level of biological complexity
+¹ considered to be positive, but only one valid study was available to the Working Group
– considered to be negative
–¹ considered to be negative, but only one valid study was available to the Working Group
? considered to be equivocal or inconclusive (e.g. there were contradictory results from different laboratories; there were confounding exposures; the results were equivocal)

Summary table of genetic and related effects of cadmium compounds

Compound	Nonmammalian systems												Mammalian systems																		
	Prokaryotes		Lower eukaryotes				Plants			Insects				In vitro												In vivo					
														Animal cells						Human cells						Animals					Humans
	D	G	D	R	G	A	D	G	C	R	G	C	A	D	G	S	M	C	A	T	D	G	S	M	C	A	T	D	G	S	M	C	A	DL	A	D	S	M	C	A
Cadmium acetate	+?	?												+¹		–¹			+		+¹				?¹	+		+¹		?. ?										
Cadmium chloride	+?	?	+	–¹	–					–			+¹	+¹	+	+?	+¹	+	+		+		+¹	+¹	–¹					+	–	+							
Cadmium nitrate										–¹				+¹		–¹																							
Cadmium oxide	–¹																																						
Cadmium sulfate	+?	?	+¹											+¹	+¹		+						–¹																
Cadmium sulfide														+¹					+¹					+¹																

A, aneuploidy; C, chromosomal aberrations; D, DNA damage; DL, dominant lethal mutation; G, gene mutation; I, inhibition of intercellular communication; M, micronuclei; R, mitotic recombination and gene conversion; S, sister chromatid exchange; T, cell transformation

In completing the tables, the following symbols indicate the consensus of the Working Group with regard to the results for each end-point:

+   considered to be positive for the specific end-point and level of biological complexity
+¹ considered to be positive, but only one valid study was available to the Working Group
–   considered to be negative
–¹ considered to be negative, but only one valid study was available to the Working Group
?   considered to be equivocal or inconclusive (e.g. there were contradictory results from different laboratories; there were confounding exposures; the results were equivocal)

Summary table of genetic and related effects of mercury and mercury compounds

	Nonmammalian systems					Mammalian, fish and amphibian systems			
	Prokaryotes	Lower eukaryotes	Plants	Insects		In vitro		In vivo	
						Animal cells	Human cells	Animals	Humans
Compound	D G	D R G A	D G	C* R G C A		D G S M C A* T I	D G S M C A* T	D G S M C DL A*	D S M C A

Compound	D	G	D	R	G	A	D	G	C*	R	G	C	A	D	G	S	M	C	A*	T	I	D	G	S	M	C	A*	T	D	G	S	M	C	DL	A*	D	S	M	C	A
Inorganic mercury																																								
Metallic mercury																																					+?	??	−	−?
Amalgams																																								
Mercuric chloride	−		??	+?				+?						+	+?	??	−?	+?	+?	+?				+?		??				??	??	+?	??	+?	−					
Mercurous chloride	+?																																							
Mercuric acetate																	+?																−							
Organomercury																																								
Methylmercury chloride[b]	+?		−?	??				+?	+?				+?	+			+?	+?	+?						+?		+		??		??	+?	??	+	+				??	??
Methylmercury hydroxide		−?					+		+	−?	+	??	+	−?			+?																		??					
Methylmercury acetate[c]																																								
Methylmercury dicyandiamide									+?																								−?							
Methoxyethyl-mercury chloride									+				−	+?						+?	+?						+?	+?												
Bis(ethylmercury) hydrogen phosphate	−?																																							
Dimethylmercury			+?														+?																							
Ethylmercury																																								
Ethylmercury chloride									+?								+?			+?							+?	+?												

Summary table of genetic and related effects of mercury and mercury compounds (contd)

	Nonmammalian systems						Mammalian, fish and amphibian systems				
	Proka-ryotes	Lower eukaryotes	Plants	Insects			In vitro			In vivo	
							Animal cells	Human cells		Animals	Humans
Compound	D G	D R G A	D G C*	R G C	A		D G S M C A* T	D G S M C A* T		D G S M C DL A*	D S M C A
Organomercury (contd)											
Butylmercury bromide			+?								
Phenylmercury	–?										?
Phenylmercury chloride			+				+?				?
Phenylmercury hydroxide			+								+? ?
Phenylmercury acetate	?		+?		+?						?
Phenylmercury nitrate					+?			+?			+? ? +?
Mercury fulminate											
Mixture of mercury compounds				?							
Fungicides											
Panogen 5[d]			+?								
Panogen 8[e]			+?								
Panogen 15[f]			+								
Ceresan[g]			+								
Agrimax M[h]				+?							
Ceresan M[i]											
Granosan[j]			+	–							
Agallol[k]											

APPENDIX 1

Summary table of genetic and related effects of mercury and mercury compounds (contd)

Compound	Nonmammalian systems														Mammalian, fish and amphibian systems																	
	Prokaryotes	Lower eukaryotes				Plants			Insects				In vitro													In vivo					Humans				
													Animal cells							Human cells						Animals								
	D	G	D	R	G	A	D	G	C*	R	G	C	A	D	G	S	M	C	A*	T	D	G	S	M	C	A*	T	I	D	G	S	M	C	DL	A*	D	S	M	C	A
Fungicides (contd)																																								
Betoxin[f]	–[1]																																							
New improved ceresan[m]									+[1]																															
Azo dye																																								
Mercury orange									+[1]																															
Alimentary sources																																								
Mercury-contaminated fish or seal																														–[1]			?				?	?	?

A, aneuploidy; C, chromosomal aberrations; D, DNA damage; DL, dominant lethal mutation; G, gene mutation; I, inhibition of intercellular communication; M, micronuclei; R, mitotic recombination and gene conversion; S, sister chromatid exchange; T, cell transformation

In completing the tables, the following symbols indicate the consensus of the Working Group with regard to the results for each end-point.

+ considered to be positive for the specific end-point and level of biological complexity
+[1] considered to be positive, but only one valid study was available to the Working Group
– considered to be negative
–[1] considered to be negative, but only one valid study was available to the Working Group
? considered to be equivocal or inconclusive (e.g. there were contradictory results from different laboratories; there were confounding exposures; the results were equivocal)

[a] Including spindle disturbances; [b] Micronuclei in plants, +; [c] Sperm head abnormality, mice in vivo, –[1]; [d] Containing methylmercury diacyandiamide (5 g Hg/L); [e] Containing methylmercury diacyandiamide (6.4 Hg/L); [f] Containing methylmercury diacyandiamide (2.3%); [g] Containing phenylmercury acetate; [h] Containing phenylmercury dinaphthylmethanedisulfonate; [i] Containing ethylmercury-p-toluenesulfanylamide; [j] Containing ethylmercury chloride; [k] Containing methoxyethylmercury chloride; [l] Containing ethylmercury halogenide (90%); [m] Containing ethylmercury phosphate

APPENDIX 2

ACTIVITY PROFILES FOR GENETIC AND RELATED EFFECTS

APPENDIX 2

ACTIVITY PROFILES FOR
GENETIC AND RELATED EFFECTS

Methods

The x-axis of the activity profile (Waters *et al.*, 1987, 1988) represents the bioassays in phylogenetic sequence by endpoint, and the values on the y-axis represent the logarithmically transformed lowest effective doses (LED) and highest ineffective doses (HID) tested. The term 'dose', as used in this report, does not take into consideration length of treatment or exposure and may therefore be considered synonymous with concentration. In practice, the concentrations used in all the in-vitro tests were converted to µg/ml, and those for in-vivo tests were expressed as mg/kg bw. Because dose units are plotted on a log scale, differences in molecular weights of compounds do not, in most cases, greatly influence comparisons of their activity profiles. Conventions for dose conversions are given below.

Profile-line height (the magnitude of each bar) is a function of the LED or HID, which is associated with the characteristics of each individual test system—such as population size, cell-cycle kinetics and metabolic competence. Thus, the detection limit of each test system is different, and, across a given activity profile, responses will vary substantially. No attempt is made to adjust or relate responses in one test system to those of another.

Line heights are derived as follows: for negative test results, the highest dose tested without appreciable toxicity is defined as the HID. If there was evidence of extreme toxicity, the next highest dose is used. A single dose tested with a negative result is considered to be equivalent to the HID. Similarly, for positive results, the LED is recorded. If the original data were analysed statistically by the author, the dose recorded is that at which the response was significant ($p < 0.05$). If the available data were not analysed statistically, the dose required to produce an effect is estimated as follows: when a dose-related positive response is observed with two or more doses, the lower of the doses is taken as the LED; a single dose resulting in a positive response is considered to be equivalent to the LED.

In order to accommodate both the wide range of doses encountered and positive and negative responses on a continuous scale, doses are transformed logarithmically, so that effective (LED) and ineffective (HID) doses are represented by positive and negative numbers, respectively. The response, or logarithmic dose unit (LDU_{ij}), for a given test system i and chemical j is represented by the expressions

$LDU_{ij} = -\log_{10}$ (dose), for HID values; LDU ≤ 0

and (1)

$LDU_{ij} = -\log_{10}$ (dose $\times$ 10^{-5}), for LED values; LDU ≥ 0.

These simple relationships define a dose range of 0 to -5 logarithmic units for ineffective doses (1–100 000 µg/ml or mg/kg bw) and 0 to $+8$ logarithmic units for effective doses (100 000–0.001 µg/ml or mg/kg bw). A scale illustrating the LDU values is shown in Figure 1. Negative responses at doses less than 1 µg/ml (mg/kg bw) are set equal to 1. Effectively, an LED value $\geq$100 000 or an HID value $\leq$1 produces an LDU = 0; no quantitative information is gained from such extreme values. The dotted lines at the levels of log dose units 1 and -1 define a 'zone of uncertainty' in which positive results are reported at such high doses (between 10 000 and 100 000 µg/ml or mg/kg bw) or negative results are reported at such low dose levels (1 to 10 µg/ml or mg/kg bw) as to call into question the adequacy of the test.

Fig. 1. Scale of log dose units used on the y-axis of activity profiles

Positive (µg/ml or mg/kg bw)		Log dose units	
0.001		8	—
0.01		7	—
0.1		6	—
1.0		5	—
10		4	—
100		3	—
1000		2	—
10 000		1	—
100 000	1	0	—
	10	-1	—
	100	-2	—
	1000	-3	—
	10 000	-4	—
	100 000	-5	—
	Negative (µg/ml or mg/kg bw)		

LED and HID are expressed as µg/ml or mg/kg bw.

In practice, an activity profile is computer generated. A data entry programme is used to store abstracted data from published reports. A sequential file (in ASCII) is created for each compound, and a record within that file consists of the name and Chemical Abstracts Service number of the compound, a three-letter code for the test system (see below), the qualitative test result (with and without an exogenous metabolic system), dose (LED or HID), citation number and additional source information. An abbreviated citation for each publication is stored in a segment of a record accessing both the test data file and the citation file. During processing of the data file, an average of the logarithmic values of the data subset is calculated, and the length of the profile line represents this average value. All dose values are plotted for each profile line, regardless of whether results are positive or negative. Results obtained in the absence of an exogenous metabolic system are indicated by a bar (–), and results obtained in the presence of an exogenous metabolic system are indicated by an upward-directed arrow (↑). When all results for a given assay are either positive or negative, the mean of the LDU values is plotted as a solid line; when conflicting data are reported for the same assay (i.e., both positive and negative results), the majority data are shown by a solid line and the minority data by a dashed line (drawn to the extreme conflicting response). In the few cases in which the numbers of positive and negative results are equal, the solid line is drawn in the positive direction and the maximal negative response is indicated with a dashed line.

Profile lines are identified by three-letter code words representing the commonly used tests. Code words for most of the test systems in current use in genetic toxicology were defined for the US Environmental Protection Agency's GENE-TOX Program (Waters, 1979; Waters & Auletta, 1981). For *IARC Monographs* Supplement 6, Volume 44 and subsequent volumes, including this publication, codes were redefined in a manner that should facilitate inclusion of additional tests. Naming conventions are described below.

Data listings are presented in the text and include endpoint and test codes, a short test code definition, results [either with (M) or without (NM) an exogenous activation system], the associated LED or HID value and a short citation. Test codes are organized phylogenetically and by endpoint from left to right across each activity profile and from top to bottom of the corresponding data listing. Endpoints are defined as follows: A, aneuploidy; C, chromosomal aberrations; D, DNA damage; F, assays of body fluids; G, gene mutation; H, host-mediated assays; I, inhibition of intercellular communication; M, micronuclei; P, sperm morphology; R, mitotic recombination or gene conversion; S, sister chromatid exchange; and T, cell transformation.

Dose conversions for activity profiles

Doses are converted to μg/ml for in-vitro tests and to mg/kg bw per day for in-vivo experiments.

1. In-vitro test systems
   (a) Weight/volume converts directly to μg/ml.
   (b) Molar (M) concentration × molecular weight = mg/ml = 10^3 μg/ml; mM concentration × molecular weight = μg/ml.
   (c) Soluble solids expressed as % concentration are assumed to be in units of mass per volume (i.e., 1% = 0.01 g/ml = 10 000 μg/ml; also, 1 ppm = 1 μg/ml).
   (d) Liquids and gases expressed as % concentration are assumed to be given in units of volume per volume. Liquids are converted to weight per volume using the density (D) of the solution (D = g/ml). Gases are converted from volume to mass using the ideal gas law, PV = nRT. For exposure at 20–37°C at standard atmospheric pressure, 1% (v/v) = 0.4 μg/ml × molecular weight of the gas. Also, 1 ppm (v/v) = 4 × 10^{-5} μg/ml × molecular weight.

(e) In microbial plate tests, it is usual for the doses to be reported as weight/plate, whereas concentrations are required to enter data on the activity profile chart. While remaining cognisant of the errors involved in the process, it is assumed that a 2-ml volume of top agar is delivered to each plate and that the test substance remains in solution within it; concentrations are derived from the reported weight/plate values by dividing by this arbitrary volume. For spot tests, a 1-ml volume is used in the calculation.

(f) Conversion of particulate concentrations given in µg/cm² are based on the area (A) of the dish and the volume of medium per dish; i.e., for a 100-mm dish: $A = \pi R^2 = \pi \times (5\ cm)^2 = 78.5\ cm^2$. If the volume of medium is 10 ml, then 78.5 cm² = 10 ml and 1 cm² = 0.13 ml.

2. In-vitro systems using in-vivo activation

For the body fluid–urine (BF–) test, the concentration used is the dose (in mg/kg bw) of the compound administered to test animals or patients.

3. In-vivo test systems

(a) Doses are converted to mg/kg bw per day of exposure, assuming 100% absorption. Standard values are used for each sex and species of rodent, including body weight and average intake per day, as reported by Gold *et al.* (1984). For example, in a test using male mice fed 50 ppm of the agent in the diet, the standard food intake per day is 12% of body weight, and the conversion is dose = 50 ppm × 12% = 6 mg/kg bw per day.

Standard values used for humans are: weight—males, 70 kg; females, 55 kg; surface area, 1.7 m²; inhalation rate, 20 l/min for light work, 30 l/min for mild exercise.

(b) When reported, the dose at the target site is used. For example, doses given in studies of lymphocytes of humans exposed *in vivo* are the measured blood concentrations in µg/ml.

Codes for test systems

For specific nonmammalian test systems, the first two letters of the three-symbol code word define the test organism (e.g., SA– for *Salmonella typhimurium*, EC– for *Escherichia coli*). If the species is not known, the convention used is –S–. The third symbol may be used to define the tester strain (e.g., SA8 for *S. typhimurium* TA1538, ECW for *E. coli* WP2*uvr*A). When strain designation is not indicated, the third letter is used to define the specific genetic endpoint under investigation (e.g., ––D for differential toxicity, ––F for forward mutation, ––G for gene conversion or genetic crossing-over, ––N for aneuploidy, ––R for reverse mutation, ––U for unscheduled DNA synthesis). The third letter may also be used to define the general endpoint under investigation when a more complete definition is not possible or relevant (e.g., ––M for mutation, ––C for chromosomal aberration).

For mammalian test systems, the first letter of the three-letter code word defines the genetic endpoint under investigation: A–– for aneuploidy, B–– for binding, C–– for chromosomal aberration, D–– for DNA strand breaks, G–– for gene mutation, I–– for inhibition of intercellular communication, M–– for micronucleus formation, R–– for DNA repair, S— for sister chromatid exchange, T— for cell transformation and U— for unscheduled DNA synthesis.

For animal (i.e., non-human) test systems *in vitro*, when the cell type is not specified, the code letters –IA are used. For such assays *in vivo*, when the animal species is not specified, the code letters –VA are used. Commonly used animal species are identified by the third letter (e.g., —C for Chinese hamster, —M for mouse, —R for rat, —S for Syrian hamster).

For test systems using human cells *in vitro*, when the cell type is not specified, the code letters –IH are used. For assays on humans *in vivo*, when the cell type is not specified, the code letters –VH are used. Otherwise, the second letter specifies the cell type under investigation (e.g., –BH for bone marrow, –LH for lymphocytes).

Some other specific coding conventions used for mammalian systems are as follows: BF– for body fluids, HM– for host-mediated, —L for leukocytes or lymphocytes *in vitro* (–AL, animals; –HL, humans), –L– for leukocytes *in vivo* (–LA, animals; –LH, humans), —T for transformed cells.

Note that these are examples of major conventions used to define the assay code words. The alphabetized listing of codes must be examined to confirm a specific code word. As might be expected from the limitation to three symbols, some codes do not fit the naming conventions precisely. In a few cases, test systems are defined by first-letter code words, for example: MST, mouse spot test; SLP, mouse specific locus test, postspermatogonia; SLO, mouse specific locus test, other stages; DLM, dominant lethal test in mice; DLR, dominant lethal test in rats; MHT, mouse heritable translocation test.

The genetic activity profiles and listings were prepared in collaboration with Environmental Health Research and Testing Inc. (EHRT) under contract to the US Environmental Protection Agency; EHRT also determined the doses used. The references cited in each genetic activity profile listing can be found in the list of references in the appropriate monograph.

References

Garrett, N.E., Stack, H.F., Gross, M.R. & Waters, M.D. (1984) An analysis of the spectra of genetic activity produced by known or suspected human carcinogens. *Mutat. Res.*, *134*, 89–111

Gold, L.S., Sawyer, C.B., Magaw, R., Backman, G.M., de Veciana, M., Levinson, R., Hooper, N.K., Havender, W.R., Bernstein, L., Peto, R., Pike, M.C. & Ames, B.N. (1984) A carcinogenic potency database of the standardized results of animal bioassays. *Environ. Health Perspect.*, *58*, 9–319

Waters, M.D. (1979) *The GENE-TOX program*. In: Hsie, A.W., O'Neill, J.P. & McElheny, V.K., eds, *Mammalian Cell Mutagenesis: The Maturation of Test Systems* (Banbury Report 2), Cold Spring Harbor, NY, CSH Press, pp. 449–467

Waters, M.D. & Auletta, A. (1981) The GENE-TOX program: genetic activity evaluation. *J. chem. Inf. comput. Sci.*, *21*, 35–38

Waters, M.D., Stack, H.F., Brady, A.L., Lohman, P.H.M., Haroun, L. & Vainio, H. (1987) Appendix 1: Activity profiles for genetic and related tests. In: *IARC Monographs on the Evaluation of the Carcinogenic Risk of Chemicals to Humans*, Suppl. 6, *Genetic and Related Effects: An Updating of Selected IARC Monographs from Volumes 1 to 42*, Lyon, IARC, pp. 687–696

Waters, M.D., Stack, H.F., Brady, A.L., Lohman, P.H.M., Haroun, L. & Vainio, H. (1988) Use of computerized data listings and activity profiles of genetic and related effects in the review of 195 compounds. *Mutat. Res.*, 205, 295-312

APPENDIX 2

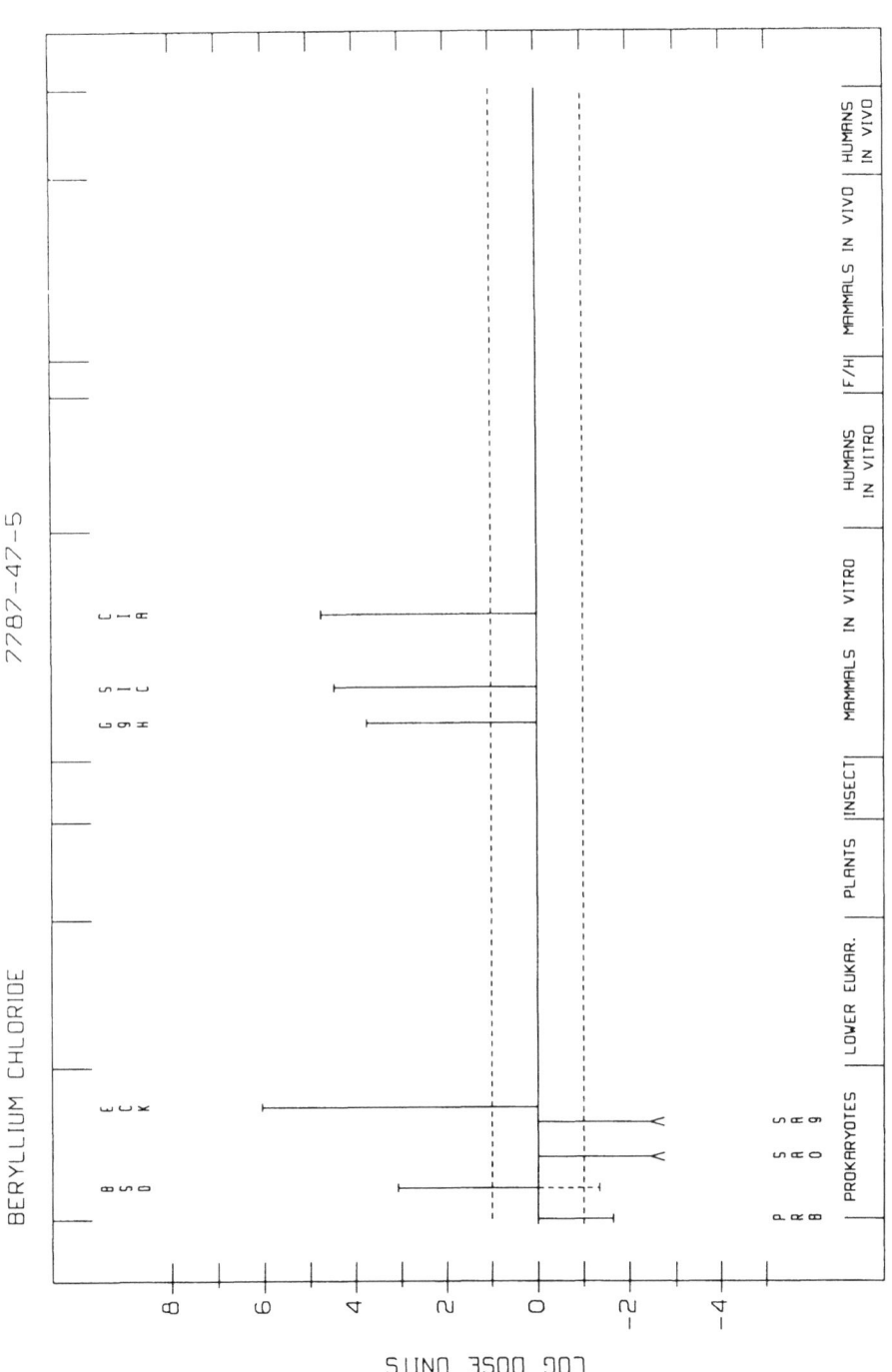

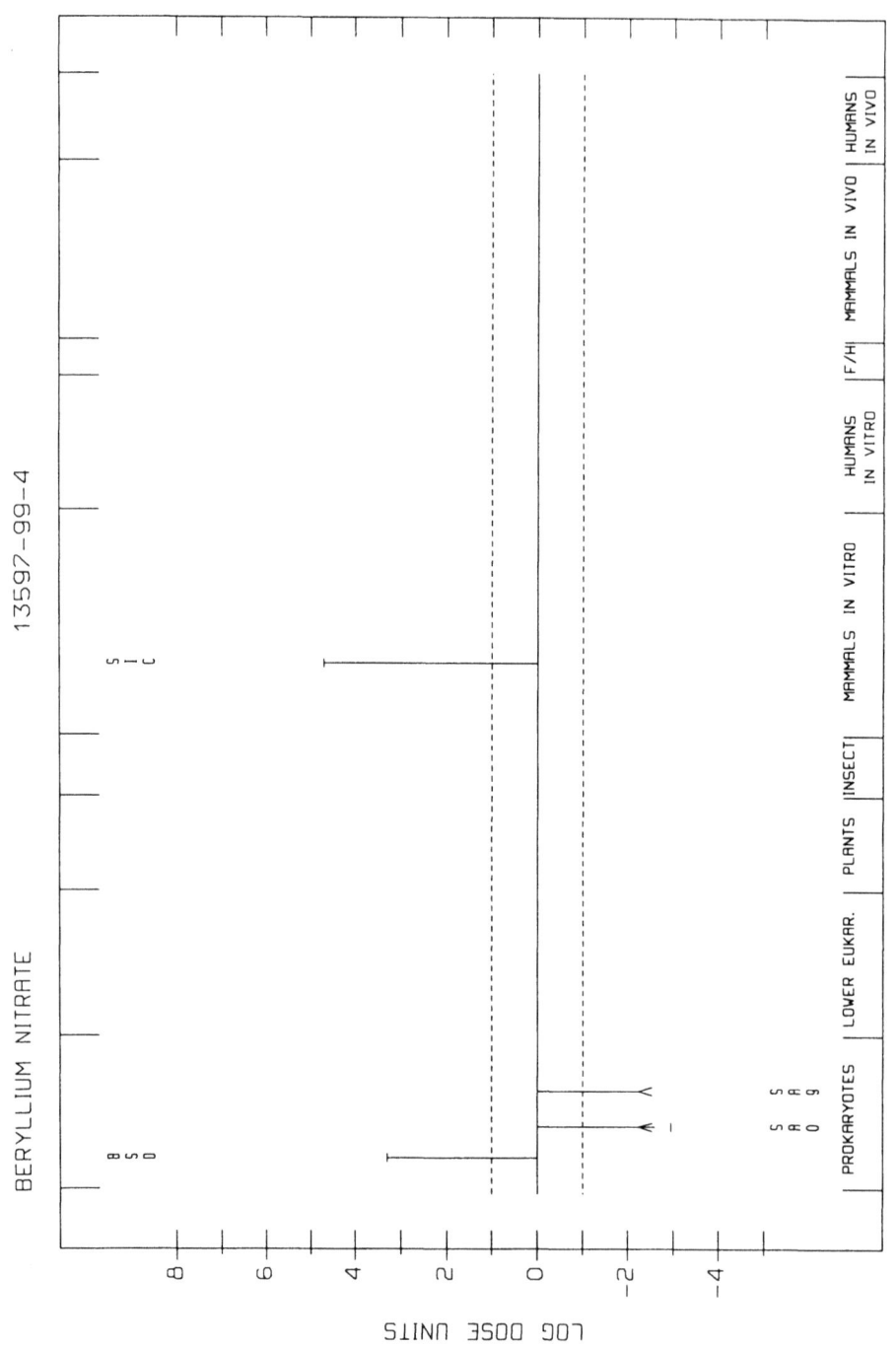

APPENDIX 2

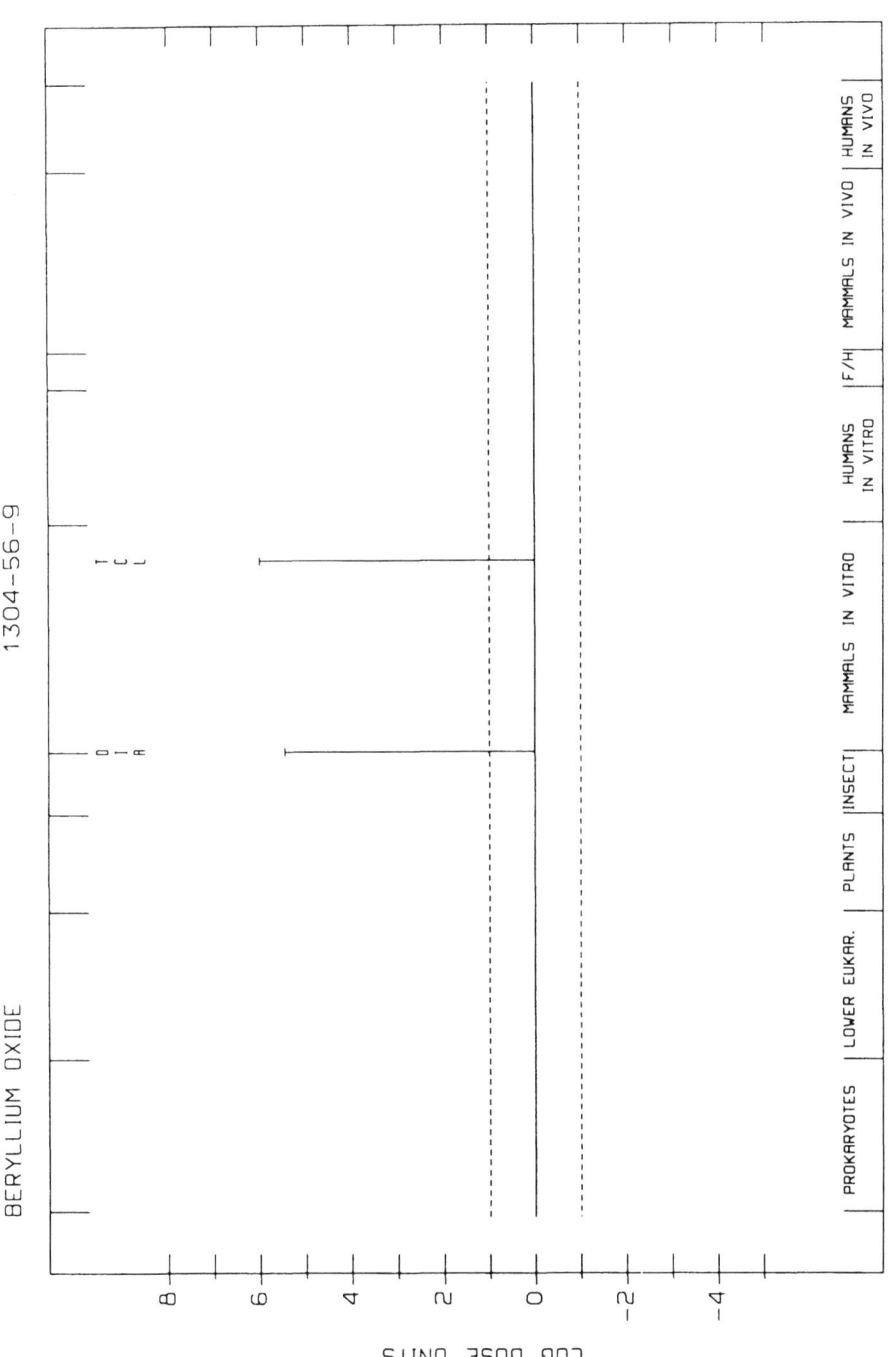

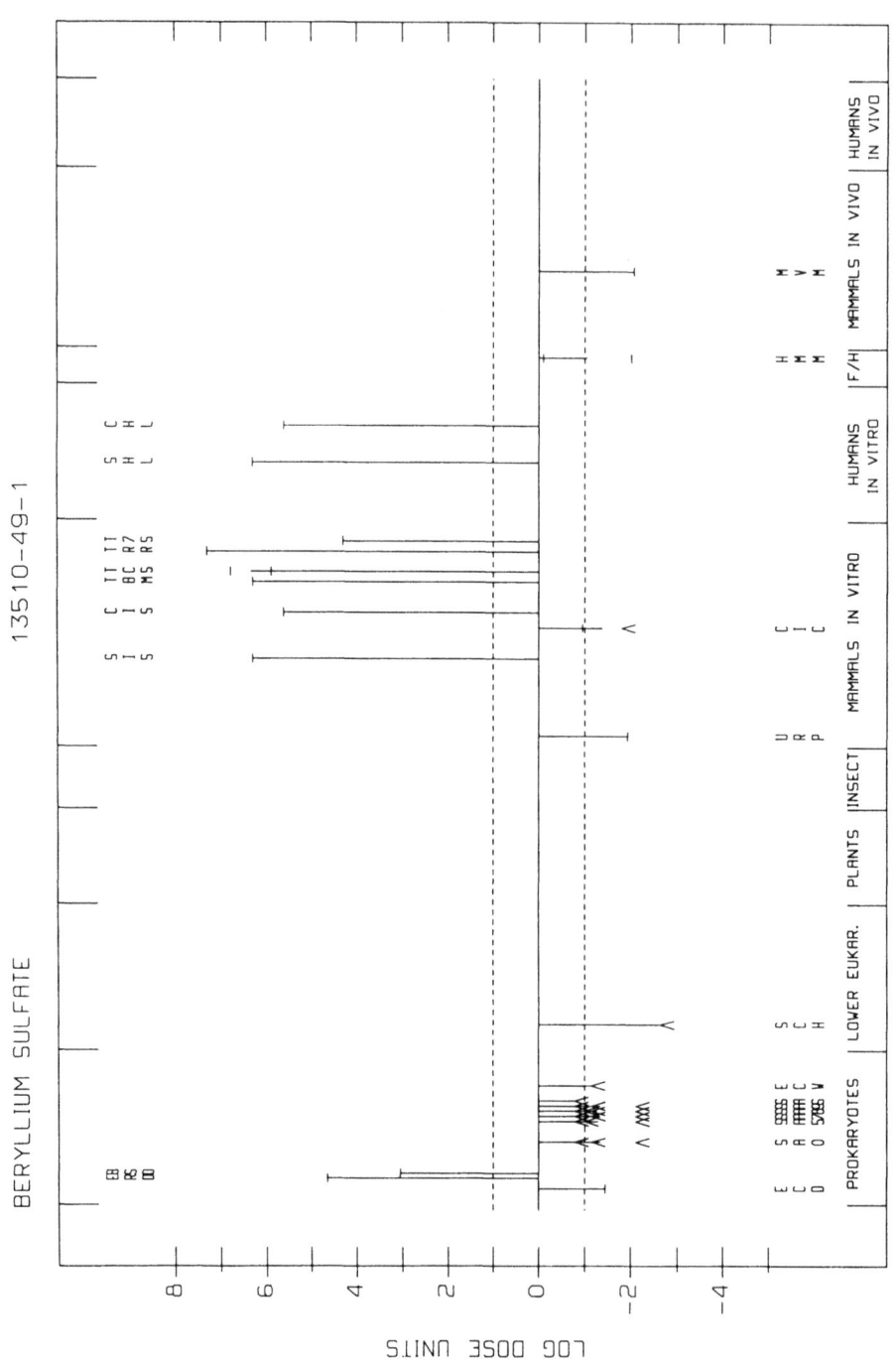

APPENDIX 2

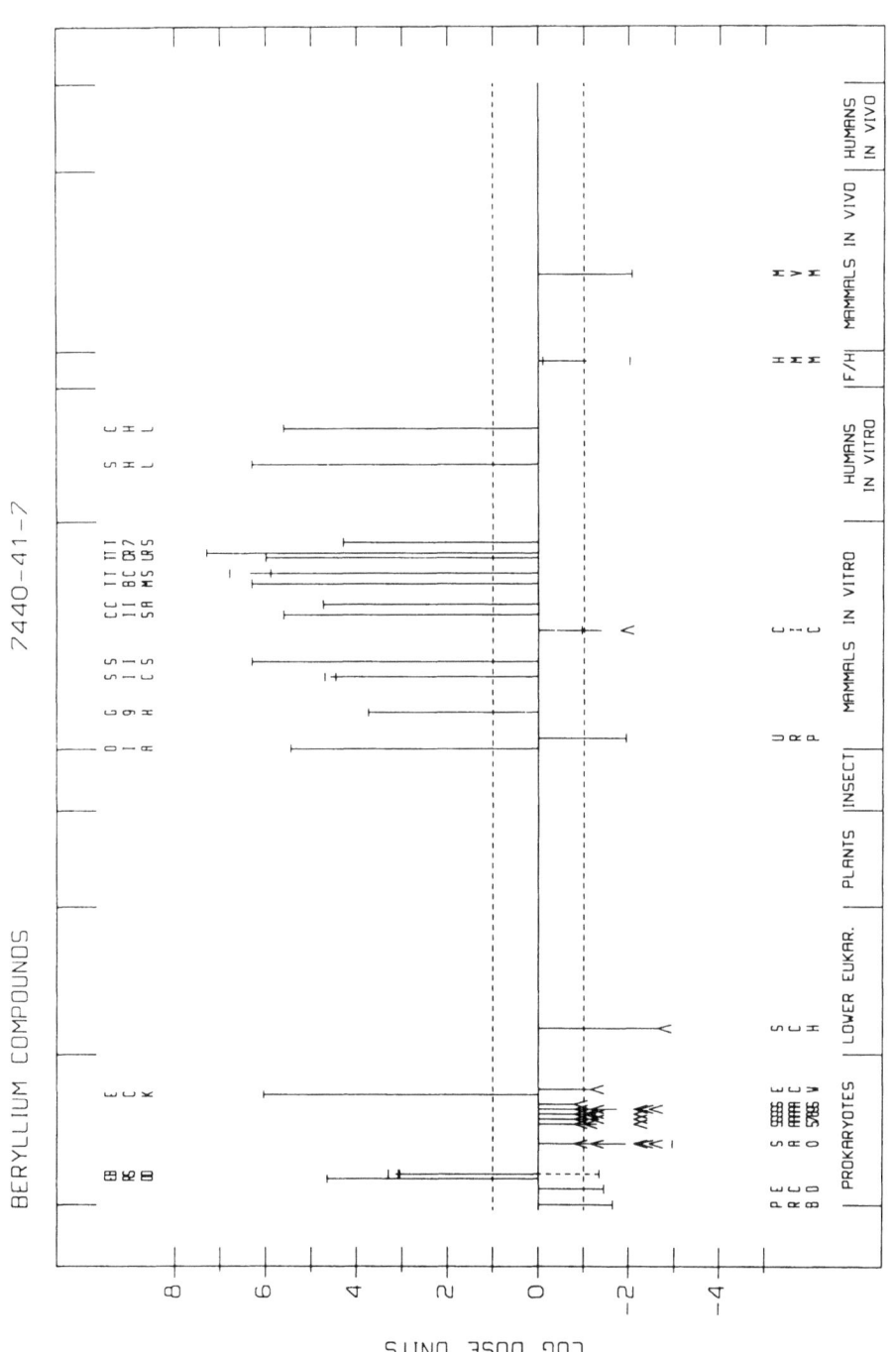

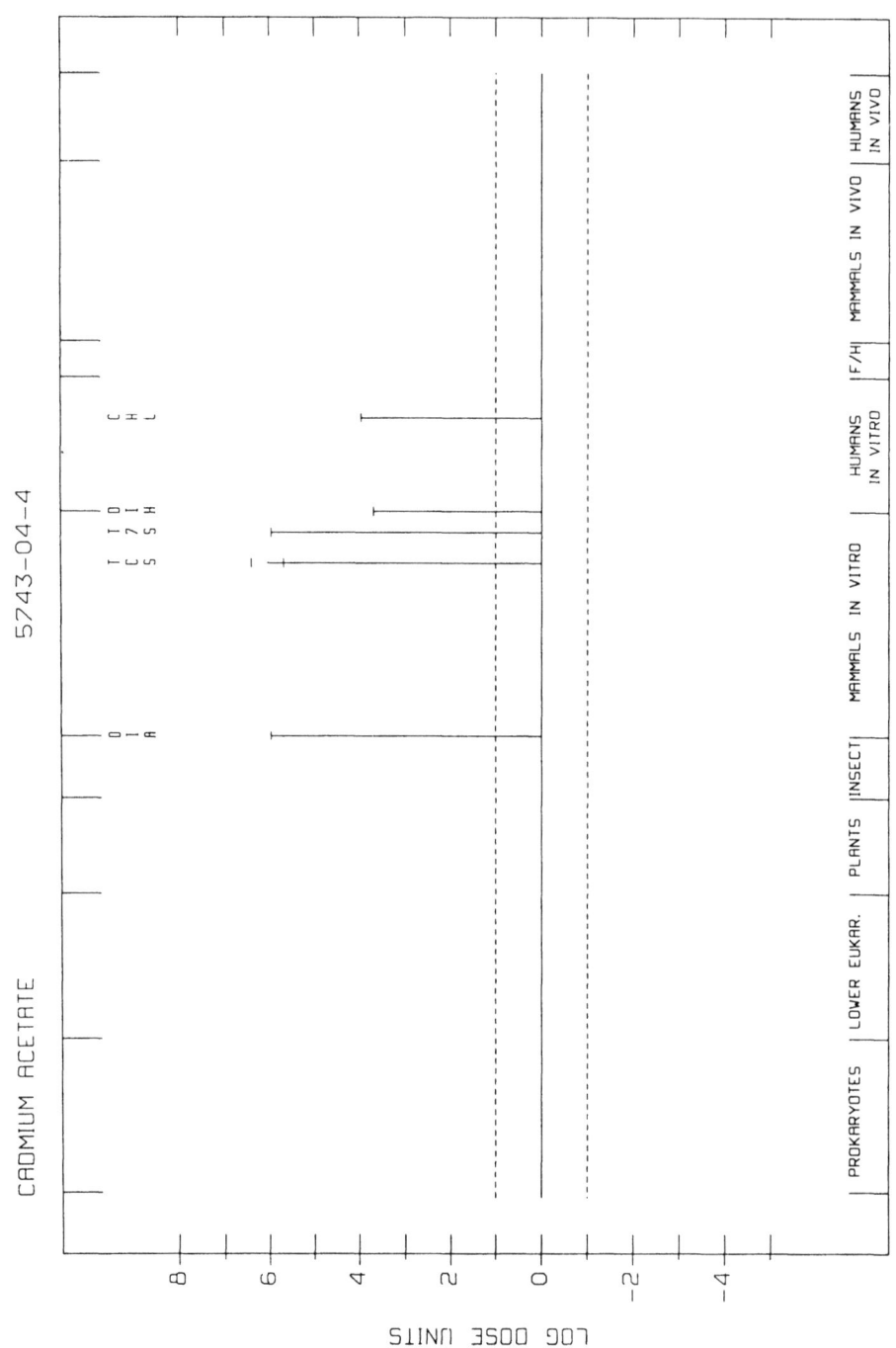

APPENDIX 2

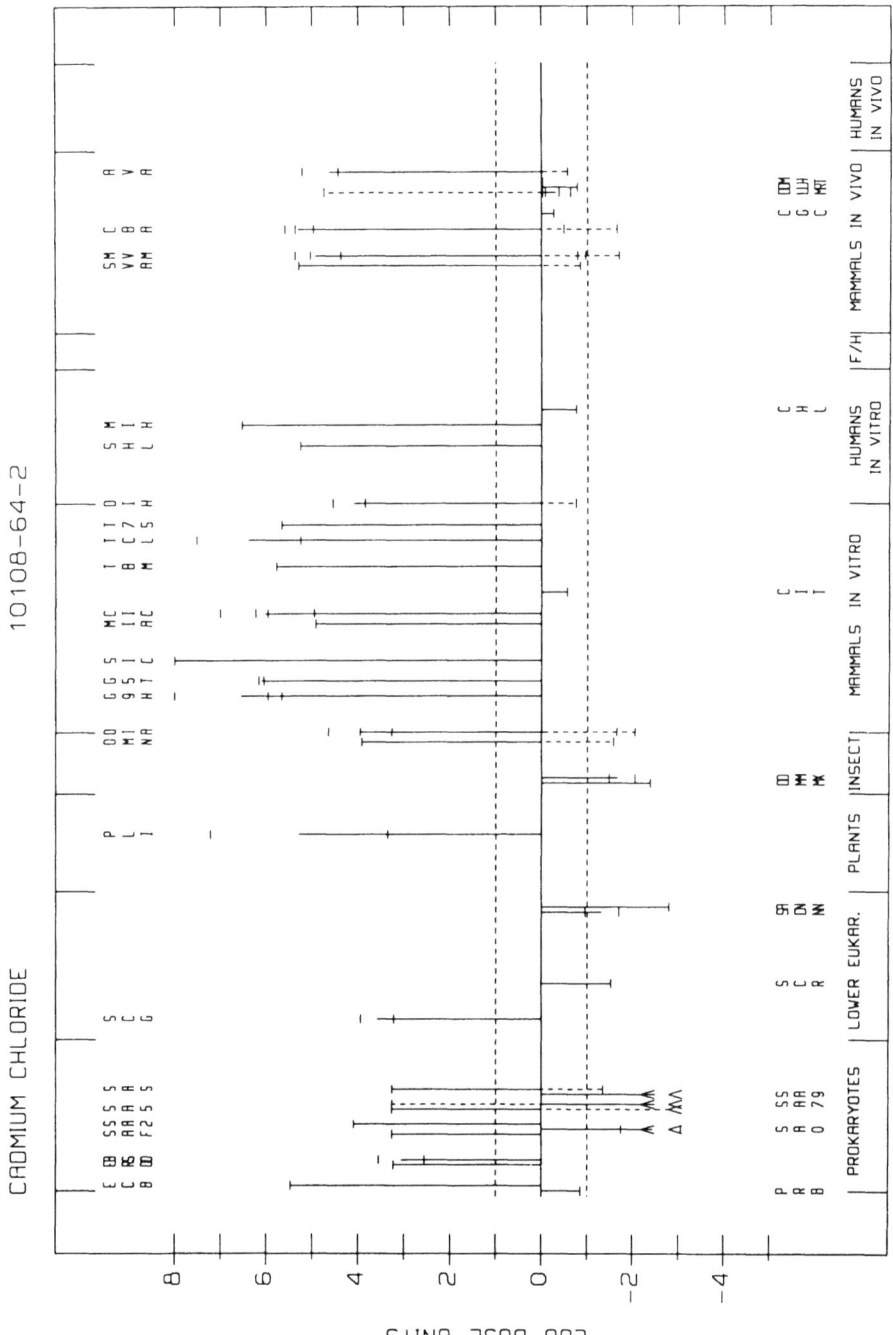

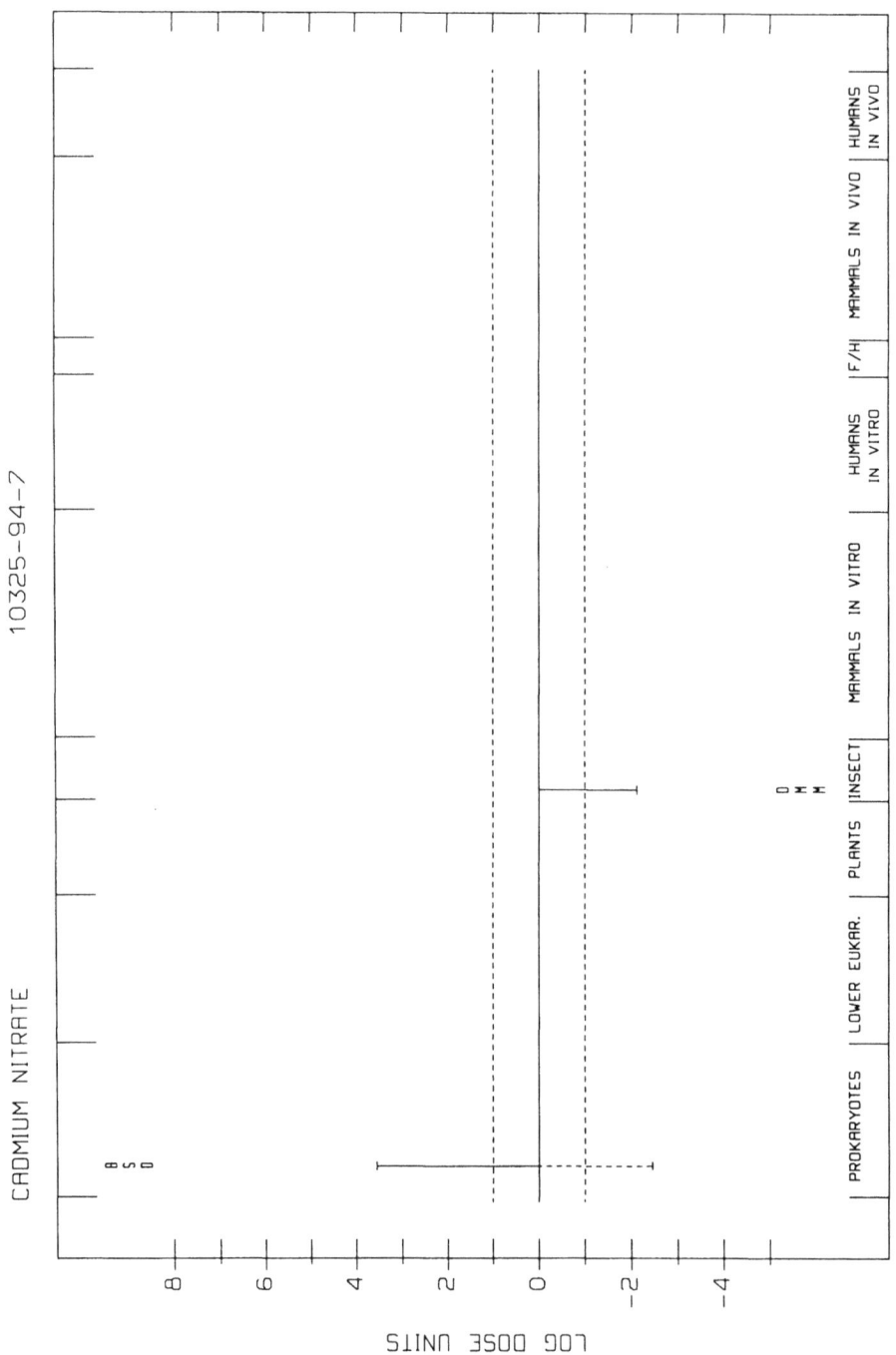

APPENDIX 2

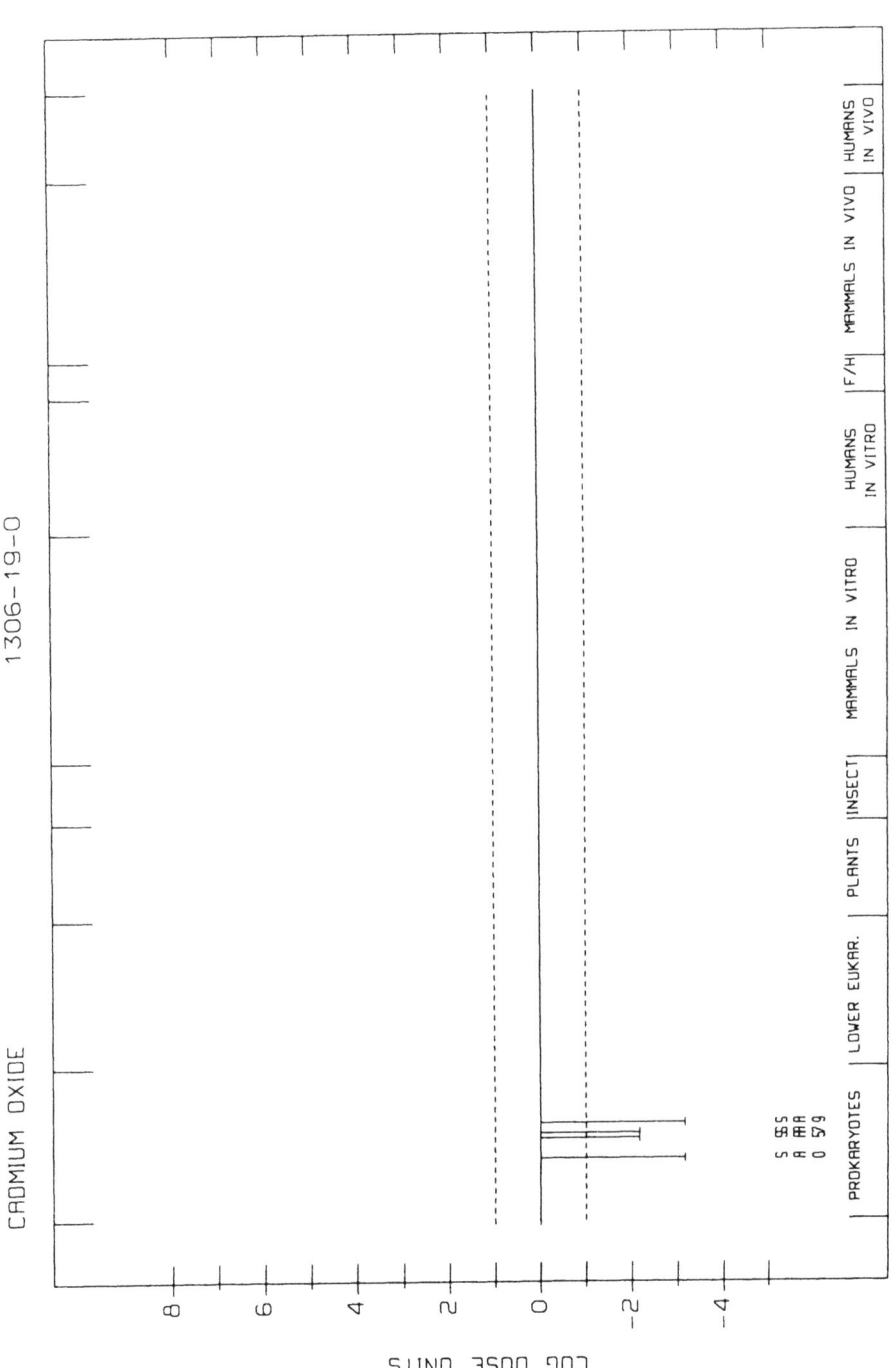

404

IARC MONOGRAPHS VOLUME 58

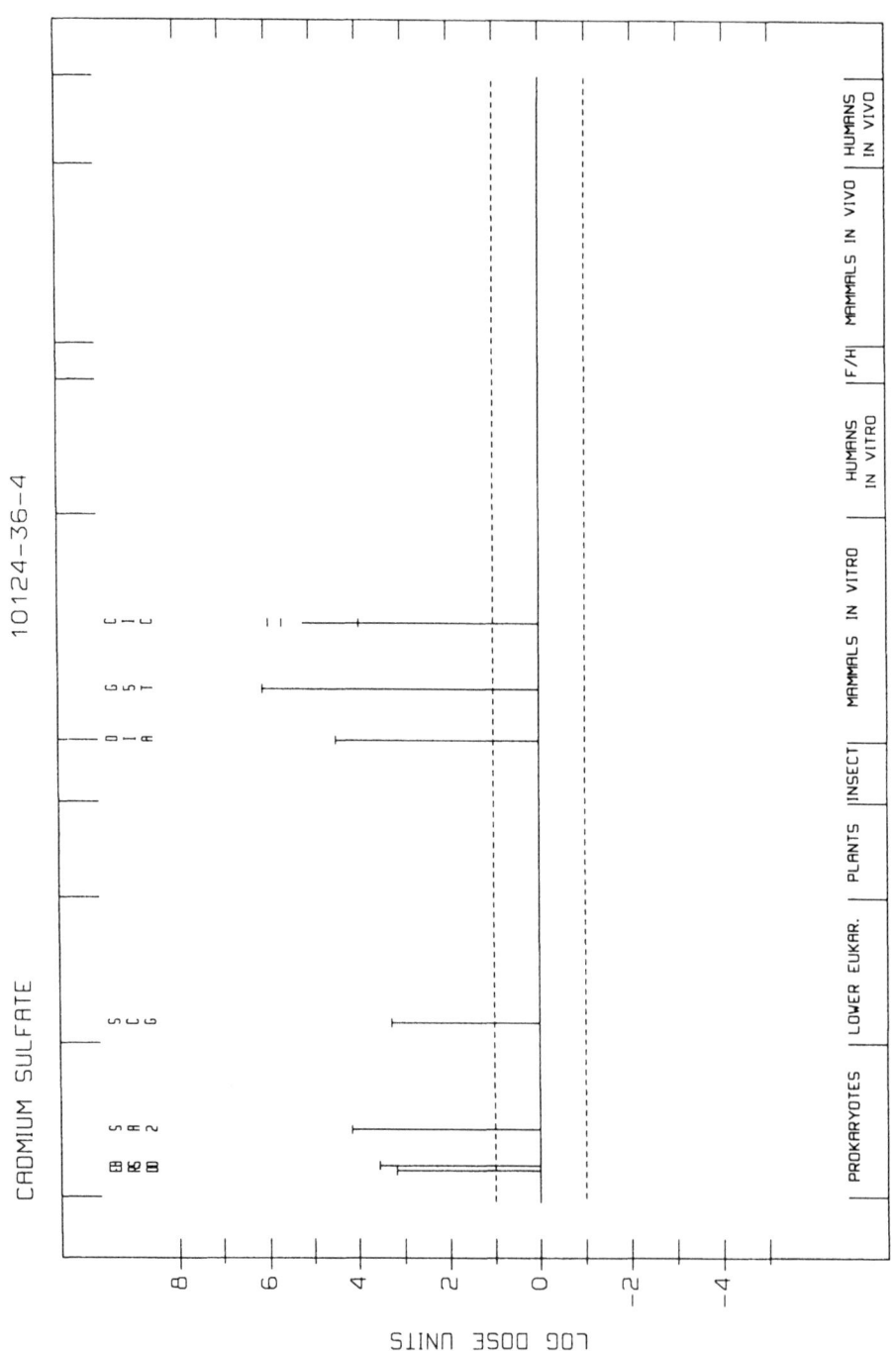

APPENDIX 2

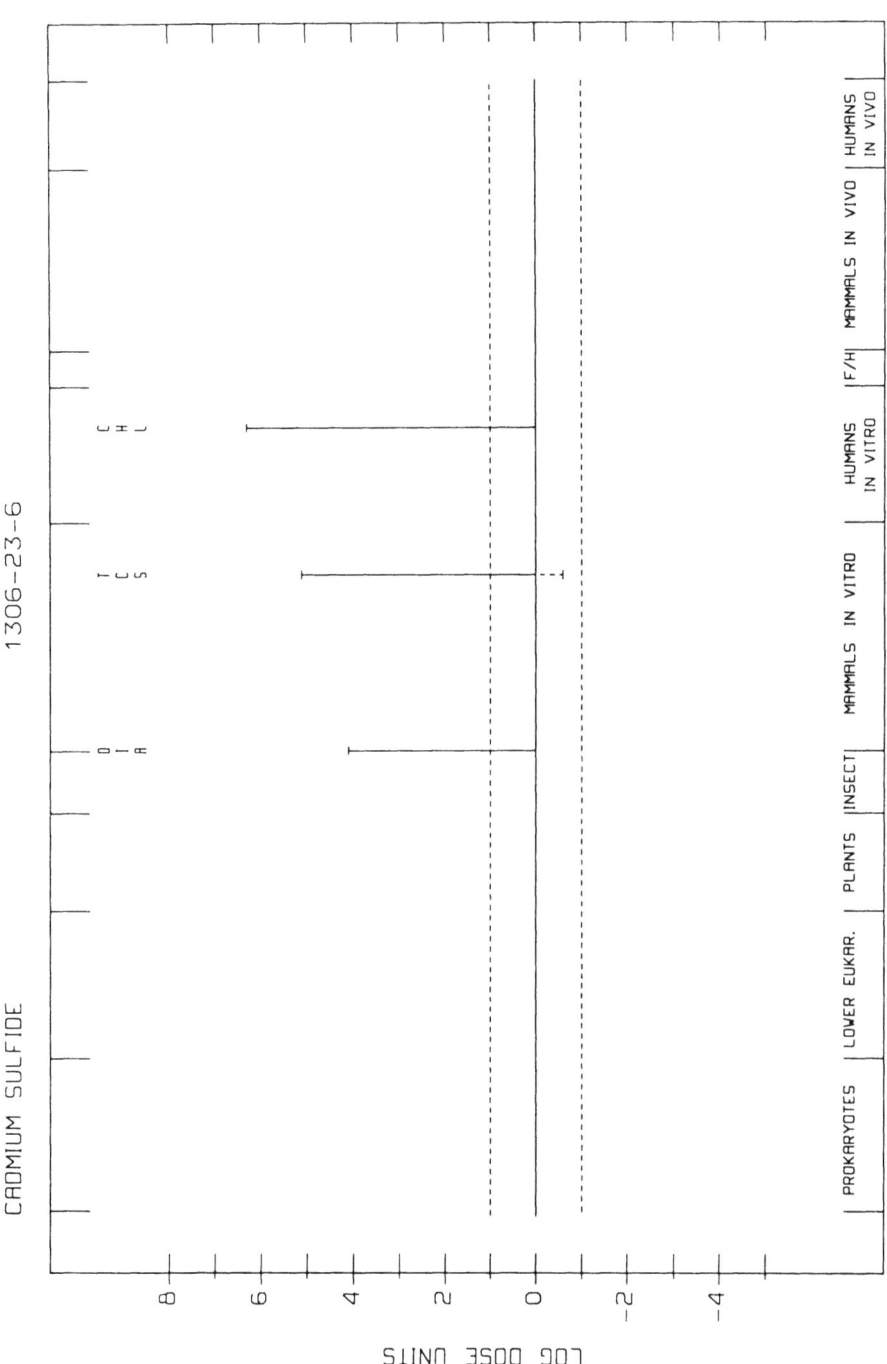

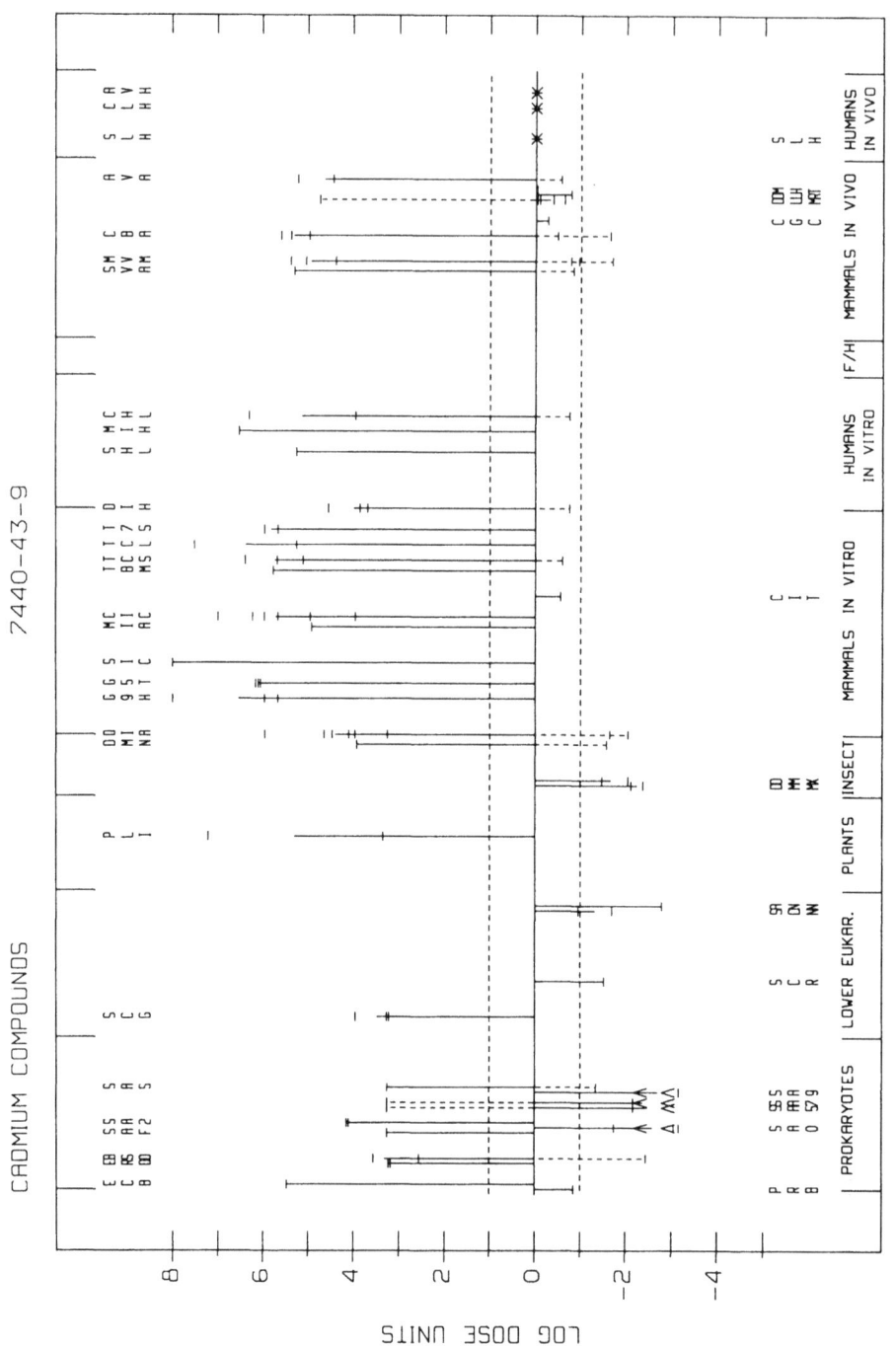

APPENDIX 2

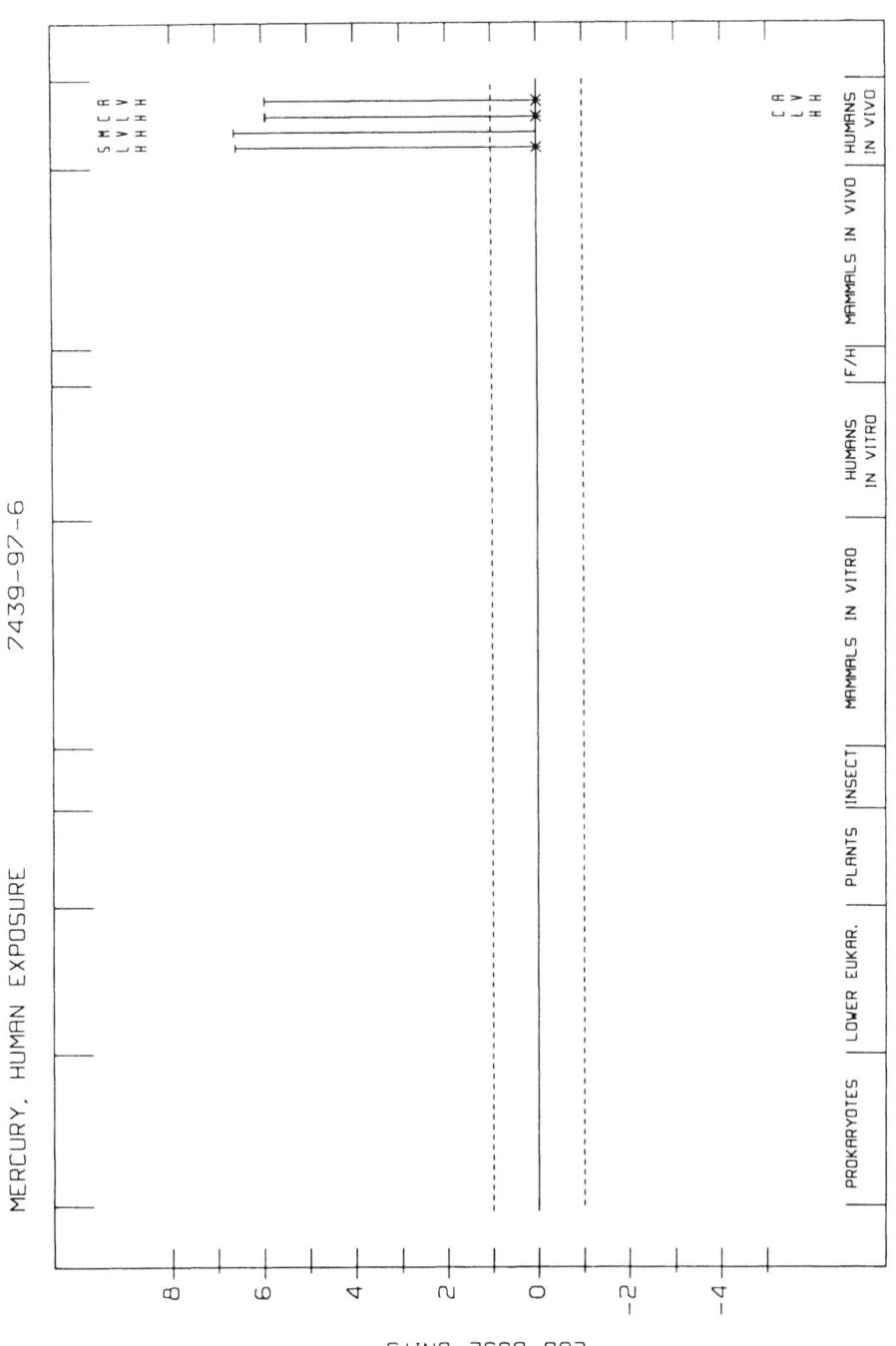

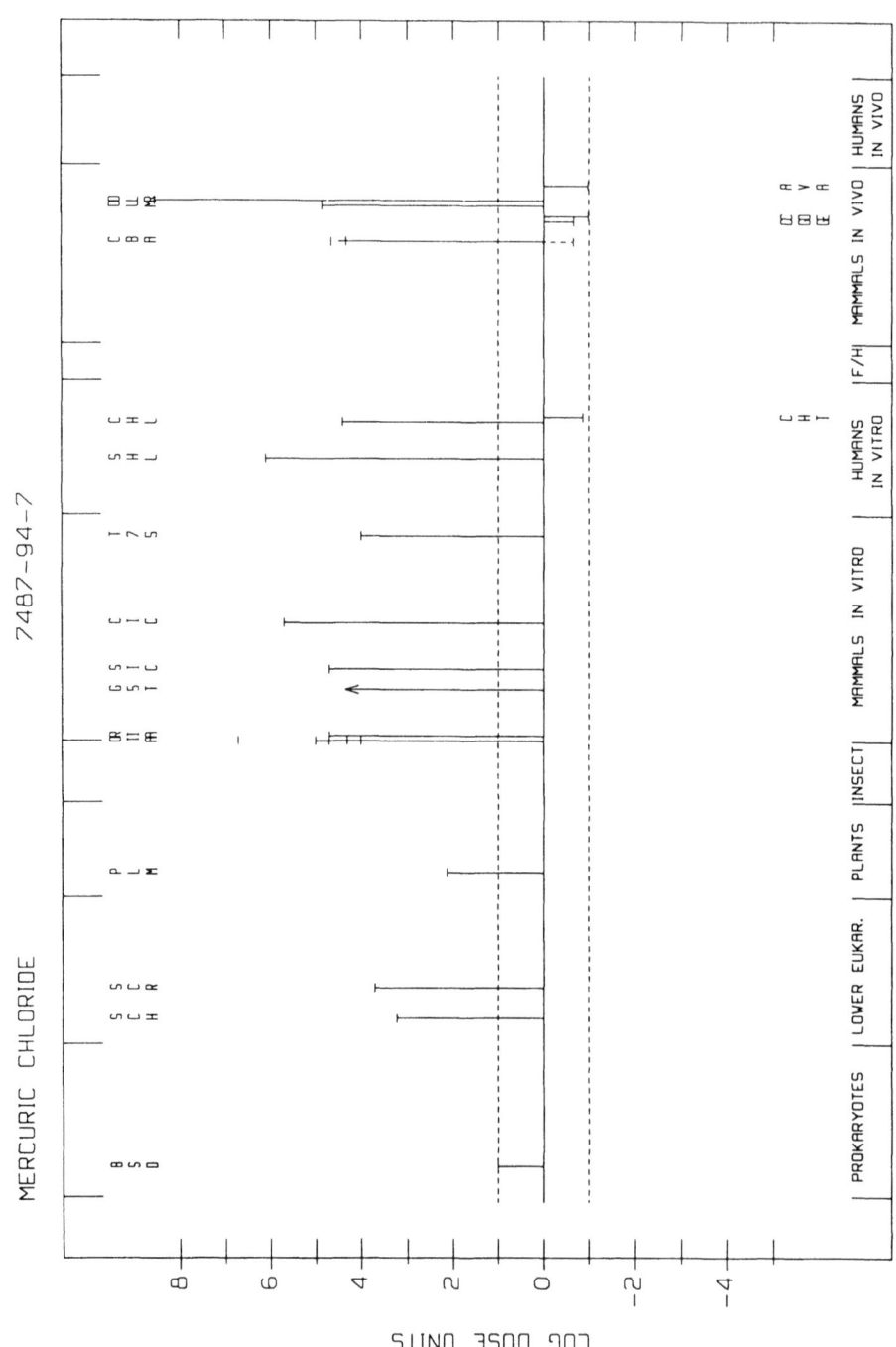

APPENDIX 2

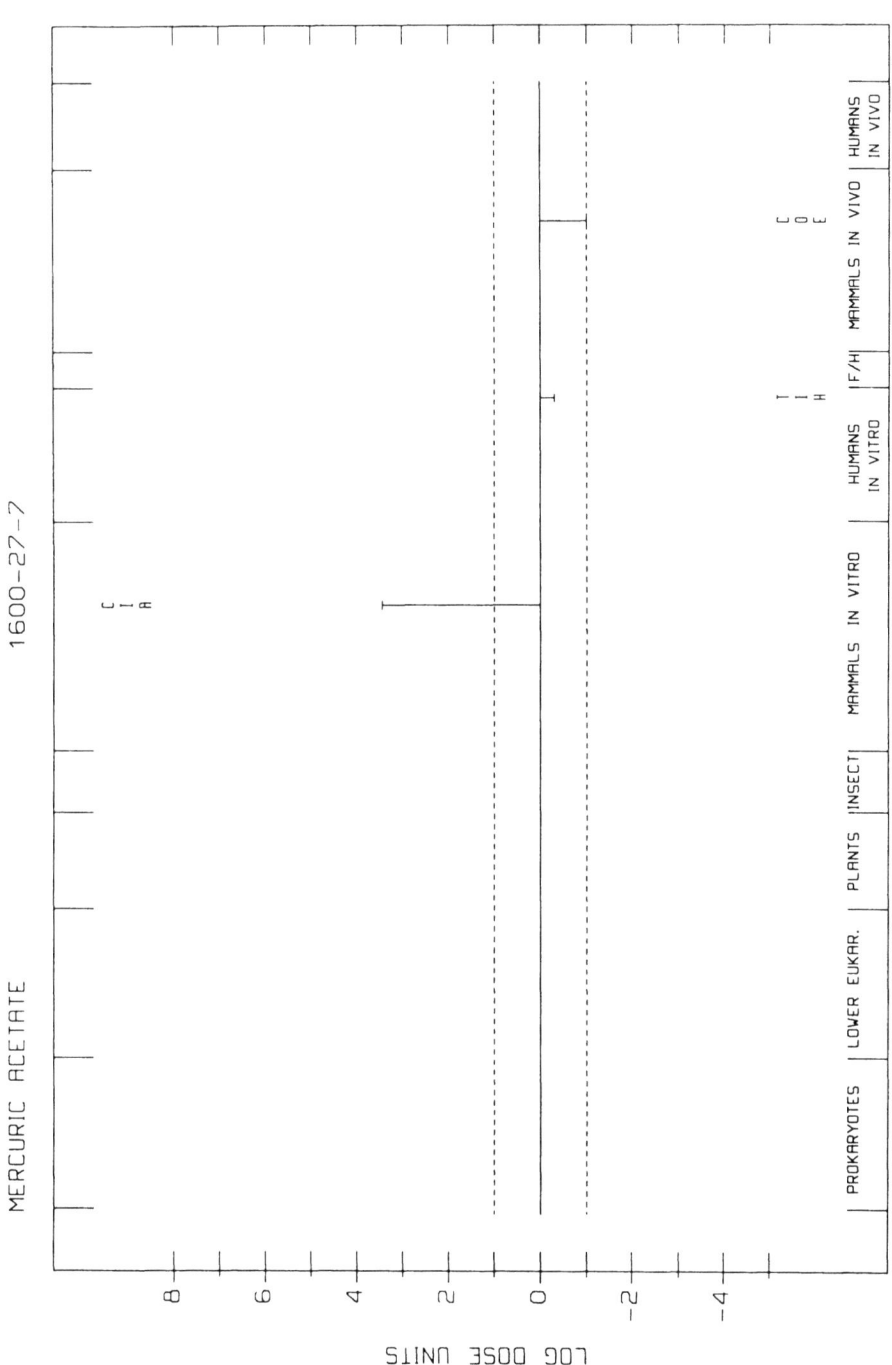

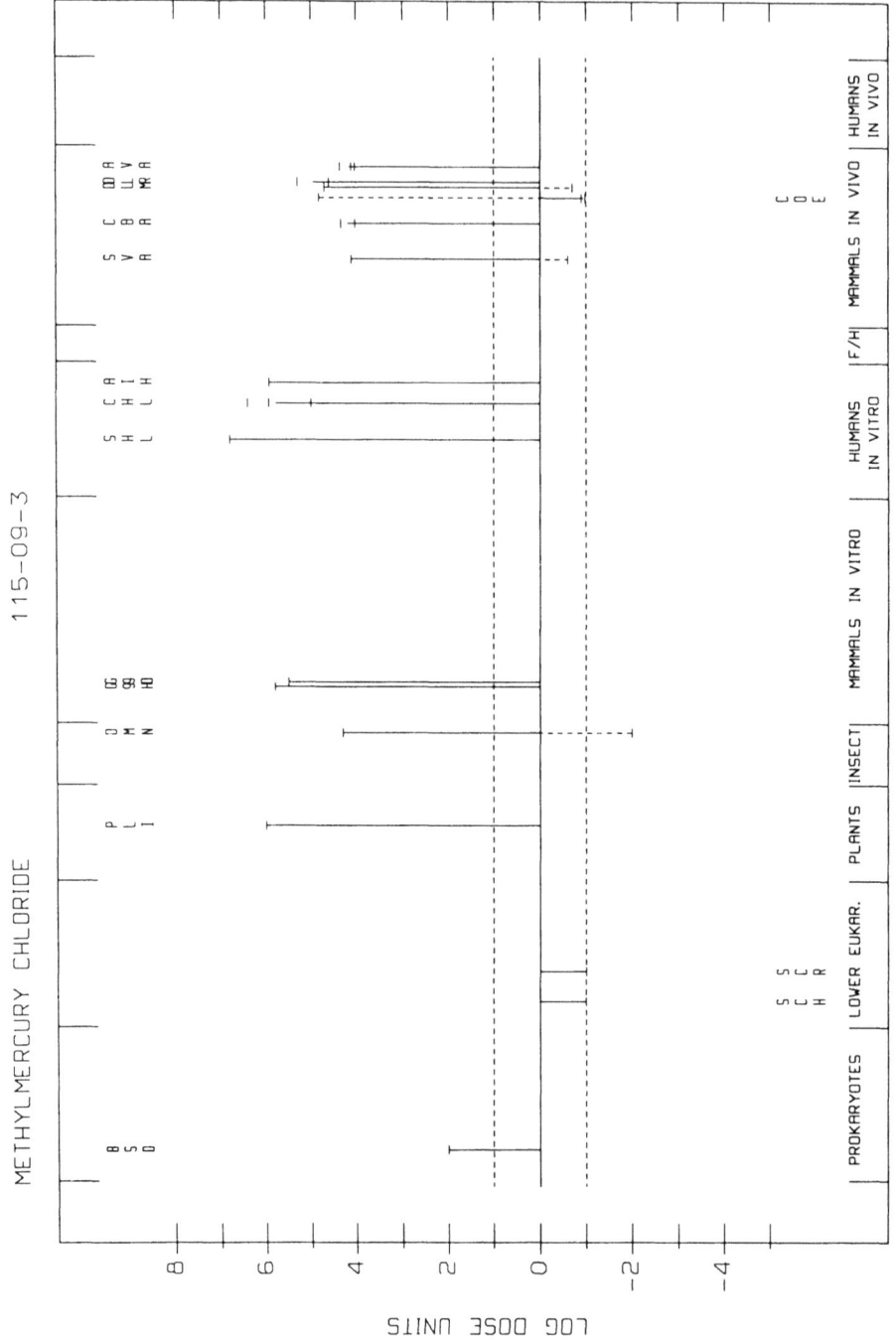

APPENDIX 2

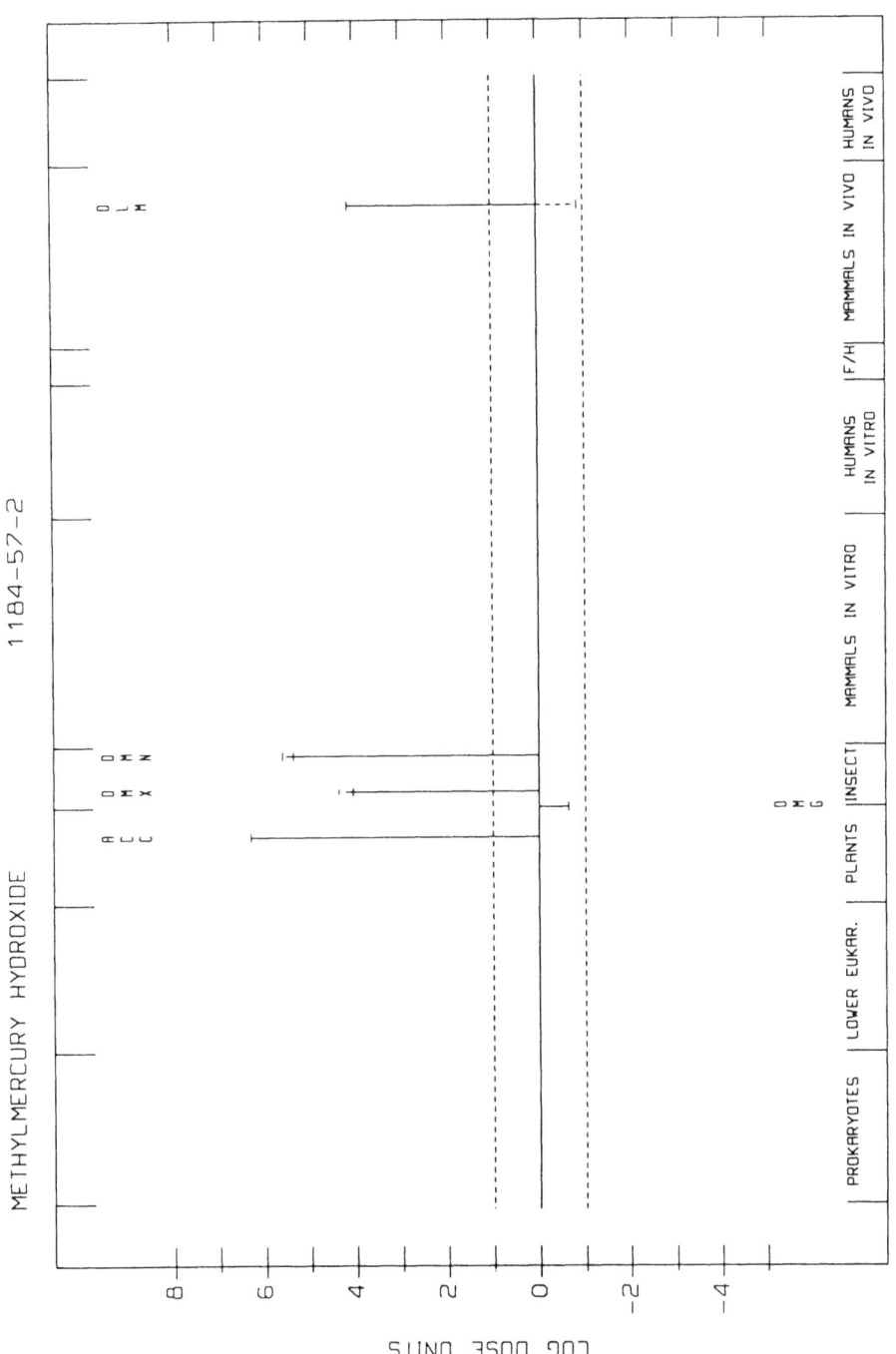

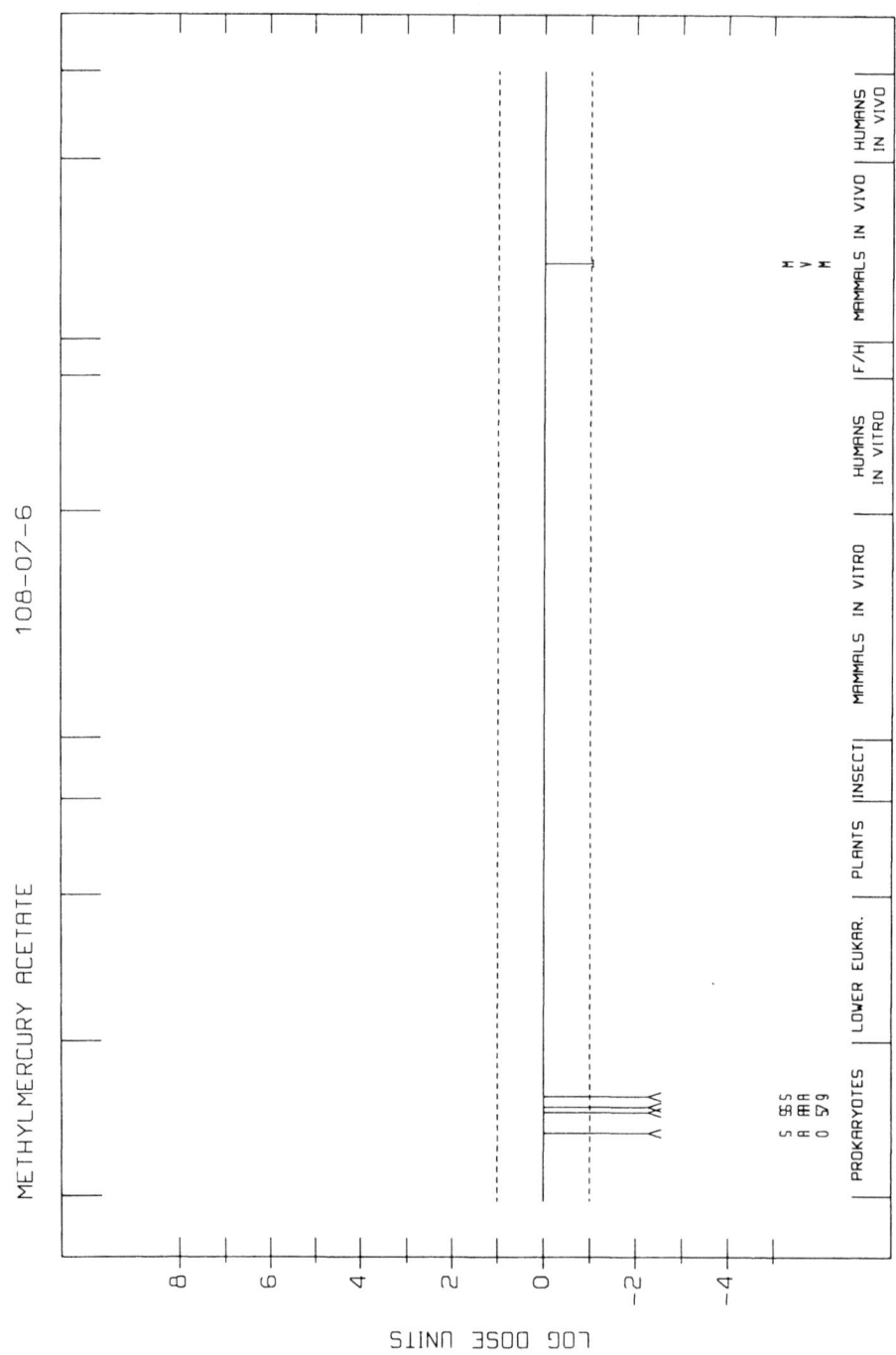

APPENDIX 2

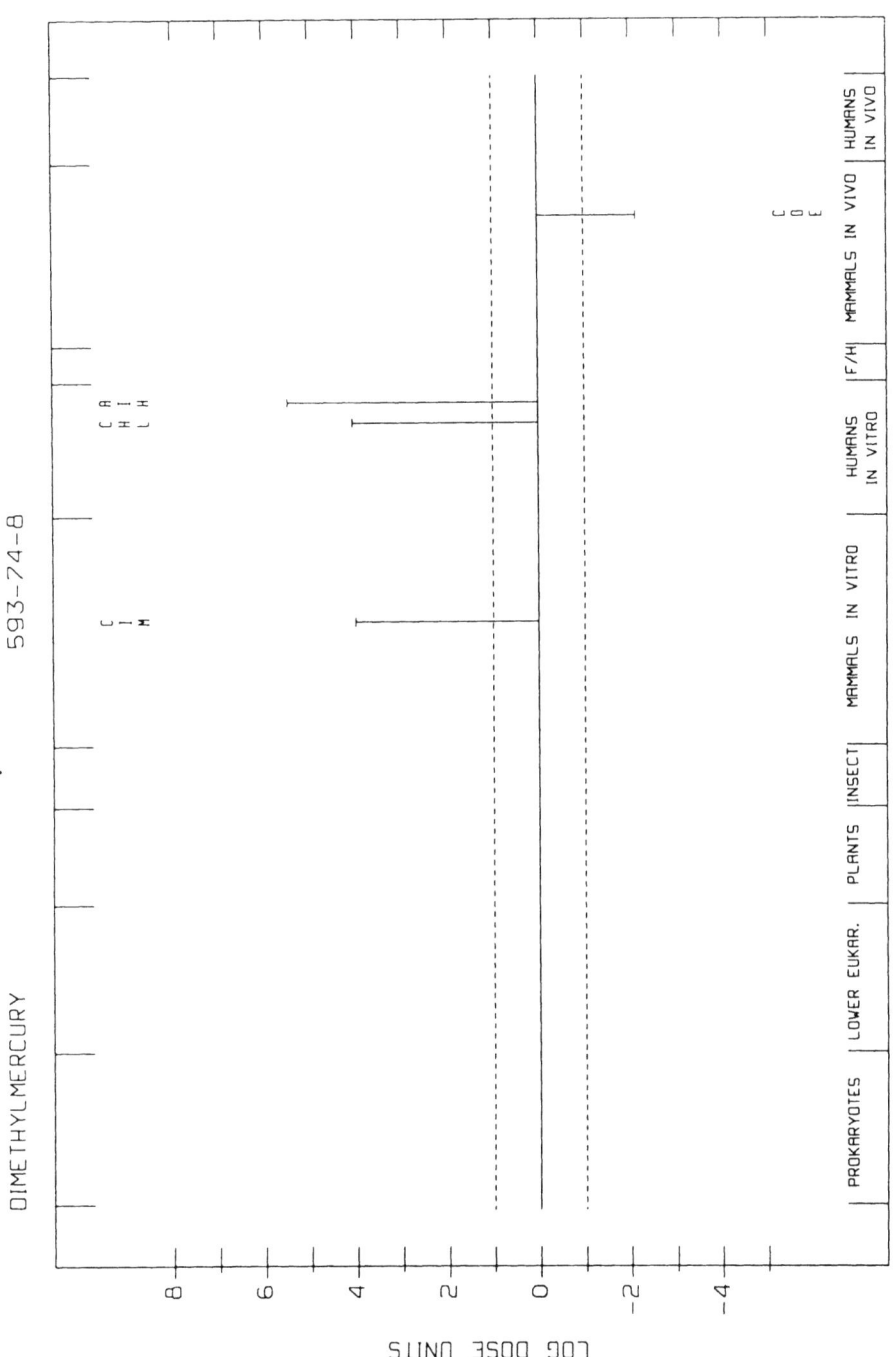

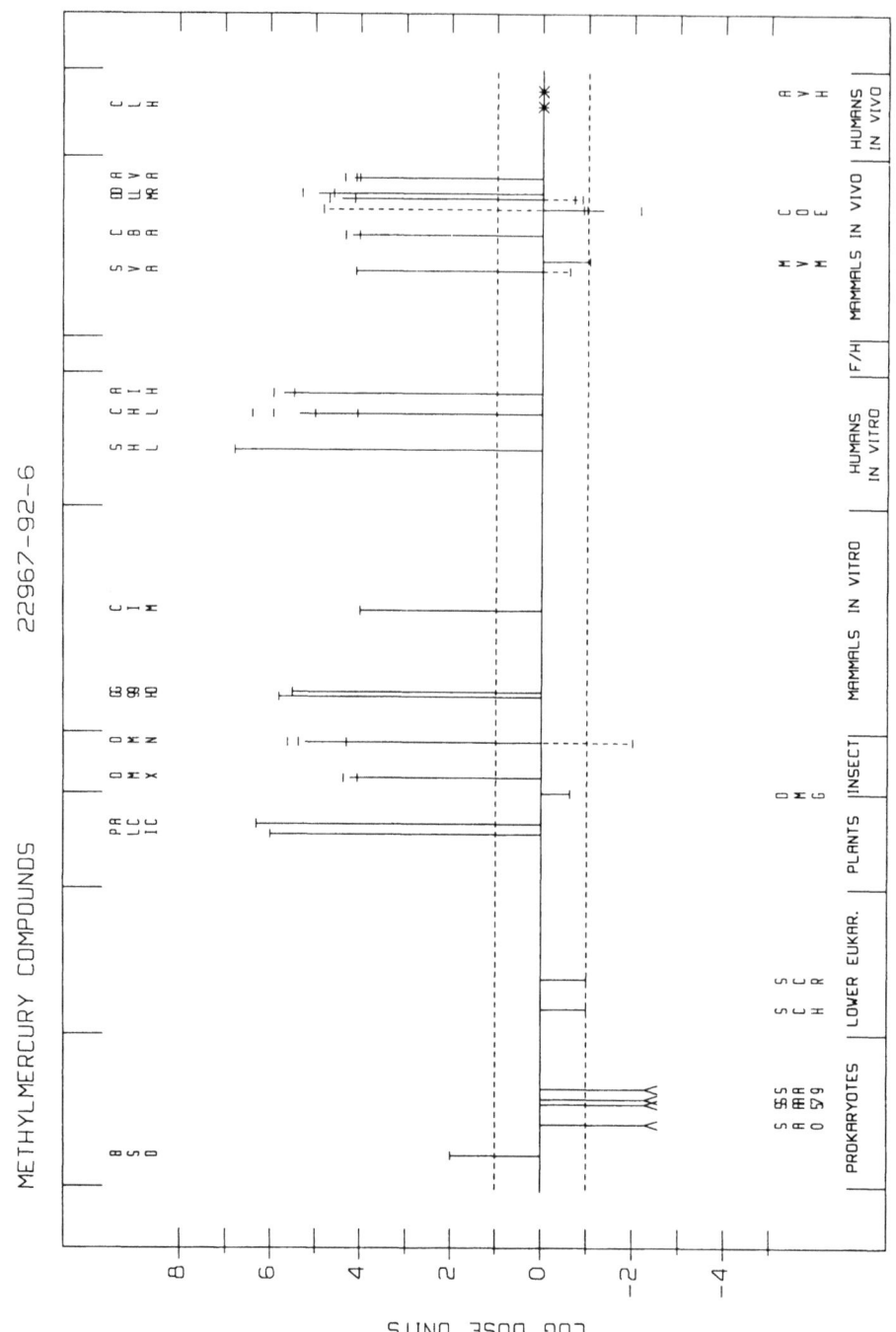

APPENDIX 2

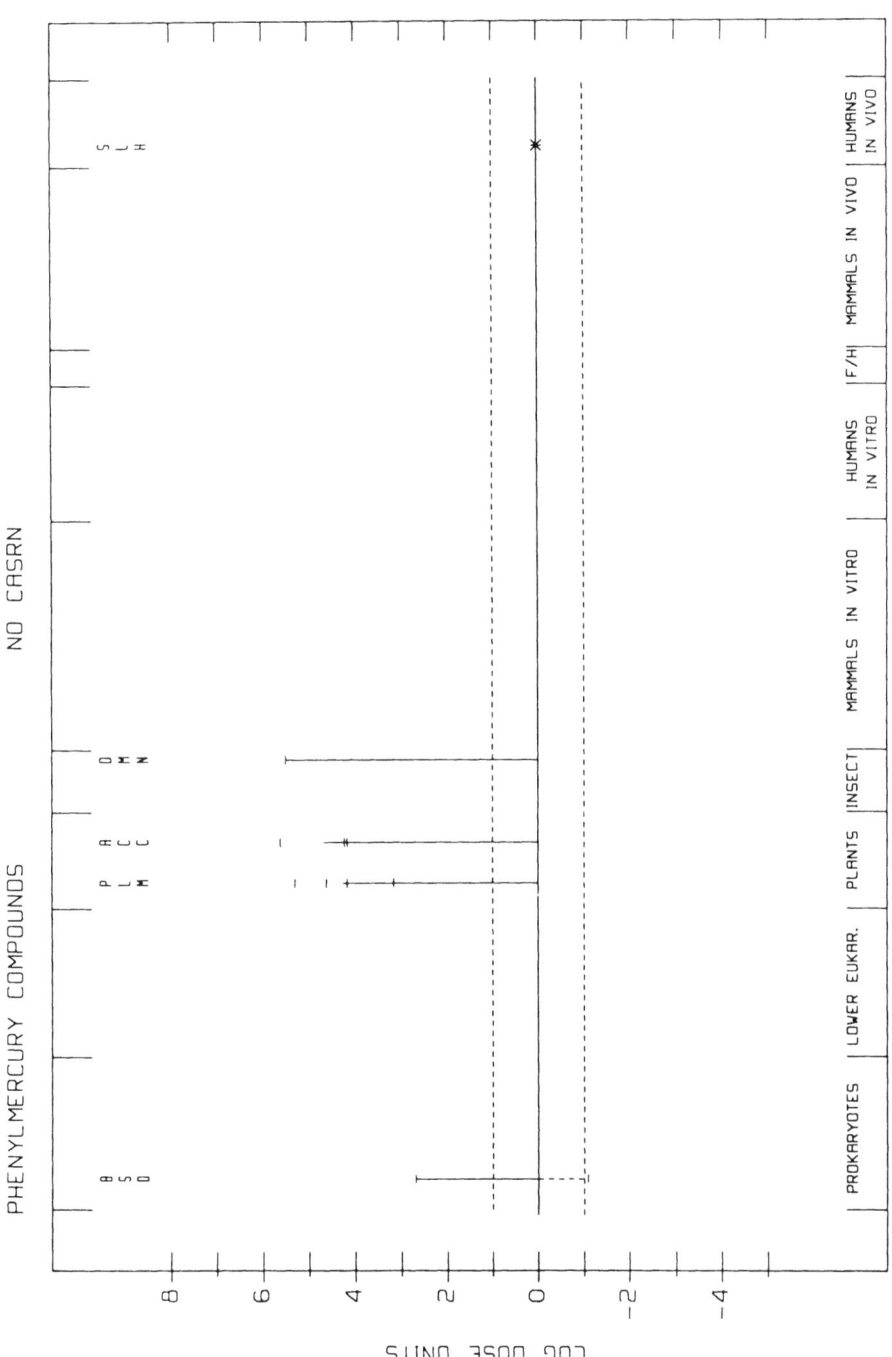

CUMULATIVE CROSS INDEX TO *IARC MONOGRAPHS ON THE EVALUATION OF CARCINOGENIC RISKS TO HUMANS*

The volume, page and year are given. References to corrigenda are given in parentheses.

A

A-α-C	*40*, 245 (1986); *Suppl. 7*, 56 (1987)
Acetaldehyde	*36*, 101 (1985) (*corr. 42*, 263); *Suppl. 7*, 77 (1987)
Acetaldehyde formylmethylhydrazone (*see* Gyromitrin)	
Acetamide	*7*, 197 (1974); *Suppl. 7*, 389 (1987)
Acetaminophen (*see* Paracetamol)	
Acridine orange	*16*, 145 (1978); *Suppl. 7*, 56 (1987)
Acriflavinium chloride	*13*, 31 (1977); *Suppl. 7*, 56 (1987)
Acrolein	*19*, 479 (1979); *36*, 133 (1985); *Suppl. 7*, 78 (1987)
Acrylamide	*39*, 41 (1986); *Suppl. 7*, 56 (1987)
Acrylic acid	*19*, 47 (1979); *Suppl. 7*, 56 (1987)
Acrylic fibres	*19*, 86 (1979); *Suppl. 7*, 56 (1987)
Acrylonitrile	*19*, 73 (1979); *Suppl. 7*, 79 (1987)
Acrylonitrile–butadiene–styrene copolymers	*19*, 91 (1979); *Suppl. 7*, 56 (1987)
Actinolite (*see* Asbestos)	
Actinomycins	*10*, 29 (1976) (*corr. 42*, 255); *Suppl. 7*, 80 (1987)
Adriamycin	*10*, 43 (1976); *Suppl. 7*, 82 (1987)
AF-2	*31*, 47 (1983); *Suppl. 7*, 56 (1987)
Aflatoxins	*1*, 145 (1972) (*corr. 42*, 251); *10*, 51 (1976); *Suppl. 7*, 83 (1987); *56*, 245 (1993)
Aflatoxin B_1 (*see* Aflatoxins)	
Aflatoxin B_2 (*see* Aflatoxins)	
Aflatoxin G_1 (*see* Aflatoxins)	
Aflatoxin G_2 (*see* Aflatoxins)	
Aflatoxin M_1 (*see* Aflatoxins)	
Agaritine	*31*, 63 (1983); *Suppl. 7*, 56 (1987)
Alcohol drinking	*44* (1988)
Aldicarb	*53*, 93 (1991)
Aldrin	*5*, 25 (1974); *Suppl. 7*, 88 (1987)
Allyl chloride	*36*, 39 (1985); *Suppl. 7*, 56 (1987)
Allyl isothiocyanate	*36*, 55 (1985); *Suppl. 7*, 56 (1987)
Allyl isovalerate	*36*, 69 (1985); *Suppl. 7*, 56 (1987)
Aluminium production	*34*, 37 (1984); *Suppl. 7*, 89 (1987)
Amaranth	*8*, 41 (1975); *Suppl. 7*, 56 (1987)

5-Aminoacenaphthene	16, 243 (1978); Suppl. 7, 56 (1987)
2-Aminoanthraquinone	27, 191 (1982); Suppl. 7, 56 (1987)
para-Aminoazobenzene	8, 53 (1975); Suppl. 7, 390 (1987)
ortho-Aminoazotoluene	8, 61 (1975) (corr. 42, 254); Suppl. 7, 56 (1987)
para-Aminobenzoic acid	16, 249 (1978); Suppl. 7, 56 (1987)
4-Aminobiphenyl	1, 74 (1972) (corr. 42, 251); Suppl. 7, 91 (1987)
2-Amino-3,4-dimethylimidazo[4,5-f]quinoline (see MeIQ)	
2-Amino-3,8-dimethylimidazo[4,5-f]quinoxaline (see MeIQx)	
3-Amino-1,4-dimethyl-5H-pyrido[4,3-b]indole (see Trp-P-1)	
2-Aminodipyrido[1,2-a:3',2'-d]imidazole (see Glu-P-2)	
1-Amino-2-methylanthraquinone	27, 199 (1982); Suppl. 7, 57 (1987)
2-Amino-3-methylimidazo[4,5-f]quinoline (see IQ)	
2-Amino-6-methyldipyrido[1,2-a:3',2'-d]imidazole (see Glu-P-1)	
2-Amino-1-methyl-6-phenylimidazo[4,5-b]pyridine (see PhIP)	
2-Amino-3-methyl-9H-pyrido[2,3-b]indole (see MeA-α-C)	
3-Amino-1-methyl-5H-pyrido[4,3-b]indole (see Trp-P-2)	
2-Amino-5-(5-nitro-2-furyl)-1,3,4-thiadiazole	7, 143 (1974); Suppl. 7, 57 (1987)
4-Amino-2-nitrophenol	16, 43 (1978); Suppl. 7, 57 (1987)
2-Amino-4-nitrophenol	57, 167 (1993)
2-Amino-5-nitrophenol	57, 177 (1993)
2-Amino-5-nitrothiazole	31, 71 (1983); Suppl. 7, 57 (1987)
2-Amino-9H-pyrido[2,3-b]indole (see A-α-C)	
11-Aminoundecanoic acid	39, 239 (1986); Suppl. 7, 57 (1987)
Amitrole	7, 31 (1974); 41, 293 (1986) (corr. 52, 513; Suppl. 7, 92 (1987)
Ammonium potassium selenide (see Selenium and selenium compounds)	
Amorphous silica (see also Silica)	42, 39 (1987); Suppl. 7, 341 (1987)
Amosite (see Asbestos)	
Ampicillin	50, 153 (1990)
Anabolic steroids (see Androgenic (anabolic) steroids)	
Anaesthetics, volatile	11, 285 (1976); Suppl. 7, 93 (1987)
Analgesic mixtures containing phenacetin (see also Phenacetin)	Suppl. 7, 310 (1987)
Androgenic (anabolic) steroids	Suppl. 7, 96 (1987)
Angelicin and some synthetic derivatives (see also Angelicins)	40, 291 (1986)
Angelicin plus ultraviolet radiation (see also Angelicin and some synthetic derivatives)	Suppl. 7, 57 (1987)
Angelicins	Suppl. 7, 57 (1987)
Aniline	4, 27 (1974) (corr. 42, 252); 27, 39 (1982); Suppl. 7, 99 (1987)
ortho-Anisidine	27, 63 (1982); Suppl. 7, 57 (1987)
para-Anisidine	27, 65 (1982); Suppl. 7, 57 (1987)
Anthanthrene	32, 95 (1983); Suppl. 7, 57 (1987)
Anthophyllite (see Asbestos)	
Anthracene	32, 105 (1983); Suppl. 7, 57 (1987)
Anthranilic acid	16, 265 (1978); Suppl. 7, 57 (1987)
Antimony trioxide	47, 291 (1989)
Antimony trisulfide	47, 291 (1989)
ANTU (see 1-Naphthylthiourea)	
Apholate	9, 31 (1975); Suppl. 7, 57 (1987)
Aramite®	5, 39 (1974); Suppl. 7, 57 (1987)

Areca nut (see Betel quid)
Arsanilic acid (see Arsenic and arsenic compounds)
Arsenic and arsenic compounds 1, 41 (1972); 2, 48 (1973); 23, 39 (1980); Suppl. 7, 100 (1987)

Arsenic pentoxide (see Arsenic and arsenic compounds)
Arsenic sulfide (see Arsenic and arsenic compounds)
Arsenic trioxide (see Arsenic and arsenic compounds)
Arsine (see Arsenic and arsenic compounds)
Asbestos 2, 17 (1973) (corr. 42, 252); 14 (1977) (corr. 42, 256); Suppl. 7, 106 (1987) (corr. 45, 283)

Atrazine 53, 441 (1991)
Attapulgite 42, 159 (1987); Suppl. 7, 117 (1987)
Auramine (technical-grade) 1, 69 (1972) (corr. 42, 251); Suppl. 7, 118 (1987)

Auramine, manufacture of (see also Auramine, technical-grade) Suppl. 7, 118 (1987)
Aurothioglucose 13, 39 (1977); Suppl. 7, 57 (1987)
Azacitidine 26, 37 (1981); Suppl. 7, 57 (1987); 50, 47 (1990)

5-Azacytidine (see Azacitidine)
Azaserine 10, 73 (1976) (corr. 42, 255); Suppl. 7, 57 (1987)

Azathioprine 26, 47 (1981); Suppl. 7, 119 (1987)
Aziridine 9, 37 (1975); Suppl. 7, 58 (1987)
2-(1-Aziridinyl)ethanol 9, 47 (1975); Suppl. 7, 58 (1987)
Aziridyl benzoquinone 9, 51 (1975); Suppl. 7, 58 (1987)
Azobenzene 8, 75 (1975); Suppl. 7, 58 (1987)

B

Barium chromate (see Chromium and chromium compounds)
Basic chromic sulfate (see Chromium and chromium compounds)
BCNU (see Bischloroethyl nitrosourea)
Benz[a]acridine 32, 123 (1983); Suppl. 7, 58 (1987)
Benz[c]acridine 3, 241 (1973); 32, 129 (1983); Suppl. 7, 58 (1987)

Benzal chloride (see also α-Chlorinated toluenes) 29, 65 (1982); Suppl. 7, 148 (1987)
Benz[a]anthracene 3, 45 (1973); 32, 135 (1983); Suppl. 7, 58 (1987)

Benzene 7, 203 (1974) (corr. 42, 254); 29, 93, 391 (1982); Suppl. 7, 120 (1987)
Benzidine 1, 80 (1972); 29, 149, 391 (1982); Suppl. 7, 123 (1987)

Benzidine-based dyes Suppl. 7, 125 (1987)
Benzo[b]fluoranthene 3, 69 (1973); 32, 147 (1983); Suppl. 7, 58 (1987)

Benzo[j]fluoranthene 3, 82 (1973); 32, 155 (1983); Suppl. 7, 58 (1987)

Benzo[k]fluoranthene 32, 163 (1983); Suppl. 7, 58 (1987)
Benzo[ghi]fluoranthene 32, 171 (1983); Suppl. 7, 58 (1987)
Benzo[a]fluorene 32, 177 (1983); Suppl. 7, 58 (1987)
Benzo[b]fluorene 32, 183 (1983); Suppl. 7, 58 (1987)

Benzo[c]fluorene	32, 189 (1983); Suppl. 7, 58 (1987)
Benzo[ghi]perylene	32, 195 (1983); Suppl. 7, 58 (1987)
Benzo[c]phenanthrene	32, 205 (1983); Suppl. 7, 58 (1987)
Benzo[a]pyrene	3, 91 (1973); 32, 211 (1983); Suppl. 7, 58 (1987)
Benzo[e]pyrene	3, 137 (1973); 32, 225 (1983); Suppl. 7, 58 (1987)
para-Benzoquinone dioxime	29, 185 (1982); Suppl. 7, 58 (1987)
Benzotrichloride (see also α-Chlorinated toluenes)	29, 73 (1982); Suppl. 7, 148 (1987)
Benzoyl chloride	29, 83 (1982) (corr. 42, 261); Suppl. 7, 126 (1987)
Benzoyl peroxide	36, 267 (1985); Suppl. 7, 58 (1987)
Benzyl acetate	40, 109 (1986); Suppl. 7, 58 (1987)
Benzyl chloride (see also α-Chlorinated toluenes)	11, 217 (1976) (corr. 42, 256); 29, 49 (1982); Suppl. 7, 148 (1987)
Benzyl violet 4B	16, 153 (1978); Suppl. 7, 58 (1987)
Bertrandite (see Beryllium and beryllium compounds)	
Beryllium and beryllium compounds	1, 17 (1972); 23, 143 (1980) (corr. 42, 260); Suppl. 7, 127 (1987); 58, 41 (1993)
Beryllium acetate (see Beryllium and beryllium compounds)	
Beryllium acetate, basic (see Beryllium and beryllium compounds)	
Beryllium–aluminium alloy (see Beryllium and beryllium compounds)	
Beryllium carbonate (see Beryllium and beryllium compounds)	
Beryllium chloride (see Beryllium and beryllium compounds)	
Beryllium–copper alloy (see Beryllium and beryllium compounds)	
Beryllium–copper–cobalt alloy (see Beryllium and beryllium compounds)	
Beryllium fluoride (see Beryllium and beryllium compounds)	
Beryllium hydroxide (see Beryllium and beryllium compounds)	
Beryllium–nickel alloy (see Beryllium and beryllium compounds)	
Beryllium oxide (see Beryllium and beryllium compounds)	
Beryllium phosphate (see Beryllium and beryllium compounds)	
Beryllium silicate (see Beryllium and beryllium compounds)	
Beryllium sulfate (see Beryllium and beryllium compounds)	
Beryl ore (see Beryllium and beryllium compounds)	
Betel quid	37, 141 (1985); Suppl. 7, 128 (1987)
Betel-quid chewing (see Betel quid)	
BHA (see Butylated hydroxyanisole)	
BHT (see Butylated hydroxytoluene)	
Bis(1-aziridinyl)morpholinophosphine sulfide	9, 55 (1975); Suppl. 7, 58 (1987)
Bis(2-chloroethyl)ether	9, 117 (1975); Suppl. 7, 58 (1987)
N,N-Bis(2-chloroethyl)-2-naphthylamine	4, 119 (1974) (corr. 42, 253); Suppl. 7, 130 (1987)
Bischloroethyl nitrosourea (see also Chloroethyl nitrosoureas)	26, 79 (1981); Suppl. 7, 150 (1987)
1,2-Bis(chloromethoxy)ethane	15, 31 (1977); Suppl. 7, 58 (1987)
1,4-Bis(chloromethoxymethyl)benzene	15, 37 (1977); Suppl. 7, 58 (1987)
Bis(chloromethyl)ether	4, 231 (1974) (corr. 42, 253); Suppl. 7, 131 (1987)
Bis(2-chloro-1-methylethyl)ether	41, 149 (1986); Suppl. 7, 59 (1987)
Bis(2,3-epoxycyclopentyl)ether	47, 231 (1989)
Bisphenol A diglycidyl ether (see Glycidyl ethers)	
Bisulfites (see Sulfur dioxide and some sulfites, bisulfites and metabisulfites)	

Bitumens	35, 39 (1985); *Suppl. 7*, 133 (1987)
Bleomycins	26, 97 (1981); *Suppl. 7*, 134 (1987)
Blue VRS	16, 163 (1978); *Suppl. 7*, 59 (1987)
Boot and shoe manufacture and repair	25, 249 (1981); *Suppl. 7*, 232 (1987)
Bracken fern	40, 47 (1986); *Suppl. 7*, 135 (1987)
Brilliant Blue FCF, disodium salt	16, 171 (1978) (*corr.* 42, 257); *Suppl. 7*, 59 (1987)
Bromochloroacetonitrile (*see* Halogenated acetonitriles)	
Bromodichloromethane	52, 179 (1991)
Bromoethane	52, 299 (1991)
Bromoform	52, 213 (1991)
1,3-Butadiene	39, 155 (1986) (*corr.* 42, 264); *Suppl. 7*, 136 (1987); 54, 237 (1992)
1,4-Butanediol dimethanesulfonate	4, 247 (1974); *Suppl. 7*, 137 (1987)
n-Butyl acrylate	39, 67 (1986); *Suppl. 7*, 59 (1987)
Butylated hydroxyanisole	40, 123 (1986); *Suppl. 7*, 59 (1987)
Butylated hydroxytoluene	40, 161 (1986); *Suppl. 7*, 59 (1987)
Butyl benzyl phthalate	29, 193 (1982) (*corr.* 42, 261); *Suppl. 7*, 59 (1987)
β-Butyrolactone	11, 225 (1976); *Suppl. 7*, 59 (1987)
γ-Butyrolactone	11, 231 (1976); *Suppl. 7*, 59 (1987)

C

Cabinet-making (*see* Furniture and cabinet-making)	
Cadmium acetate (*see* Cadmium and cadmium compounds)	
Cadmium and cadmium compounds	2, 74 (1973); 11, 39 (1976) (*corr.* 42, 255); *Suppl. 7*, 139 (1987); 58, 119 (1993)
Cadmium chloride (*see* Cadmium and cadmium compounds)	
Cadmium oxide (*see* Cadmium and cadmium compounds)	
Cadmium sulfate (*see* Cadmium and cadmium compounds)	
Cadmium sulfide (*see* Cadmium and cadmium compounds)	
Caffeic acid	56, 115 (1993)
Caffeine	51, 291 (1991)
Calcium arsenate (*see* Arsenic and arsenic compounds)	
Calcium chromate (*see* Chromium and chromium compounds)	
Calcium cyclamate (*see* Cyclamates)	
Calcium saccharin (*see* Saccharin)	
Cantharidin	10, 79 (1976); *Suppl. 7*, 59 (1987)
Caprolactam	19, 115 (1979) (*corr.* 42, 258); 39, 247 (1986) (*corr.* 42, 264); *Suppl. 7*, 390 (1987)
Captafol	53, 353 (1991)
Captan	30, 295 (1983); *Suppl. 7*, 59 (1987)
Carbaryl	12, 37 (1976); *Suppl. 7*, 59 (1987)
Carbazole	32, 239 (1983); *Suppl. 7*, 59 (1987)
3-Carbethoxypsoralen	40, 317 (1986); *Suppl. 7*, 59 (1987)
Carbon blacks	3, 22 (1973); 33, 35 (1984); *Suppl. 7*, 142 (1987)
Carbon tetrachloride	1, 53 (1972); 20, 371 (1979); *Suppl. 7*, 143 (1987)

Carmoisine	8, 83 (1975); *Suppl.* 7, 59 (1987)
Carpentry and joinery	25, 139 (1981); *Suppl.* 7, 378 (1987)
Carrageenan	10, 181 (1976) (*corr.* 42, 255); 31, 79 (1983); *Suppl.* 7, 59 (1987)
Catechol	15, 155 (1977); *Suppl.* 7, 59 (1987)
CCNU (*see* 1-(2-Chloroethyl)-3-cyclohexyl-1-nitrosourea)	
Ceramic fibres (*see* Man-made mineral fibres)	
Chemotherapy, combined, including alkylating agents (*see* MOPP and other combined chemotherapy including alkylating agents)	
Chlorambucil	9, 125 (1975); 26, 115 (1981); *Suppl.* 7, 144 (1987)
Chloramphenicol	10, 85 (1976); *Suppl.* 7, 145 (1987); 50, 169 (1990)
Chlordane (*see also* Chlordane/Heptachlor)	20, 45 (1979) (*corr.* 42, 258)
Chlordane/Heptachlor	*Suppl.* 7, 146 (1987); 53, 115 (1991)
Chlordecone	20, 67 (1979); *Suppl.* 7, 59 (1987)
Chlordimeform	30, 61 (1983); *Suppl.* 7, 59 (1987)
Chlorendic acid	48, 45 (1990)
Chlorinated dibenzodioxins (other than TCDD)	15, 41 (1977); *Suppl.* 7, 59 (1987)
Chlorinated drinking-water	52, 45 (1991)
Chlorinated paraffins	48, 55 (1990)
α-Chlorinated toluenes	*Suppl.* 7, 148 (1987)
Chlormadinone acetate (*see also* Progestins; Combined oral contraceptives)	6, 149 (1974); 21, 365 (1979)
Chlornaphazine (*see* N,N-Bis(2-chloroethyl)-2-naphthylamine)	
Chloroacetonitrile (*see* Halogenated acetonitriles)	
para-Chloroaniline	57, 305 (1993)
Chlorobenzilate	5, 75 (1974); 30, 73 (1983); *Suppl.* 7, 60 (1987)
Chlorodibromomethane	52, 243 (1991)
Chlorodifluoromethane	41, 237 (1986) (*corr.* 51, 483); *Suppl.* 7, 149 (1987)
Chloroethane	52, 315 (1991)
1-(2-Chloroethyl)-3-cyclohexyl-1-nitrosourea (*see also* Chloroethyl nitrosoureas)	26, 137 (1981) (*corr.* 42, 260); *Suppl.* 7, 150 (1987)
1-(2-Chloroethyl)-3-(4-methylcyclohexyl)-1-nitrosourea (*see also* Chloroethyl nitrosoureas)	*Suppl.* 7, 150 (1987)
Chloroethyl nitrosoureas	*Suppl.* 7, 150 (1987)
Chlorofluoromethane	41, 229 (1986); *Suppl.* 7, 60 (1987)
Chloroform	1, 61 (1972); 20, 401 (1979); *Suppl.* 7, 152 (1987)
Chloromethyl methyl ether (technical-grade) (*see also* Bis(chloromethyl)ether)	4, 239 (1974); *Suppl.* 7, 131 (1987)
(4-Chloro-2-methylphenoxy)acetic acid (*see* MCPA)	
Chlorophenols	*Suppl.* 7, 154 (1987)
Chlorophenols (occupational exposures to)	41, 319 (1986)
Chlorophenoxy herbicides	*Suppl.* 7, 156 (1987)
Chlorophenoxy herbicides (occupational exposures to)	41, 357 (1986)
4-Chloro-*ortho*-phenylenediamine	27, 81 (1982); *Suppl.* 7, 60 (1987)
4-Chloro-*meta*-phenylenediamine	27, 82 (1982); *Suppl.* 7, 60 (1987)
Chloroprene	19, 131 (1979); *Suppl.* 7, 160 (1987)
Chloropropham	12, 55 (1976); *Suppl.* 7, 60 (1987)

Chloroquine	13, 47 (1977); *Suppl. 7*, 60 (1987)
Chlorothalonil	30, 319 (1983); *Suppl. 7*, 60 (1987)
para-Chloro-*ortho*-toluidine and its strong acid salts (*see also* Chlordimeform)	16, 277 (1978); 30, 65 (1983); *Suppl. 7*, 60 (1987); 48, 123 (1990)
Chlorotrianisene (*see also* Nonsteroidal oestrogens)	21, 139 (1979)
2-Chloro-1,1,1-trifluoroethane	41, 253 (1986); *Suppl. 7*, 60 (1987)
Chlorozotocin	50, 65 (1990)
Cholesterol	10, 99 (1976); 31, 95 (1983); *Suppl. 7*, 161 (1987)
Chromic acetate (*see* Chromium and chromium compounds)	
Chromic chloride (*see* Chromium and chromium compounds)	
Chromic oxide (*see* Chromium and chromium compounds)	
Chromic phosphate (*see* Chromium and chromium compounds)	
Chromite ore (*see* Chromium and chromium compounds)	
Chromium and chromium compounds	2, 100 (1973); 23, 205 (1980); *Suppl. 7*, 165 (1987); 49, 49 (1990) (*corr.* 51, 483)
Chromium carbonyl (*see* Chromium and chromium compounds)	
Chromium potassium sulfate (*see* Chromium and chromium compounds)	
Chromium sulfate (*see* Chromium and chromium compounds)	
Chromium trioxide (*see* Chromium and chromium compounds)	
Chrysazin (*see* Dantron)	
Chrysene	3, 159 (1973); 32, 247 (1983); *Suppl. 7*, 60 (1987)
Chrysoidine	8, 91 (1975); *Suppl. 7*, 169 (1987)
Chrysotile (*see* Asbestos)	
CI Acid Orange 3	57, 121 (1993)
CI Acid Red 114	57, 247 (1993)
CI Basic Red 9	57, 215 (1993)
Ciclosporin	50, 77 (1990)
CI Direct Blue 15	57, 235 (1993)
CI Disperse Yellow 3 (*see* Disperse Yellow 3)	
Cimetidine	50, 235 (1990)
Cinnamyl anthranilate	16, 287 (1978); 31, 133 (1983); *Suppl. 7*, 60 (1987)
CI Pigment Red 3	57, 259 (1993)
CI Pigment Red 53:1 (*see* D&C Red No. 9)	
Cisplatin	26, 151 (1981); *Suppl. 7*, 170 (1987)
Citrinin	40, 67 (1986); *Suppl. 7*, 60 (1987)
Citrus Red No. 2	8, 101 (1975) (*corr.* 42, 254); *Suppl. 7*, 60 (1987)
Clofibrate	24, 39 (1980); *Suppl. 7*, 171 (1987)
Clomiphene citrate	21, 551 (1979); *Suppl. 7*, 172 (1987)
Coal gasification	34, 65 (1984); *Suppl. 7*, 173 (1987)
Coal-tar pitches (*see also* Coal-tars)	35, 83 (1985); *Suppl. 7*, 174 (1987)
Coal-tars	35, 83 (1985); *Suppl. 7*, 175 (1987)
Cobalt[III] acetate (*see* Cobalt and cobalt compounds)	
Cobalt–aluminium–chromium spinel (*see* Cobalt and cobalt compounds)	
Cobalt and cobalt compounds	52, 363 (1991)
Cobalt[II] chloride (*see* Cobalt and cobalt compounds)	

Cobalt–chromium alloy (see Chromium and chromium
  compounds)
Cobalt–chromium–molybdenum alloys (see Cobalt and cobalt compounds)
Cobalt metal powder (see Cobalt and cobalt compounds)
Cobalt naphthenate (see Cobalt and cobalt compounds)
Cobalt[II] oxide (see Cobalt and cobalt compounds)
Cobalt[II,III] oxide (see Cobalt and cobalt compounds)
Cobalt[II] sulfide (see Cobalt and cobalt compounds)
Coffee   51, 41 (1991) (corr. 52, 513)
Coke production   34, 101 (1984); Suppl. 7, 176 (1987)
Combined oral contraceptives (see also Oestrogens, progestins   Suppl. 7, 297 (1987)
  and combinations)
Conjugated oestrogens (see also Steroidal oestrogens)   21, 147 (1979)
Contraceptives, oral (see Combined oral contraceptives;
  Sequential oral contraceptives)
Copper 8-hydroxyquinoline   15, 103 (1977); Suppl. 7, 61 (1987)
Coronene   32, 263 (1983); Suppl. 7, 61 (1987)
Coumarin   10, 113 (1976); Suppl. 7, 61 (1987)
Creosotes (see also Coal-tars)   35, 83 (1985); Suppl. 7, 177 (1987)
meta-Cresidine   27, 91 (1982); Suppl. 7, 61 (1987)
para-Cresidine   27, 92 (1982); Suppl. 7, 61 (1987)
Crocidolite (see Asbestos)
Crude oil   45, 119 (1989)
Crystalline silica (see also Silica)   42, 39 (1987); Suppl. 7, 341 (1987)
Cycasin   1, 157 (1972) (corr. 42, 251); 10,
  121 (1976); Suppl. 7, 61 (1987)
Cyclamates   22, 55 (1980); Suppl. 7, 178 (1987)
Cyclamic acid (see Cyclamates)
Cyclochlorotine   10, 139 (1976); Suppl. 7, 61 (1987)
Cyclohexanone   47, 157 (1989)
Cyclohexylamine (see Cyclamates)
Cyclopenta[cd]pyrene   32, 269 (1983); Suppl. 7, 61 (1987)
Cyclopropane (see Anaesthetics, volatile)
Cyclophosphamide   9, 135 (1975); 26, 165 (1981);
  Suppl. 7, 182 (1987)

D

2,4-D (see also Chlorophenoxy herbicides; Chlorophenoxy   15, 111 (1977)
  herbicides, occupational exposures to)
Dacarbazine   26, 203 (1981); Suppl. 7, 184 (1987)
Dantron   50, 265 (1990)
D&C Red No. 9   8, 107 (1975); Suppl. 7, 61 (1987);
  57, 203 (1993)
Dapsone   24, 59 (1980); Suppl. 7, 185 (1987)
Daunomycin   10, 145 (1976); Suppl. 7, 61 (1987)
DDD (see DDT)
DDE (see DDT)
DDT   5, 83 (1974) (corr. 42, 253);
  Suppl. 7, 186 (1987); 53, 179 (1991)
Decabromodiphenyl oxide   48, 73 (1990)
Deltamethrin   53, 251 (1991)

Deoxynivalenol (*see* Toxins derived from *Fusarium graminearum, F. culmorum* and *F. crookwellense*)
Diacetylaminoazotoluene 8, 113 (1975); *Suppl.* 7, 61 (1987)
N,N'-Diacetylbenzidine 16, 293 (1978); *Suppl.* 7, 61 (1987)
Diallate 12, 69 (1976); 30, 235 (1983); *Suppl.* 7, 61 (1987)
2,4-Diaminoanisole 16, 51 (1978); 27, 103 (1982); *Suppl.* 7, 61 (1987)
4,4'-Diaminodiphenyl ether 16, 301 (1978); 29, 203 (1982); *Suppl.* 7, 61 (1987)
1,2-Diamino-4-nitrobenzene 16, 63 (1978); *Suppl.* 7, 61 (1987)
1,4-Diamino-2-nitrobenzene 16, 73 (1978); *Suppl.* 7, 61 (1987); 57, 185 (1993)
2,6-Diamino-3-(phenylazo)pyridine (*see* Phenazopyridine hydrochloride)
2,4-Diaminotoluene (*see also* Toluene diisocyanates) 16, 83 (1978); *Suppl.* 7, 61 (1987)
2,5-Diaminotoluene (*see also* Toluene diisocyanates) 16, 97 (1978); *Suppl.* 7, 61 (1987)
ortho-Dianisidine (*see* 3,3'-Dimethoxybenzidine)
Diazepam 13, 57 (1977); *Suppl.* 7, 189 (1987)
Diazomethane 7, 223 (1974); *Suppl.* 7, 61 (1987)
Dibenz[*a,h*]acridine 3, 247 (1973); 32, 277 (1983); *Suppl.* 7, 61 (1987)
Dibenz[*a,j*]acridine 3, 254 (1973); 32, 283 (1983); *Suppl.* 7, 61 (1987)
Dibenz[*a,c*]anthracene 32, 289 (1983) (*corr.* 42, 262); *Suppl.* 7, 61 (1987)
Dibenz[*a,h*]anthracene 3, 178 (1973) (*corr.* 43, 261); 32, 299 (1983); *Suppl.* 7, 61 (1987)
Dibenz[*a,j*]anthracene 32, 309 (1983); *Suppl.* 7, 61 (1987)
7H-Dibenzo[*c,g*]carbazole 3, 260 (1973); 32, 315 (1983); *Suppl.* 7, 61 (1987)
Dibenzodioxins, chlorinated (other than TCDD) [*see* Chlorinated dibenzodioxins (other than TCDD)]
Dibenzo[*a,e*]fluoranthene 32, 321 (1983); *Suppl.* 7, 61 (1987)
Dibenzo[*h,rst*]pentaphene 3, 197 (1973); *Suppl.* 7, 62 (1987)
Dibenzo[*a,e*]pyrene 3, 201 (1973); 32, 327 (1983); *Suppl.* 7, 62 (1987)
Dibenzo[*a,h*]pyrene 3, 207 (1973); 32, 331 (1983); *Suppl.* 7, 62 (1987)
Dibenzo[*a,i*]pyrene 3, 215 (1973); 32, 337 (1983); *Suppl.* 7, 62 (1987)
Dibenzo[*a,l*]pyrene 3, 224 (1973); 32, 343 (1983); *Suppl.* 7, 62 (1987)
Dibromoacetonitrile (*see* Halogenated acetonitriles)
1,2-Dibromo-3-chloropropane 15, 139 (1977); 20, 83 (1979); *Suppl.* 7, 191 (1987)
Dichloroacetonitrile (*see* Halogenated acetonitriles)
Dichloroacetylene 39, 369 (1986); *Suppl.* 7, 62 (1987)
ortho-Dichlorobenzene 7, 231 (1974); 29, 213 (1982); *Suppl.* 7, 192 (1987)
para-Dichlorobenzene 7, 231 (1974); 29, 215 (1982); *Suppl.* 7, 192 (1987)

3,3'-Dichlorobenzidine	4, 49 (1974); 29, 239 (1982); Suppl. 7, 193 (1987)
trans-1,4-Dichlorobutene	15, 149 (1977); Suppl. 7, 62 (1987)
3,3'-Dichloro-4,4'-diaminodiphenyl ether	16, 309 (1978); Suppl. 7, 62 (1987)
1,2-Dichloroethane	20, 429 (1979); Suppl. 7, 62 (1987)
Dichloromethane	20, 449 (1979); 41, 43 (1986); Suppl. 7, 194 (1987)
2,4-Dichlorophenol (see Chlorophenols; Chlorophenols, occupational exposures to)	
(2,4-Dichlorophenoxy)acetic acid (see 2,4-D)	
2,6-Dichloro-para-phenylenediamine	39, 325 (1986); Suppl. 7, 62 (1987)
1,2-Dichloropropane	41, 131 (1986); Suppl. 7, 62 (1987)
1,3-Dichloropropene (technical-grade)	41, 113 (1986); Suppl. 7, 195 (1987)
Dichlorvos	20, 97 (1979); Suppl. 7, 62 (1987); 53, 267 (1991)
Dicofol	30, 87 (1983); Suppl. 7, 62 (1987)
Dicyclohexylamine (see Cyclamates)	
Dieldrin	5, 125 (1974); Suppl. 7, 196 (1987)
Dienoestrol (see also Nonsteroidal oestrogens)	21, 161 (1979)
Diepoxybutane	11, 115 (1976) (corr. 42, 255); Suppl. 7, 62 (1987)
Diesel and gasoline engine exhausts	46, 41 (1989)
Diesel fuels	45, 219 (1989) (corr. 47, 505)
Diethyl ether (see Anaesthetics, volatile)	
Di(2-ethylhexyl)adipate	29, 257 (1982); Suppl. 7, 62 (1987)
Di(2-ethylhexyl)phthalate	29, 269 (1982) (corr. 42, 261); Suppl. 7, 62 (1987)
1,2-Diethylhydrazine	4, 153 (1974); Suppl. 7, 62 (1987)
Diethylstilboestrol	6, 55 (1974); 21, 173 (1979) (corr. 42, 259); Suppl. 7, 273 (1987)
Diethylstilboestrol dipropionate (see Diethylstilboestrol)	
Diethyl sulfate	4, 277 (1974); Suppl. 7, 198 (1987); 54, 213 (1992)
Diglycidyl resorcinol ether	11, 125 (1976); 36, 181 (1985); Suppl. 7, 62 (1987)
Dihydrosafrole	1, 170 (1972); 10, 233 (1976); Suppl. 7, 62 (1987)
1,8-Dihydroxyanthraquinone (see Dantron)	
Dihydroxybenzenes (see Catechol; Hydroquinone; Resorcinol)	
Dihydroxymethylfuratrizine	24, 77 (1980); Suppl. 7, 62 (1987)
Diisopropyl sulfate	54, 229 (1992)
Dimethisterone (see also Progestins; Sequential oral contraceptives)	6, 167 (1974); 21, 377 (1979)
Dimethoxane	15, 177 (1977); Suppl. 7, 62 (1987)
3,3'-Dimethoxybenzidine	4, 41 (1974); Suppl. 7, 198 (1987)
3,3'-Dimethoxybenzidine-4,4'-diisocyanate	39, 279 (1986); Suppl. 7, 62 (1987)
para-Dimethylaminoazobenzene	8, 125 (1975); Suppl. 7, 62 (1987)
para-Dimethylaminoazobenzenediazo sodium sulfonate	8, 147 (1975); Suppl. 7, 62 (1987)
trans-2-[(Dimethylamino)methylimino]-5-[2-(5-nitro-2-furyl)-vinyl]-1,3,4-oxadiazole	7, 147 (1974) (corr. 42, 253); Suppl. 7, 62 (1987)
4,4'-Dimethylangelicin plus ultraviolet radiation (see also Angelicin and some synthetic derivatives)	Suppl. 7, 57 (1987)

4,5'-Dimethylangelicin plus ultraviolet radiation (*see also* Angelicin and some synthetic derivatives)	*Suppl. 7*, 57 (1987)
2,6-Dimethylaniline	*57*, 323 (1993)
N,N-Dimethylaniline	*57*, 337 (1993)
Dimethylarsinic acid (*see* Arsenic and arsenic compounds)	
3,3'-Dimethylbenzidine	*1*, 87 (1972); *Suppl. 7*, 62 (1987)
Dimethylcarbamoyl chloride	*12*, 77 (1976); *Suppl. 7*, 199 (1987)
Dimethylformamide	*47*, 171 (1989)
1,1-Dimethylhydrazine	*4*, 137 (1974); *Suppl. 7*, 62 (1987)
1,2-Dimethylhydrazine	*4*, 145 (1974) (*corr. 42*, 253); *Suppl. 7*, 62 (1987)
Dimethyl hydrogen phosphite	*48*, 85 (1990)
1,4-Dimethylphenanthrene	*32*, 349 (1983); *Suppl. 7*, 62 (1987)
Dimethyl sulfate	*4*, 271 (1974); *Suppl. 7*, 200 (1987)
3,7-Dinitrofluoranthene	*46*, 189 (1989)
3,9-Dinitrofluoranthene	*46*, 195 (1989)
1,3-Dinitropyrene	*46*, 201 (1989)
1,6-Dinitropyrene	*46*, 215 (1989)
1,8-Dinitropyrene	*33*, 171 (1984); *Suppl. 7*, 63 (1987); *46*, 231 (1989)
Dinitrosopentamethylenetetramine	*11*, 241 (1976); *Suppl. 7*, 63 (1987)
1,4-Dioxane	*11*, 247 (1976); *Suppl. 7*, 201 (1987)
2,4'-Diphenyldiamine	*16*, 313 (1978); *Suppl. 7*, 63 (1987)
Direct Black 38 (*see also* Benzidine-based dyes)	*29*, 295 (1982) (*corr. 42*, 261)
Direct Blue 6 (*see also* Benzidine-based dyes)	*29*, 311 (1982)
Direct Brown 95 (*see also* Benzidine-based dyes)	*29*, 321 (1982)
Disperse Blue 1	*48*, 139 (1990)
Disperse Yellow 3	*8*, 97 (1975); *Suppl. 7*, 60 (1987); *48*, 149 (1990)
Disulfiram	*12*, 85 (1976); *Suppl. 7*, 63 (1987)
Dithranol	*13*, 75 (1977); *Suppl. 7*, 63 (1987)
Divinyl ether (*see* Anaesthetics, volatile)	
Dulcin	*12*, 97 (1976); *Suppl. 7*, 63 (1987)

E

Endrin	*5*, 157 (1974); *Suppl. 7*, 63 (1987)
Enflurane (*see* Anaesthetics, volatile)	
Eosin	*15*, 183 (1977); *Suppl. 7*, 63 (1987)
Epichlorohydrin	*11*, 131 (1976) (*corr. 42*, 256); *Suppl. 7*, 202 (1987)
1,2-Epoxybutane	*47*, 217 (1989)
1-Epoxyethyl-3,4-epoxycyclohexane	*11*, 141 (1976); *Suppl. 7*, 63 (1987)
3,4-Epoxy-6-methylcyclohexylmethyl-3,4-epoxy-6-methyl-cyclohexane carboxylate	*11*, 147 (1976); *Suppl. 7*, 63 (1987)
cis-9,10-Epoxystearic acid	*11*, 153 (1976); *Suppl. 7*, 63 (1987)
Erionite	*42*, 225 (1987); *Suppl. 7*, 203 (1987)
Ethinyloestradiol (*see also* Steroidal oestrogens)	*6*, 77 (1974); *21*, 233 (1979)
Ethionamide	*13*, 83 (1977); *Suppl. 7*, 63 (1987)
Ethyl acrylate	*19*, 57 (1979); *39*, 81 (1986); *Suppl. 7*, 63 (1987)
Ethylene	*19*, 157 (1979); *Suppl. 7*, 63 (1987)

Ethylene dibromide	15, 195 (1977); *Suppl. 7*, 204 (1987)
Ethylene oxide	11, 157 (1976); 36, 189 (1985) (*corr.* 42, 263); *Suppl. 7*, 205 (1987)
Ethylene sulfide	11, 257 (1976); *Suppl. 7*, 63 (1987)
Ethylene thiourea	7, 45 (1974); *Suppl. 7*, 207 (1987)
Ethyl methanesulfonate	7, 245 (1974); *Suppl. 7*, 63 (1987)
N-Ethyl-N-nitrosourea	1, 135 (1972); 17, 191 (1978); *Suppl. 7*, 63 (1987)
Ethyl selenac (*see also* Selenium and selenium compounds)	12, 107 (1976); *Suppl. 7*, 63 (1987)
Ethyl tellurac	12, 115 (1976); *Suppl. 7*, 63 (1987)
Ethynodiol diacetate (*see also* Progestins; Combined oral contraceptives)	6, 173 (1974); 21, 387 (1979)
Eugenol	36, 75 (1985); *Suppl. 7*, 63 (1987)
Evans blue	8, 151 (1975); *Suppl. 7*, 63 (1987)

F

Fast Green FCF	16, 187 (1978); *Suppl. 7*, 63 (1987)
Fenvalerate	53, 309 (1991)
Ferbam	12, 121 (1976) (*corr.* 42, 256); *Suppl. 7*, 63 (1987)
Ferric oxide	1, 29 (1972); *Suppl. 7*, 216 (1987)
Ferrochromium (*see* Chromium and chromium compounds)	
Fluometuron	30, 245 (1983); *Suppl. 7*, 63 (1987)
Fluoranthene	32, 355 (1983); *Suppl. 7*, 63 (1987)
Fluorene	32, 365 (1983); *Suppl. 7*, 63 (1987)
Fluorescent lighting (exposure to) (*see* Ultraviolet radiation)	
Fluorides (inorganic, used in drinking-water)	27, 237 (1982); *Suppl. 7*, 208 (1987)
5-Fluorouracil	26, 217 (1981); *Suppl. 7*, 210 (1987)
Fluorspar (*see* Fluorides)	
Fluosilicic acid (*see* Fluorides)	
Fluroxene (*see* Anaesthetics, volatile)	
Formaldehyde	29, 345 (1982); *Suppl. 7*, 211 (1987)
2-(2-Formylhydrazino)-4-(5-nitro-2-furyl)thiazole	7, 151 (1974) (*corr.* 42, 253); *Suppl. 7*, 63 (1987)
Frusemide (*see* Furosemide)	
Fuel oils (heating oils)	45, 239 (1989) (*corr.* 47, 505)
Fumonisin B$_1$ (*see* Toxins derived from *Fusarium moniliforme*)	
Fumonisin B$_2$ (*see* Toxins derived from *Fusarium moniliforme*)	
Furazolidone	31, 141 (1983); *Suppl. 7*, 63 (1987)
Furniture and cabinet-making	25, 99 (1981); *Suppl. 7*, 380 (1987)
Furosemide	50, 277 (1990)
2-(2-Furyl)-3-(5-nitro-2-furyl)acrylamide (*see* AF-2)	
Fusarenon-X (*see* Toxins derived from *Fusarium graminearum, F. culmorum* and *F. crookwellense*)	
Fusarenone-X (*see* Toxins derived from *Fusarium graminearum, F. culmorum* and *F. crookwellense*)	
Fusarin C (*see* Toxins derived from *Fusarium moniliforme*)	

G

Gasoline	45, 159 (1989) (*corr.* 47, 505)

Gasoline engine exhaust (*see* Diesel and gasoline engine exhausts)	
Glass fibres (*see* Man-made mineral fibres)	
Glass manufacturing industry, occupational exposures in	*58*, 347 (1993)
Glasswool (*see* Man-made mineral fibres)	
Glass filaments (*see* Man-made mineral fibres)	
Glu-P-1	*40*, 223 (1986); *Suppl. 7*, 64 (1987)
Glu-P-2	*40*, 235 (1986); *Suppl. 7*, 64 (1987)
L-Glutamic acid, 5-[2-(4-hydroxymethyl)phenylhydrazide] (*see* Agaritine)	
Glycidaldehyde	*11*, 175 (1976); *Suppl. 7*, 64 (1987)
Glycidyl ethers	*47*, 237 (1989)
Glycidyl oleate	11, 183 (1976); *Suppl. 7*, 64 (1987)
Glycidyl stearate	*11*, 187 (1976); *Suppl. 7*, 64 (1987)
Griseofulvin	*10*, 153 (1976); *Suppl. 7*, 391 (1987)
Guinea Green B	*16*, 199 (1978); *Suppl. 7*, 64 (1987)
Gyromitrin	*31*, 163 (1983); *Suppl. 7*, 391 (1987)

H

Haematite	*1*, 29 (1972); *Suppl. 7*, 216 (1987)
Haematite and ferric oxide	*Suppl. 7*, 216 (1987)
Haematite mining, underground, with exposure to radon	*1*, 29 (1972); *Suppl. 7*, 216 (1987)
Hairdressers and barbers (occupational exposure as)	*57*, 43 (1993)
Hair dyes, epidemiology of	*16*, 29 (1978); *27*, 307 (1982);
Halogenated acetonitriles	*52*, 269 (1991)
Halothane (*see* Anaesthetics, volatile)	
HC Blue No. 1	*57*, 129 (1993)
HC Blue No. 2	*57*, 143 (1993)
α-HCH (*see* Hexachlorocyclohexanes)	
β-HCH (*see* Hexachlorocyclohexanes)	
γ-HCH (*see* Hexachlorocyclohexanes)	
HC Red No. 3	*57*, 153 (1993)
HC Yellow No. 4	*57*, 159 (1993)
Heating oils (*see* Fuel oils)	
Heptachlor (*see also* Chlordane/Heptachlor)	*5*, 173 (1974); *20*, 129 (1979)
Hexachlorobenzene	*20*, 155 (1979); *Suppl. 7*, 219 (1987)
Hexachlorobutadiene	*20*, 179 (1979); *Suppl. 7*, 64 (1987)
Hexachlorocyclohexanes	*5*, 47 (1974); *20*, 195 (1979) (*corr. 42*, 258); *Suppl. 7*, 220 (1987)
Hexachlorocyclohexane, technical-grade (*see* Hexachlorocyclohexanes)	
Hexachloroethane	*20*, 467 (1979); *Suppl. 7*, 64 (1987)
Hexachlorophene	*20*, 241 (1979); *Suppl. 7*, 64 (1987)
Hexamethylphosphoramide	*15*, 211 (1977); *Suppl. 7*, 64 (1987)
Hexoestrol (*see* Nonsteroidal oestrogens)	
Hycanthone mesylate	*13*, 91 (1977); *Suppl. 7*, 64 (1987)
Hydralazine	*24*, 85 (1980); *Suppl. 7*, 222 (1987)
Hydrazine	*4*, 127 (1974); *Suppl. 7*, 223 (1987)
Hydrochloric acid	*54*, 189 (1992)
Hydrochlorothiazide	*50*, 293 (1990)
Hydrogen peroxide	*36*, 285 (1985); *Suppl. 7*, 64 (1987)
Hydroquinone	*15*, 155 (1977); *Suppl. 7*, 64 (1987)

4-Hydroxyazobenzene   8, 157 (1975); Suppl. 7, 64 (1987)
17α-Hydroxyprogesterone caproate (see also Progestins)   21, 399 (1979) (corr. 42, 259)
8-Hydroxyquinoline   13, 101 (1977); Suppl. 7, 64 (1987)
8-Hydroxysenkirkine   10, 265 (1976); Suppl. 7, 64 (1987)
Hypochlorite salts   52, 159 (1991)

I

Indeno[1,2,3-cd]pyrene   3, 229 (1973); 32, 373 (1983);
                                                                 Suppl. 7, 64 (1987)

Inorganic acids (see Sulfuric acid and other strong inorganic acids,
    occupational exposures to mists and vapours from)
Insecticides, occupational exposures in spraying and application of   53, 45 (1991)
IQ   40, 261 (1986); Suppl. 7, 64 (1987);
                                                                 56, 165 (1993)
Iron and steel founding   34, 133 (1984); Suppl. 7, 224 (1987)
Iron-dextran complex   2, 161 (1973); Suppl. 7, 226 (1987)
Iron-dextrin complex   2, 161 (1973) (corr. 42, 252);
                                                                 Suppl. 7, 64 (1987)

Iron oxide (see Ferric oxide)
Iron oxide, saccharated (see Saccharated iron oxide)
Iron sorbitol–citric acid complex   2, 161 (1973); Suppl. 7, 64 (1987)
Isatidine   10, 269 (1976); Suppl. 7, 65 (1987)
Isoflurane (see Anaesthetics, volatile)
Isoniazid (see Isonicotinic acid hydrazide)
Isonicotinic acid hydrazide   4, 159 (1974); Suppl. 7, 227 (1987)
Isophosphamide   26, 237 (1981); Suppl. 7, 65 (1987)
Isopropyl alcohol   15, 223 (1977); Suppl. 7, 229 (1987)
Isopropyl alcohol manufacture (strong-acid process)   Suppl. 7, 229 (1987)
    (see also Isopropyl alcohol; Sulfuric acid and other strong inorganic
    acids, occupational exposures to mists and vapours from)
Isopropyl oils   15, 223 (1977); Suppl. 7, 229 (1987)
Isosafrole   1, 169 (1972); 10, 232 (1976);
                                                                 Suppl. 7, 65 (1987)

J

Jacobine   10, 275 (1976); Suppl. 7, 65 (1987)
Jet fuel   45, 203 (1989)
Joinery (see Carpentry and joinery)

K

Kaempferol   31, 171 (1983); Suppl. 7, 65 (1987)
Kepone (see Chlordecone)

L

Lasiocarpine   10, 281 (1976); Suppl. 7, 65 (1987)
Lauroyl peroxide   36, 315 (1985); Suppl. 7, 65 (1987)
Lead acetate (see Lead and lead compounds)

Lead and lead compounds	*1*, 40 (1972) (*corr. 42*, 251); *2*, 52, 150 (1973); *12*, 131 (1976); *23*, 40, 208, 209, 325 (1980); *Suppl. 7*, 230 (1987)
Lead arsenate (*see* Arsenic and arsenic compounds)	
Lead carbonate (*see* Lead and lead compounds)	
Lead chloride (*see* Lead and lead compounds)	
Lead chromate (*see* Chromium and chromium compounds)	
Lead chromate oxide (*see* Chromium and chromium compounds)	
Lead naphthenate (*see* Lead and lead compounds)	
Lead nitrate (*see* Lead and lead compounds)	
Lead oxide (*see* Lead and lead compounds)	
Lead phosphate (*see* Lead and lead compounds)	
Lead subacetate (*see* Lead and lead compounds)	
Lead tetroxide (*see* Lead and lead compounds)	
Leather goods manufacture	*25*, 279 (1981); *Suppl. 7*, 235 (1987)
Leather industries	*25*, 199 (1981); *Suppl. 7*, 232 (1987)
Leather tanning and processing	*25*, 201 (1981); *Suppl. 7*, 236 (1987)
Ledate (*see also* Lead and lead compounds)	*12*, 131 (1976)
Light Green SF	*16*, 209 (1978); *Suppl. 7*, 65 (1987)
d-Limonene	*56*, 135 (1993)
Lindane (*see* Hexachlorocyclohexanes)	
The lumber and sawmill industries (including logging)	*25*, 49 (1981); *Suppl. 7*, 383 (1987)
Luteoskyrin	*10*, 163 (1976); *Suppl. 7*, 65 (1987)
Lynoestrenol (*see also* Progestins; Combined oral contraceptives)	*21*, 407 (1979)

M

Magenta	*4*, 57 (1974) (*corr. 42*, 252); *Suppl. 7*, 238 (1987); *57*, 215 (1993)
Magenta, manufacture of (*see also* Magenta)	*Suppl. 7*, 238 (1987)
Malathion	*30*, 103 (1983); *Suppl. 7*, 65 (1987)
Maleic hydrazide	*4*, 173 (1974) (*corr. 42*, 253); *Suppl. 7*, 65 (1987)
Malonaldehyde	*36*, 163 (1985); *Suppl. 7*, 65 (1987)
Maneb	*12*, 137 (1976); *Suppl. 7*, 65 (1987)
Man-made mineral fibres	*43*, 39 (1988)
Mannomustine	*9*, 157 (1975); *Suppl. 7*, 65 (1987)
Mate	*51*, 273 (1991)
MCPA (*see also* Chlorophenoxy herbicides; Chlorophenoxy herbicides, occupational exposures to)	*30*, 255 (1983)
MeA-α-C	*40*, 253 (1986); *Suppl. 7*, 65 (1987)
Medphalan	*9*, 168 (1975); *Suppl. 7*, 65 (1987)
Medroxyprogesterone acetate	*6*, 157 (1974); *21*, 417 (1979) (*corr. 42*, 259); *Suppl. 7*, 289 (1987)
Megestrol acetate (*see* also Progestins; Combined oral contraceptives)	
MeIQ	*40*, 275 (1986); *Suppl. 7*, 65 (1987); *56*, 197 (1993)
MeIQx	*40*, 283 (1986); *Suppl. 7*, 65 (1987) *56*, 211 (1993)
Melamine	*39*, 333 (1986); *Suppl. 7*, 65 (1987)

Melphalan	9, 167 (1975); Suppl. 7, 239 (1987)
6-Mercaptopurine	26, 249 (1981); Suppl. 7, 240 (1987)
Mercuric chloride (see Mercury and mercury compounds)	
Mercury and mercury compounds	58, 239 (1993)
Merphalan	9, 169 (1975); Suppl. 7, 65 (1987)
Mestranol (see also Steroidal oestrogens)	6, 87 (1974); 21, 257 (1979) (corr. 42, 259)
Metabisulfites (see Sulfur dioxide and some sulfites, bisulfites and metabisulfites)	
Metallic mercury (see Mercury and mercury compounds)	
Methanearsonic acid, disodium salt (see Arsenic and arsenic compounds)	
Methanearsonic acid, monosodium salt (see Arsenic and arsenic compounds)	
Methotrexate	26, 267 (1981); Suppl. 7, 241 (1987)
Methoxsalen (see 8-Methoxypsoralen)	
Methoxychlor	5, 193 (1974); 20, 259 (1979); Suppl. 7, 66 (1987)
Methoxyflurane (see Anaesthetics, volatile)	
5-Methoxypsoralen	40, 327 (1986); Suppl. 7, 242 (1987)
8-Methoxypsoralen (see also 8-Methoxypsoralen plus ultraviolet radiation)	24, 101 (1980)
8-Methoxypsoralen plus ultraviolet radiation	Suppl. 7, 243 (1987)
Methyl acrylate	19, 52 (1979); 39, 99 (1986); Suppl. 7, 66 (1987)
5-Methylangelicin plus ultraviolet radiation (see also Angelicin and some synthetic derivatives)	Suppl. 7, 57 (1987)
2-Methylaziridine	9, 61 (1975); Suppl. 7, 66 (1987)
Methylazoxymethanol acetate	1, 164 (1972); 10, 131 (1976); Suppl. 7, 66 (1987)
Methyl bromide	41, 187 (1986) (corr. 45, 283); Suppl. 7, 245 (1987)
Methyl carbamate	12, 151 (1976); Suppl. 7, 66 (1987)
Methyl-CCNU [see 1-(2-Chloroethyl)-3-(4-methylcyclohexyl)-1-nitrosourea]	
Methyl chloride	41, 161 (1986); Suppl. 7, 246 (1987)
1-, 2-, 3-, 4-, 5- and 6-Methylchrysenes	32, 379 (1983); Suppl. 7, 66 (1987)
N-Methyl-N,4-dinitrosoaniline	1, 141 (1972); Suppl. 7, 66 (1987)
4,4'-Methylene bis(2-chloroaniline)	4, 65 (1974) (corr. 42, 252); Suppl. 7, 246 (1987); 57, 271 (1993)
4,4'-Methylene bis(N,N-dimethyl)benzenamine	27, 119 (1982); Suppl. 7, 66 (1987)
4,4'-Methylene bis(2-methylaniline)	4, 73 (1974); Suppl. 7, 248 (1987)
4,4'-Methylenedianiline	4, 79 (1974) (corr. 42, 252); 39, 347 (1986); Suppl. 7, 66 (1987)
4,4'-Methylenediphenyl diisocyanate	19, 314 (1979); Suppl. 7, 66 (1987)
2-Methylfluoranthene	32, 399 (1983); Suppl. 7, 66 (1987)
3-Methylfluoranthene	32, 399 (1983); Suppl. 7, 66 (1987)
Methylglyoxal	51, 443 (1991)
Methyl iodide	15, 245 (1977); 41, 213 (1986); Suppl. 7, 66 (1987)
Methylmercury chloride (see Mercury and mercury compounds)	
Methylmercury compounds (see Mercury and mercury compounds)	

Methyl methacrylate	*19*, 187 (1979); *Suppl. 7*, 66 (1987)
Methyl methanesulfonate	*7*, 253 (1974); *Suppl. 7*, 66 (1987)
2-Methyl-1-nitroanthraquinone	*27*, 205 (1982); *Suppl. 7*, 66 (1987)
N-Methyl-N'-nitro-N-nitrosoguanidine	*4*, 183 (1974); *Suppl. 7*, 248 (1987)
3-Methylnitrosaminopropionaldehyde [*see* 3-(N-Nitrosomethylamino)-propionaldehyde]	
3-Methylnitrosaminopropionitrile [*see* 3-(N-Nitrosomethylamino)-propionitrile]	
4-(Methylnitrosamino)-4-(3-pyridyl)-1-butanal [*see* 4-(N-Nitrosomethylamino)-4-(3-pyridyl)-1-butanal]	
4-(Methylnitrosamino)-1-(3-pyridyl)-1-butanone [*see* 4-(N-Nitrosomethylamino)-1-(3-pyridyl)-1-butanone]	
N-Methyl-N-nitrosourea	*1*, 125 (1972); *17*, 227 (1978); *Suppl. 7*, 66 (1987)
N-Methyl-N-nitrosourethane	*4*, 211 (1974); *Suppl. 7*, 66 (1987)
Methyl parathion	*30*, 131 (1983); *Suppl. 7*, 392 (1987)
1-Methylphenanthrene	*32*, 405 (1983); *Suppl. 7*, 66 (1987)
7-Methylpyrido[3,4-c]psoralen	*40*, 349 (1986); *Suppl. 7*, 71 (1987)
Methyl red	*8*, 161 (1975); *Suppl. 7*, 66 (1987)
Methyl selenac (*see also* Selenium and selenium compounds)	*12*, 161 (1976); *Suppl. 7*, 66 (1987)
Methylthiouracil	*7*, 53 (1974); *Suppl. 7*, 66 (1987)
Metronidazole	*13*, 113 (1977); *Suppl. 7*, 250 (1987)
Mineral oils	*3*, 30 (1973); *33*, 87 (1984) (*corr. 42*, 262); *Suppl. 7*, 252 (1987)
Mirex	*5*, 203 (1974); *20*, 283 (1979) (*corr. 42*, 258); *Suppl. 7*, 66 (1987)
Mitomycin C	*10*, 171 (1976); *Suppl. 7*, 67 (1987)
MNNG [*see* N-Methyl-N'-nitro-N-nitrosoguanidine]	
MOCA [*see* 4,4'-Methylene bis(2-chloroaniline)]	
Modacrylic fibres	*19*, 86 (1979); *Suppl. 7*, 67 (1987)
Monocrotaline	*10*, 291 (1976); *Suppl. 7*, 67 (1987)
Monuron	*12*, 167 (1976); *Suppl. 7*, 67 (1987); *53*, 467 (1991)
MOPP and other combined chemotherapy including alkylating agents	*Suppl. 7*, 254 (1987)
Morpholine	*47*, 199 (1989)
5-(Morpholinomethyl)-3-[(5-nitrofurfurylidene)amino]-2-oxazolidinone	*7*, 161 (1974); *Suppl. 7*, 67 (1987)
Mustard gas	*9*, 181 (1975) (*corr. 42*, 254); *Suppl. 7*, 259 (1987)
Myleran (*see* 1,4-Butanediol dimethanesulfonate)	

N

Nafenopin	*24*, 125 (1980); *Suppl. 7*, 67 (1987)
1,5-Naphthalenediamine	*27*, 127 (1982); *Suppl. 7*, 67 (1987)
1,5-Naphthalene diisocyanate	*19*, 311 (1979); *Suppl. 7*, 67 (1987)
1-Naphthylamine	*4*, 87 (1974) (*corr. 42*, 253); *Suppl. 7*, 260 (1987)
2-Naphthylamine	*4*, 97 (1974); *Suppl. 7*, 261 (1987)
1-Naphthylthiourea	*30*, 347 (1983); *Suppl. 7*, 263 (1987)
Nickel acetate (*see* Nickel and nickel compounds)	

Nickel ammonium sulfate (*see* Nickel and nickel compounds)	
Nickel and nickel compounds	2, 126 (1973) (*corr.* 42, 252); 11, 75 (1976); *Suppl.* 7, 264 (1987) (*corr.* 45, 283); 49, 257 (1990)
Nickel carbonate (*see* Nickel and nickel compounds)	
Nickel carbonyl (*see* Nickel and nickel compounds)	
Nickel chloride (*see* Nickel and nickel compounds)	
Nickel–gallium alloy (*see* Nickel and nickel compounds)	
Nickel hydroxide (*see* Nickel and nickel compounds)	
Nickelocene (*see* Nickel and nickel compounds)	
Nickel oxide (*see* Nickel and nickel compounds)	
Nickel subsulfide (*see* Nickel and nickel compounds)	
Nickel sulfate (*see* Nickel and nickel compounds)	
Niridazole	13, 123 (1977); *Suppl.* 7, 67 (1987)
Nithiazide	31, 179 (1983); *Suppl.* 7, 67 (1987)
Nitrilotriacetic acid and its salts	48, 181 (1990)
5-Nitroacenaphthene	16, 319 (1978); *Suppl.* 7, 67 (1987)
5-Nitro-*ortho*-anisidine	27, 133 (1982); *Suppl.* 7, 67 (1987)
9-Nitroanthracene	33, 179 (1984); *Suppl.* 7, 67 (1987)
7-Nitrobenz[*a*]anthracene	46, 247 (1989)
6-Nitrobenzo[*a*]pyrene	33, 187 (1984); *Suppl.* 7, 67 (1987); 46, 255 (1989)
4-Nitrobiphenyl	4, 113 (1974); *Suppl.* 7, 67 (1987)
6-Nitrochrysene	33, 195 (1984); *Suppl.* 7, 67 (1987); 46, 267 (1989)
Nitrofen (technical-grade)	30, 271 (1983); *Suppl.* 7, 67 (1987)
3-Nitrofluoranthene	33, 201 (1984); *Suppl.* 7, 67 (1987)
2-Nitrofluorene	46, 277 (1989)
Nitrofural	7, 171 (1974); *Suppl.* 7, 67 (1987); 50, 195 (1990)
5-Nitro-2-furaldehyde semicarbazone (*see* Nitrofural)	
Nitrofurantoin	50, 211 (1990)
Nitrofurazone (*see* Nitrofural)	
1-[(5-Nitrofurfurylidene)amino]-2-imidazolidinone	7, 181 (1974); *Suppl.* 7, 67 (1987)
N-[4-(5-Nitro-2-furyl)-2-thiazolyl]acetamide	1, 181 (1972); 7, 185 (1974); *Suppl.* 7, 67 (1987)
Nitrogen mustard	9, 193 (1975); *Suppl.* 7, 269 (1987)
Nitrogen mustard *N*-oxide	9, 209 (1975); *Suppl.* 7, 67 (1987)
1-Nitronaphthalene	46, 291 (1989)
2-Nitronaphthalene	46, 303 (1989)
3-Nitroperylene	46, 313 (1989)
2-Nitro-*para*-phenylenediamine (*see* 1,4-Diamino-2-nitrobenzene)	
2-Nitropropane	29, 331 (1982); *Suppl.* 7, 67 (1987)
1-Nitropyrene	33, 209 (1984); *Suppl.* 7, 67 (1987); 46, 321 (1989)
2-Nitropyrene	46, 359 (1989)
4-Nitropyrene	46, 367 (1989)
N-Nitrosatable drugs	24, 297 (1980) (*corr.* 42, 260)
N-Nitrosatable pesticides	30, 359 (1983)
N'-Nitrosoanabasine	37, 225 (1985); *Suppl.* 7, 67 (1987)
N'-Nitrosoanatabine	37, 233 (1985); *Suppl.* 7, 67 (1987)

N-Nitrosodi-n-butylamine	4, 197 (1974); 17, 51 (1978); Suppl. 7, 67 (1987)
N-Nitrosodiethanolamine	17, 77 (1978); Suppl. 7, 67 (1987)
N-Nitrosodiethylamine	1, 107 (1972) (corr. 42, 251); 17, 83 (1978) (corr. 42, 257); Suppl. 7, 67 (1987)
N-Nitrosodimethylamine	1, 95 (1972); 17, 125 (1978) (corr. 42, 257); Suppl. 7, 67 (1987)
N-Nitrosodiphenylamine	27, 213 (1982); Suppl. 7, 67 (1987)
para-Nitrosodiphenylamine	27, 227 (1982) (corr. 42, 261); Suppl. 7, 68 (1987)
N-Nitrosodi-n-propylamine	17, 177 (1978); Suppl. 7, 68 (1987)
N-Nitroso-N-ethylurea (see N-Ethyl-N-nitrosourea)	
N-Nitrosofolic acid	17, 217 (1978); Suppl. 7, 68 (1987)
N-Nitrosoguvacine	37, 263 (1985); Suppl. 7, 68 (1987)
N-Nitrosoguvacoline	37, 263 (1985); Suppl. 7, 68 (1987)
N-Nitrosohydroxyproline	17, 304 (1978); Suppl. 7, 68 (1987)
3-(N-Nitrosomethylamino)propionaldehyde	37, 263 (1985); Suppl. 7, 68 (1987)
3-(N-Nitrosomethylamino)propionitrile	37, 263 (1985); Suppl. 7, 68 (1987)
4-(N-Nitrosomethylamino)-4-(3-pyridyl)-1-butanal	37, 205 (1985); Suppl. 7, 68 (1987)
4-(N-Nitrosomethylamino)-1-(3-pyridyl)-1-butanone	37, 209 (1985); Suppl. 7, 68 (1987)
N-Nitrosomethylethylamine	17, 221 (1978); Suppl. 7, 68 (1987)
N-Nitroso-N-methylurea (see N-Methyl-N-nitrosourea)	
N-Nitroso-N-methylurethane (see N-Methyl-N-methylurethane)	
N-Nitrosomethylvinylamine	17, 257 (1978); Suppl. 7, 68 (1987)
N-Nitrosomorpholine	17, 263 (1978); Suppl. 7, 68 (1987)
N'-Nitrosonornicotine	17, 281 (1978); 37, 241 (1985); Suppl. 7, 68 (1987)
N-Nitrosopiperidine	17, 287 (1978); Suppl. 7, 68 (1987)
N-Nitrosoproline	17, 303 (1978); Suppl. 7, 68 (1987)
N-Nitrosopyrrolidine	17, 313 (1978); Suppl. 7, 68 (1987)
N-Nitrososarcosine	17, 327 (1978); Suppl. 7, 68 (1987)
Nitrosoureas, chloroethyl (see Chloroethyl nitrosoureas)	
5-Nitro-ortho-toluidine	48, 169 (1990)
Nitrous oxide (see Anaesthetics, volatile)	
Nitrovin	31, 185 (1983); Suppl. 7, 68 (1987)
Nivalenol (see Toxins derived from Fusarium graminearum, F. culmorum and F. crookwellense)	
NNA [see 4-(N-Nitrosomethylamino)-4-(3-pyridyl)-1-butanal]	
NNK [see 4-(N-Nitrosomethylamino)-1-(3-pyridyl)-1-butanone]	
Nonsteroidal oestrogens (see also Oestrogens, progestins and combinations)	Suppl. 7, 272 (1987)
Norethisterone (see also Progestins; Combined oral contraceptives)	6, 179 (1974); 21, 461 (1979)
Norethynodrel (see also Progestins; Combined oral contraceptives	6, 191 (1974); 21, 461 (1979) (corr. 42, 259)
Norgestrel (see also Progestins, Combined oral contraceptives)	6, 201 (1974); 21, 479 (1979)
Nylon 6	19, 120 (1979); Suppl. 7, 68 (1987)

O

Ochratoxin A	10, 191 (1976); 31, 191 (1983) (corr. 42, 262); Suppl. 7, 271 (1987); 56, 489 (1993)
Oestradiol-17β (see also Steroidal oestrogens)	6, 99 (1974); 21, 279 (1979)
Oestradiol 3-benzoate (see Oestradiol-17β)	
Oestradiol dipropionate (see Oestradiol-17β)	
Oestradiol mustard	9, 217 (1975)
Oestradiol-17β-valerate (see Oestradiol-17β)	
Oestriol (see also Steroidal oestrogens)	6, 117 (1974); 21, 327 (1979)
Oestrogen–progestin combinations (see Oestrogens, progestins and combinations)	
Oestrogen–progestin replacement therapy (see also Oestrogens, progestins and combinations)	Suppl. 7, 308 (1987)
Oestrogen replacement therapy (see also Oestrogens, progestins and combinations)	Suppl. 7, 280 (1987)
Oestrogens (see Oestrogens, progestins and combinations)	
Oestrogens, conjugated (see Conjugated oestrogens)	
Oestrogens, nonsteroidal (see Nonsteroidal oestrogens)	
Oestrogens, progestins and combinations	6 (1974); 21 (1979); Suppl. 7, 272 (1987)
Oestrogens, steroidal (see Steroidal oestrogens)	
Oestrone (see also Steroidal oestrogens)	6, 123 (1974); 21, 343 (1979) (corr. 42, 259)
Oestrone benzoate (see Oestrone)	
Oil Orange SS	8, 165 (1975); Suppl. 7, 69 (1987)
Oral contraceptives, combined (see Combined oral contraceptives)	
Oral contraceptives, investigational (see Combined oral contraceptives)	
Oral contraceptives, sequential (see Sequential oral contraceptives)	
Orange I	8, 173 (1975); Suppl. 7, 69 (1987)
Orange G	8, 181 (1975); Suppl. 7, 69 (1987)
Organolead compounds (see also Lead and lead compounds)	Suppl. 7, 230 (1987)
Oxazepam	13, 58 (1977); Suppl. 7, 69 (1987)
Oxymetholone [see also Androgenic (anabolic) steroids]	13, 131 (1977)
Oxyphenbutazone	13, 185 (1977); Suppl. 7, 69 (1987)

P

Paint manufacture and painting (occupational exposures in)	47, 329 (1989)
Panfuran S (see also Dihydroxymethylfuratrizine)	24, 77 (1980); Suppl. 7, 69 (1987)
Paper manufacture (see Pulp and paper manufacture)	
Paracetamol	50, 307 (1990)
Parasorbic acid	10, 199 (1976) (corr. 42, 255); Suppl. 7, 69 (1987)
Parathion	30, 153 (1983); Suppl. 7, 69 (1987)
Patulin	10, 205 (1976); 40, 83 (1986); Suppl. 7, 69 (1987)
Penicillic acid	10, 211 (1976); Suppl. 7, 69 (1987)
Pentachloroethane	41, 99 (1986); Suppl. 7, 69 (1987)
Pentachloronitrobenzene (see Quintozene)	

Pentachlorophenol (*see also* Chlorophenols; Chlorophenols, occupational exposures to)	*20*, 303 (1979); *53*, 371 (1991)
Permethrin	*53*, 329 (1991)
Perylene	*32*, 411 (1983); *Suppl. 7*, 69 (1987)
Petasitenine	*31*, 207 (1983); *Suppl. 7*, 69 (1987)
Petasites japonicus (*see* Pyrrolizidine alkaloids)	
Petroleum refining (occupational exposures in)	*45*, 39 (1989)
Some petroleum solvents	*47*, 43 (1989)
Phenacetin	*13*, 141 (1977); *24*, 135 (1980); *Suppl. 7*, 310 (1987)
Phenanthrene	*32*, 419 (1983); *Suppl. 7*, 69 (1987)
Phenazopyridine hydrochloride	*8*, 117 (1975); *24*, 163 (1980) (*corr. 42*, 260); *Suppl. 7*, 312 (1987)
Phenelzine sulfate	*24*, 175 (1980); *Suppl. 7*, 312 (1987)
Phenicarbazide	*12*, 177 (1976); *Suppl. 7*, 70 (1987)
Phenobarbital	*13*, 157 (1977); *Suppl. 7*, 313 (1987)
Phenol	*47*, 263 (1989) (*corr. 50*, 385)
Phenoxyacetic acid herbicides (*see* Chlorophenoxy herbicides)	
Phenoxybenzamine hydrochloride	*9*, 223 (1975); *24*, 185 (1980); *Suppl. 7*, 70 (1987)
Phenylbutazone	*13*, 183 (1977); *Suppl. 7*, 316 (1987)
meta-Phenylenediamine	*16*, 111 (1978); *Suppl. 7*, 70 (1987)
para-Phenylenediamine	*16*, 125 (1978); *Suppl. 7*, 70 (1987)
Phenyl glycidyl ether (*see* Glycidyl ethers)	
N-Phenyl-2-naphthylamine	*16*, 325 (1978) (*corr. 42*, 257); *Suppl. 7*, 318 (1987)
ortho-Phenylphenol	*30*, 329 (1983); *Suppl. 7*, 70 (1987)
Phenytoin	*13*, 201 (1977); *Suppl. 7*, 319 (1987)
PhIP	*56*, 229 (1993)
Pickled vegetables	*56*, 83 (1993)
Picloram	*53*, 481 (1991)
Piperazine oestrone sulfate (*see* Conjugated oestrogens)	
Piperonyl butoxide	*30*, 183 (1983); *Suppl. 7*, 70 (1987)
Pitches, coal-tar (*see* Coal-tar pitches)	
Polyacrylic acid	*19*, 62 (1979); *Suppl. 7*, 70 (1987)
Polybrominated biphenyls	*18*, 107 (1978); *41*, 261 (1986); *Suppl. 7*, 321 (1987)
Polychlorinated biphenyls	*7*, 261 (1974); *18*, 43 (1978) (*corr. 42*, 258); *Suppl. 7*, 322 (1987)
Polychlorinated camphenes (*see* Toxaphene)	
Polychloroprene	*19*, 141 (1979); *Suppl. 7*, 70 (1987)
Polyethylene	*19*, 164 (1979); *Suppl. 7*, 70 (1987)
Polymethylene polyphenyl isocyanate	*19*, 314 (1979); *Suppl. 7*, 70 (1987)
Polymethyl methacrylate	*19*, 195 (1979); *Suppl. 7*, 70 (1987)
Polyoestradiol phosphate (*see* Oestradiol-17β)	
Polypropylene	*19*, 218 (1979); *Suppl. 7*, 70 (1987)
Polystyrene	*19*, 245 (1979); *Suppl. 7*, 70 (1987)
Polytetrafluoroethylene	*19*, 288 (1979); *Suppl. 7*, 70 (1987)
Polyurethane foams	*19*, 320 (1979); *Suppl. 7*, 70 (1987)
Polyvinyl acetate	*19*, 346 (1979); *Suppl. 7*, 70 (1987)
Polyvinyl alcohol	*19*, 351 (1979); *Suppl. 7*, 70 (1987)

Polyvinyl chloride	7, 306 (1974); *19*, 402 (1979); *Suppl. 7*, 70 (1987)
Polyvinyl pyrrolidone	*19*, 463 (1979); *Suppl. 7*, 70 (1987)
Ponceau MX	*8*, 189 (1975); *Suppl. 7*, 70 (1987)
Ponceau 3R	*8*, 199 (1975); *Suppl. 7*, 70 (1987)
Ponceau SX	*8*, 207 (1975); *Suppl. 7*, 70 (1987)
Potassium arsenate (*see* Arsenic and arsenic compounds)	
Potassium arsenite (*see* Arsenic and arsenic compounds)	
Potassium bis(2-hydroxyethyl)dithiocarbamate	*12*, 183 (1976); *Suppl. 7*, 70 (1987)
Potassium bromate	*40*, 207 (1986); *Suppl. 7*, 70 (1987)
Potassium chromate (*see* Chromium and chromium compounds)	
Potassium dichromate (*see* Chromium and chromium compounds)	
Prednimustine	*50*, 115 (1990)
Prednisone	*26*, 293 (1981); *Suppl. 7*, 326 (1987)
Procarbazine hydrochloride	*26*, 311 (1981); *Suppl. 7*, 327 (1987)
Proflavine salts	*24*, 195 (1980); *Suppl. 7*, 70 (1987)
Progesterone (*see also* Progestins; Combined oral contraceptives)	*6*, 135 (1974); *21*, 491 (1979) (*corr. 42*, 259)
Progestins (*see also* Oestrogens, progestins and combinations)	*Suppl. 7*, 289 (1987)
Pronetalol hydrochloride	*13*, 227 (1977) (*corr. 42*, 256); *Suppl. 7*, 70 (1987)
1,3-Propane sultone	*4*, 253 (1974) (*corr. 42*, 253); *Suppl. 7*, 70 (1987)
Propham	*12*, 189 (1976); *Suppl. 7*, 70 (1987)
β-Propiolactone	*4*, 259 (1974) (*corr. 42*, 253); *Suppl. 7*, 70 (1987)
n-Propyl carbamate	*12*, 201 (1976); *Suppl. 7*, 70 (1987)
Propylene	*19*, 213 (1979); *Suppl. 7*, 71 (1987)
Propylene oxide	*11*, 191 (1976); *36*, 227 (1985) (*corr. 42*, 263); *Suppl. 7*, 328 (1987)
Propylthiouracil	*7*, 67 (1974); *Suppl. 7*, 329 (1987)
Ptaquiloside (*see also* Bracken fern)	*40*, 55 (1986); *Suppl. 7*, 71 (1987)
Pulp and paper manufacture	*25*, 157 (1981); *Suppl. 7*, 385 (1987)
Pyrene	*32*, 431 (1983); *Suppl. 7*, 71 (1987)
Pyrido[3,4-*c*]psoralen	*40*, 349 (1986); *Suppl. 7*, 71 (1987)
Pyrimethamine	*13*, 233 (1977); *Suppl. 7*, 71 (1987)
Pyrrolizidine alkaloids (*see* Hydroxysenkirkine; Isatidine; Jacobine; Lasiocarpine; Monocrotaline; Retrorsine; Riddelliine; Seneciphylline; Senkirkine)	

Q

Quercetin (*see also* Bracken fern)	*31*, 213 (1983); *Suppl. 7*, 71 (1987)
para-Quinone	*15*, 255 (1977); *Suppl. 7*, 71 (1987)
Quintozene	*5*, 211 (1974); *Suppl. 7*, 71 (1987)

R

Radon	*43*, 173 (1988) (*corr. 45*, 283)
Reserpine	*10*, 217 (1976); *24*, 211 (1980) (*corr. 42*, 260); *Suppl. 7*, 330 (1987)
Resorcinol	*15*, 155 (1977); *Suppl. 7*, 71 (1987)

Retrorsine	*10*, 303 (1976); *Suppl. 7*, 71 (1987)
Rhodamine B	*16*, 221 (1978); *Suppl. 7*, 71 (1987)
Rhodamine 6G	*16*, 233 (1978); *Suppl. 7*, 71 (1987)
Riddelliine	*10*, 313 (1976); *Suppl. 7*, 71 (1987)
Rifampicin	*24*, 243 (1980); *Suppl. 7*, 71 (1987)
Rockwool (*see* Man-made mineral fibres)	
The rubber industry	*28* (1982) (*corr. 42*, 261); *Suppl. 7*, 332 (1987)
Rugulosin	*40*, 99 (1986); *Suppl. 7*, 71 (1987)

S

Saccharated iron oxide	*2*, 161 (1973); *Suppl. 7*, 71 (1987)
Saccharin	*22*, 111 (1980) (*corr. 42*, 259); *Suppl. 7*, 334 (1987)
Safrole	*1*, 169 (1972); *10*, 231 (1976); *Suppl. 7*, 71 (1987)
Salted fish	*56*, 41 (1993)
The sawmill industry (including logging) [*see* The lumber and sawmill industry (including logging)]	
Scarlet Red	*8*, 217 (1975); *Suppl. 7*, 71 (1987)
Selenium and selenium compounds	*9*, 245 (1975) (*corr. 42*, 255); *Suppl. 7*, 71 (1987)
Selenium dioxide (*see* Selenium and selenium compounds)	
Selenium oxide (*see* Selenium and selenium compounds)	
Semicarbazide hydrochloride	*12*, 209 (1976) (*corr. 42*, 256); *Suppl. 7*, 71 (1987)
Senecio jacobaea L. (*see* Pyrrolizidine alkaloids)	
Senecio longilobus (*see* Pyrrolizidine alkaloids)	
Seneciphylline	*10*, 319, 335 (1976); *Suppl. 7*, 71 (1987)
Senkirkine	*10*, 327 (1976); *31*, 231 (1983); *Suppl. 7*, 71 (1987)
Sepiolite	*42*, 175 (1987); *Suppl. 7*, 71 (1987)
Sequential oral contraceptives (*see also* Oestrogens, progestins and combinations)	*Suppl. 7*, 296 (1987)
Shale-oils	*35*, 161 (1985); *Suppl. 7*, 339 (1987)
Shikimic acid (*see also* Bracken fern)	*40*, 55 (1986); *Suppl. 7*, 71 (1987)
Shoe manufacture and repair (*see* Boot and shoe manufacture and repair)	
Silica (*see also* Amorphous silica; Crystalline silica)	*42*, 39 (1987)
Simazine	*53*, 495 (1991)
Slagwool (*see* Man-made mineral fibres)	
Sodium arsenate (*see* Arsenic and arsenic compounds)	
Sodium arsenite (*see* Arsenic and arsenic compounds)	
Sodium cacodylate (*see* Arsenic and arsenic compounds)	
Sodium chlorite	*52*, 145 (1991)
Sodium chromate (*see* Chromium and chromium compounds)	
Sodium cyclamate (*see* Cyclamates)	
Sodium dichromate (*see* Chromium and chromium compounds)	
Sodium diethyldithiocarbamate	*12*, 217 (1976); *Suppl. 7*, 71 (1987)
Sodium equilin sulfate (*see* Conjugated oestrogens)	

Sodium fluoride (see Fluorides)
Sodium monofluorophosphate (see Fluorides)
Sodium oestrone sulfate (see Conjugated oestrogens)
Sodium *ortho*-phenylphenate (see also *ortho*-Phenylphenol)   30, 329 (1983); *Suppl. 7*, 392 (1987)
Sodium saccharin (see Saccharin)
Sodium selenate (see Selenium and selenium compounds)
Sodium selenite (see Selenium and selenium compounds)
Sodium silicofluoride (see Fluorides)
Solar radiation   55 (1992)
Soots   3, 22 (1973); 35, 219 (1985); *Suppl. 7*, 343 (1987)
Spironolactone   24, 259 (1980); *Suppl. 7*, 344 (1987)
Stannous fluoride (see Fluorides)
Steel founding (see Iron and steel founding)
Sterigmatocystin   1, 175 (1972); 10, 245 (1976); *Suppl. 7*, 72 (1987)
Steroidal oestrogens (see also Oestrogens, progestins and combinations)   *Suppl. 7*, 280 (1987)
Streptozotocin   4, 221 (1974); 17, 337 (1978); *Suppl. 7*, 72 (1987)
Strobane® (see Terpene polychlorinates)
Strontium chromate (see Chromium and chromium compounds)
Styrene   19, 231 (1979) (corr. 42, 258); *Suppl. 7*, 345 (1987)
Styrene-acrylonitrile copolymers   19, 97 (1979); *Suppl. 7*, 72 (1987)
Styrene-butadiene copolymers   19, 252 (1979); *Suppl. 7*, 72 (1987)
Styrene oxide   11, 201 (1976); 19, 275 (1979); 36, 245 (1985); *Suppl. 7*, 72 (1987)
Succinic anhydride   15, 265 (1977); *Suppl. 7*, 72 (1987)
Sudan I   8, 225 (1975); *Suppl. 7*, 72 (1987)
Sudan II   8, 233 (1975); *Suppl. 7*, 72 (1987)
Sudan III   8, 241 (1975); *Suppl. 7*, 72 (1987)
Sudan Brown RR   8, 249 (1975); *Suppl. 7*, 72 (1987)
Sudan Red 7B   8, 253 (1975); *Suppl. 7*, 72 (1987)
Sulfafurazole   24, 275 (1980); *Suppl. 7*, 347 (1987)
Sulfallate   30, 283 (1983); *Suppl. 7*, 72 (1987)
Sulfamethoxazole   24, 285 (1980); *Suppl. 7*, 348 (1987)
Sulfites (see Sulfur dioxide and some sulfites, bisulfites and metabisulfites)
Sulfur dioxide and some sulfites, bisulfites and metabisulfites   54, 131 (1992)
Sulfur mustard (see Mustard gas)
Sulfuric acid and other strong inorganic acids, occupational exposures to mists and vapours from   54, 41 (1992)
Sulfur trioxide   54, 121 (1992)
Sulphisoxazole (see Sulfafurazole)
Sunset Yellow FCF   8, 257 (1975); *Suppl. 7*, 72 (1987)
Symphytine   31, 239 (1983); *Suppl. 7*, 72 (1987)

T

2,4,5-T (see also Chlorophenoxy herbicides; Chlorophenoxy herbicides, occupational exposures to)   15, 273 (1977)
Talc   42, 185 (1987); *Suppl. 7*, 349 (1987)

Tannic acid	*10*, 253 (1976) (*corr. 42*, 255); *Suppl. 7*, 72 (1987)
Tannins (*see also* Tannic acid)	*10*, 254 (1976); *Suppl. 7*, 72 (1987)
TCDD (*see* 2,3,7,8-Tetrachlorodibenzo-*para*-dioxin)	
TDE (*see* DDT)	
Tea	*51*, 207 (1991)
Terpene polychlorinates	*5*, 219 (1974); *Suppl. 7*, 72 (1987)
Testosterone (*see also* Androgenic (anabolic) steroids)	*6*, 209 (1974); *21*, 519 (1979)
Testosterone oenanthate (*see* Testosterone)	
Testosterone propionate (*see* Testosterone)	
2,2',5,5'-Tetrachlorobenzidine	*27*, 141 (1982); *Suppl. 7*, 72 (1987)
2,3,7,8-Tetrachlorodibenzo-*para*-dioxin	*15*, 41 (1977); *Suppl. 7*, 350 (1987)
1,1,1,2-Tetrachloroethane	*41*, 87 (1986); *Suppl. 7*, 72 (1987)
1,1,2,2-Tetrachloroethane	*20*, 477 (1979); *Suppl. 7*, 354 (1987)
Tetrachloroethylene	*20*, 491 (1979); *Suppl. 7*, 355 (1987)
2,3,4,6-Tetrachlorophenol (*see* Chlorophenols; Chlorophenols, occupational exposures to)	
Tetrachlorvinphos	*30*, 197 (1983); *Suppl. 7*, 72 (1987)
Tetraethyllead (*see* Lead and lead compounds)	
Tetrafluoroethylene	*19*, 285 (1979); *Suppl. 7*, 72 (1987)
Tetrakis(hydroxymethyl) phosphonium salts	*48*, 95 (1990)
Tetramethyllead (*see* Lead and lead compounds)	
Textile manufacturing industry, exposures in	*48*, 215 (1990) (*corr. 51*, 483)
Theobromine	*51*, 421 (1991)
Theophylline	*51*, 391 (1991)
Thioacetamide	*7*, 77 (1974); *Suppl. 7*, 72 (1987)
4,4'-Thiodianiline	*16*, 343 (1978); *27*, 147 (1982); *Suppl. 7*, 72 (1987)
Thiotepa	*9*, 85 (1975); *Suppl. 7*, 368 (1987); *50*, 123 (1990)
Thiouracil	*7*, 85 (1974); *Suppl. 7*, 72 (1987)
Thiourea	*7*, 95 (1974); *Suppl. 7*, 72 (1987)
Thiram	*12*, 225 (1976); *Suppl. 7*, 72 (1987); *53*, 403 (1991)
Titanium dioxide	*47*, 307 (1989)
Tobacco habits other than smoking (*see* Tobacco products, smokeless)	
Tobacco products, smokeless	*37* (1985) (*corr. 42*, 263; *52*, 513); *Suppl. 7*, 357 (1987)
Tobacco smoke	*38* (1986) (*corr. 42*, 263); *Suppl. 7*, 357 (1987)
Tobacco smoking (*see* Tobacco smoke)	
ortho-Tolidine (*see* 3,3'-Dimethylbenzidine)	
2,4-Toluene diisocyanate (*see also* Toluene diisocyanates)	*19*, 303 (1979); *39*, 287 (1986)
2,6-Toluene diisocyanate (*see also* Toluene diisocyanates)	*19*, 303 (1979); *39*, 289 (1986)
Toluene	*47*, 79 (1989)
Toluene diisocyanates	*39*, 287 (1986) (*corr. 42*, 264); *Suppl. 7*, 72 (1987)
Toluenes, α-chlorinated (*see* α-Chlorinated toluenes)	
ortho-Toluenesulfonamide (*see* Saccharin)	
ortho-Toluidine	*16*, 349 (1978); *27*, 155 (1982); *Suppl. 7*, 362 (1987)

Toxaphene	20, 327 (1979); Suppl. 7, 72 (1987)
T-2 Toxin (see Toxins derived from *Fusarium sporotrichioides*)	
Toxins derived from *Fusarium graminearum*, *F. culmorum* and *F. crookwellense*	11, 169 (1976); 31, 153, 279 (1983); Suppl. 7, 64, 74 (1987); 56, 397 (1993)
Toxins derived from *Fusarium moniliforme*	56, 445 (1993)
Toxins derived from *Fusarium sporotrichioides*	31, 265 (1983); Suppl. 7, 73 (1987); 56, 467 (1993)
Tremolite (see Asbestos)	
Treosulfan	26, 341 (1981); Suppl. 7, 363 (1987)
Triaziquone [see Tris(aziridinyl)-*para*-benzoquinone]	
Trichlorfon	30, 207 (1983); Suppl. 7, 73 (1987)
Trichlormethine	9, 229 (1975); Suppl. 7, 73 (1987); 50, 143 (1990)
Trichloroacetonitrile (see Halogenated acetonitriles)	
1,1,1-Trichloroethane	20, 515 (1979); Suppl. 7, 73 (1987)
1,1,2-Trichloroethane	20, 533 (1979); Suppl. 7, 73 (1987); 52, 337 (1991)
Trichloroethylene	11, 263 (1976); 20, 545 (1979); Suppl. 7, 364 (1987)
2,4,5-Trichlorophenol (see also Chlorophenols; Chlorophenols occupational exposures to)	20, 349 (1979)
2,4,6-Trichlorophenol (see also Chlorophenols; Chlorophenols, occupational exposures to)	20, 349 (1979)
(2,4,5-Trichlorophenoxy)acetic acid (see 2,4,5-T)	
Trichlorotriethylamine hydrochloride (see Trichlormethine)	
T$_2$-Trichothecene (see Toxins derived from *Fusarium sporotrichioides*)	
Triethylene glycol diglycidyl ether	11, 209 (1976); Suppl. 7, 73 (1987)
Trifluralin	53, 515 (1991)
4,4',6-Trimethylangelicin plus ultraviolet radiation (see also Angelicin and some synthetic derivatives)	Suppl. 7, 57 (1987)
2,4,5-Trimethylaniline	27, 177 (1982); Suppl. 7, 73 (1987)
2,4,6-Trimethylaniline	27, 178 (1982); Suppl. 7, 73 (1987)
4,5',8-Trimethylpsoralen	40, 357 (1986); Suppl. 7, 366 (1987)
Trimustine hydrochloride (see Trichlormethine)	
Triphenylene	32, 447 (1983); Suppl. 7, 73 (1987)
Tris(aziridinyl)-*para*-benzoquinone	9, 67 (1975); Suppl. 7, 367 (1987)
Tris(1-aziridinyl)phosphine oxide	9, 75 (1975); Suppl. 7, 73 (1987)
Tris(1-aziridinyl)phosphine sulphide (see Thiotepa)	
2,4,6-Tris(1-aziridinyl)-*s*-triazine	9, 95 (1975); Suppl. 7, 73 (1987)
Tris(2-chloroethyl) phosphate	48, 109 (1990)
1,2,3-Tris(chloromethoxy)propane	15, 301 (1977); Suppl. 7, 73 (1987)
Tris(2,3-dibromopropyl)phosphate	20, 575 (1979); Suppl. 7, 369 (1987)
Tris(2-methyl-1-aziridinyl)phosphine oxide	9, 107 (1975); Suppl. 7, 73 (1987)
Trp-P-1	31, 247 (1983); Suppl. 7, 73 (1987)
Trp-P-2	31, 255 (1983); Suppl. 7, 73 (1987)
Trypan blue	8, 267 (1975); Suppl. 7, 73 (1987)
Tussilago farfara L. (see Pyrrolizidine alkaloids)	

U

Ultraviolet radiation	40, 379 (1986); 55 (1992)
Underground haematite mining with exposure to radon	1, 29 (1972); Suppl. 7, 216 (1987)

Uracil mustard	9, 235 (1975); *Suppl. 7*, 370 (1987)
Urethane	7, 111 (1974); *Suppl. 7*, 73 (1987)

V

Vat Yellow 4	*48*, 161 (1990)
Vinblastine sulfate	*26*, 349 (1981) (*corr. 42*, 261); *Suppl. 7*, 371 (1987)
Vincristine sulfate	*26*, 365 (1981); *Suppl. 7*, 372 (1987)
Vinyl acetate	*19*, 341 (1979); *39*, 113 (1986); *Suppl. 7*, 73 (1987)
Vinyl bromide	*19*, 367 (1979); *39*, 133 (1986); *Suppl. 7*, 73 (1987)
Vinyl chloride	7, 291 (1974); *19*, 377 (1979) (*corr. 42*, 258); *Suppl. 7*, 373 (1987)
Vinyl chloride–vinyl acetate copolymers	7, 311 (1976); *19*, 412 (1979) (*corr. 42*, 258); *Suppl. 7*, 73 (1987)
4-Vinylcyclohexene	*11*, 277 (1976); *39*, 181 (1986); *Suppl. 7*, 73 (1987)
Vinyl fluoride	*39*, 147 (1986); *Suppl. 7*, 73 (1987)
Vinylidene chloride	*19*, 439 (1979); *39*, 195 (1986); *Suppl. 7*, 376 (1987)
Vinylidene chloride–vinyl chloride copolymers	*19*, 448 (1979) (*corr. 42*, 258); *Suppl. 7*, 73 (1987)
Vinylidene fluoride	*39*, 227 (1986); *Suppl. 7*, 73 (1987)
N-Vinyl-2-pyrrolidone	*19*, 461 (1979); *Suppl. 7*, 73 (1987)

W

Welding	*49*, 447 (1990) (*corr. 52*, 513)
Wollastonite	*42*, 145 (1987); *Suppl. 7*, 377 (1987)
Wood industries	*25* (1981); *Suppl. 7*, 378 (1987)

X

Xylene	*47*, 125 (1989)
2,4-Xylidine	*16*, 367 (1978); *Suppl. 7*, 74 (1987)
2,5-Xylidine	*16*, 377 (1978); *Suppl. 7*, 74 (1987)
2,6-Xylidine (*see* 2,6-Dimethylaniline)	

Y

Yellow AB	*8*, 279 (1975); *Suppl. 7*, 74 (1987)
Yellow OB	*8*, 287 (1975); *Suppl. 7*, 74 (1987)

Z

Zearalenone (*see* Toxins derived from *Fusarium graminearum, F. culmorum* and *F. crookwellense*)	
Zectran	*12*, 237 (1976); *Suppl. 7*, 74 (1987)
Zinc beryllium silicate (*see* Beryllium and beryllium compounds)	

Zinc chromate (*see* Chromium and chromium compounds)
Zinc chromate hydroxide (*see* Chromium and chromium compounds)
Zinc potassium chromate (*see* Chromium and chromium compounds)
Zinc yellow (*see* Chromium and chromium compounds)
Zineb   *12*, 245 (1976); *Suppl. 7*, 74 (1987)
Ziram   *12*, 259 (1976); *Suppl. 7*, 74 (1987); *53*, 423 (1991)

PUBLICATIONS OF THE INTERNATIONAL AGENCY FOR RESEARCH ON CANCER

Scientific Publications Series

(Available from Oxford University Press through local bookshops)

No. 1 **Liver Cancer**
1971; 176 pages (*out of print*)

No. 2 **Oncogenesis and Herpesviruses**
Edited by P.M. Biggs, G. de-Thé and L.N. Payne
1972; 515 pages (*out of print*)

No. 3 **N-Nitroso Compounds: Analysis and Formation**
Edited by P. Bogovski, R. Preussman and E.A. Walker
1972; 140 pages (*out of print*)

No. 4 **Transplacental Carcinogenesis**
Edited by L. Tomatis and U. Mohr
1973; 181 pages (*out of print*)

No. 5/6 **Pathology of Tumours in Laboratory Animals, Volume 1, Tumours of the Rat**
Edited by V.S. Turusov
1973/1976; 533 pages (*out of print*)

No. 7 **Host Environment Interactions in the Etiology of Cancer in Man**
Edited by R. Doll and I. Vodopija
1973; 464 pages (*out of print*)

No. 8 **Biological Effects of Asbestos**
Edited by P. Bogovski, J.C. Gilson, V. Timbrell and J.C. Wagner
1973; 346 pages (*out of print*)

No. 9 **N-Nitroso Compounds in the Environment**
Edited by P. Bogovski and E.A. Walker
1974; 243 pages (*out of print*)

No. 10 **Chemical Carcinogenesis Essays**
Edited by R. Montesano and L. Tomatis
1974: 230 pages (*out of print*)

No. 11 **Oncogenesis and Herpesviruses II**
Edited by G. de-Thé, M.A. Epstein and H. zur Hausen
1975; Part I: 511 pages
Part II: 403 pages (*out of print*)

No. 12 **Screening Tests in Chemical Carcinogenesis**
Edited by R. Montesano, H. Bartsch and L. Tomatis
1976; 666 pages (*out of print*)

No. 13 **Environmental Pollution and Carcinogenic Risks**
Edited by C. Rosenfeld and W. Davis
1975; 441 pages (*out of print*)

No. 14 **Environmental N-Nitroso Compounds. Analysis and Formation**
Edited by E.A. Walker, P. Bogovski and L. Griciute
1976; 512 pages (*out of print*)

No. 15 **Cancer Incidence in Five Continents, Volume III**
Edited by J.A.H. Waterhouse, C. Muir, P. Correa and J. Powell
1976; 584 pages (*out of print*)

No. 16 **Air Pollution and Cancer in Man**
Edited by U. Mohr, D. Schmähl and L. Tomatis
1977; 328 pages (*out of print*)

No. 17 **Directory of On-going Research in Cancer Epidemiology 1977**
Edited by C.S. Muir and G. Wagner
1977; 599 pages (*out of print*)

No. 18 **Environmental Carcinogens. Selected Methods of Analysis. Volume 1: Analysis of Volatile Nitrosamines in Food**
Editor-in-Chief: H. Egan
1978; 212 pages (*out of print*)

No. 19 **Environmental Aspects of N-Nitroso Compounds**
Edited by E.A. Walker, M. Castegnaro, L. Griciute and R.E. Lyle
1978; 561 pages (*out of print*)

No. 20 **Nasopharyngeal Carcinoma: Etiology and Control**
Edited by G. de-Thé and Y. Ito
1978; 606 pages (*out of print*)

No. 21 **Cancer Registration and its Techniques**
Edited by R. MacLennan, C. Muir, R. Steinitz and A. Winkler
1978; 235 pages (*out of print*)

No. 22 **Environmental Carcinogens. Selected Methods of Analysis. Volume 2: Methods for the Measurement of Vinyl Chloride in Poly(vinyl chloride), Air, Water and Foodstuffs**
Editor-in-Chief: H. Egan
1978; 142 pages (*out of print*)

No. 23 **Pathology of Tumours in Laboratory Animals. Volume II: Tumours of the Mouse**
Editor-in-Chief: V.S. Turusov
1979; 669 pages (*out of print*)

No. 24 **Oncogenesis and Herpesviruses III**
Edited by G. de-Thé, W. Henle and F. Rapp
1978; Part I: 580 pages, Part II: 512 pages (*out of print*)

Prices, valid for September 1993, are subject to change without notice

List of IARC Publications

No. 25 Carcinogenic Risk. Strategies for Intervention
Edited by W. Davis and
C. Rosenfeld
1979; 280 pages (*out of print*)

No. 26 Directory of On-going Research in Cancer Epidemiology 1978
Edited by C.S. Muir and G. Wagner
1978; 550 pages (*out of print*)

No. 27 Molecular and Cellular Aspects of Carcinogen Screening Tests
Edited by R. Montesano,
H. Bartsch and L. Tomatis
1980; 372 pages £30.00

No. 28 Directory of On-going Research in Cancer Epidemiology 1979
Edited by C.S. Muir and G. Wagner
1979; 672 pages (*out of print*)

No. 29 Environmental Carcinogens. Selected Methods of Analysis. Volume 3: Analysis of Polycyclic Aromatic Hydrocarbons in Environmental Samples
Editor-in-Chief: H. Egan
1979; 240 pages (*out of print*)

No. 30 Biological Effects of Mineral Fibres
Editor-in-Chief: J.C. Wagner
1980; **Volume 1**: 494 pages **Volume 2**: 513 pages (*out of print*)

No. 31 N-Nitroso Compounds: Analysis, Formation and Occurrence
Edited by E.A. Walker, L. Griciute, M. Castegnaro and M. Börzsönyi
1980; 835 pages (*out of print*)

No. 32 Statistical Methods in Cancer Research. Volume 1. The Analysis of Case-control Studies
By N.E. Breslow and N.E. Day
1980; 338 pages £18.00

No. 33 Handling Chemical Carcinogens in the Laboratory
Edited by R. Montesano *et al.*
1979; 32 pages (*out of print*)

No. 34 Pathology of Tumours in Laboratory Animals. Volume III. Tumours of the Hamster
Editor-in-Chief: V.S. Turusov
1982; 461 pages (*out of print*)

No. 35 Directory of On-going Research in Cancer Epidemiology 1980
Edited by C.S. Muir and G. Wagner
1980; 660 pages (*out of print*)

No. 36 Cancer Mortality by Occupation and Social Class 1851-1971
Edited by W.P.D. Logan
1982; 253 pages (*out of print*)

No. 37 Laboratory Decontamination and Destruction of Aflatoxins B_1, B_2, G_1, G_2 in Laboratory Wastes
Edited by M. Castegnaro *et al.*
1980; 56 pages (*out of print*)

No. 38 Directory of On-going Research in Cancer Epidemiology 1981
Edited by C.S. Muir and G. Wagner
1981; 696 pages (*out of print*)

No. 39 Host Factors in Human Carcinogenesis
Edited by H. Bartsch and
B. Armstrong
1982; 583 pages (*out of print*)

No. 40 Environmental Carcinogens. Selected Methods of Analysis. Volume 4: Some Aromatic Amines and Azo Dyes in the General and Industrial Environment
Edited by L. Fishbein,
M. Castegnaro, I.K. O'Neill and
H. Bartsch
1981; 347 pages (*out of print*)

No. 41 N-Nitroso Compounds: Occurrence and Biological Effects
Edited by H. Bartsch, I.K. O'Neill, M. Castegnaro and M. Okada
1982; 755 pages £50.00

No. 42 Cancer Incidence in Five Continents, Volume IV
Edited by J. Waterhouse, C. Muir, K. Shanmugaratnam and J. Powell
1982; 811 pages (*out of print*)

No. 43 Laboratory Decontamination and Destruction of Carcinogens in Laboratory Wastes: Some N-Nitrosamines
Edited by M. Castegnaro *et al.*
1982; 73 pages £7.50

No. 44 Environmental Carcinogens. Selected Methods of Analysis. Volume 5: Some Mycotoxins
Edited by L. Stoloff, M. Castegnaro, P. Scott, I.K. O'Neill and H. Bartsch
1983; 455 pages £32.50

No. 45 Environmental Carcinogens. Selected Methods of Analysis. Volume 6: N-Nitroso Compounds
Edited by R. Preussmann, I.K. O'Neill, G. Eisenbrand, B. Spiegelhalder and H. Bartsch
1983; 508 pages £32.50

No. 46 Directory of On-going Research in Cancer Epidemiology 1982
Edited by C.S. Muir and G. Wagner
1982; 722 pages (*out of print*)

No. 47 Cancer Incidence in Singapore 1968-1977
Edited by K. Shanmugaratnam, H.P. Lee and N.E. Day
1983; 171 pages (*out of print*)

No. 48 Cancer Incidence in the USSR (2nd Revised Edition)
Edited by N.P. Napalkov,
G.F. Tserkovny, V.M. Merabishvili, D.M. Parkin, M. Smans and
C.S. Muir
1983; 75 pages (*out of print*)

No. 49 Laboratory Decontamination and Destruction of Carcinogens in Laboratory Wastes: Some Polycyclic Aromatic Hydrocarbons
Edited by M. Castegnaro *et al.*
1983; 87 pages (*out of print*)

No. 50 Directory of On-going Research in Cancer Epidemiology 1983
Edited by C.S. Muir and G. Wagner
1983; 731 pages (*out of print*)

No. 51 Modulators of Experimental Carcinogenesis
Edited by V. Turusov and R. Montesano
1983; 307 pages (*out of print*)

* Available from booksellers through the network of WHO Sales agents.

† Available directly from IARC

List of IARC Publications

No. 52 Second Cancers in Relation to Radiation Treatment for Cervical Cancer: Results of a Cancer Registry Collaboration
Edited by N.E. Day and J.C. Boice, Jr
1984; 207 pages (*out of print*)

No. 53 Nickel in the Human Environment
Editor-in-Chief: F.W. Sunderman, Jr
1984; 529 pages (*out of print*)

No. 54 Laboratory Decontamination and Destruction of Carcinogens in Laboratory Wastes: Some Hydrazines
Edited by M. Castegnaro et al.
1983; 87 pages (*out of print*)

No. 55 Laboratory Decontamination and Destruction of Carcinogens in Laboratory Wastes: Some N-Nitrosamides
Edited by M. Castegnaro et al.
1984; 66 pages (*out of print*)

No. 56 Models, Mechanisms and Etiology of Tumour Promotion
Edited by M. Börzsönyi, N.E. Day, K. Lapis and H. Yamasaki
1984; 532 pages (*out of print*)

No. 57 N-Nitroso Compounds: Occurrence, Biological Effects and Relevance to Human Cancer
Edited by I.K. O'Neill, R.C. von Borstel, C.T. Miller, J. Long and H. Bartsch
1984; 1013 pages (*out of print*)

No. 58 Age-related Factors in Carcinogenesis
Edited by A. Likhachev, V. Anisimov and R. Montesano
1985; 288 pages (*out of print*)

No. 59 Monitoring Human Exposure to Carcinogenic and Mutagenic Agents
Edited by A. Berlin, M. Draper, K. Hemminki and H. Vainio
1984; 457 pages (*out of print*)

No. 60 Burkitt's Lymphoma: A Human Cancer Model
Edited by G. Lenoir, G. O'Conor and C.L.M. Olweny
1985; 484 pages (*out of print*)

No. 61 Laboratory Decontamination and Destruction of Carcinogens in Laboratory Wastes: Some Haloethers
Edited by M. Castegnaro et al.
1985; 55 pages (*out of print*)

No. 62 Directory of On-going Research in Cancer Epidemiology 1984
Edited by C.S. Muir and G. Wagner
1984; 717 pages (*out of print*)

No. 63 Virus-associated Cancers in Africa
Edited by A.O. Williams, G.T. O'Conor, G.B. de-Thé and C.A. Johnson
1984; 773 pages (*out of print*)

No. 64 Laboratory Decontamination and Destruction of Carcinogens in Laboratory Wastes: Some Aromatic Amines and 4-Nitrobiphenyl
Edited by M. Castegnaro et al.
1985; 84 pages (*out of print*)

No. 65 Interpretation of Negative Epidemiological Evidence for Carcinogenicity
Edited by N.J. Wald and R. Doll
1985; 232 pages (*out of print*)

No. 66 The Role of the Registry in Cancer Control
Edited by D.M. Parkin, G. Wagner and C.S. Muir
1985; 152 pages £10.00

No. 67 Transformation Assay of Established Cell Lines: Mechanisms and Application
Edited by T. Kakunaga and H. Yamasaki
1985; 225 pages (*out of print*)

No. 68 Environmental Carcinogens. Selected Methods of Analysis. Volume 7. Some Volatile Halogenated Hydrocarbons
Edited by L. Fishbein and I.K. O'Neill
1985; 479 pages (*out of print*)

No. 69 Directory of On-going Research in Cancer Epidemiology 1985
Edited by C.S. Muir and G. Wagner
1985; 745 pages (*out of print*)

No. 70 The Role of Cyclic Nucleic Acid Adducts in Carcinogenesis and Mutagenesis
Edited by B. Singer and H. Bartsch
1986; 467 pages (*out of print*)

No. 71 Environmental Carcinogens. Selected Methods of Analysis. Volume 8: Some Metals: As, Be, Cd, Cr, Ni, Pb, Se, Zn
Edited by I.K. O'Neill, P. Schuller and L. Fishbein
1986; 485 pages (*out of print*)

No. 72 Atlas of Cancer in Scotland, 1975–1980. Incidence and Epidemiological Perspective
Edited by I. Kemp, P. Boyle, M. Smans and C.S. Muir
1985; 285 pages (*out of print*)

No. 73 Laboratory Decontamination and Destruction of Carcinogens in Laboratory Wastes: Some Antineoplastic Agents
Edited by M. Castegnaro et al.
1985; 163 pages £12.50

No. 74 Tobacco: A Major International Health Hazard
Edited by D. Zaridze and R. Peto
1986; 324 pages £22.50

No. 75 Cancer Occurrence in Developing Countries
Edited by D.M. Parkin
1986; 339 pages £22.50

No. 76 Screening for Cancer of the Uterine Cervix
Edited by M. Hakama, A.B. Miller and N.E. Day
1986; 315 pages £30.00

No. 77 Hexachlorobenzene: Proceedings of an International Symposium
Edited by C.R. Morris and J.R.P. Cabral
1986; 668 pages (*out of print*)

No. 78 Carcinogenicity of Alkylating Cytostatic Drugs
Edited by D. Schmähl and J.M. Kaldor
1986; 337 pages (*out of print*)

No. 79 Statistical Methods in Cancer Research. Volume III: The Design and Analysis of Long-term Animal Experiments
By J.J. Gart, D. Krewski, P.N. Lee, R.E. Tarone and J. Wahrendorf
1986; 213 pages £22.00

List of IARC Publications

No. 80 Directory of On-going Research in Cancer Epidemiology 1986
Edited by C.S. Muir and G. Wagner
1986; 805 pages (*out of print*)

No. 81 Environmental Carcinogens: Methods of Analysis and Exposure Measurement. Volume 9: Passive Smoking
Edited by I.K. O'Neill, K.D. Brunnemann, B. Dodet and D. Hoffmann
1987; 383 pages £35.00

No. 82 Statistical Methods in Cancer Research. Volume II: The Design and Analysis of Cohort Studies
By N.E. Breslow and N.E. Day
1987; 404 pages £25.00

No. 83 Long-term and Short-term Assays for Carcinogens: A Critical Appraisal
Edited by R. Montesano, H. Bartsch, H. Vainio, J. Wilbourn and H. Yamasaki
1986; 575 pages £35.00

No. 84 The Relevance of N-Nitroso Compounds to Human Cancer: Exposure and Mechanisms
Edited by H. Bartsch, I.K. O'Neill and R. Schulte-Hermann
1987; 671 pages (*out of print*)

No. 85 Environmental Carcinogens: Methods of Analysis and Exposure Measurement. Volume 10: Benzene and Alkylated Benzenes
Edited by L. Fishbein and I.K. O'Neill
1988; 327 pages £40.00

No. 86 Directory of On-going Research in Cancer Epidemiology 1987
Edited by D.M. Parkin and J. Wahrendorf
1987; 676 pages (*out of print*)

No. 87 International Incidence of Childhood Cancer
Edited by D.M. Parkin, C.A. Stiller, C.A. Bieber, G.J. Draper, B. Terracini and J.L. Young
1988; 401 pages £35.00

No. 88 Cancer Incidence in Five Continents Volume V
Edited by C. Muir, J. Waterhouse, T. Mack, J. Powell and S. Whelan
1987; 1004 pages £55.00

No. 89 Method for Detecting DNA Damaging Agents in Humans: Applications in Cancer Epidemiology and Prevention
Edited by H. Bartsch, K. Hemminki and I.K. O'Neill
1988; 518 pages £50.00

No. 90 Non-occupational Exposure to Mineral Fibres
Edited by J. Bignon, J. Peto and R. Saracci
1989; 500 pages £50.00

No. 91 Trends in Cancer Incidence in Singapore 1968–1982
Edited by H.P. Lee, N.E. Day and K. Shanmugaratnam
1988; 160 pages (*out of print*)

No. 92 Cell Differentiation, Genes and Cancer
Edited by T. Kakunaga, T. Sugimura, L. Tomatis and H. Yamasaki
1988; 204 pages £27.50

No. 93 Directory of On-going Research in Cancer Epidemiology 1988
Edited by M. Coleman and J. Wahrendorf
1988; 662 pages (*out of print*)

No. 94 Human Papillomavirus and Cervical Cancer
Edited by N. Muñoz, F.X. Bosch and O.M. Jensen
1989; 154 pages £22.50

No. 95 Cancer Registration: Principles and Methods
Edited by O.M. Jensen, D.M. Parkin, R. MacLennan, C.S. Muir and R. Skeet
1991; 288 pages £28.00

No. 96 Perinatal and Multigeneration Carcinogenesis
Edited by N.P. Napalkov, J.M. Rice, L. Tomatis and H. Yamasaki
1989; 436 pages £50.00

No. 97 Occupational Exposure to Silica and Cancer Risk
Edited by L. Simonato, A.C. Fletcher, R. Saracci and T. Thomas
1990; 124 pages £22.50

No. 98 Cancer Incidence in Jewish Migrants to Israel, 1961–1981
Edited by R. Steinitz, D.M. Parkin, J.L. Young, C.A. Bieber and L. Katz
1989; 320 pages £35.00

No. 99 Pathology of Tumours in Laboratory Animals, Second Edition, Volume 1, Tumours of the Rat
Edited by V.S. Turusov and U. Mohr
740 pages £85.00

No. 100 Cancer: Causes, Occurrence and Control
Editor-in-Chief L. Tomatis
1990; 352 pages £24.00

No. 101 Directory of On-going Research in Cancer Epidemiology 1989/90
Edited by M. Coleman and J. Wahrendorf
1989; 818 pages £36.00

No. 102 Patterns of Cancer in Five Continents
Edited by S.L. Whelan, D.M. Parkin & E. Masuyer
1990; 162 pages £25.00

No. 103 Evaluating Effectiveness of Primary Prevention of Cancer
Edited by M. Hakama, V. Beral, J.W. Cullen and D.M. Parkin
1990; 250 pages £32.00

No. 104 Complex Mixtures and Cancer Risk
Edited by H. Vainio, M. Sorsa and A.J. McMichael
1990; 442 pages £38.00

No. 105 Relevance to Human Cancer of N-Nitroso Compounds, Tobacco Smoke and Mycotoxins
Edited by I.K. O'Neill, J. Chen and H. Bartsch
1991; 614 pages £70.00

No. 106 Atlas of Cancer Incidence in the Former German Democratic Republic
Edited by W.H. Mehnert, M. Smans, C.S. Muir, M. Möhner & D. Schön
1992; 384 pages £55.00

* Available from booksellers through the network of WHO Sales agents.

† Available directly from IARC

List of IARC Publications

No. 107 Atlas of Cancer Mortality in the European Economic Community
Edited by M. Smans, C.S. Muir and P. Boyle
1992; 280 pages £35.00

No. 108 Environmental Carcinogens: Methods of Analysis and Exposure Measurement. Volume 11: Polychlorinated Dioxins and Dibenzofurans
Edited by C. Rappe, H.R. Buser, B. Dodet and I.K. O'Neill
1991; 426 pages £45.00

No. 109 Environmental Carcinogens: Methods of Analysis and Exposure Measurement. Volume 12: Indoor Air Contaminants
Edited by B. Seifert, H. van de Wiel, B. Dodet and I.K. O'Neill
1993; 384 pages £45.00

No. 110 Directory of On-going Research in Cancer Epidemiology 1991
Edited by M. Coleman and J. Wahrendorf
1991; 753 pages £38.00

No. 111 Pathology of Tumours in Laboratory Animals, Second Edition, Volume 2, Tumours of the Mouse
Edited by V.S. Turusov and U. Mohr
1993; 776 pages; £90.00

No. 112 Autopsy in Epidemiology and Medical Research
Edited by E. Riboli and M. Delendi
1991; 288 pages £25.00

No. 113 Laboratory Decontamination and Destruction of Carcinogens in Laboratory Wastes: Some Mycotoxins
Edited by M. Castegnaro, J. Barek, J.-M. Frémy, M. Lafontaine, M. Miraglia, E.B. Sansone and G.M. Telling
1991; 64 pages £11.00

No. 114 Laboratory Decontamination and Destruction of Carcinogens in Laboratory Wastes: Some Polycyclic Heterocyclic Hydrocarbons
Edited by M. Castegnaro, J. Barek J. Jacob, U. Kirso, M. Lafontaine, E.B. Sansone, G.M. Telling and T. Vu Duc
1991; 50 pages £8.00

No. 115 Mycotoxins, Endemic Nephropathy and Urinary Tract Tumours
Edited by M. Castegnaro, R. Plestina, G. Dirheimer, I.N. Chernozemsky and H Bartsch
1991; 340 pages £45.00

No. 116 Mechanisms of Carcinogenesis in Risk Identification
Edited by H. Vainio, P.N. Magee, D.B. McGregor & A.J. McMichael
1992; 616 pages £65.00

No. 117 Directory of On-going Research in Cancer Epidemiology 1992
Edited by M. Coleman, J. Wahrendorf & E. Démaret
1992; 773 pages £42.00

No. 118 Cadmium in the Human Environment: Toxicity and Carcinogenicity
Edited by G.F. Nordberg, R.F.M. Herber & L. Alessio
1992; 470 pages £60.00

No. 119 The Epidemiology of Cervical Cancer and Human Papillomavirus
Edited by N. Muñoz, F.X. Bosch, K.V. Shah & A. Meheus
1992; 288 pages £28.00

No. 120 Cancer Incidence in Five Continents, Volume VI
Edited by D.M. Parkin, C.S. Muir, S.L. Whelan, Y.T. Gao, J. Ferlay & J.Powell
1992; 1080 pages £120.00

No. 121 Trends in Cancer Incidence and Mortality
M.P. Coleman, J. Estève, P. Damiecki, A. Arslan and H. Renard
1993; 806 pages, £120.00

No. 122 International Classification of Rodent Tumours. Part 1. The Rat
Editor-in-Chief: U. Mohr
1992/93; 10 fascicles of 60-100 pages, £120.00

No. 123 Cancer in Italian Migrant Populations
Edited by M. Geddes, D.M. Parkin, M. Khlat, D. Balzi and E. Buiatti
1993; 292 pages, £40.00

No. 124 Postlabelling Methods for Detection of DNA Adducts
Edited by D.H. Phillips, M. Castegnaro and H. Bartsch
1993; 392 pages; £46.00

No. 125 DNA Adducts: Identification and Biological Significance.
Edited by K. Hemminki, A. Dipple, D. Shuker, F.F. Kadlubar, D. Segerbäck and H. Bartsch
1993; 480 pages; £52.00

No. 127 Butadiene and Styrene: Assessment of Health Hazards.
Edited by M. Sorsa, K. Peltonen, H. Vainio and K. Hemminki
1993; 412 pages; £46.00

No. 130 Directory of On-going Research in Cancer Epidemiology 1994
Edited by R. Sankaranarayanan, J. Wahrendorf and E. Démaret
1994; approx. 800 pages, £46.00

List of IARC Publications

IARC MONOGRAPHS ON THE EVALUATION OF CARCINOGENIC RISKS TO HUMANS

(Available from booksellers through the network of WHO Sales Agents)

Volume 1 Some Inorganic Substances, Chlorinated Hydrocarbons, Aromatic Amines, *N*-Nitroso Compounds, and Natural Products
1972; 184 pages (*out of print*)

Volume 2 Some Inorganic and Organometallic Compounds
1973; 181 pages (*out of print*)

Volume 3 Certain Polycyclic Aromatic Hydrocarbons and Heterocyclic Compounds
1973; 271 pages (*out of print*)

Volume 4 Some Aromatic Amines, Hydrazine and Related Substances, *N*-Nitroso Compounds and Miscellaneous Alkylating Agents
1974; 286 pages Sw. fr. 18.–

Volume 5 Some Organochlorine Pesticides
1974; 241 pages (*out of print*)

Volume 6 Sex Hormones
1974; 243 pages (*out of print*)

Volume 7 Some Anti-Thyroid and Related Substances, Nitrofurans and Industrial Chemicals
1974; 326 pages (*out of print*)

Volume 8 Some Aromatic Azo Compounds
1975; 357 pages Sw. fr. 36.–

Volume 9 Some Aziridines, *N*-, *S*- and *O*-Mustards and Selenium
1975; 268 pages Sw.fr. 27.–

Volume 10 Some Naturally Occurring Substances
1976; 353 pages (*out of print*)

Volume 11 Cadmium, Nickel, Some Epoxides, Miscellaneous Industrial Chemicals and General Considerations on Volatile Anaesthetics
1976; 306 pages (*out of print*)

Volume 12 Some Carbamates, Thiocarbamates and Carbazides
1976; 282 pages Sw. fr. 34.–

Volume 13 Some Miscellaneous Pharmaceutical Substances
1977; 255 pages Sw. fr. 30.–

Volume 14 Asbestos
1977; 106 pages (*out of print*)

Volume 15 Some Fumigants, The Herbicides 2,4-D and 2,4,5-T, Chlorinated Dibenzodioxins and Miscellaneous Industrial Chemicals
1977; 354 pages Sw. fr. 50.–

Volume 16 Some Aromatic Amines and Related Nitro Compounds - Hair Dyes, Colouring Agents and Miscellaneous Industrial Chemicals
1978; 400 pages Sw. fr. 50.–

Volume 17 Some *N*-Nitroso Compounds
1978; 365 pages Sw. fr. 50.–

Volume 18 Polychlorinated Biphenyls and Polybrominated Biphenyls
1978; 140 pages Sw. fr. 20.–

Volume 19 Some Monomers, Plastics and Synthetic Elastomers, and Acrolein
1979; 513 pages (*out of print*)

Volume 20 Some Halogenated Hydrocarbons
1979; 609 pages (*out of print*)

Volume 21 Sex Hormones (II)
1979; 583 pages Sw. fr. 60.–

Volume 22 Some Non-Nutritive Sweetening Agents
1980; 208 pages Sw. fr. 25.–

Volume 23 Some Metals and Metallic Compounds
1980; 438 pages (*out of print*)

Volume 24 Some Pharmaceutical Drugs
1980; 337 pages Sw. fr. 40.–

Volume 25 Wood, Leather and Some Associated Industries
1981; 412 pages Sw. fr. 60.–

Volume 26 Some Antineoplastic and Immunosuppressive Agents
1981; 411 pages Sw. fr. 62.–

Volume 27 Some Aromatic Amines, Anthraquinones and Nitroso Compounds, and Inorganic Fluorides Used in Drinking Water and Dental Preparations
1982; 341 pages Sw. fr. 40.–

Volume 28 The Rubber Industry
1982; 486 pages Sw. fr. 70.–

Volume 29 Some Industrial Chemicals and Dyestuffs
1982; 416 pages Sw. fr. 60.–

Volume 30 Miscellaneous Pesticides
1983; 424 pages Sw. fr. 60.–

Volume 31 Some Food Additives, Feed Additives and Naturally Occurring Substances
1983; 314 pages Sw. fr. 60.–

Volume 32 Polynuclear Aromatic Compounds, Part 1: Chemical, Environmental and Experimental Data
1983; 477 pages Sw. fr. 60.–

Volume 33 Polynuclear Aromatic Compounds, Part 2: Carbon Blacks, Mineral Oils and Some Nitroarenes
1984; 245 pages Sw. fr. 50.–

Volume 34 Polynuclear Aromatic Compounds, Part 3: Industrial Exposures in Aluminium Production, Coal Gasification, Coke Production, and Iron and Steel Founding
1984; 219 pages Sw. fr. 48.–

Volume 35 Polynuclear Aromatic Compounds, Part 4: Bitumens, Coal-tars and Derived Products, Shale-oils and Soots
1985; 271 pages Sw. fr. 70.–

* Available from booksellers through the network of WHO Sales agents.

† Available directly from IARC

List of IARC Publications

Volume 36 Allyl Compounds, Aldehydes, Epoxides and Peroxides
1985; 369 pages Sw. fr. 70.-

Volume 37 Tobacco Habits Other than Smoking: Betel-quid and Areca-nut Chewing; and some Related Nitrosamines
1985; 291 pages Sw. fr. 70.-

Volume 38 Tobacco Smoking
1986; 421 pages Sw. fr. 75.-

Volume 39 Some Chemicals Used in Plastics and Elastomers
1986; 403 pages Sw. fr. 60.-

Volume 40 Some Naturally Occurring and Synthetic Food Components, Furocoumarins and Ultraviolet Radiation
1986; 444 pages Sw. fr. 65.-

Volume 41 Some Halogenated Hydrocarbons and Pesticide Exposures
1986; 434 pages Sw. fr. 65.-

Volume 42 Silica and Some Silicates
1987; 289 pages Sw. fr. 65.

Volume 43 Man-Made Mineral Fibres and Radon
1988; 300 pages Sw. fr. 65.-

Volume 44 Alcohol Drinking
1988; 416 pages Sw. fr. 65.

Volume 45 Occupational Exposures in Petroleum Refining; Crude Oil and Major Petroleum Fuels
1989; 322 pages Sw. fr. 65.-

Volume 46 Diesel and Gasoline Engine Exhausts and Some Nitroarenes
1989; 458 pages Sw. fr. 65.-

Volume 47 Some Organic Solvents, Resin Monomers and Related Compounds, Pigments and Occupational Exposures in Paint Manufacture and Painting
1989; 536 pages Sw. fr. 85.-

Volume 48 Some Flame Retardants and Textile Chemicals, and Exposures in the Textile Manufacturing Industry
1990; 345 pages Sw. fr. 65.-

Volume 49 Chromium, Nickel and Welding
1990; 677 pages Sw. fr. 95.-

Volume 50 Pharmaceutical Drugs
1990; 415 pages Sw. fr. 65.-

Volume 51 Coffee, Tea, Mate, Methylxanthines and Methylglyoxal
1991; 513 pages Sw. fr. 80.-

Volume 52 Chlorinated Drinking-water; Chlorination By-products; Some Other Halogenated Compounds; Cobalt and Cobalt Compounds
1991; 544 pages Sw. fr. 80.-

Volume 53 Occupational Exposures in Insecticide Application and some Pesticides
1991; 612 pages Sw. fr. 95.-

Volume 54 Occupational Exposures to Mists and Vapours from Strong Inorganic Acids; and Other Industrial Chemicals
1992; 336 pages Sw. fr. 65.-

Volume 55 Solar and Ultraviolet Radiation
1992; 316 pages Sw. fr. 65.-

Volume 56 Some Naturally Occurring Substances: Food Items and Constituents, Heterocyclic Aromatic Amines and Mycotoxins
1993; 600 pages Sw. fr. 95.-

Volume 57 Occupational Exposures of Hairdressers and Barbers and Personal Use of Hair Colourants; Some Hair Dyes, Cosmetic Colourants, Industrial Dyestuffs and Aromatic Amines
1993; 428 pages Sw. fr. 75.-

Volume 58 Beryllium, Cadmium, Mercury and Exposures in the Glass Manufacturing Industry
1993; 426 pages Sw. fr. 75.-

Supplement No. 1
Chemicals and Industrial Processes Associated with Cancer in Humans (IARC Monographs, Volumes 1 to 20)
1979; 71 pages (*out of print*)

Supplement No. 2
Long-term and Short-term Screening Assays for Carcinogens: A Critical Appraisal
1980; 426 pages Sw. fr. 40.-

Supplement No. 3
Cross Index of Synonyms and Trade Names in Volumes 1 to 26
1982; 199 pages (*out of print*)

Supplement No. 4
Chemicals, Industrial Processes and Industries Associated with Cancer in Humans (IARC Monographs, Volumes 1 to 29)
1982; 292 pages (*out of print*)

Supplement No. 5
Cross Index of Synonyms and Trade Names in Volumes 1 to 36
1985; 259 pages (*out of print*)

Supplement No. 6
Genetic and Related Effects: An Updating of Selected IARC Monographs from Volumes 1 to 42
1987; 729 pages Sw. fr. 80.-

Supplement No. 7
Overall Evaluations of Carcinogenicity: An Updating of IARC Monographs Volumes 1-42
1987; 440 pages Sw. fr. 65.-

Supplement No. 8
Cross Index of Synonyms and Trade Names in Volumes 1 to 46
1990; 346 pages Sw. fr. 60.-

List of IARC Publications

IARC TECHNICAL REPORTS*

No. 1 **Cancer in Costa Rica**
Edited by R. Sierra,
R. Barrantes, G. Muñoz Leiva, D.M. Parkin, C.A. Bieber and
N. Muñoz Calero
1988; 124 pages Sw. fr. 30.-

No. 2 **SEARCH: A Computer Package to Assist the Statistical Analysis of Case-control Studies**
Edited by G.J. Macfarlane,
P. Boyle and P. Maisonneuve
1991; 80 pages (*out of print*)

No. 3 **Cancer Registration in the European Economic Community**
Edited by M.P. Coleman and
E. Démaret
1988; 188 pages Sw. fr. 30.-

No. 4 **Diet, Hormones and Cancer: Methodological Issues for Prospective Studies**
Edited by E. Riboli and
R. Saracci
1988; 156 pages Sw. fr. 30.-

No. 5 **Cancer in the Philippines**
Edited by A.V. Laudico,
D. Esteban and D.M. Parkin
1989; 186 pages Sw. fr. 30.-

No. 6 **La genèse du Centre International de Recherche sur le Cancer**
Par R. Sohier et A.G.B. Sutherland
1990; 104 pages Sw. fr. 30.-

No. 7 **Epidémiologie du cancer dans les pays de langue latine**
1990; 310 pages Sw. fr. 30.-

No. 8 **Comparative Study of Anti-smoking Legislation in Countries of the European Economic Community**
Edited by A. Sasco, P. Dalla Vorgia and P. Van der Elst
1992; 82 pages Sw. fr. 30.-

No. 9 **Epidemiologie du cancer dans les pays de langue latine**
1991 346 pages Sw. fr. 30.-

No. 11 **Nitroso Compounds: Biological Mechanisms, Exposures and Cancer Etiology**
1991; 346 pages Sw. fr. 30.-
Edited by I.K. O'Neill & H. Bartsch
1992; 149 pages Sw. fr. 30.-

No. 12 **Epidémiologie du cancer dans les pays de langue latine**
1992; 375 pages Sw. fr. 30.-

No. 13 **Health, Solar UV Radiation and Environmental Change**
Edited by A. Kricker, B.K. Armstrong, M.E. Jones and R.C. Burton
1993; 216 pages Sw.fr. 30.-

No. 14 **Epidémiologie du cancer dans les pays de langue latine**
1993; 385 pages Sw. fr. 30.-

No. 15 **Cancer in the African Population of Bulawayo, Zimbabwe, 1963-1977: Incidence, Time Trends and Risk Factors**
By M.E.G. Skinner, D.M. Parkin, A.P. Vizcaino and A. Ndhlovu
1993; 123 pages Sw. fr. 30.-

No. 16 **Cancer in Thailand, 1988-1991**
By V. Vatanasapt, N. Martin, H. Sriplung, K. Vindavijak, S. Sontipong, S. Sriamporn, D.M. Parkin and J. Ferlay
1993; 164 pages Sw. fr. 30.-

DIRECTORY OF AGENTS BEING TESTED FOR CARCINOGENICITY (Until Vol. 13 Information Bulletin on the Survey of Chemicals Being Tested for Carcinogenicity)*

No. 8 Edited by M.-J. Ghess,
H. Bartsch and L. Tomatis
1979; 604 pages Sw. fr. 40.-

No. 9 Edited by M.-J. Ghess,
J.D. Wilbourn, H. Bartsch and
L. Tomatis
1981; 294 pages Sw. fr. 41.-

No. 10 Edited by M.-J. Ghess,
J.D. Wilbourn and H. Bartsch
1982; 362 pages Sw. fr. 42.-

No. 11 Edited by M.-J. Ghess,
J.D. Wilbourn, H. Vainio and
H. Bartsch
1984; 362 pages Sw. fr. 50.-

No. 12 Edited by M.-J. Ghess,
J.D. Wilbourn, A. Tossavainen and
H. Vainio
1986; 385 pages Sw. fr. 50.-

No. 13 Edited by M.-J. Ghess,
J.D. Wilbourn and A. Aitio 1988;
404 pages Sw. fr. 43.-

No. 14 Edited by M.-J. Ghess,
J.D. Wilbourn and H. Vainio
1990; 370 pages Sw. fr. 45.-

No. 15 Edited by M.-J. Ghess, J.D. Wilbourn and H. Vainio
1992; 318 pages Sw. fr. 45.-

NON-SERIAL PUBLICATIONS

Alcool et Cancer†
By A. Tuyns (in French only)
1978; 42 pages Fr. fr. 35.-

Cancer Morbidity and Causes of Death Among Danish Brewery Workers†
By O.M. Jensen
1980; 143 pages Fr. fr. 75.-

Directory of Computer Systems Used in Cancer Registries†
By H.R. Menck and D.M. Parkin
1986; 236 pages Fr. fr. 50.-

Facts and Figures of Cancer in the European Community*
Edited by J. Estève, A. Kricker, J. Ferlay and D.M. Parkin
1993; 52 pages Sw. fr. 10.-

---

* Available from booksellers through the network of WHO Sales agents.

† Available directly from IARC

www.ingramcontent.com/pod-product-compliance
Ingram Content Group UK Ltd.
Pitfield, Milton Keynes, MK11 3LW, UK
UKHW051258180426
11947UKWH00020B/1773